Exploring Life and Career

Martha Dunn-Strohecker, Ph.D., CFCS
Author of Family and Consumer
Sciences Textbooks
and Management Consultant
Marblehead, Massachusetts

Deborah Tunstall Tippett, Ph.D., CFCS
Professor and Head
Department of Human Environmental Sciences
Meredith College
Raleigh, North Carolina

Publisher
The Goodheart-Willcox Company, Inc.
Tinley Park, Illinois
www.g-w.com

Previously published as *Teen Life! Living/Learning/Caring*
Formerly published as *You: Living, Learning, and Caring*
Previous editions copyright 2008, 2006, 1999, 1997, 1992

Manufactured in the United States of America.

Library of Congress Catalog Card Number 2006041070

ISBN 978-1-60525-615-3

1 2 3 4 5 6 7 8 9 – 12 – 17 16 15 14 13 12 11

Library of Congress Cataloging-in-Publication Data

Dunn-Strohecker, Martha.
Exploring life and career / Martha Dunn-Strohecker, Deborah Tunstall Tippett.
p. cm.
Includes index.
"Previous editions copyright 2008 and 2006 published as Teen Life! Living/Learning/Caring."
ISBN 978-1-60525-615-3
1. Teenagers--Life skills guides. 2. Teenagers--Conduct of life. I. Tippett, Deborah Tunstall. II. Dunn-Strohecker, Martha. Teen life!. III. Title.
HQ796.D765 2012
646.700835--dc22

2011013842

Cover Image: Christopher Futcher/GettyImages

Introduction

Exploring Life and Career is a book about you. It's about understanding yourself. It's about being a responsible member of your family and community. It's about managing your resources. It's about the foods you eat, the clothes you wear, and the job you may choose in the future.

You are a special person. You are growing, developing, and learning responsibility. You are also learning about life. This book will teach you skills that can make a difference in your life and the lives of others.

This book will also help you enjoy your life because you will feel more confident about making decisions. Your life is affected by the decisions you make each day. You will learn to make decisions concerning yourself, others, and your environment. You will also learn how your decisions affect others and the world in which you live.

Life is an adventure! This book will help you enjoy, understand, and value life's adventure.

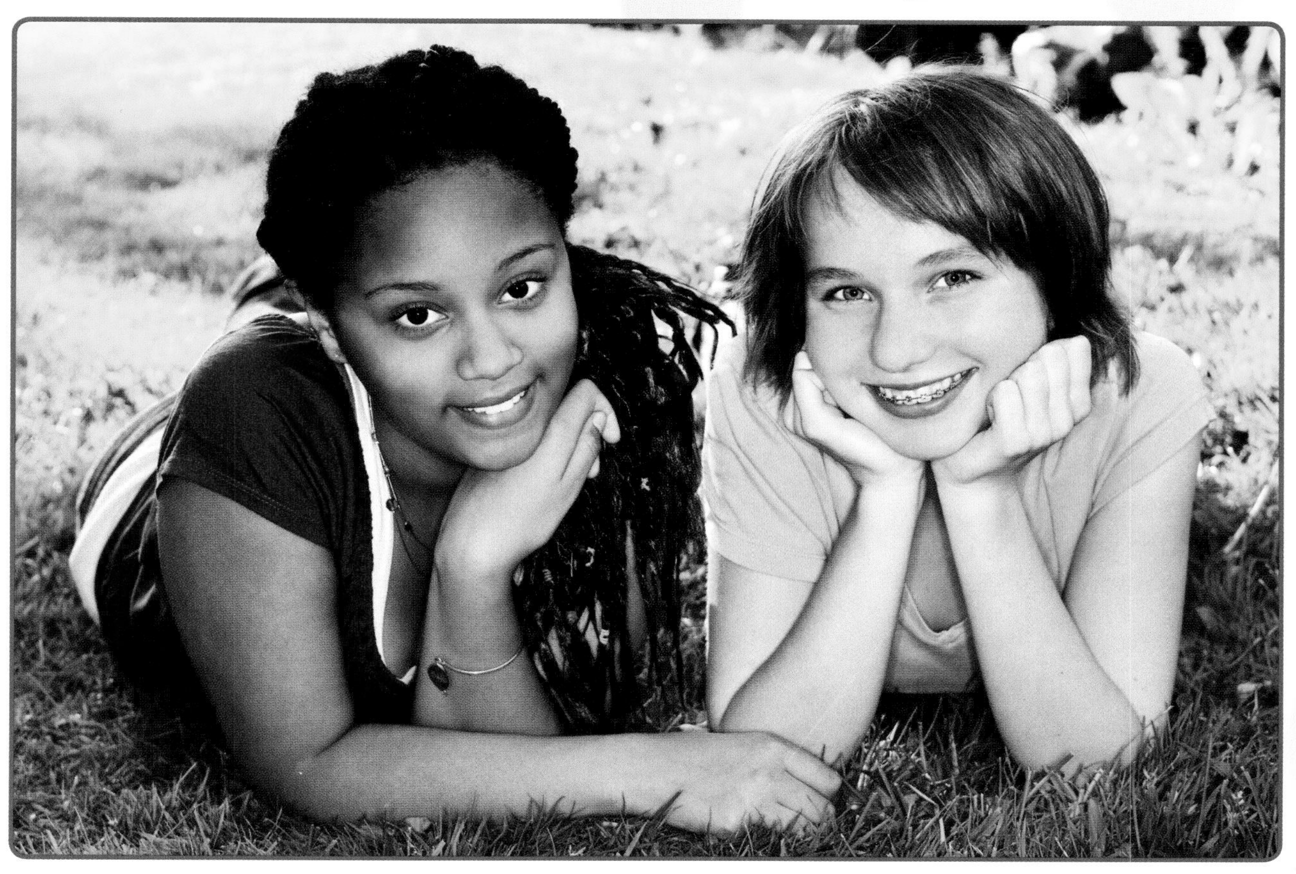

About the Authors

Martha Dunn-Strohecker's professional background includes secondary and higher education teaching, public management practice, and community service in nonprofit and religious organizations. Martha's extensive career combines family and consumer sciences, community nutrition, and public service focused on helping individuals and families use their resources more effectively and efficiently.

Martha presently serves as a consultant in management and diversity training. Among her numerous honors, she received Ohio State University's highest award, the Centennial Award, and also Ohio State's Outstanding Leadership Recognition for services to families. Further, she has been listed in *Who's Who of American Women*, and received volunteer service awards from Goodwill Industries and the American Red Cross. Martha is presently a faculty member in Gerontology at North Shore Community College where she developed the first online course in gerontology. She also does freelance writing, consulting work in management, and diversity training.

Deborah Tunstall Tippett's background includes 12 years as a family and consumer sciences teacher at the middle school level and as a teacher educator at both the University of North Carolina at Greensboro and at Meredith College. She is currently a professor and Department Head of the Human Environmental Sciences Department at Meredith College. She has published research and presented workshops and courses on middle school family and consumer sciences.

Dr. Tippett served as a national officer of the Family and Consumer Sciences Education Association, the Kappa Omicron Nu Honor Society, and the U.S./International Federation of Home Economics. She has won such awards as honorary membership on North Carolina's FCCLA, the Professional of the Year of the North Carolina Association of Family and Consumer Sciences, the Presidential Award for Outstanding Service at Meredith College, and the Excellence in Teaching Award at Meredith College. As a public school teacher, she was recognized as the local, county, and regional teacher of the year. She is listed in *Who's Who in Education* and *Who's Who of American Women*.

Acknowledgments

The authors and Goodheart-Willcox Publisher would like to thank the following professionals who provided valuable input:

Reviewers

Sandra R. Jones
Family and Consumer Sciences District Program Coordinator
Fairfax County Public Schools
Falls Church, Virginia

Lynn Murray
Family and Consumer Sciences Educator, Retired
Hauppauge Middle School
Hauppauge, New York

Lynne M. Turner
Family and Consumer Sciences Educator
Jane Macon Middle School
Brunswick, Georgia

Technical Reviewers

Steven Benko, Ph.D.
Assistant Professor
Department of Religious and Ethical Studies
Meredith College
Raleigh, North Carolina

Mitzi Cook
Assistant Professor Apparel and Textiles
Department of Family and Consumer Sciences
Appalachian State University
Boone, North Carolina

Laura Fieselman
Sustainability Coordinator
Meredith College
Raleigh, North Carolina

Denise Jones
Family and Consumer Sciences Educator
East Wake Middle School
Wake County Public Schools
Raleigh, North Carolina

Chelsea McGlaughlin
Development Tester
SAS Institute
Cary, North Carolina

Organized for Successful Learning

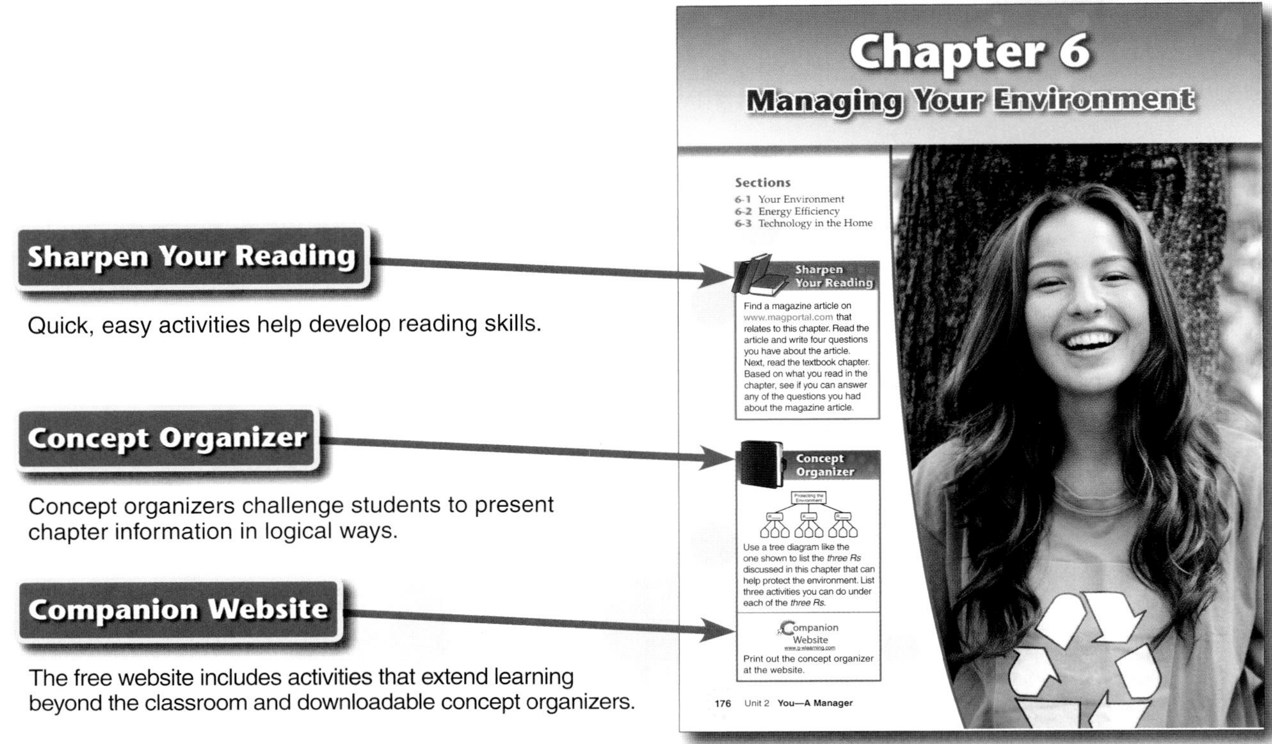

Chapter 6
Managing Your Environment
Sections
6-1 Your Environment
6-2 Energy Efficiency
6-3 Technology in the Home
Sharpen Your Reading
Find a magazine article on www.magportal.com that relates to this chapter. Read the article and write four questions you have about the article. Next, read the textbook chapter. Based on what you read in the chapter, see if you can answer any of the questions you had about the magazine article.
Concept Organizer
Use a tree diagram like the one shown to list the three Rs discussed in this chapter that can help protect the environment. List three activities you can do under each of the three Rs.
Companion Website
Print out the concept organizer at the website.
176 Unit 2 You—A Manager

Sharpen Your Reading

Quick, easy activities help develop reading skills.

Concept Organizer

Concept organizers challenge students to present chapter information in logical ways.

Companion Website

The free website includes activities that extend learning beyond the classroom and downloadable concept organizers.

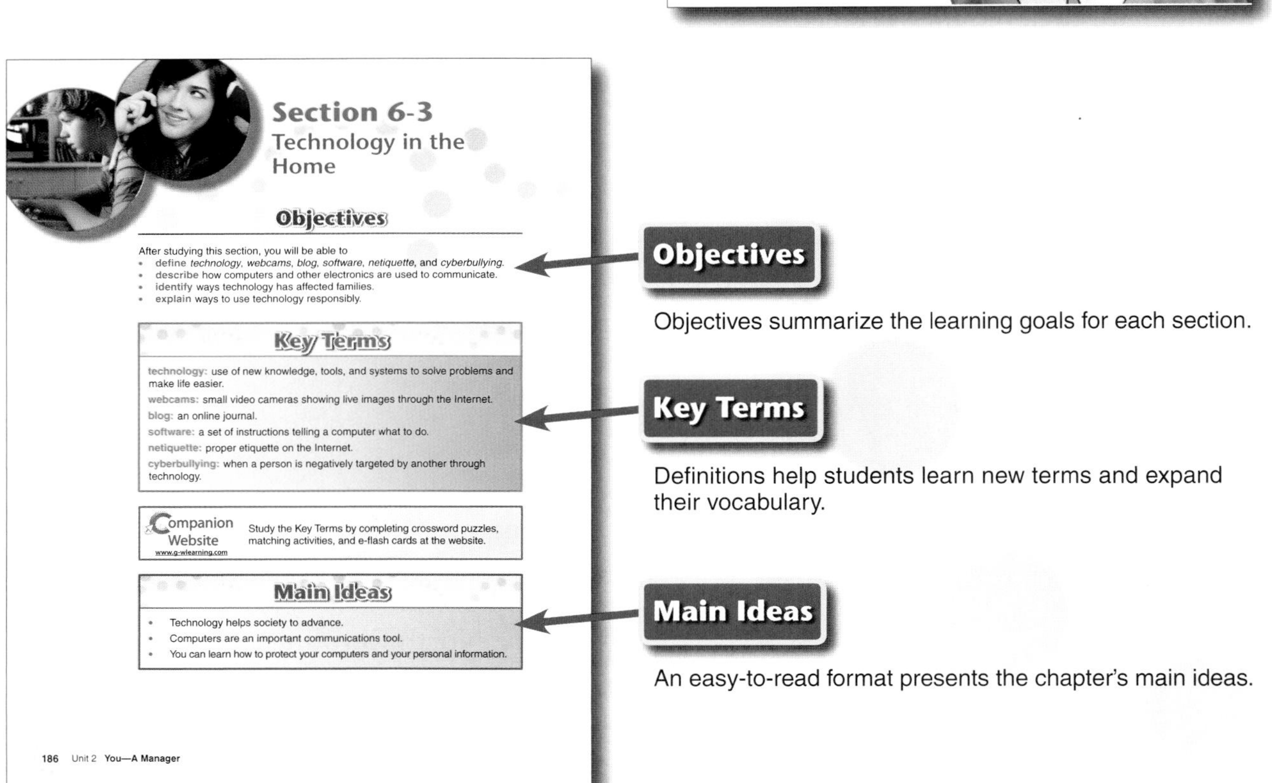

Section 6-3
Technology in the Home
Objectives
After studying this section, you will be able to
define technology, webcams, blog, software, netiquette, and cyberbullying.
describe how computers and other electronics are used to communicate.
identify ways technology has affected families.
explain ways to use technology responsibly.
Key Terms
technology: use of new knowledge, tools, and systems to solve problems and make life easier.
webcams: small video cameras showing live images through the Internet.
blog: an online journal.
software: a set of instructions telling a computer what to do.
netiquette: proper etiquette on the Internet.
cyberbullying: when a person is negatively targeted by another through technology.
Companion Website
www.g-wlearning.com
Study the Key Terms by completing crossword puzzles, matching activities, and e-flash cards at the website.
Main Ideas
Technology helps society to advance.
Computers are an important communications tool.
You can learn how to protect your computers and your personal information.
186 Unit 2 You—A Manager

Objectives

Objectives summarize the learning goals for each section.

Key Terms

Definitions help students learn new terms and expand their vocabulary.

Main Ideas

An easy-to-read format presents the chapter's main ideas.

Activities Enhance and Extend Learning

Chapter Review

Questions reinforce recall of chapter content.

Life Skills

Activities encourage real-life application of skills discussed in the text.

Technology

Students apply various technologies to explore chapter topics and complete activities.

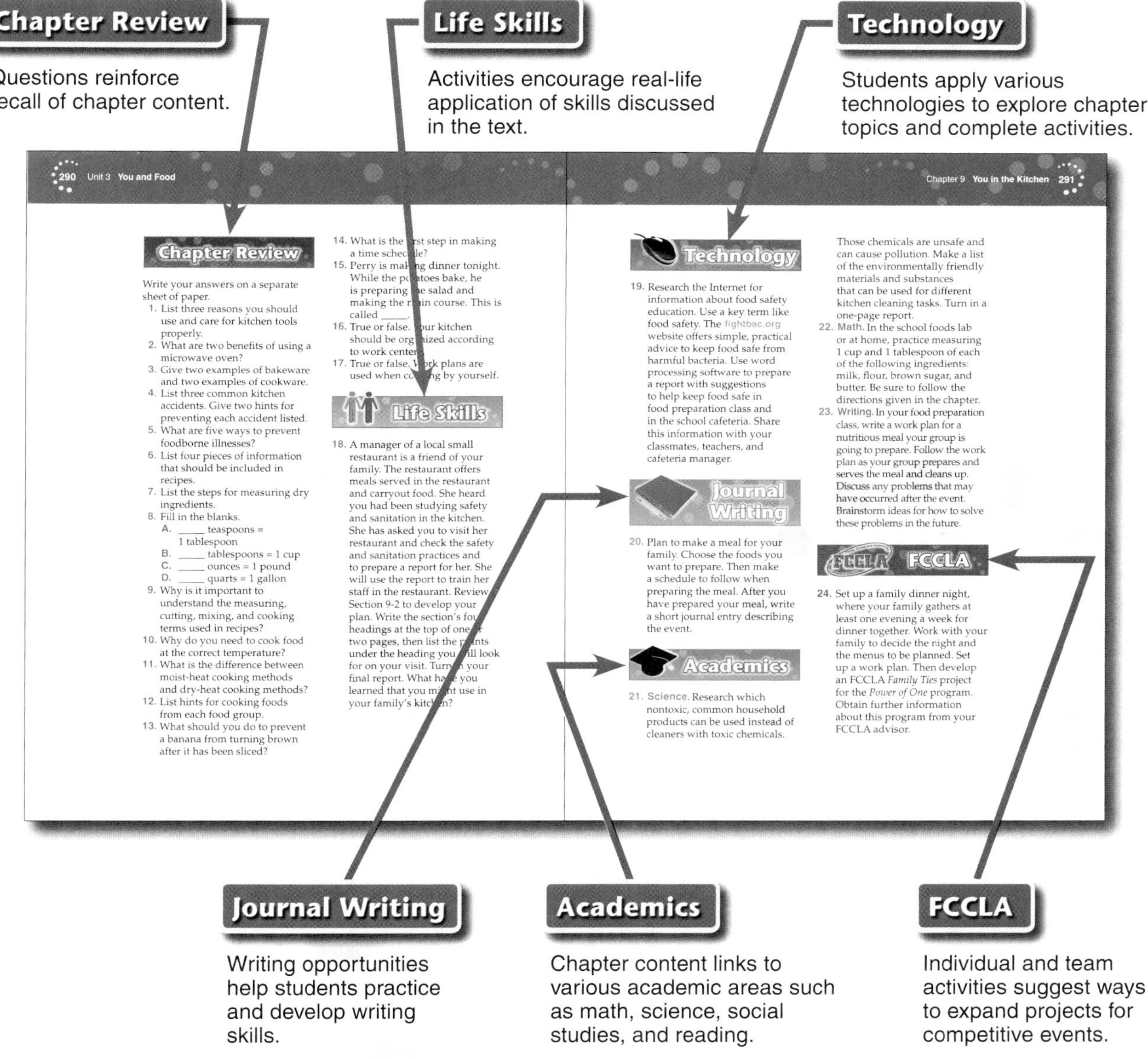

290 Unit 3 You and Food

Chapter Review

Write your answers on a separate sheet of paper.

1. List three reasons you should use and care for kitchen tools properly.
2. What are two benefits of using a microwave oven?
3. Give two examples of bakeware and two examples of cookware.
4. List three common kitchen accidents. Give two hints for preventing each accident listed.
5. What are five ways to prevent foodborne illnesses?
6. List four pieces of information that should be included in recipes.
7. List the steps for measuring dry ingredients.
8. Fill in the blanks.
   A. _____ teaspoons = 1 tablespoon
   B. _____ tablespoons = 1 cup
   C. _____ ounces = 1 pound
   D. _____ quarts = 1 gallon
9. Why is it important to understand the measuring, cutting, mixing, and cooking terms used in recipes?
10. Why do you need to cook food at the correct temperature?
11. What is the difference between moist-heat cooking methods and dry-heat cooking methods?
12. List hints for cooking foods from each food group.
13. What should you do to prevent a banana from turning brown after it has been sliced?
14. What is the first step in making a time schedule?
15. Perry is making dinner tonight. While the potatoes bake, he is preparing the salad and making the main course. This is called _____.
16. True or false. Your kitchen should be organized according to work centers.
17. True or false. Work plans are used when cooking by yourself.

Life Skills

18. A manager of a local small restaurant is a friend of your family. The restaurant offers meals served in the restaurant and carryout food. She heard you had been studying safety and sanitation in the kitchen. She has asked you to visit her restaurant and check the safety and sanitation practices and to prepare a report for her. She will use the report to train her staff in the restaurant. Review Section 9-2 to develop your plan. Write the section's four headings at the top of one or two pages, then list the points under the heading you will look for on your visit. Turn in your final report. What have you learned that you might use in your family's kitchen?

Chapter 9 You in the Kitchen 291

Technology

19. Research the Internet for information about food safety education. Use a key term like food safety. The fightbac.org website offers simple, practical advice to keep food safe from harmful bacteria. Use word processing software to prepare a report with suggestions to help keep food safe in food preparation class and in the school cafeteria. Share this information with your classmates, teachers, and cafeteria manager.

Journal Writing

20. Plan to make a meal for your family. Choose the foods you want to prepare. Then make a schedule to follow when preparing the meal. After you have prepared your meal, write a short journal entry describing the event.

Academics

21. Science. Research which nontoxic, common household products can be used instead of cleaners with toxic chemicals. Those chemicals are unsafe and can cause pollution. Make a list of the environmentally friendly materials and substances that can be used for different kitchen cleaning tasks. Turn in a one-page report.
22. Math. In the school foods lab or at home, practice measuring 1 cup and 1 tablespoon of each of the following ingredients: milk, flour, brown sugar, and butter. Be sure to follow the directions given in the chapter.
23. Writing. In your food preparation class, write a work plan for a nutritious meal your group is going to prepare. Follow the work plan as your group prepares and serves the meal and cleans up. Discuss any problems that may have occurred after the event. Brainstorm ideas for how to solve these problems in the future.

FCCLA

24. Set up a family dinner night, where your family gathers at least one evening a week for dinner together. Work with your family to decide the night and the menus to be planned. Set up a work plan. Then develop an FCCLA *Family Ties* project for the *Power of One* program. Obtain further information about this program from your FCCLA advisor.

Journal Writing

Writing opportunities help students practice and develop writing skills.

Academics

Chapter content links to various academic areas such as math, science, social studies, and reading.

FCCLA

Individual and team activities suggest ways to expand projects for competitive events.

Lively Features and Charts

Succeed in Life

Explore life skills that promote success now and in the future.

Succeed in Life

Managing Your Stress

There are other actions you can take to manage your stress. You can practice good time management skills. You can prepare for events ahead of time. If getting ready for school is stressful, choose your clothes the night before. If you are worried about being in a new place, learn as much about it ahead of time as possible.

Take time to relax and have fun. Physical activity can help you cope with stress. Solving puzzles, playing games, and reading can take your mind off your stress. Many people tell their problems to their pets. Sometimes, just taking a walk will make you feel better. Many teens like listening to music when they are feeling stressed. Hobbies can be relaxing, too. What actions can you take to better manage your stress?

Handling Stress

Some people set too many goals. They do not have enough time and energy to meet their goals. This can cause stress. **Stress** is emotional, mental, or physical tension felt when faced with change. You can feel stress when you are in a new setting. Stress can also be caused by having too much to do.

When you are feeling stressed, your hands may become sweaty. Your heart may beat rapidly. You may even feel dizzy. These are all physical signs of stress. There are also emotional signs of stress. They include crying easily or acting bored, cranky, or depressed. People react differently to stress.

The leading cause of stress is change. When you are in a new setting, it is normal to feel uncomfortable. Moving to a new school or neighborhood is very stressful for many teens. Divorce, death, and illness can also cause stress. These events may cause changes in your family. A change in your family can be very hard to accept.

Following a healthful lifestyle can help reduce stress. You will be better able to cope with problems and changes if you feel your best. When you are tired, do not have enough energy, or do not eat right, situations may seem worse than they really are. Everyday problems may seem bigger. They may not be as easy for you

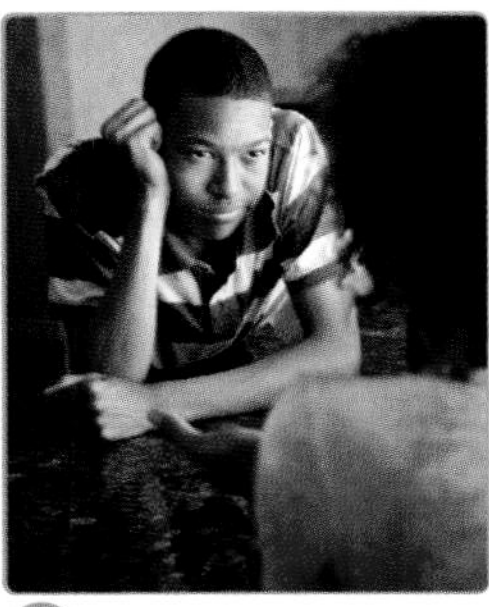

4-8 Talking with someone you trust can help you deal with stress.

Think Green

Environmental features suggest ways to raise student awareness.

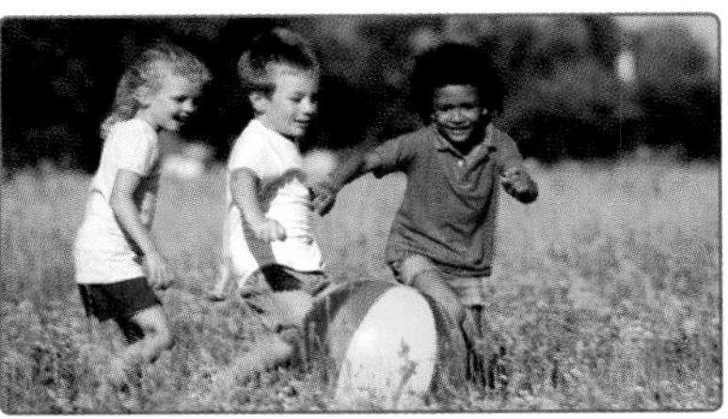

2-14 During the preschooler stage, children grow taller.

Preschoolers are children between the ages of three and five years. During this time, preschoolers are gaining greater independence moving about, talking, playing with others, and expressing emotions. Their bodies grow and develop in many different ways. See **2-14**. They gain greater ability to think, reason, and use language. Preschoolers tend to be more social and agreeable than toddlers. They are better able to express their emotions.

Physical Development

Preschoolers do not grow as fast as infants and toddlers. They gain weight slowly while growing taller. This makes them look slimmer.

The larger muscles of the arms and legs grow stronger during the preschool years. This allows preschoolers to enjoy active play. Preschoolers can climb trees or run up and down sidewalks. They can ride tricycles and use swings. These activities help preschoolers learn to control use of their large muscles.

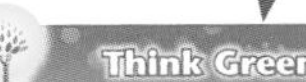

Think Green

Eco-friendly Play Dough

Making homemade play dough is not only a fun activity for young children, but it saves money, contains nothing toxic, and is biodegradable.

Ingredients
1 cup flour
1 cup warm water
½ cup salt
1 tablespoon vegetable oil
2 tablespoons cream of tartar
a few drops of food coloring

Mix all ingredients together, and stir over low heat. The dough will begin to thicken and look like mashed potatoes. Remove the pan from heat when dough pulls away from the sides and clumps. Allow it to cool enough to handle. Knead the dough on waxed paper until smooth and add food coloring. Always wash your hands before working with the dough. Store in airtight container in refrigerator.

Charts

Colorful charts bring chapter content to life and make concepts clearer.

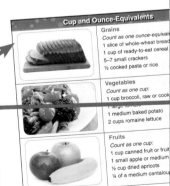

Cup and Ounce-Equivalents

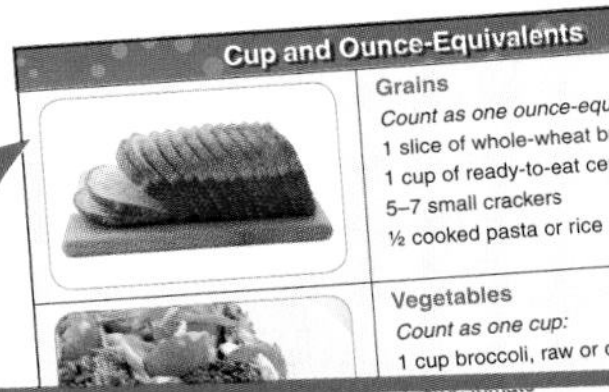

Grains
Count as one ounce-equival
1 slice of whole-wheat bread
1 cup of ready-to-eat cereal
5–7 small crackers
½ cooked pasta or rice

Vegetables
Count as one cup:
1 cup broccoli, raw or cook
1 medium baked potato
2 cups romaine lettuce

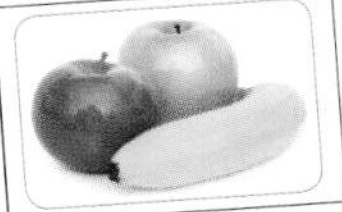

Fruits
Count as one cup:
1 cup canned fruit or fruit
1 small apple or medium
½ cup dried apricots
¼ of a medium cantalou

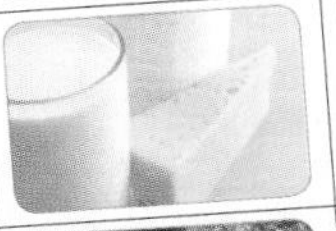

Dairy
Count as one cup:
1 cup fat-free or low-fat
1½ ounces natural che
2 ounces processed (A
⅓ cup shredded chees

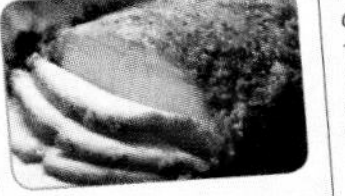

Protein
Count as one ounce-e
1 ounce cooked lean
1 egg
½ ounce of nuts
1 tablespoon peanut
¼ cup dried beans o
½ ounce sunflower s

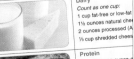

7-8 You need to know how to count the foods you eat ... groups in MyPlate.

The Nutrients

Functions	Sources
Proteions	
• Needed for growth and repair of body tissues. • Help body organs function and stay in good condition. • Supply energy.	Meat, eggs, poultry, fish, legumes, peanuts, nuts, seeds, milk, cheese, and yogurt.
Carbohydrates	
• Supply energy. • Provide fiber to aid in digestion and remove body wastes.	Breads, cereals, rice, pasta, fruits, vegetables, legumes, and sugar and other sweets.
Fats	
• Provide energy. • Insulate the body. • Cushion body organs. • Help promote growth and healthy skin.	Oil, butter, margarine, salad dressing, meat, poultry, eggs, cheese, nuts, and peanut butter.
Vitamins	
Vitamin A • Helps with normal vision. • Helps keep body tissues healthy. • Helps with growth.	Dark green vegetables, deep yellow or orange vegetables and fruits, and eggs.
B Vitamins (thiamin, riboflavin, niacin) • Help your body use other nutrients in food for energy. • Help keep skin, hair, muscles, and nerves healthy. • Help keep appetite and digestion normal. • Help your body use oxygen more efficiently.	Meat, poultry, fish, eggs, whole-grain and enriched breads and cereals, milk, cheese, yogurt, and ice cream.
Vitamin C • Helps keep gums healthy. • Helps cuts and bruises heal. • Helps your body fight infections. • Helps with growth.	Oranges, grapefruit, lemons, limes, tangerines, berries, papaya, melons, broccoli, spinach, peppers, kale, collards, mustard greens, turnip greens, potatoes, tomatoes, and cabbage.
Minerals	
Calcium • Helps build strong, healthy bones and teeth. • Helps the heart beat properly. • Helps muscles move.	Milk, cheese, yogurt, ice cream, leafy green vegetables, and fish with tiny bones.
Iron • Helps blood carry oxygen. • Helps cells use oxygen.	Meat, eggs, liver, legumes, and whole-grain and enriched breads and cereals.
Water	
• Carries nutrients to the cells and wastes away from cells. • Helps regulate body processes such as digestion. • Helps maintain normal body temperature. • Helps cells operate.	Milk, juices, soups, drinking water, juicy fruits and vegetables, and some solid foods.

7-1 Knowing the functions and sources of nutrients can help you eat nutritiously.

Concepts Presented Simply

Link

These features relate chapter content to academic skills, health and safety, and community involvement:

Community Link	Reading Link	Think Green
Financial Literacy Link	Safety Link	Writing Link
Health Link	Science Link	
Math Link	Social Studies Link	

36 Unit 1 You and Others

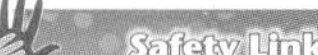

Safety Link

Prevent Bullying

Acting like a bully is an unhealthy form of communication. Bullying can be the use of written, verbal, or electronic expression, or a physical act or gesture. Some schools have guidelines to prevent bullying. If you experience bullying, share the details with an adult, such as a parent or teacher. Always use healthy communication.

You enjoy being with other people. Healthy communication means letting people know how you really feel. When you do, they can better understand you.

Try to express positive thoughts and feelings about other people. Do not assume people know you care about them. There are many ways to let them know. You can tell them in person. Write a letter or poem. Show how you feel by using nonverbal communication. You can make a drawing or give someone a hug or a smile.

Healthy communication often occurs when you feel good about yourself, and then you share that with others. There are times, however, when you do not feel good about yourself. You may take this out on other people. You may use harsh words to hurt them or ignore them. You may act like a bully. A **bully** is a person who uses strength or power to persuade or pressure others (using force or fear) to do something. These are unhealthy forms of communication that can hurt people.

When people feel hurt, healthy communication can still be present. If people are aware of others' moods, they can help. For instance, your mother may sense when you feel hurt, and respond lovingly. Your teacher may know you work hard in class, and offer praise.

Talk about your negative feelings. For instance, when your parents buy you new clothes, thank them. If you do not like the clothes, let them know. Explain why you do not like the clothes. Ask your parents if you can return them and choose what you like. Your parents should try to understand. When they tell you why they chose the clothes, you will better understand them.

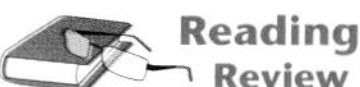

Reading Review

1. What are some benefits of healthy communication?
2. How can you let people know you care about them?
3. What are some signs of unhealthy communication?

96 Unit 2 You—A Manager

Community Link

Learning Values from Others

You learn values from what others say and do. For instance, young children are strongly affected by their parents' values. They notice how their parents act and what they say. For instance, when parents volunteer to help with a food drive, children often learn to value community involvement. Some children are also influenced by the values of their religious training.

As children get older, they have more experiences outside the home. Their friends and teachers may have values different from their parents. Children may consider these values. They may then accept some of the values, and reject others.

What is most important to you in life? What do you hope to do today and in the future? The answers to these questions are determined by your values and goals. **Values** are strong beliefs and ideas about what is important. **Goals** are what you want to achieve. Your values and goals affect the life you lead.

Values

Your values are part of you. See 3-6. They serve as guides for how you live your life. They provide direction for your actions. Knowing your values can help you make satisfying decisions.

You can have many different values. A few examples are freedom, service to others, and strong family ties. You and your family's views on religion, education, health, and security are also values. Your values affect what you want and how you act. They also affect how you use your resources and the decisions you make, or choose not to make. For instance, you may value being healthy. To maintain a healthful lifestyle, you choose to be physically active and eat healthful foods.

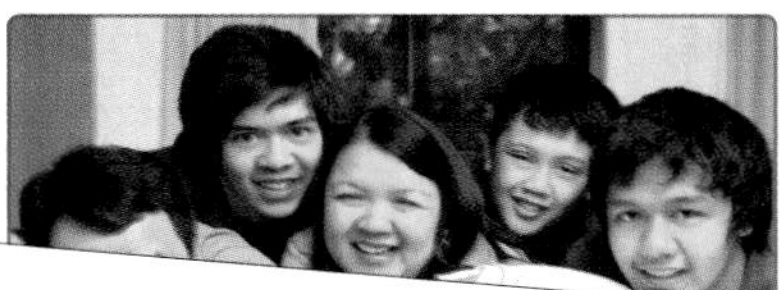

Chapter 7 The Foods You Eat 203

Cultural and Social Influences

Another strong influence on your choice of food is your ethnic or cultural heritage. When people talk about their culture, they often describe special foods that are part of their background. Throughout the world, people enjoy foods that reflect their local cultures. In England, people might dine on fish and chips. In Italy, pasta dishes are part of the culture. In the Middle East, people often eat hummus, which is a food made from chickpeas. See 7-3.

A wide variety of foods is part of the culture in the United States. People from many different cultures contributed these foods. Native Americans were one of these cultural groups. Hundreds of years ago, Native Americans raised corn, beans, pumpkins, and squash. These foods are still part of the culture in the United States.

Each cultural group that settled in the United States brought its own eating habits and food customs. For instance, people from China brought the cooking technique of stir-frying. People from Mexico brought foods such as tacos and burritos.

Sometimes people could not find foods from their culture. Therefore, they adapted available foods to their ways of cooking. They also created new ways to prepare these foods. For instance, French people in Louisiana developed Cajun cooking.

As the United States grew, many people moved from one region to another. They again brought their food customs with them. As a result, you can now find many cultural foods throughout the United States.

Traditions are customs passed from one generation to another. Family traditions affect foods children learn to like and enjoy. Typical breads on your family table may be bagels, biscuits, or tortillas. Special meats, fish, or baked goods may be prepared for family celebrations. Some families adapt traditional foods to meet the changing likes and dislikes of family members. Some families and individuals follow vegetarian meal patterns. See 7-4.

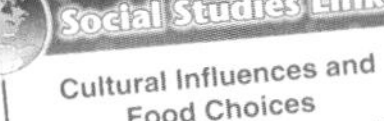

Social Studies Link

Cultural Influences and Food Choices

Some of the foods your family eats may relate to your culture. They may be foods your relatives brought from another country. The region where you live is also part of your culture. Some of the foods you enjoy may be special to your region. Southern fried chicken and New England clam chowder are examples.

Bring a special family food to class and have a *tasting party*. Along with the food, include a brief summary of the origin of the food and the recipe. Bring enough copies of the recipe to share with the class.

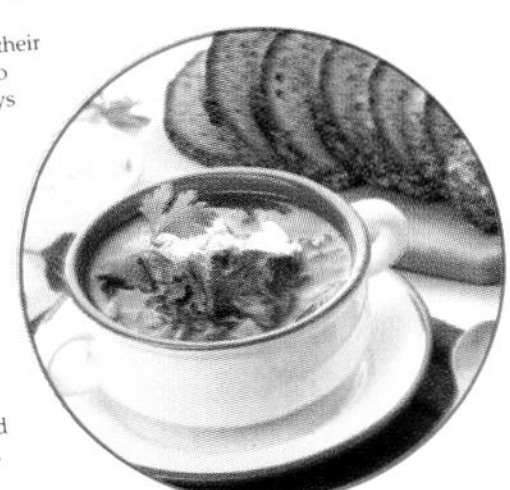

7-3 Borscht, a beet soup, is popular in Russian culture.

Chapter 7 The Foods You Eat 215

Most teens want to look and feel their best. Every person's natural size is different. There is no one size that is *better* than another. You may, however, want to gain or lose a few pounds. You may want to maintain your current weight. To manage your weight, you need to learn how to balance the healthful foods you eat with physical activity.

Health Link

Planning a Healthful Diet

When planning a diet, remember to choose foods from the five main groups in MyPlate. You should also eat regular meals that include a variety of foods. Be sure to choose lower calorie foods and eat smaller amounts to lose weight. If you want to gain weight, choose nutritious higher calorie foods and eat larger amounts. Be sure to check with a doctor, nutritionist, or school nurse before beginning any diet program.

Calories

Energy is the capacity for doing work. The energy you get from food helps you stay alive, work, play, grow, and be healthy. **Calories** are units of energy provided by proteins, carbohydrates, and fats. For instance, an orange has around 60 calories. This means it will supply your body with that much energy for activity. You need to eat a certain number of calories each day. They provide your body with the energy it needs to function.

You need to learn about calories. Your MyPlate plan tells you how many calories you need. This amount depends on your age, sex, and level of physical activity. See 7-9. Physical activity helps you use calories.

You should also find out how many calories are in the foods you eat. Some cookbooks and nutrition books have calorie charts. You can record your physical activity and the food you eat on choose**MyPlate**.gov. It will keep track of your calories for you.

Reading Review

1. Why might you and your friends have different calorie needs?
2. How can you find out how many calories are in your favorite foods?

Calories and Weight

The food you eat provides your body with the calories it needs. If you eat a balanced diet and are at a healthy weight for your body build, you are probably eating the right number of calories. This means your body uses all the calories you take in from

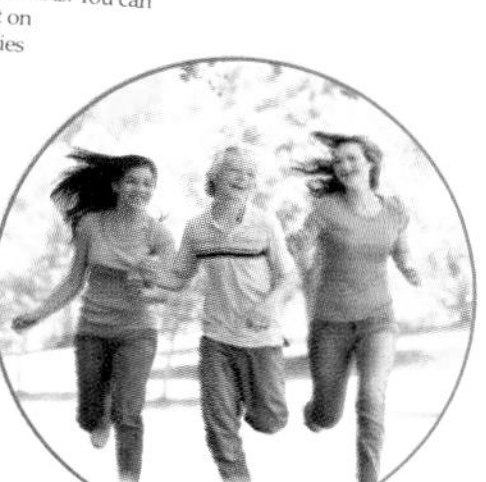

7-9 Your body needs more calories to run than it does to watch TV.

Career Options to Plan for the Future

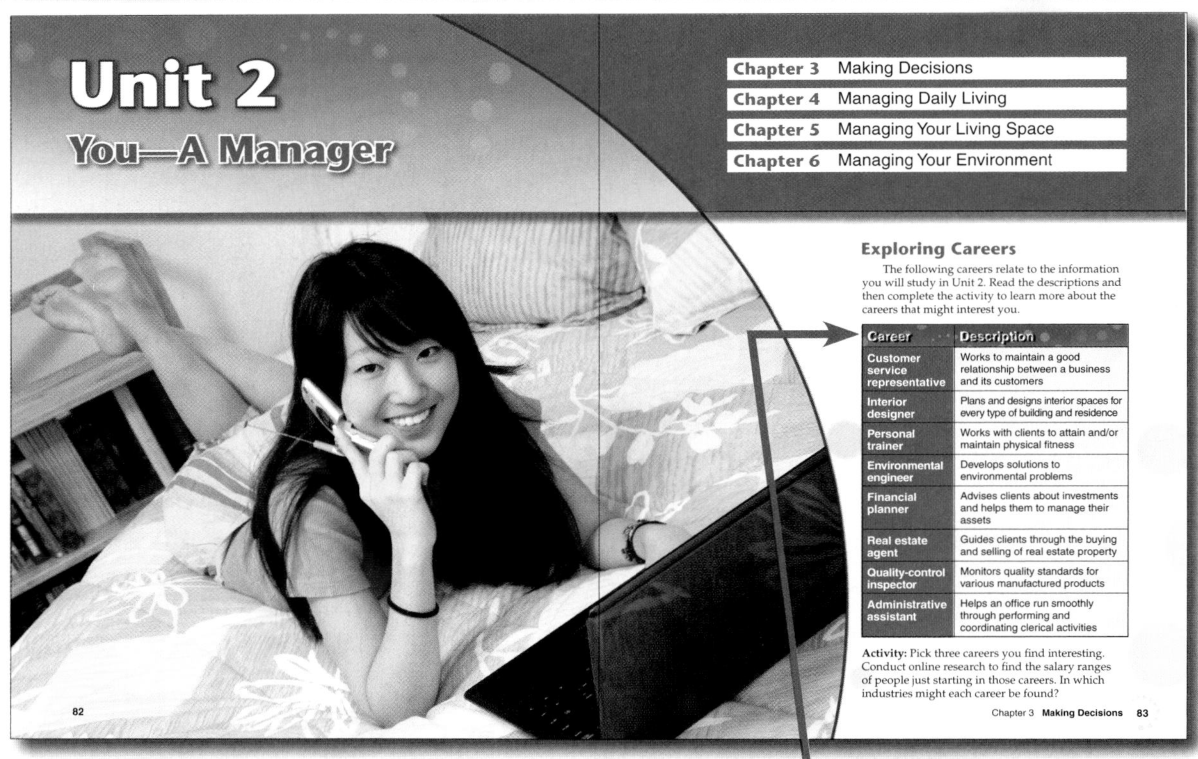
Unit 2
You—A Manager

Chapter 3 Making Decisions
Chapter 4 Managing Daily Living
Chapter 5 Managing Your Living Space
Chapter 6 Managing Your Environment

Exploring Careers

The following careers relate to the information you will study in Unit 2. Read the descriptions and then complete the activity to learn more about the careers that might interest you.

Career	Description
Customer service representative	Works to maintain a good relationship between a business and its customers
Interior designer	Plans and designs interior spaces for every type of building and residence
Personal trainer	Works with clients to attain and/or maintain physical fitness
Environmental engineer	Develops solutions to environmental problems
Financial planner	Advises clients about investments and helps them to manage their assets
Real estate agent	Guides clients through the buying and selling of real estate property
Quality-control inspector	Monitors quality standards for various manufactured products
Administrative assistant	Helps an office run smoothly through performing and coordinating clerical activities

Activity: Pick three careers you find interesting. Conduct online research to find the salary ranges of people just starting in those careers. In which industries might each career be found?

82

Chapter 3 **Making Decisions** 83

Exploring Careers

On each unit opener, career snapshots relate to the information you will study. Complete the activities to learn about more career options available.

Unit 5
The World of Work

Chapter 12
Learning About Work
- Section 12-1 Questions About Work
- Section 12-2 Researching Careers
- Section 12-3 Heading for a Career
- Section 12-4 Career Options

Chapter 13
Preparing for Work
- Section 13-1 Getting Your First Job
- Section 13-2 Getting Ready for Job Success

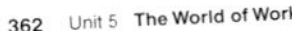

362 Unit 5 The World of Work

you have an aptitude for music, you may quickly develop the abili... play an instrument. If you have a low aptitude, however, you may... practice much more to learn the skill.

Learning about your interests, aptitudes, and abilities can p... you to careers you will enjoy. Your guidance counselor can give... interest inventory or an aptitude test. These tests are often avail... take online, too.

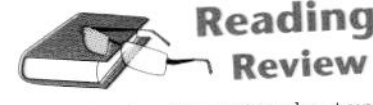

Reading Review

1. Why should learning about yourself be the first step in de... career?
2. What is one of your aptitudes? What job might let you use...

The Career Clusters

The **career clusters** are 16 groups of career specialties. ... cluster includes jobs that require similar knowledge and ski... *knowledge and skills*. When you explore each cluster, you wi...

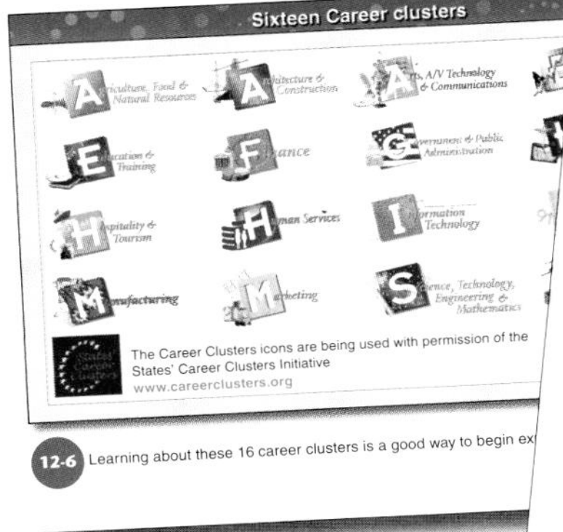

Sixteen Career clusters
The Career Clusters icons are being used with permission of the States' Career Clusters Initiative
www.careerclusters.org

12-6 Learning about these 16 career clusters is a good way to begin ex...

Chapter 12 Learning About Work 377

Family and Consumer Sciences

Major Categories	Postsecondary Training and / or Associate's Degree	Bachelor's Degree or Higher
Food Science, Nutrition, and Wellness	Banquet manager Caterer Chef or chief cook Cook's helper Executive chef Personal trainer Restaurant owner Short-order cook	Athletic trainer Dietitian Food service manager Food technologist Product developer Quality control supervisor Sanitation supervisor
Housing and Interior Design	Designer's aide Drapery/slipcover maker Home furnishings salesperson Home lighting assistant Upholstery assistant	Facilities planner Home furnishings buyer Home lighting designer Home planning specialist Interior designer Kitchen and bath designer
Textiles and Apparel	Alterationist Clothing consultant Display artist Dry cleaner Fashion or textile designer Store manager Tailor/reweaver	Apparel historian Apparel marketing specialist Merchandise manager Textile market analyst Textile scientist
Child and Human Development	Child care teacher Designer of children's clothing, toys, or furniture Parent's helper Scout leader Teacher's aide	Child care center or preschool administrator Early childhood educator Parent educator Recreation director
Family Relations	Home companions Counseling paraprofessional Homemaker services director Hot line counselor Older adult living facilities aide	Crisis center counselor Family health counselor Family/marriage therapist Youth services specialist
Personal and Family Finance	Bank teller Collection agent Consumer product specialist Consumer service representative Credit bureau clerk Loan officer assistant	Consumer affairs director Credit counselor Financial planner Loan officer Money investment advisor Retail credit manager
Education and Communications	4-H leader Journalism intern Teacher's aide	Cooperative extension agent Family and consumer sciences teacher or college professor

12-17 Family and consumer sciences offers a wide range of job opportunities.

Chapter 12

Chapter 12 introduces and summarizes the 16 career clusters. It also shows examples of the many Family and Consumer Sciences career choices available.

Chapter 13

Chapter 13 describes the skills you need to get your first job and how to be successful in the workplace.

Chapter 13 Preparing for Work 385

Applying for Jobs

You can apply for a job in person, by telephone, by mail, or online. Carefully follow the directions given by the jobs that interest you. The employer may ask you to submit a résumé, letter of application, and references.

A **résumé** is a written description of a person's education, qualifications, and work experience. See 13-2. Your résumé will help employers learn more about you. Some employers may want you to submit an *electronic résumé*. This is a text-only file with any special formatting removed.

Jennifer L. Wright
1603 Main Street
Parker, Iowa 50992
(555) 555-7474
jenwright@provider.com

Objective	Seeking a summer camp assistant counselor position.
Education	Parkview High School, Parker, Iowa, 20XX to present. Focus on human services, with an emphasis in child development. Graduating in June, 20XX.
Experience	Activities Volunteer, Ronald McDonald House (RMDH), 20XX to present. Responsible for preparing snacks and planning and running activities for the families staying at RMDH while their children are hospitalized far from home. Babysitter, 20XX to present. Providing quality child care for three families with children ages ten months to nine years.
Computer skills	Proficient in keyboarding and Microsoft Word, Excel, and PowerPoint.
Honors and Activities	Parkview High School honor roll, 20XX. Member, Family, Career and Community Leaders of America (FCCLA), Parkview High School chapter, 20XX to present. Member, Parkview High School creative writing club, 20XX to present. Captain, Parkview High School JV volleyball team, 20XX.

13-2 The information on your résumé helps employers decide if you will be a good fit for their company.

Unit 5 The World of Work

Sometimes when applying for a job, you may need to submit a letter of application. A **letter of application** is a document you send with your résumé to give more information about your skills. See 13-3.

Many employers also want you to give references when applying for jobs. A **reference** is a name of a person who can be contacted about you and your work habits. Always ask people if they will give you

1603 Main Street
Parker, Iowa 50992
April 10, 20XX

Ms. Britta Nelson
Program Director
Twin Pines Camp
Rural Route 1
Big Bear Lake, Iowa 51119

Dear Ms. Nelson:

I am interested in working as a counselor-in-training at Twin Pines this summer. My guidance counselor at Parkview High School, Mr. Brandon, suggested I write you and explain my qualifications. I am currently a junior and have already taken two child development classes, with another planned next year.

I went to Twin Pines' camp for three years and really loved it. So I am very familiar with the camp and its policies and procedures. In addition to babysitting for the past five years, I also volunteer four hours a week at the Ronald McDonald House, a charity through McDonald's Corporation that keeps families together while their child is receiving critical medical treatment far from home. My duties involve planning a variety of activities for the families, such as crafts, games, and snacks. I enjoy being with children and helping them learn. My long-term career goal is to open my own child care center when I graduate from college.

I have enclosed my résumé and would appreciate the opportunity to meet for an interview. Please contact me at (555) 555-7474 or at jenwright@provider.com. I look forward to further discussion about Twin Pines' counselors-in-training program. Thank you for your time and consideration.

Sincerely,

Jennifer L. Wright

Jennifer L. Wright

13-3 A letter of application introduces your résumé and highlights specific skills.

Contents in Brief

Contents

Unit 1
You and Others

Chapter 1

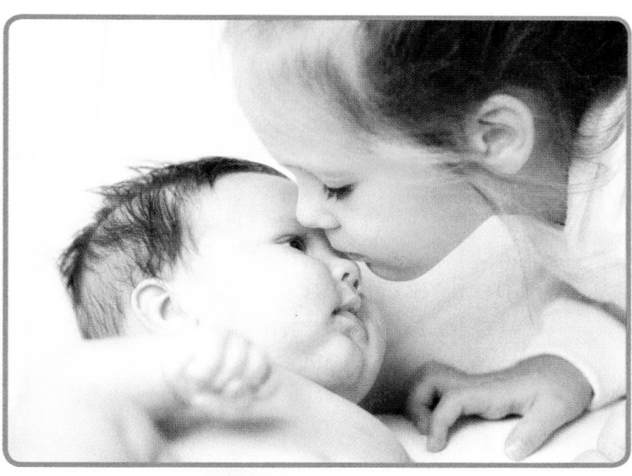

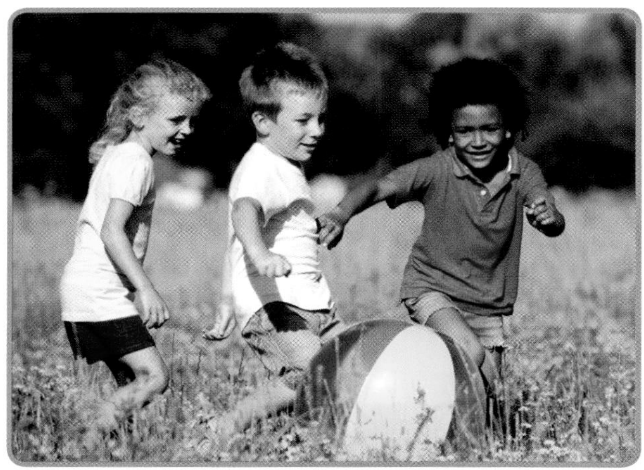

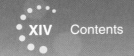

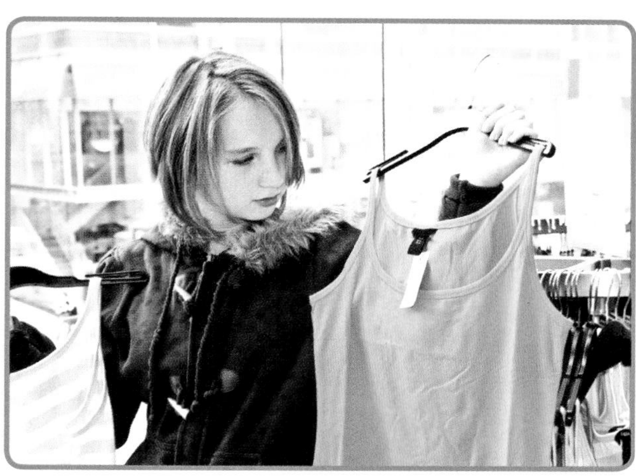

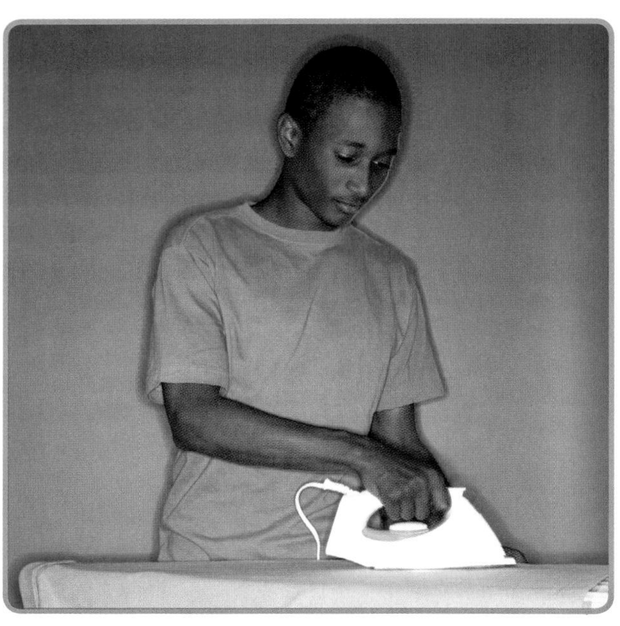

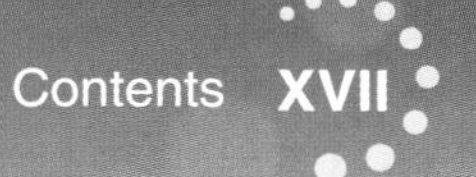

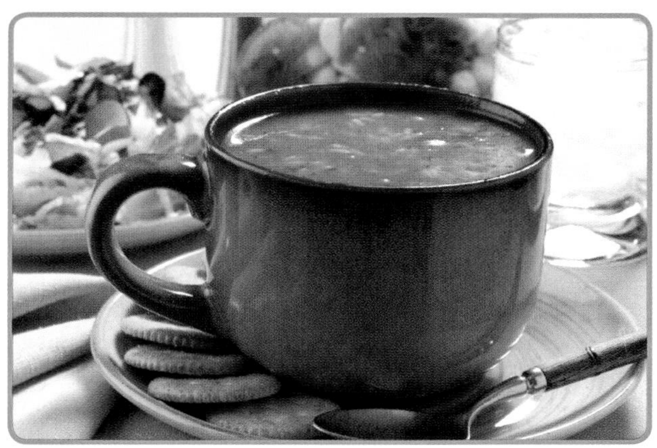

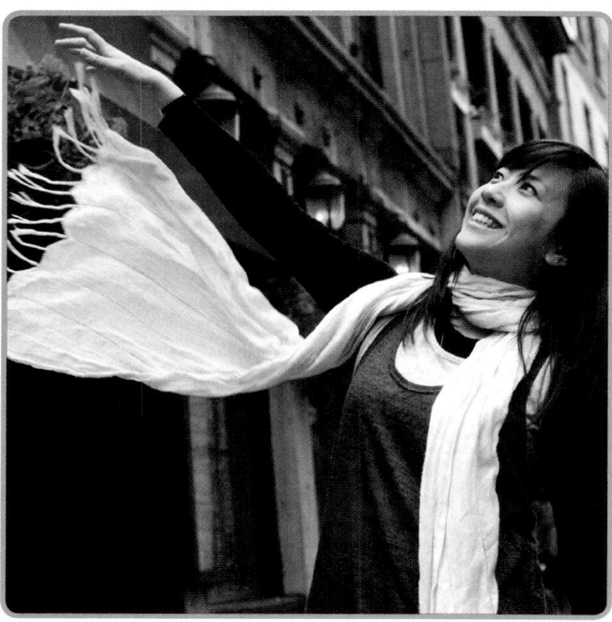

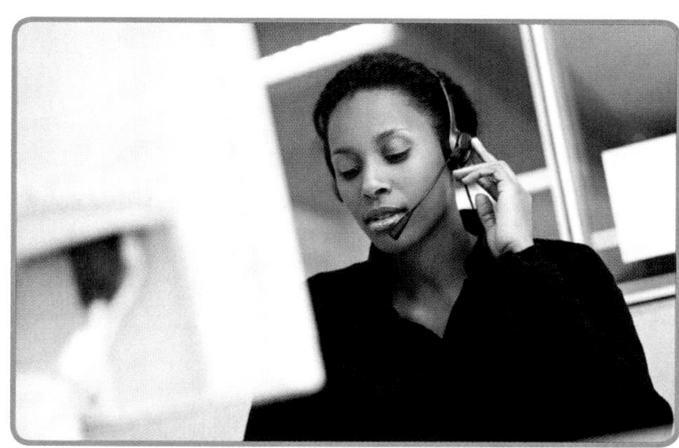

Features

Succeed in Life

Community Link

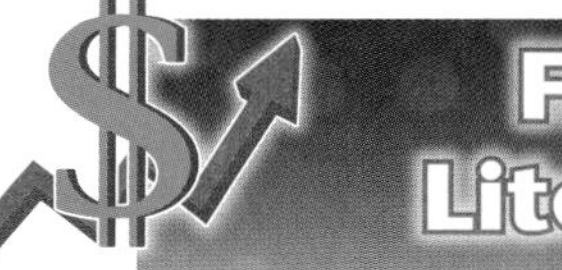

Financial Literacy Link

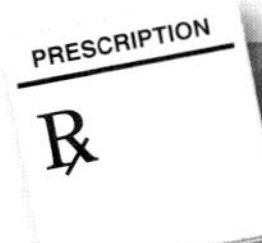

Health Link

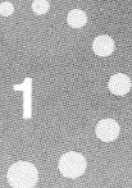

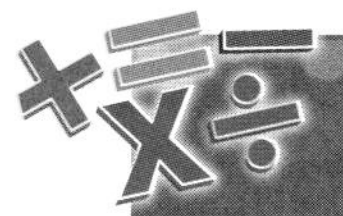

Math Link

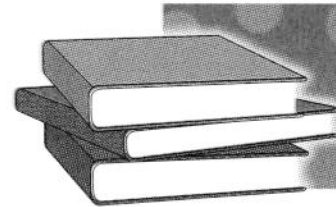

Reading Link

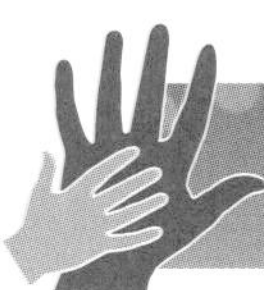

Safety Link

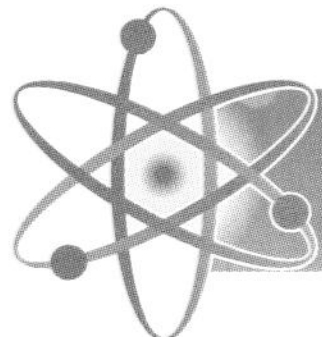

Science Link

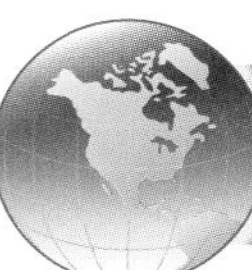

Social Studies Link

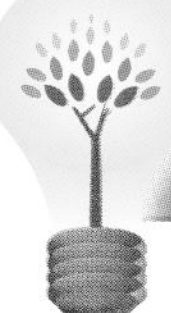

Think Green

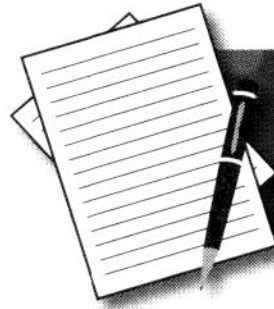

Writing Link

Unit 1
You and Others

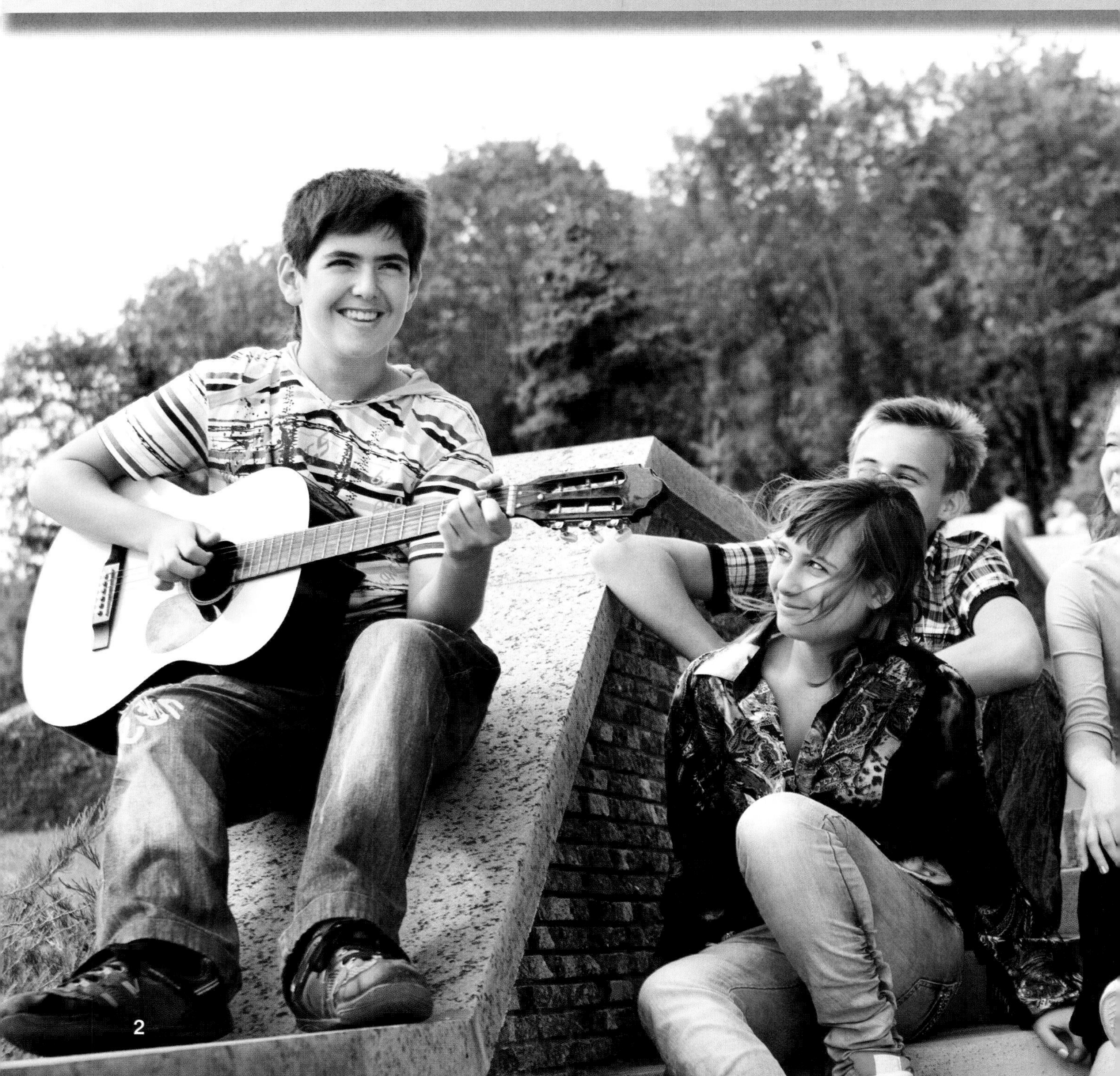

Chapter 1 Learning About You

Chapter 2 Learning About Children

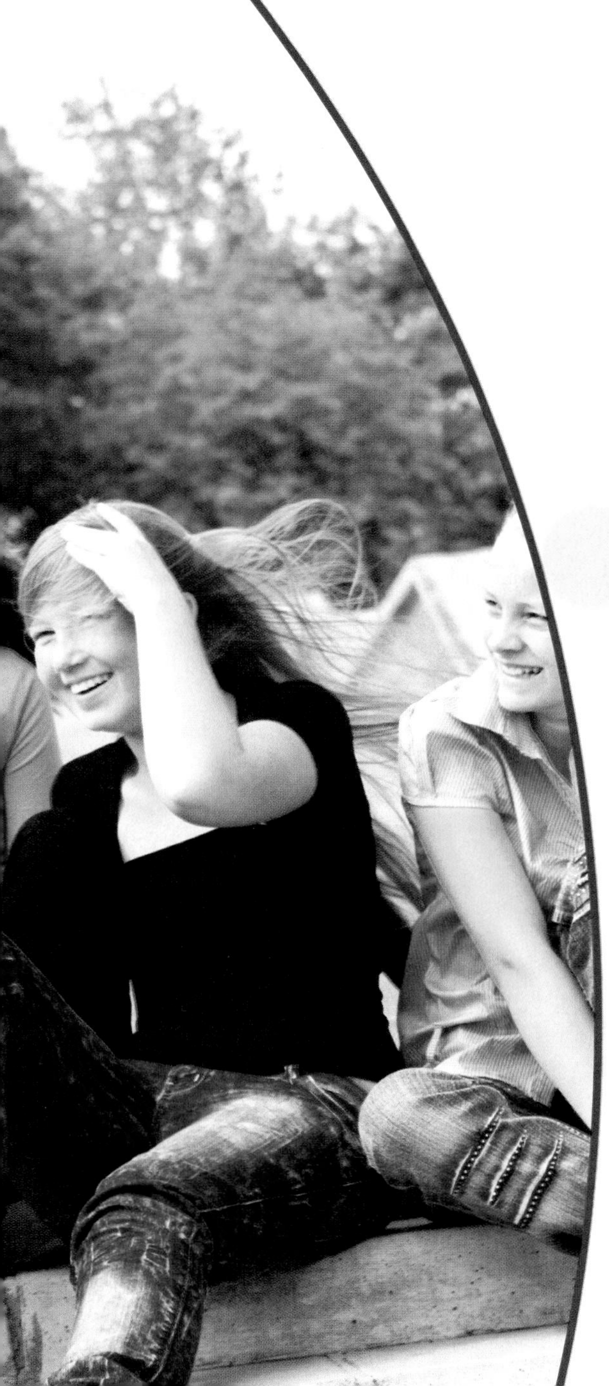

Exploring Careers

The following careers relate to the information you will study in Unit 1. Read the descriptions and then complete the activity to learn more about the careers that might interest you.

Career	Description
Family therapist	Promotes healthier family functioning
Activity specialist	Provides instruction in specialties such as art, music, and drama
Toy designer	Develops products suitable for use by children
Child care worker	Provides for the physical and emotional needs of children
Camp counselor	Leads and instructs children and teens in various forms of recreation
Social worker	Helps people deal with various personal and family problems
Guidance counselor	Helps students deal with social, behavioral, and personal problems
Preschool teacher	Helps children learn basic concepts and improve social skills

Activity: Choose two careers from the list that interest you. Use online or print sources to find out about the training and education needed for each career. Make a list of classes you may need to take to prepare for these careers.

Chapter 1
Learning About You

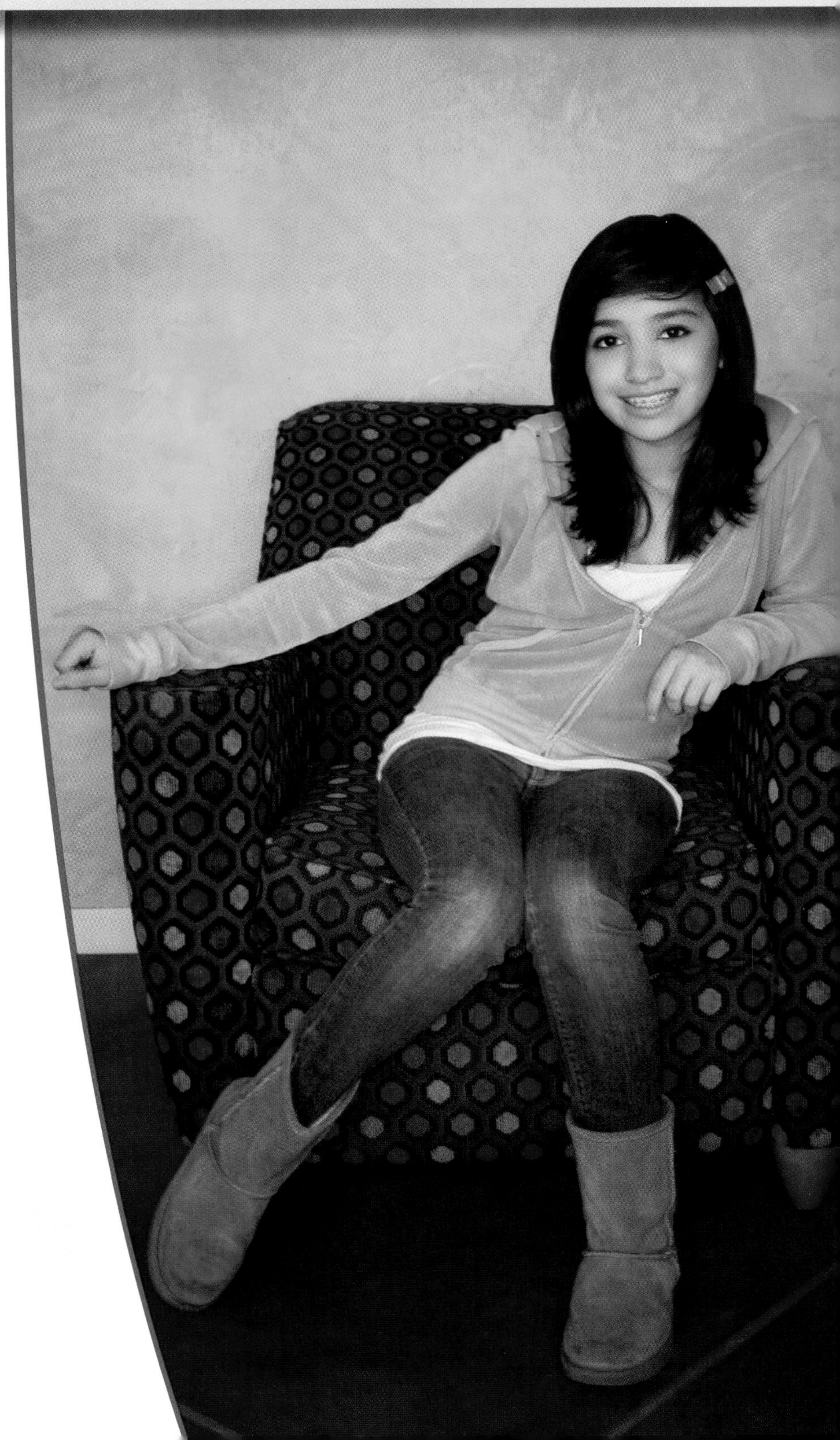

Sections

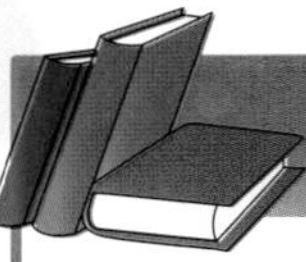

Sharpen Your Reading

Before you read the chapter, read all chart and photo captions. What do you learn about the material covered in this chapter just from reading the captions?

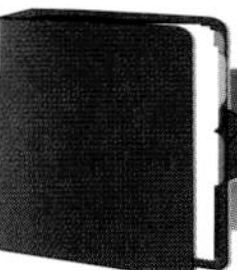

Concept Organizer

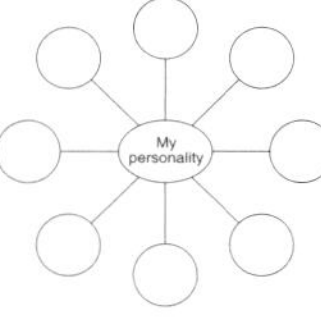

Use a star diagram like the one shown to identify the traits that best describe your personality. How does your personality influence what your family and friends think of you?

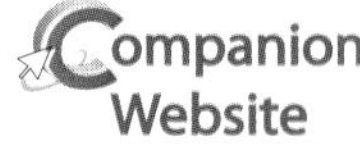

Print out the concept organizer at the website.

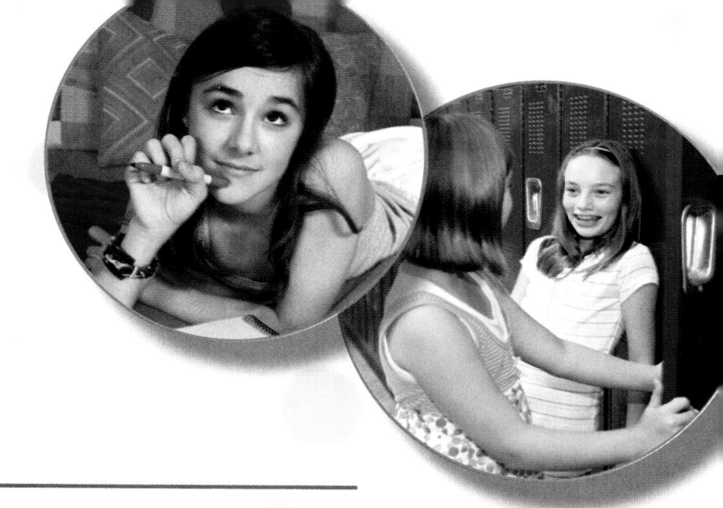

Section 1-1
Looking at Yourself

Objectives

After studying this section, you will be able to
- **define** *traits*, *personality*, *heredity*, *environment*, *self-concept*, *self-esteem*, and *self-confidence*.
- **describe** how traits identify a person.
- **explain** how you can change your physical traits and personality.

Key Terms

traits: distinguishing characteristics of a person.

personality: the group of traits that makes each person a unique individual.

heredity: the result of receiving traits from parents or ancestors.

environment: the conditions, objects, places, and people that are all around a person.

self-concept: the way a person sees himself or herself.

self-esteem: the way a person feels about his or her self-concept.

self-confidence: the feeling of being sure of yourself and your abilities.

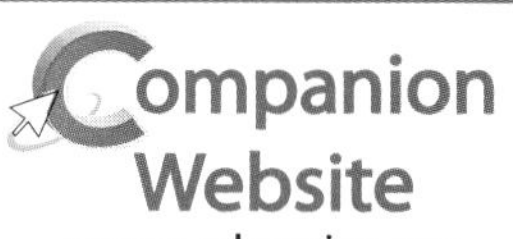

Study the Key Terms by completing crossword puzzles, matching activities, and e-flash cards at the website.

Main Ideas

- The personality of each person is unique.
- The physical traits and personality of each person are influenced by heredity and environment.
- Learning how to become the person you want to be is important in growth and development.

Have you ever looked in a mirror and asked, "Who am I?" It can be fun and exciting to do that sometimes. When you gaze in the mirror, you may think about the person you want to become. You are an individual, a special person. No other human being in the whole world is just like you. See **1-1**.

Personality

The way you act and feel makes you unique. Your feelings and actions are influenced by your **traits**, or your distinguishing characteristics. They start developing early in life. Throughout your life, they continue to grow and develop. Your traits combine in a way that makes you one of a kind.

Your **personality** is made up of the group of traits that makes you unique. Reflect on your personality for a moment. The way you look, think, and behave are all part of your personality. Your personality should reveal who you are, not what others think you should be.

How you get along with people reflects your personality. Your personality also influences what your family and friends think of you. Words such as *friendly*, *nice*, *thoughtful*, *pleasant*, and *witty* may describe you. Perhaps you use different words to describe yourself and the personalities of other people.

You may wonder why a person has a certain personality. Two factors affect personality: heredity and environment.

1-1 Taking a close look at yourself can help you identify all your special qualities.

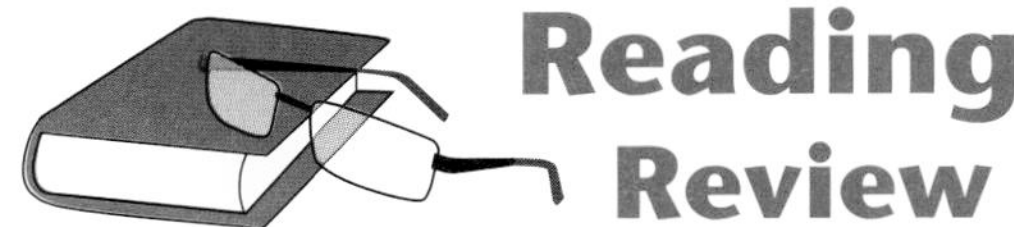

Reading Review

1. What causes each person to have a unique personality?
2. Name two factors that affect personality.

Heredity and Environment

Your development is the result of both heredity and environment. **Heredity** is the result of receiving traits from parents or ancestors. Heredity helps determine your physical traits. *Physical traits* are the distinguishing characteristics of your body. They are the characteristics that people can see, such as your height and body build. The color of your eyes, hair, and skin are also physical traits. You received these traits from your parents and grandparents. They are *inherited*.

Of course, certain other factors affect the physical traits you inherit. One is the way you live. For instance, if you are usually active, you can more easily maintain your desired weight. This affects the appearance of your inherited body build. Another factor is how you change your features. An example is changing the color of your hair. Your diet can affect your physical traits, too. The food you eat can influence your weight and your height. It also affects the appearance of your hair and the condition of your skin.

Heredity

In some families, brothers and sisters look alike. In other families, the children may not look like each other or their parents. Sometimes, children begin to look more like their parents as they grow older. The reason people look like other family members is heredity.

Look at pictures of yourself at various ages. Compare these pictures with those of other family members. In what ways do you look like the rest of your family? How are you different?

The other factor that influences your personality is environment. Your **environment** is your surroundings and the people in your life. Your environment includes your home, neighborhood, and school. It also includes family members, neighbors, classmates, and teachers.

All the people and places in your life affect you in your environment. Your family and friends, however, probably have the greatest effect on you. They are closer to you than anyone else. They are part of your environment every day. See **1-2**.

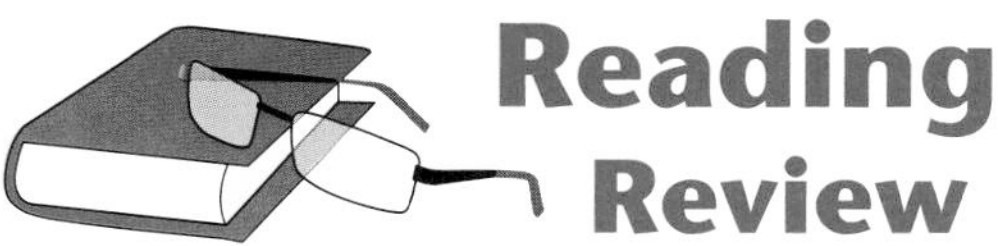

1. What are some physical traits you inherit from your parents?
2. What factors can influence the physical traits you inherit?
3. How do the people and places in your life affect you in your environment?

Self-Concept

Your **self-concept** is the way you see yourself. This includes the way you think about yourself. For instance, the feelings you have about your appearance are part of your self-concept.

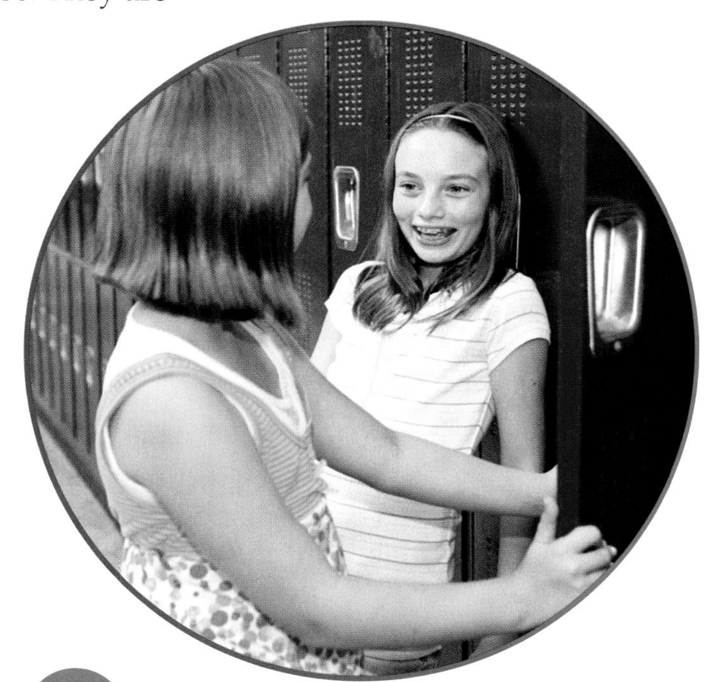

1-2 Your friends at school are part of your environment.

The feelings others have about you are reflected in your self-concept. The trust your parents have in you influences your self-concept. You feel confident and good about yourself when others trust you. The respect of your friends shapes your self-concept as well.

Self-Esteem

Think for a moment about your self-concept. Do you think about yourself in positive ways? Do you feel good about your appearance? Do you feel proud about your accomplishments? These feelings are part of your self-esteem. How you feel about your self-concept is called **self-esteem**.

People with healthy self-esteem feel good about themselves and enjoy life. They see themselves as able to do things. They accept and respect themselves and others.

Self-Confidence

Having a positive self-concept and healthy self-esteem creates **self-confidence**. You feel sure of yourself. You believe in yourself and your abilities. This gives you the courage to deal with new experiences and people in positive ways. As a result, you will feel that your actions are worthwhile. You will do better in school, and trying new activities will seem more fun.

You can boost the self-confidence of your family members and friends. Make them feel appreciated, worthwhile, and loved.

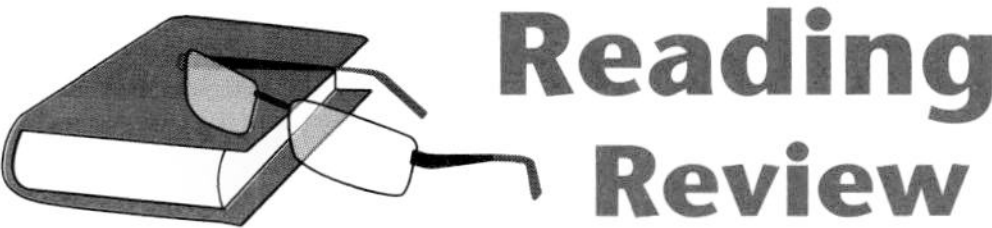

1. How can the feelings others have about you affect your self-concept?
2. Why do people with healthy self-esteem enjoy life?
3. How is your school performance affected by your self-confidence?

How You Can Change

Do you like the person you are? Are you happy with your appearance and your personality? People who have positive feelings about themselves enjoy life. Other people like them and enjoy being with them.

Suppose you are not happy with the way you look. You may wish you could change. There are ways you can do this. Exercise can help tone your muscles and make you feel more energetic. You can change your appearance by updating your wardrobe, wearing contact lenses, or changing your hairstyle.

You can also make changes if you do not feel good about your personality. Making changes may not be easy, but they are possible. You have control over who you are.

Who Am I?

- Am I happy with my appearance, weight, hairstyle, complexion, and posture? Why or why not? How can I make changes?
- Am I doing things I like to do, or doing things only because my friends do them? How do I feel about this?
- Do I talk a lot, or am I quiet much of the time? Do I talk a lot about myself, or do I try to learn about other people? How does this make me feel?
- Do I enjoy being with other people? Do others enjoy being with me? How does this make me feel?
- Am I comfortable spending time alone, or do I always have to be with other people? How do I feel about this?

1-3 Spend a few private moments thinking about who you are and how you feel.

Ask yourself the questions in Figure **1-3**. You may think of others. Some of your answers may please you, and some may not. Your answers, however, should be honest. These answers will give you a true picture of your own personality. Then you are ready to plan for changes.

Some changes you can work on alone. For others, you may need the help and advice of other people. Ask your parents, teachers, or other adults what they think about your ideas. Their comments may help you as you try to understand yourself. Try to be patient as you work on improving your personality and your appearance. Remember that changes do not happen at once. They take time.

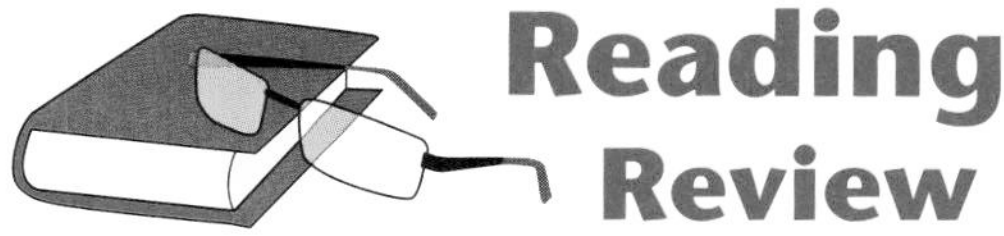

Reading Review

1. What are some physical traits that are possible to change? Explain your answer.
2. What are some ways you can change personality traits?

Section Summary

- Your development is the result of both heredity and environment.
- The traits and personality of each person are unique.
- Personality develops and changes as a person grows and matures.
- Some physical traits are inherited.
- Self-concept is the way a person sees himself or herself.
- Self-esteem is how a person feels about his or her self-concept. Having a positive self-concept creates self-confidence.
- A person can change his or her appearance and personality.

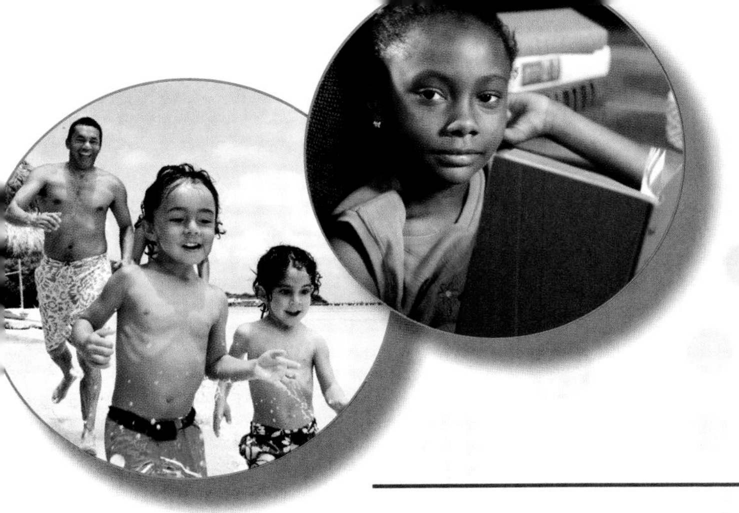

Section 1-2
Changing and Growing

Objectives

After studying this section, you will be able to
- **define** *growth*, *development*, *accept*, *developmental tasks*, *independence*, *adolescence*, *character*, and *responsibility*.
- **give examples** of ways people continually grow and develop.
- **explain** how adolescence prepares you to become an adult.

Key Terms

growth: specific body changes that can be measured.

development: age-related changes that are orderly and directional (moves toward greater complexity).

accept: to view as normal or proper.

developmental tasks: skills or behavior patterns people should accomplish at certain stages of their lives.

independence: the freedom to decide, act, and care for yourself.

adolescence: the stage of growth between childhood and adulthood.

character: the traits that guide you in deciding right from wrong.

responsibility: a task you are expected or trusted to do.

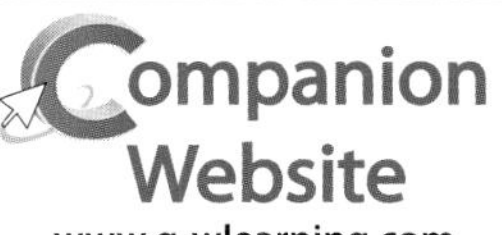

Study the Key Terms by completing crossword puzzles, matching activities, and e-flash cards at the website.

Main Ideas

- The process of growth and development continues throughout life.
- Adolescence is a period of time between childhood and adulthood.
- Adolescence is a stage of life that prepares you for greater responsibilities and independence as an adult.

Life is a constant process of growth and development. From birth to death, people grow and change in many ways. You know that you have changed in many ways since childhood. You will keep on changing and growing during adolescence and adulthood.

Your Growth and Development

Experts in human development study the growth and development of people. **Growth** includes specific body changes that can be measured. **Development** refers to age-related changes that are orderly and directional (moves toward greater complexity). Experts usually agree on four major types of growth and development. They are physical, intellectual, social, and emotional.

Physical growth and development involves body changes. For instance, you grow taller as you grow from childhood to adulthood. Your body shape changes. Actual growth stops in the late teens or early twenties. Physical changes, however, continue through adulthood until death.

Intellectual growth and development refers to learning. It includes developing the ability to think and reason. It also involves using language and forming ideas. When children learn to read and tell time, they are growing intellectually. Young people begin to question ideas they learned earlier in life. They debate points of view and search for facts. They try performing tasks in different ways. Adults keep growing intellectually through classes, reading, and contact with other people.

Social growth and development includes forming friendships and getting along with others. It also includes demonstrating positive social character traits such as sharing, kindness, and generosity. A sign of social growth in young children is learning to share. In older children, obeying rules without being reminded is an example of social growth. What are some other examples? See **1-4**.

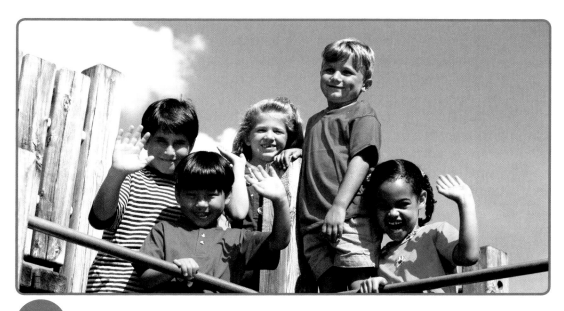

1-4 Part of social growth is making friends and learning to get along with others.

Emotional growth and development involves feelings. People learn to recognize and respect their feelings. They **accept** their feelings, or view them as normal and proper. They find ways to express feelings that do not hurt themselves or others. For instance, a child learns to express anger through talking rather than a temper tantrum. This is a sign of emotional growth. Trying to understand ideas from a different point of view is another sign of emotional growth.

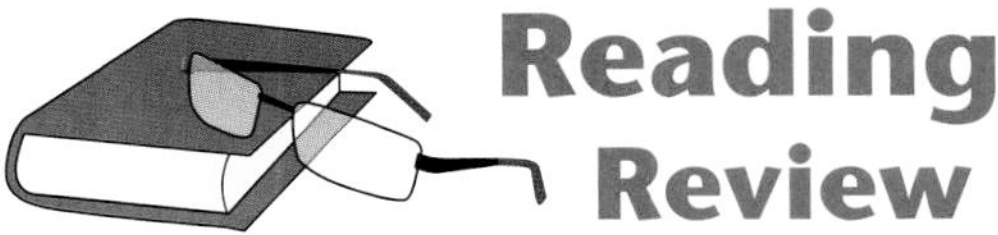

Reading Review

1. Explain the following statement: "Life is a constant process of growth and development."
2. What are the four major types of growth and development?
3. Which of these four types of growth and development can you influence? Give examples.

Stages of Growth and Development

A normal life span has three main stages of growth and development. These are *childhood*, *adolescence*, and *adulthood*. Some experts divide these stages into smaller stages. For instance, they may divide adolescence into early and late adolescence.

People change during each life stage. They grow and develop physically, intellectually, socially, and emotionally. These types of growth and development are closely related. More than one type of growth can occur at a time. As your body grows, so do your abilities. You are able to learn new ideas. You also get along with others and are better able to show emotions.

Experts in human development have identified developmental tasks for each stage of life. **Developmental tasks** are skills or behavior patterns most people will achieve at certain stages of their lives. You can think of developmental tasks as goals of growth. Some examples are learning to stand, walk, talk, and care about others. Another example is making career choices.

People need to achieve the tasks in each stage of development. If they do not, they may have problems reaching the goals of the next stage. For instance, learning to share is a developmental task of childhood. Forming mature relationships is a developmental task of the teen years. Very young children need to form close relationships with their parents or caregivers. Then, when they become teens, they will be better able to form positive peer relationships.

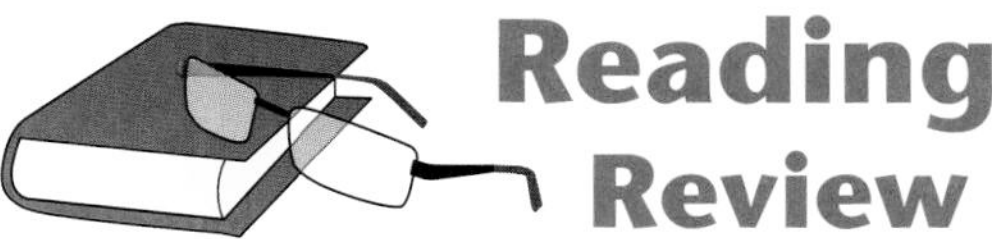

Reading Review

1. What are the three different stages of growth and development?
2. Why is it important to achieve the developmental tasks during each stage of development?

Childhood

Childhood is the stage of growth from birth to adolescence. A great deal of growth and development happens during this stage. Babies learn to sit, crawl, walk, and talk. Later, children learn to play with other children and share their toys. An important goal of childhood is for children to learn to talk and use language to express their ideas, opinions, and desires. They begin developing ideas about what is right and what is wrong. They also start learning about their emotions and how to deal with them. These are just some of the goals of growth during early childhood. Learning how to read and write, and learning to accept responsibilities at home and school are also goals. See **1-5**.

1-5 Learning to read independently is an important goal of childhood.

Beginning to develop independence is another goal of childhood. **Independence** is the freedom to decide, act, and care for yourself. For instance, babies depend on others to meet all their needs. Others must feed, dress, and try to soothe them when they are upset. As children grow, they learn how to perform many tasks for themselves. They learn to become more independent. This prepares them for adolescence and adulthood.

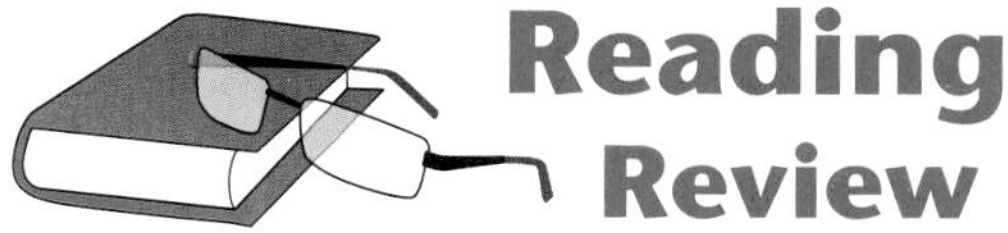

Reading Review

1. What are some important goals of development in childhood?
2. How do children begin to show their independence? Give examples.

Adolescence

Adolescence is the stage of growth between childhood and adulthood. People in this stage of growth are called *adolescents*. Adolescence begins when a person's body starts to develop into an adult size and shape.

During adolescence, many changes occur. Adolescents are more aware of themselves. They are trying to better understand themselves. They begin to

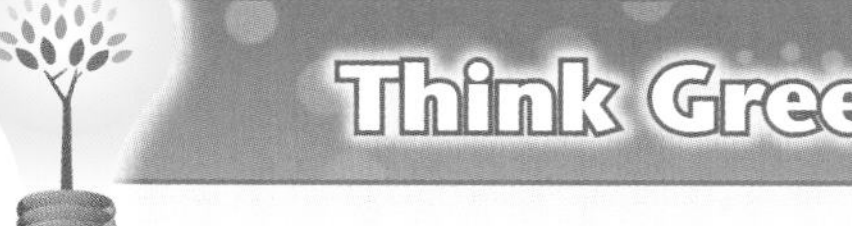

Volunteer to Plant a Tree

You can improve your environment simply by planting a tree. In addition to making an area look nice, trees produce oxygen. Trees also help clean the air by reducing the amount of air pollution. They can even make some of the air pollutants less harmful. Check for organizations in your community that plant trees and spend some time volunteering.

think more about the direction of their lives and ask important questions. Feelings about families and friends become more intense.

Many young people develop strong interests during adolescence. They may begin to work on causes for other people by joining volunteer programs. They may become active in clubs, sports, or religious groups. These interests may change, or they may last for a long time.

As an adolescent, you may not act as you feel. You may act bold, but feel scared inside. You may say you do not need love, but inside you desire love. You may claim to be grown up, but seek out adults who praise you. You may not act upset when you make a mistake, but feel embarrassed inside.

All these feelings are typical. Each year will bring new growth and development for you. Adolescence is the time when you are moving from childhood to adulthood. You must allow yourself time to move through this period of your life.

Your character is a product of growth and development. It develops during adolescence. **Character** is made up of the traits that guide you in deciding right from wrong. Your beliefs about what is important help form your character. The strong beliefs about right and wrong that guide your conduct are called *ethics*. The ways you behave express your character and ethics to others.

Another goal of adolescence is to become more independent from adults. You want more freedom to think, act, and care for yourself. This takes time, as you must reach smaller goals first. You need to learn how to get along with others. You begin to think about a career and find your identity.

One of the best ways to show you are ready to be more independent is to become responsible for yourself and your actions. A **responsibility** is a task you are expected or trusted to do. You may have responsibilities at home. Your family may expect you to keep your room clean. They may expect you to do other chores, too. You have responsibilities at school. Teachers expect you to get to class on time and do your homework. You have responsibilities to your friends. They expect you to be thoughtful, patient, and honest.

One of the important goals of adolescence is fulfilling your responsibilities. You need to show others they can count on you. This will let them know you are ready to accept even more responsibilities as an adult.

Meeting the goals of becoming an adolescent takes work. You need to think about the type of person you want to become. Set goals and plan steps to achieve these goals. This effort helps prepare you for adulthood.

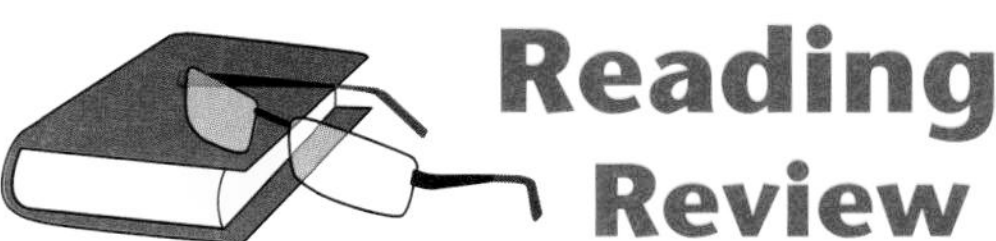

Reading Review

1. What are some of the changes that occur in each person's life during adolescence?
2. Why is it important for adolescents to become more independent from adults?

Succeed in Life

Your Character and Ethics

Answer the following questions honestly. Then think about how developing these traits would make you a more caring friend, family member, and community member.

- ***Are you trustworthy?*** Being trustworthy means you are honest and reliable. You have the courage to do the right thing.
- ***Do you assume responsibility?*** Being responsible is doing what you are expected to do. You keep on trying and always do your best.
- ***Do you show respect?*** Showing respect means you are considerate of the feelings of others. You accept that others are different from you. Using good manners is important to you.
- ***Do you act with fairness?*** Acting with fairness is listening to others and being open-minded. You play by the rules, take turns, and share.
- ***Are you a caring person?*** Being a caring person includes being kind and compassionate. You take time to say thank you and help people in need.
- ***Do you practice good citizenship?*** Being a good citizen means you do your share to make your community a better place. You obey laws and rules and respect authority. You help protect the environment.

Developmental Needs of Young Adolescents

The ages between eleven and fourteen are sometimes called *early adolescence*. If you are in this age group, you may be having many new feelings. You may feel family members, teachers, and friends are suddenly expecting a lot from you.

You may wonder whether your friends have some of the same feelings and thoughts. You may feel that people expect more of you than they expect of others. It may seem that everyone is watching to see how you perform. You have many needs during this time of your life. Your parents and teachers are trying to help you meet those needs.

What are the needs of young adolescents? The basic needs are listed in Figure **1-6**. You should be aware of these needs so you can better understand yourself and your peers.

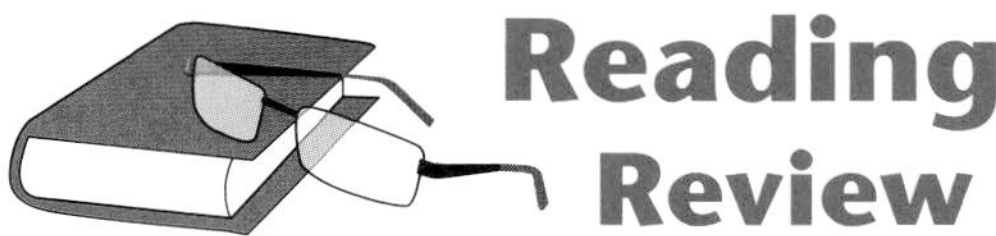

Reading Review

1. List the four developmental needs of young adolescents you think are most important.
2. How can you use what you learn at school in community projects?
3. What physical activity would you like to learn to do well?

Basic Needs of Young Adolescents

- ***To understand yourself.*** You want to learn about yourself, your interests, and your capabilities.
- ***To have many different experiences.*** Your interests and concerns may vary from day to day. You want to explore the world around you. The knowledge you gain will be used at home, at school, and in the neighborhood.
- ***To have meaningful relationships.*** You will be building relationships with people in your family, your school, and the community.
- ***To have positive relationships with peers.*** You want to have time for casual conversations with your peers. Spending time with your friends is important.
- ***To be successful.*** Gaining skills will help you achieve more goals. You will want to receive praise and rewards for doing tasks well.
- ***To become physically fit and healthy.*** The body grows and develops rapidly during early adolescence. Your nutritional needs increase to help muscles and bones develop.
- ***To have opportunities for physical activity.*** During adolescence, you have a lot of energy. Your body needs to move and get exercise. Physical activities are enjoyable and help you learn new skills.

1-6 As a young adolescent, you have these needs.

Adulthood

Adulthood is the stage of growth following adolescence. This stage begins as people gain greater independence. They do not depend on parents or other adults all the time. Adults support themselves by holding a job. They take care of problems without becoming upset easily. They are able to develop good relationships with many people. Adults enjoy being with family members and friends. They know what they want from life. They know how to properly express their emotions. They value communication.

Physical growth levels off during adulthood. Other types of growth and development, however, will continue. Many people marry and have children. This adds responsibilities and calls for more learning to take place. See **1-7**. If the goals of adolescence have not been reached, adults may have problems dealing with marriage and a family. They may not be willing, or able, to make needed changes.

At times, life may be confusing for adults. Although adults are more mature than teens, they may sometimes feel as they did during adolescence. Adults may question who they really are. They may feel confused about what they want from life. Some adults find growing old hard to understand and accept. They may try to act younger than their age. This type of behavior can sometimes cause problems. Aging, however, is a normal part of life.

People in their twenties are in early adulthood. The major goal of early adulthood centers on finding a place in society. Every person wants to become the best person he or she can be. This goal may be achieved through choosing a certain job or way of life.

People in their thirties and forties try to fit the goals they had as young adults into their current goals. As young adults, these people may have chosen careers and started families. Now, focus may change to advancing careers and raising children. Striving to reach these goals adds purpose and meaning to their lives.

People in their fifties and sixties continue working toward their goals. They also begin to think about retirement. Preparing for the later years in life is an important task. Adults need to feel useful and stay active. They need to develop interests to pursue after they retire.

People today live longer than ever before. Many people in their seventies, eighties, and nineties enjoy good health and remain physically active. Some keep learning new hobbies and developing relationships with family and friends during these later years.

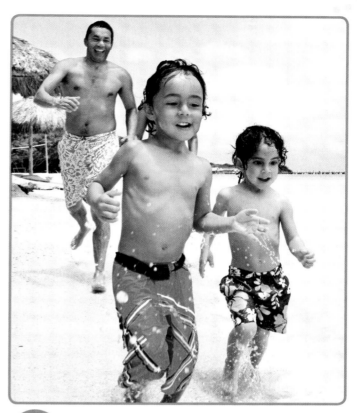

1-7 Adults who choose to become parents must accept the responsibilities of caring for children.

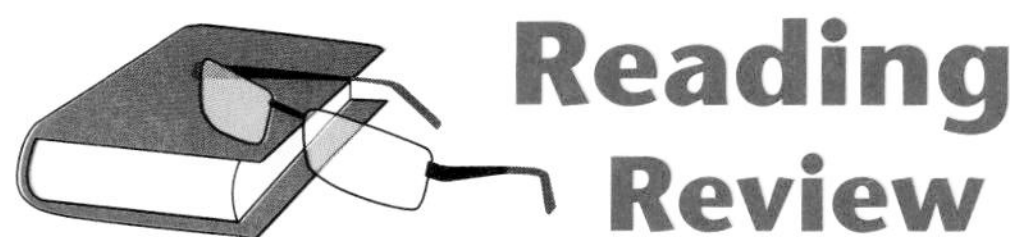

Reading Review

1. What are three traits that can be used to describe adults?
2. What is the major goal of early adulthood, and how can it be met during the adult years?

Section Summary

- The four areas of growth and development are physical, intellectual, social, and emotional.
- The three main stages of growth and development for each person are childhood, adolescence, and adulthood.
- Developmental tasks are necessary for a person to develop to his or her fullest potential.
- The adolescent years are the time when a young person is moving from childhood toward adulthood.
- Certain goals of growth and development must be accomplished during adolescence in order to better meet added responsibilities during adulthood.

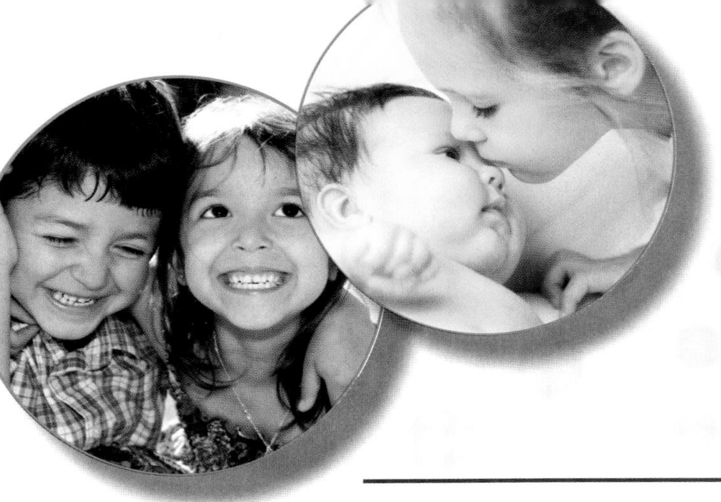

Section 1-3
You and Your Family

Objectives

After studying this section, you will be able to

- **define** *relationship*, *socialization*, *culture*, *family*, *generation*, *family type*, *role*, *siblings*, *affection*, and *respect*.
- **explain** why the relationship between children and parents is important.
- **give examples** of how brothers and sisters can learn to get along with one another.
- **describe** how people can stay active and independent as they grow older.

Key Terms

relationship: a pattern of interaction with one or more persons over time.

socialization: teaching the ways and customs of a culture to others.

culture: the beliefs and customs of a certain racial, religious, or social group.

family: a group of people related to one another by blood (birth), marriage, or adoption.

generation: all the people who are born and live in about the same time span.

family type: the makeup of a family.

role: a person's place in a group.

siblings: brothers and sisters.

affection: a feeling of fondness.

respect: a high or special regard for someone.

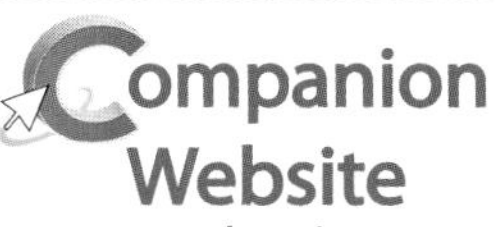

Study the Key Terms by completing crossword puzzles, matching activities, and e-flash cards at the website.

Main Ideas

- Family types vary.
- Communication among family members is important, especially among children and parents.
- Brothers and sisters need to learn how to get along with one another.
- Older relatives living with a family need to be treated with love and respect.

Families exist around the world. You are part of a family. Your relationships with your family members are important. A **relationship** is a pattern of interaction with one or more persons over time.

You also need relationships outside the family. Friendships may start because you share common interests. Relationships with neighbors may form because you live on the same street.

Family relationships, however, are likely to have the greatest effect on you. Family members help meet your needs. They teach you proper behavior. This is part of socialization. **Socialization** is teaching the ways and customs of a culture to others. **Culture** is the beliefs and customs of a certain racial, religious, or social group.

The Family

A family is the basic unit of society. A **family** is a group of people related to one another by blood (birth), marriage, or adoption. This group may include a mother, a father, and one or more children. Sometimes, other relatives are part of the family group that lives together. Also, a family may care for children who are not related to family members.

Family members make up different generations. A **generation** is all the people who are born and live in about the same time span. You and your brothers and sisters are part of one generation. Your parents, aunts, and uncles make up a second generation. Your grandparents are part of a third generation. See **1-8**.

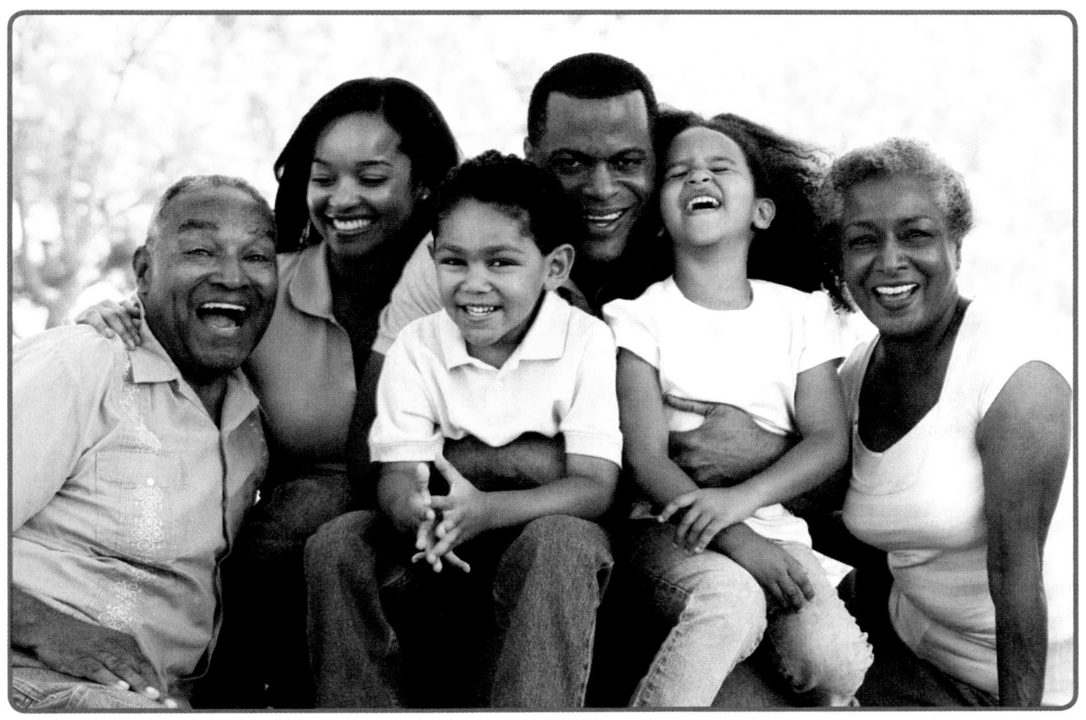

1-8 This family photo shows three generations.

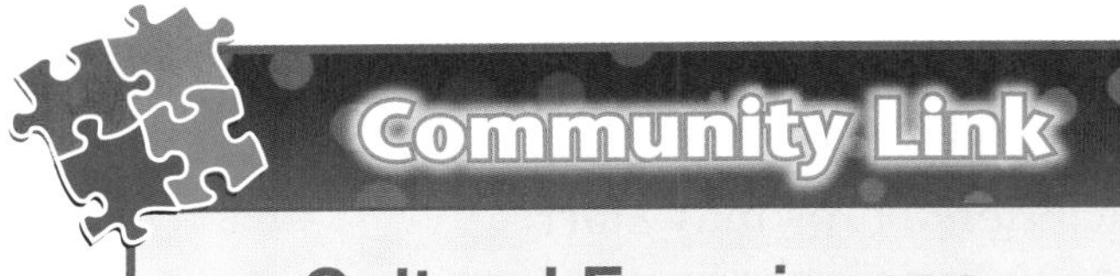

Cultural Experiences

Learn more about a culture other than your own. What is the common language? What are the main food dishes? What is the modern way of dress? How are holidays and special family events celebrated? Think about how you can use this information to improve your community relationships.

Family Types

Not all families are the same. **Family type** refers to the makeup of a family. Each family type provides its members with the love, support, and attention they need.

- A *nuclear family* consists of a married man and woman and their biological children. Parents share the duties of raising their children. They also share the duties of earning income. Both parents help care for the home.
- A *single-parent family* consists of one adult who is raising one or more children. The single parent may be separated or divorced. The adult's spouse may have died. The adult may never have married. The single parent must care for the family and provide income and support.
- A *stepfamily* forms when a single parent marries. The husband, the wife, or both have children from other marriages. Some stepfamilies include two mothers and two fathers. Members of this family type are called *stepparents* and *stepchildren*. All family members must adjust to these new relationships. This type of family is also called a *blended family*.
- An *extended family* has several generations of relatives living together. Grandparents, aunts, uncles, and cousins might live as part of an extended family. Everyone in the family must deal with many people in the home. There are also more family members to help care for children, earn money, and complete household tasks.
- A *foster family* cares for children who are not related to other family members. These children may need a temporary home. Family members must work together to adjust to these new relationships.
- An *adoptive family* forms when a couple, or a single person, chooses to raise another person's child as their own. Adoptive parents must legally be granted responsibility for the child by a state court. The child then becomes a permanent part of the family.
- A *childless family* is a couple without children. Some couples choose not to have children. Others are not able to have children. They may focus their life on each other and their careers. They may also be able to spend time with the children of friends and relatives.
- A *guardian* may be chosen by a family to take responsibility for a child if the parents are no longer able to provide care. A guardian is often someone who has a relationship with the family. For instance, a close relative or friend. A guardian must legally be appointed by a state court.

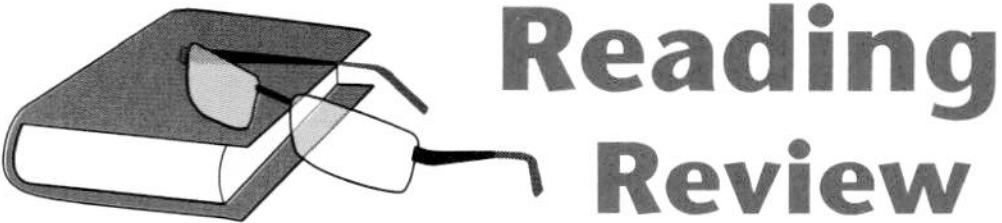

1. How many living generations are there in your family?
2. Describe the different family types.

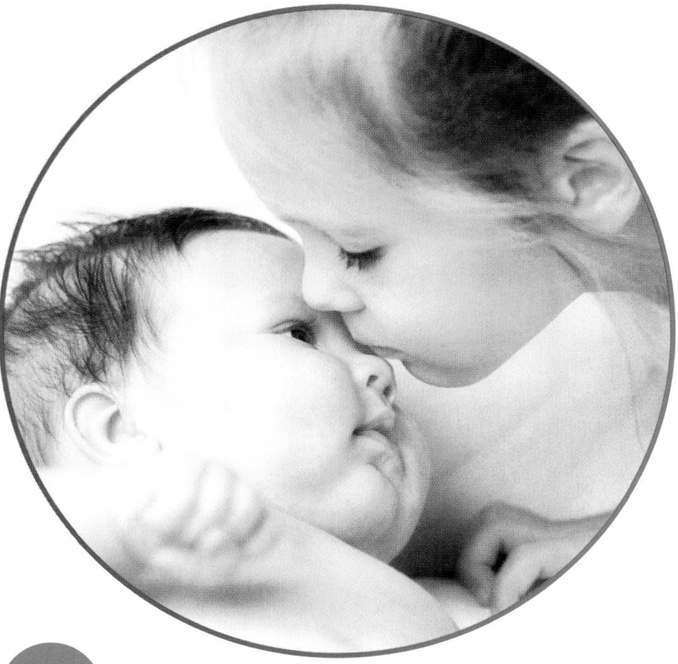

1-9 In addition to having the role of daughter, this young girl also has the role of sister.

Your Roles

As a member of a family, you have several roles. A **role** is your place in a group. You have responsibilities in each of your roles. In your family group, you have the role of son, daughter, stepdaughter, or stepson. In this role, one of your responsibilities is to obey your parents. Other family roles you may have include grandchild, niece or nephew, and brother or sister. See. **1-9**. Roles in groups outside your family may include student, friend, team member, and worker.

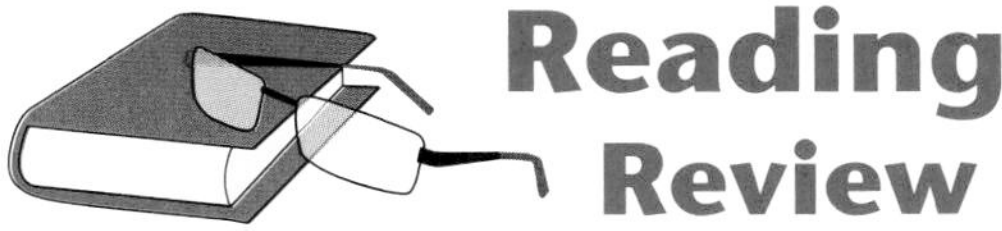

1. What roles do you have within your family?
2. Name some roles you have outside your family.

Parents

Children are affected throughout their lives by many adults. Children, however, have a special relationship with their parents. Mothers, fathers, foster parents, and guardians are responsible for the growth and development of their children. They care for and protect their children. They help their children to be the best they can be.

Relationships with their parents affect teens' growth and development. Parents care about their children. They are concerned about what happens to them today and in the future. They offer advice based on their life experiences. They hope their advice will be helpful.

Teens may not always agree with their parents. They may feel their parents do not understand their feelings or friends. They may wonder why their parents act as they do.

Having these thoughts and feelings is normal. Teens should share them with their parents. Communication with parents is important. By talking to parents, teens can learn to understand and respect their parents' feelings.

Parents and children sometimes disagree. Living in close contact sometimes causes problems. Differences may occur because teens are starting to become more independent. They may not want to follow some of their parents' rules. Teens may have trouble realizing their parents are still responsible for them.

Parents and children can love and care for one another and still have differences. This is part of a healthy relationship. Communication can help settle differences and make relationships stronger.

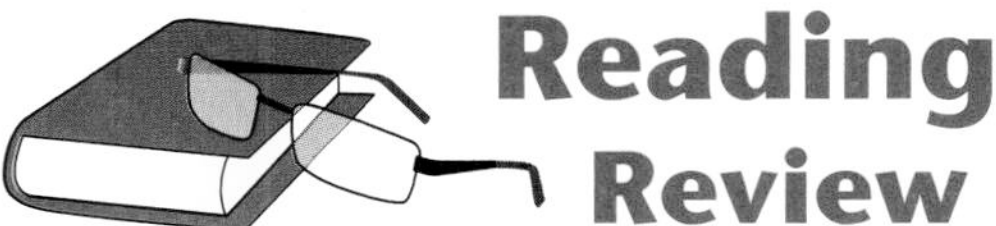

Reading Review

1. Describe the relationship among parents and children.
2. Why do regular conversations between a parent and a child help build a good relationship?
3. What are some reasons parents and children may disagree?

Brothers and Sisters

If you have the role of brother, stepbrother, sister, or stepsister, one of your responsibilities is to get along with your siblings. **Siblings**, or brothers and sisters, get along differently in each family. In many families, they support one another. Siblings, however, sometimes argue. They become jealous. They tease one another.

These actions are normal, but they can still hurt. A child who is teased may develop feelings of resentment. These feelings are not easy to overcome. They can create problems in relationships with other people.

Teens should develop a sense of humor. They should learn not to take themselves, or others, too seriously. This will help them ignore some of the teasing that comes from brothers and sisters.

Siblings should be able to settle their differences. This is part of growing up. Brothers and sisters cannot expect their parents or other adults to always tell them how to handle disputes.

Getting along is based on understanding and respect. Spending time talking and laughing together can help brothers and sisters get to know one another better. This will help them realize they share many of the same needs. It will also help them develop the patience and understanding needed to form kind, caring relationships. See **1-10**.

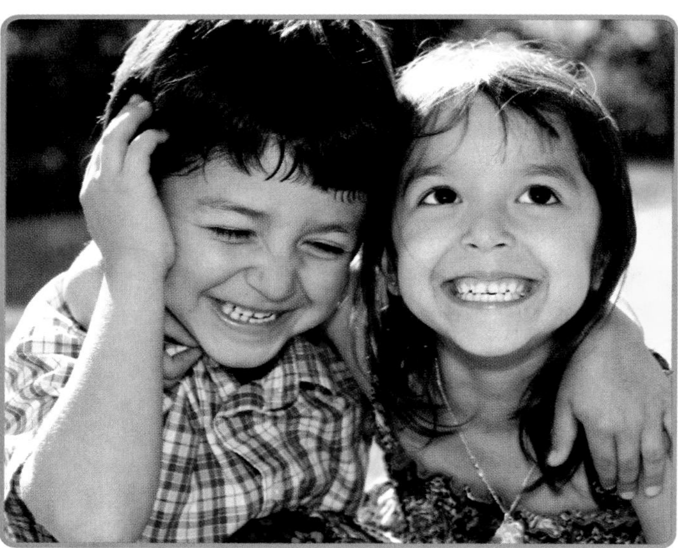

1-10 Brothers and sisters can care for each other and have fun together.

Brothers and sisters can show love and affection for one another in many ways. (**Affection** is a feeling of fondness.) They can offer to help one another. They can give advice. Brothers and sisters can also be willing listeners. This shows they care about one another's problems.

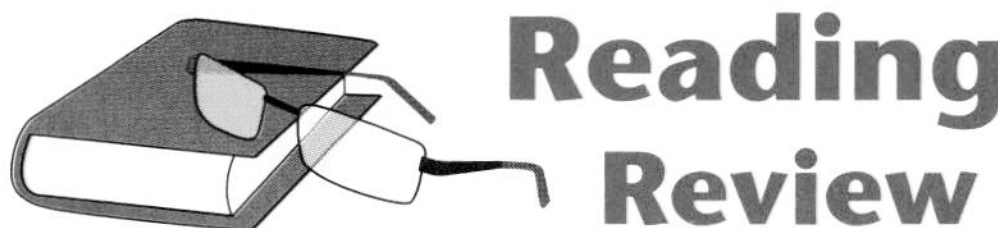

Reading Review

1. Why is it important for brothers and sisters to learn how to get along with one another?
2. What can brothers and sisters do to get along with one another better?
3. How can brothers and sisters show affection for one another?

The Older Generation

Grandparents are often the third generation of a family. Most grandparents want their family members to love and respect them. **Respect** is a high or special regard for someone.

Older adults need love and affection as much as every other age group. Most people need someone to care about them. Older adults have feelings just like you. They appreciate it when family members are thoughtful, considerate, and cheerful toward them. Family members show love and respect if they consider the needs of grandparents when making family plans.

Older adults also need to feel useful and wanted. In some families, they are not only useful, but are also a big help. Some parents depend on grandparents to care for children. See **1-11**.

Family members may also rely on grandparents to help with other tasks. Family members should not take this help for granted. They should let grandparents know how important they are.

Most older adults have many interests besides their families. They may have hobbies. They may take part in community activities. They may plan social gatherings with friends. Interests inside and outside the home help keep older adults active, alert, and happy.

Older adults also need to be as independent as possible. They need privacy and time to be alone when they live with other family members. There should be a time and place where they can take care of their own interests and hobbies. They need a place to keep mail and store personal papers. They need to have their own spending money and not account to anyone for it.

Older adults want to be healthy and enjoy life. They want to be able to take care of themselves. Changes occur in the human body, however, as people age. These changes may be hard for family members to accept.

As people grow older, their bodies are not as strong as earlier in life. Certain movements are more difficult; such as lifting, bending, kneeling, and walking. Older adults sometimes become forgetful. If this happens, family members need to be patient, understanding, and willing to help when needed.

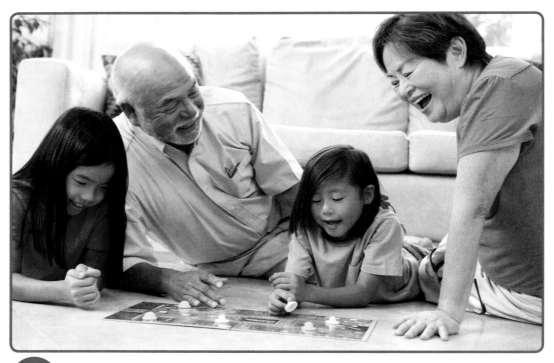

1-11 This older couple enjoys babysitting for their grandchildren.

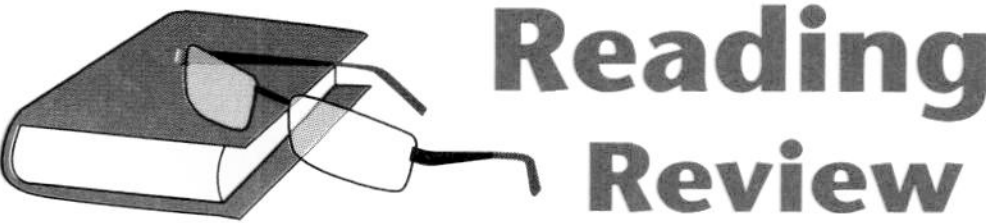

Reading Review

1. What are some needs of older adults? How are these different from a younger person's needs? How are they the same?
2. How can younger family members help older adults feel useful and wanted?

Section Summary

- Families vary in size. They include people from different generations.
- Family members need to support one another.
- Family types describe the makeup of a family.
- Parents care for, and are responsible for, the growth and development of their children.
- It is important that parents and children talk to one another about how they feel.
- Brothers and sisters sometimes have disagreements and tease one another. Learning to get along depends on caring for and respecting one another.
- Older adults need to feel useful and loved. They also need to be independent, healthy, and respected. At times, however, older adults may need help taking care of themselves.

Section 1-4
Friends

Objectives

After studying this lesson, you will be able to

- **define** *friend*, *trust*, *share*, *peers*, *peer pressure*, *reputation*, and *group dating*.
- **explain** what it means to be a good friend.
- **describe** how your peers influence you.
- **recognize** why your family cares about the friends you choose.
- **give examples** of how you can help your family and friends get to know one another.

Key Terms

friend: someone you care about, trust, and respect.

trust: to believe a person is honest and reliable.

share: to experience or enjoy with others.

peers: people who belong to the same age group.

peer pressure: the influence people's peers have on them.

reputation: what others think of a person.

group dating: when several people of both sexes meet for an activity.

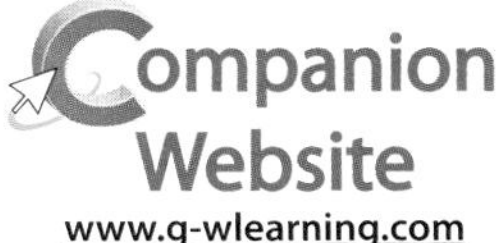

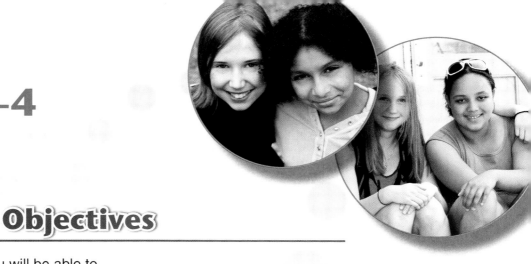

Study the Key Terms by completing crossword puzzles, matching activities, and e-flash cards at the website.

Main Ideas

- A good friend is someone you care about, trust, and respect.
- Peers can provide you with a sense of belonging.
- You can learn skills to manage peer pressure.
- Skills for making new friends can be used throughout your life.
- You can find ways to help your family and friends know and like one another.

A **friend** is someone you care about, trust, and respect. When you **trust** someone, you believe he or she is honest and reliable. Having friends is part of your growth and development. See **1-12**. They help you grow. They are part of your support system.

Being a Friend

A good friend is someone with whom you share ideas, thoughts, and dreams. (**Share** means to experience or enjoy with others.) Good friends talk with one another. They laugh and have fun together. They make one another feel good about themselves. You can enjoy both being a friend and having friends.

Friends have certain qualities. They understand one another. They are able to help one another with problems. They care about each other instead of just themselves. Friends are also dependable. You can count on your friends to be there when you need them. You should also be there when they need you.

Good friends like to spend a lot of time together. Sometimes, however, they need time apart from one another. Most people need time alone to do what they want. Let your friends know you respect their need for privacy by giving them time to themselves.

Another quality of a friend is being *trustworthy*. Friends often share secrets. If your friend tells you a secret, do not tell others. Your friend trusts you to keep that information private. (On the other hand, secrets that involve health risks or danger should not be kept secret. You can help a friend more by telling a responsible adult if you are afraid a friend could be in trouble.)

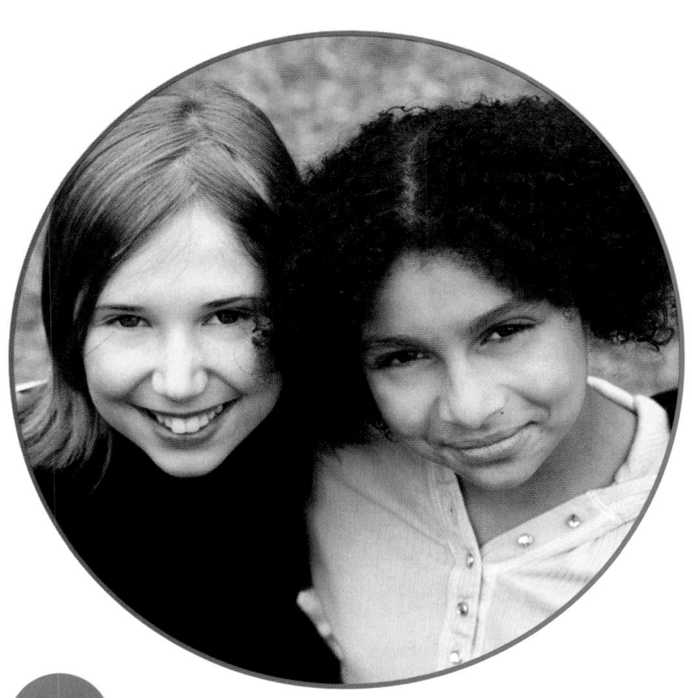

1-12 Friendships you develop when you are young can continue throughout your life.

Reading Review

1. How do you share with your friends? Give examples.
2. What qualities do good friends have? Give examples.

Making Friends

When you were a young child, your parents often chose your friends. They may have been from families your parents knew. They may have lived in your neighborhood.

As you grow older, you become more independent. You join new social groups. You begin making your own friends. This can be an exciting time. See **1-13**.

You will meet many new people during your life. You may meet them at school, social events, or when you visit friends. You

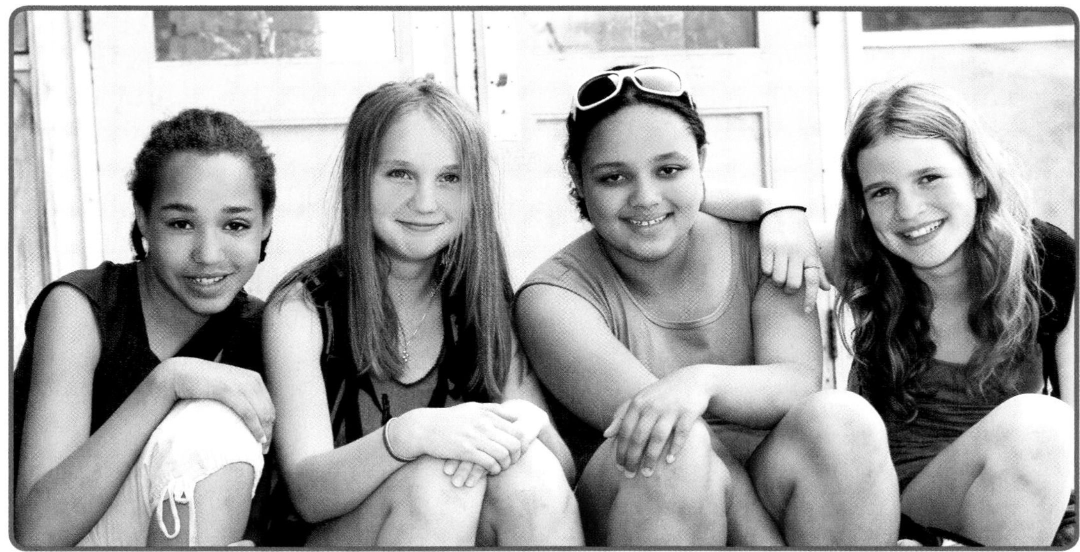

1-13 As you get older, you will make friends at school and in other groups to which you belong.

will meet some people and become good friends with them. Other people you may like, but you will not become good friends.

Someday you may find yourself in a situation where you do not know many people. You may want to introduce yourself to people. Do not wait for them to make the first move. This is a good skill to have. You will find it helpful when you meet new people at school, club meetings, or on the job.

Being open and friendly with people makes them friendlier toward you. Greet people with a warm smile. This is important when making new friends.

Also, get to know people before you form an opinion about them. People sometimes change after you get to know them better. First impressions are not always correct.

The number of friends you have is not as important as the quality of your friendships. A few close friends may be right for you.

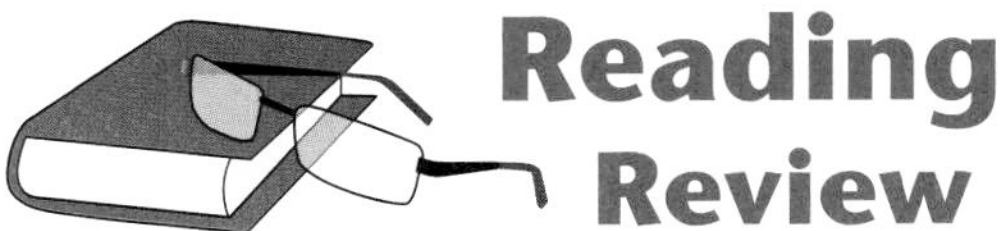

Reading Review

1. Where can you meet new people?
2. How can you show someone you want to be friends?
3. What should you do when you meet people for the first time?

Peers

Peers are people who belong to the same age group. They have similar experiences and interests. Your peer group includes your classmates and close friends.

Peers serve an important purpose in your life. They provide you with friendships that make you feel wanted and give you a sense of belonging.

This feeling of belonging is important, especially during your school years. Having friends your own age helps you feel secure. You and your friends can go places together. Peers listen to one another's problems and plans. You can talk about your opinions, ideas, likes, and dislikes with your peers.

You may want to look and act like your peers. You fit into a group if you look and act like the other members. Some of your peers may feel they have to buy certain clothes or have certain hairstyles to be "in." There is nothing wrong with wanting to look and act like your peers. This can give you a feeling of security.

Sometimes, however, peers try to influence you to make decisions. This influence is called **peer pressure**. If the influence is not right for you, it is called *negative peer pressure*. An example is when a friend tells you to ignore the time your parents told you to be home.

If peers influence you to do something that is good for you, it is called *positive peer pressure*. An example is when a friend urges you to go home on time to show respect for your parents.

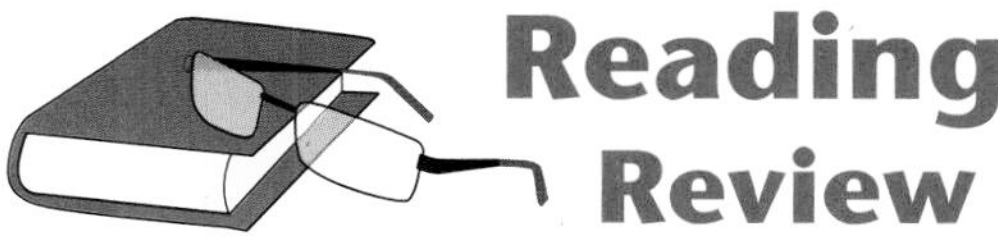

1. What important purposes do peers serve in your life?
2. Explain negative peer pressure. Give some examples.
3. Why should you always be honest with your peers?

Families and Friends

When your friends visit your home for the first time, introduce them to your family. Your family is interested in meeting your friends. Family members care about the friends you choose because they care about you.

Succeed in Life

Handling Peer Pressure

It is not easy to handle negative peer pressure. The way others act may not reflect your beliefs. Stand up for what you believe is right. You must think about what actions are right for you. Talk to adults you trust about peer pressure you feel from friends.

Being honest with your feelings is a good way to deal with peer pressure. Sometimes friends disagree. Though friends say *yes*, you can say *no*. Tell them about your beliefs. Tell them how your thoughts are different from theirs. Good friends respect one another's differences.

Let your family and friends have a chance to talk to one another. Getting to know your family may help your friends relax. They may feel more at home when they visit you. If your parents know more about your friends, they will feel better when you go out with your friends.

Sometimes you may invite a person to your home who does not act as you expected. After the person has left, let your parents know how you feel. Tell them you are disappointed in this person's behavior. This shows your parents you are learning to use good judgment about people. Your parents like to know you can share your feelings and make wise decisions.

Talking with your parents is important. Conflicts may arise over choices of good friends. See **1-14**. When you and your parents have a good relationship, you can more easily discuss conflicts. You can help your parents to better understand your friends. Your parents can let you know about their concerns.

If you have a friend who does not get along with your family, try to find out why. It could be you are wrong about your friend. Perhaps you have not tried to help your family understand your friend. Talk and try to reach an understanding. Respect one another's opinions.

A **reputation** is what others think of a person. If you are friends with someone who does not have a good reputation, your family may object. People do not always see a person the same way. Your family may not see your friends the way you see them.

You may also think your family unfairly criticizes your friends. This may be true. Your family, however, may just be trying to help you. Observe how your friends behave. Are they disrespectful toward others? Do they

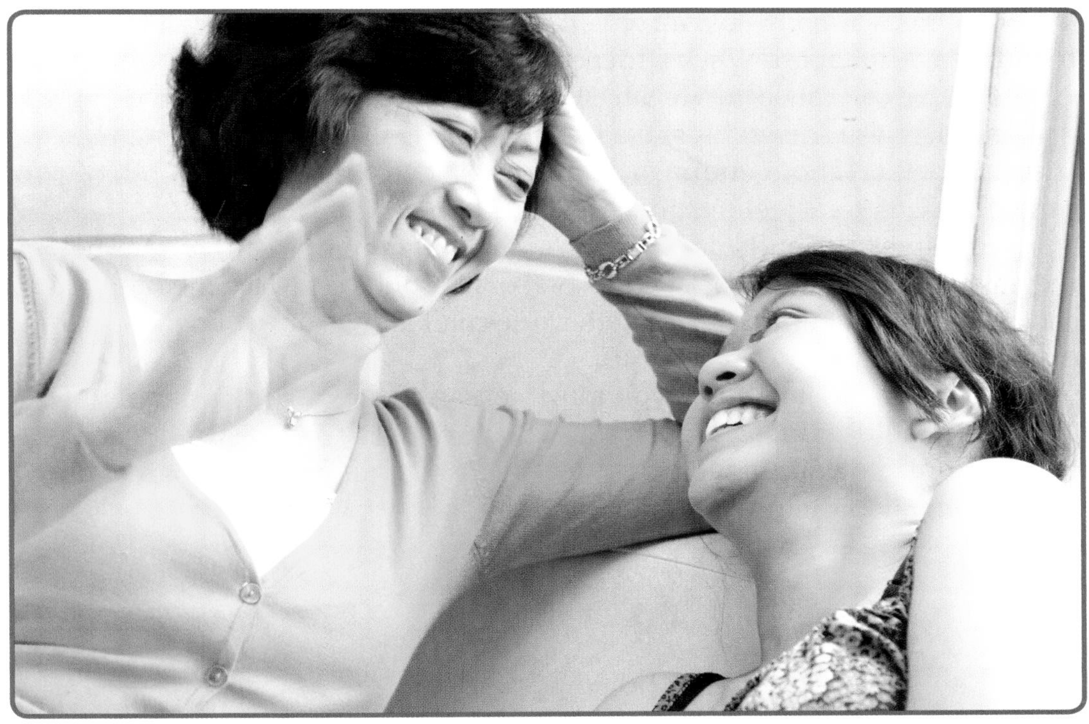

1-14 When you and your parents have a good relationship, you can more easily discuss conflicts.

put their feet on the furniture? Are they destructive? Do they smoke or use profane language? Do they act in other ways that might upset your family? These are concerns that may cause your family to worry about the friends you choose.

Friendships also produce dating experiences. Group dating is often a teen's first dating experience. **Group dating** occurs when a number of people of both sexes meet for an activity, such as attending a movie. Each teen can get to know all the members of the group and not feel pressure to be close to just one person. After feeling confident in a group, most people are ready for casual dating. *Casual dating* involves being part of a couple.

Spending time with dating partners helps you learn about yourself. You learn how to give and take in personal relationships. You learn about members of the opposite sex. Spending time with dating partners helps to prepare people for marriage.

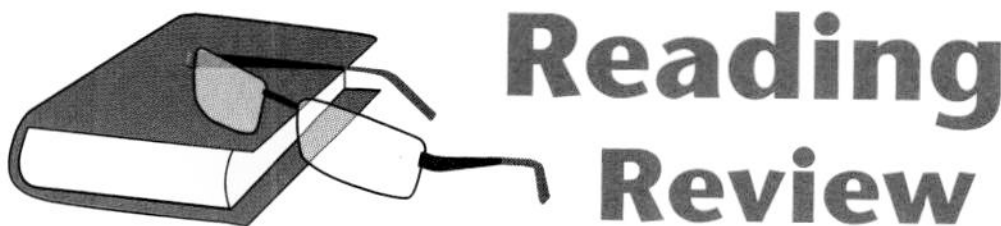

Reading Review

1. Why should you introduce your friends to your family?
2. Why is it good for you to talk to your parents about your friends?
3. What may make your family worry about your choice of friends?

Ending a Friendship

Sometimes, friendships can end. If your interests change, you and your friends may drift apart. When a friend moves away, it is painful for both of you. An argument can cause hurt feelings, and possibly damage your friendship.

Ending close friendships in a healthy way is important. Talking to a friend in person about ending a friendship is helpful. This way, both of you can talk about your feelings together. See **1-15**.

Sometimes a friendship ends through a letter, phone call, or Internet message. These methods are not as personal as a face-to-face meeting. This can create hurt feelings. Also, a letter or e-mail allows only one person to express feelings.

When a friendship ends, you may feel sad and cry. That is healthy. This experience helps you learn about what is important to you. It can teach you to communicate your values to another person. Talking with a parent about your feelings can help you understand them.

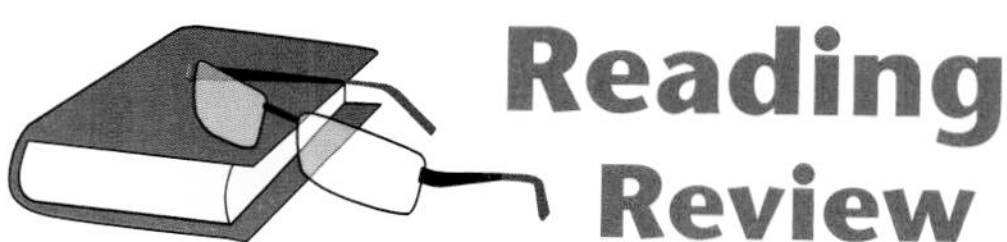

Reading Review

1. What may cause you to end a friendship?
2. What do you think is the best way to end a friendship? Why?

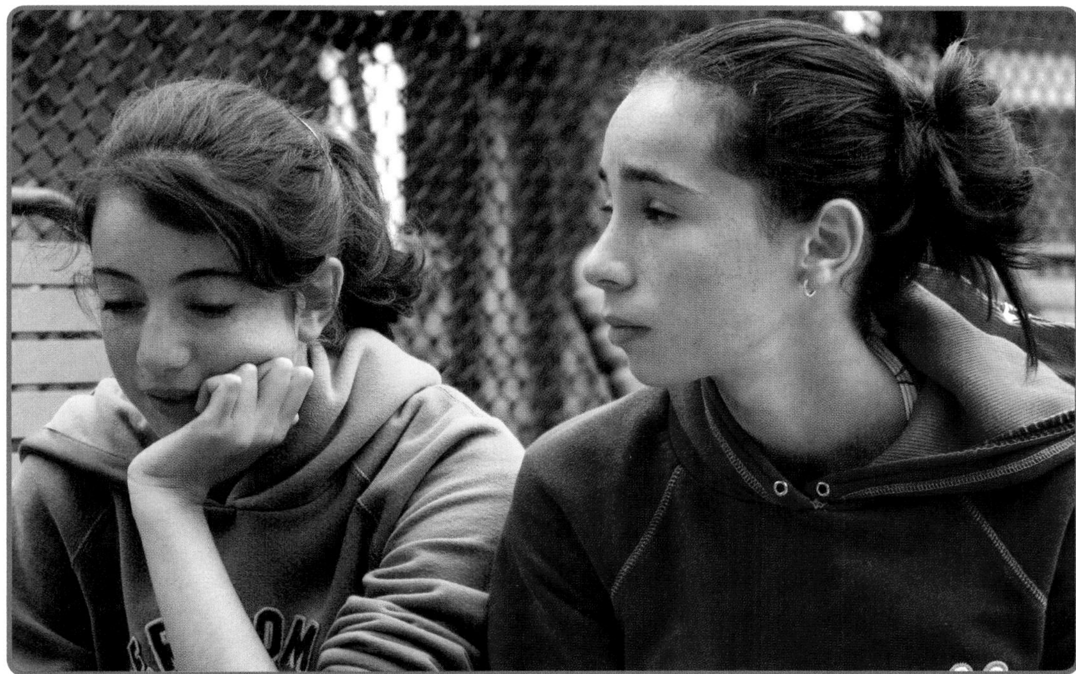

1-15 Ending a friendship is not easy. Talking about your feelings can make it less painful.

Section Summary

- Having friends is an important part of growth and development.
- A good friend is someone you care about, trust, and respect.
- You will make many new friends during your life. Being open and friendly is helpful.
- Peers can give you a sense of belonging.
- You can learn skills to manage peer pressure.
- You need to help your family and friends know and understand one another.
- Group dating is often the first dating experience.
- When ending a friendship, discuss your feelings with your friend.

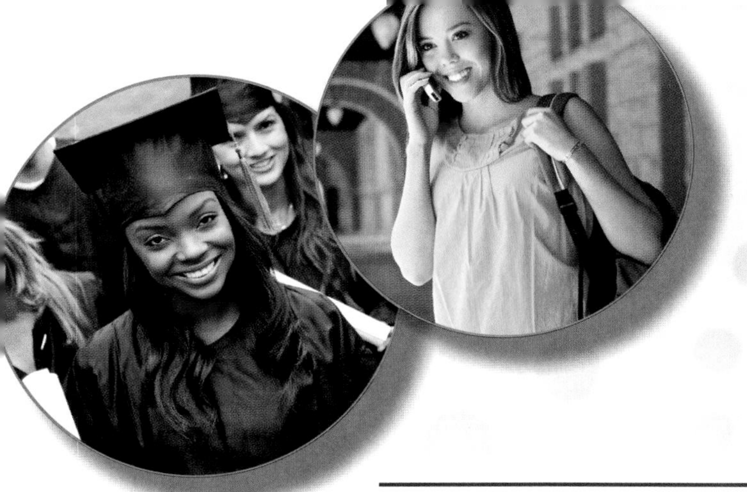

Section 1-5
Communicating with Others

Objectives

After studying this lesson, you will be able to

- **define** *communication*, *verbal communication*, *nonverbal communication*, *active listening*, *feedback*, and *bully*.
- **state** how you can develop effective communication skills.
- **explain** the importance of using feedback when communicating.
- **describe** healthy communication among individuals.

Key Terms

communication: sending or receiving information, signals, or messages.

verbal communication: the use of words to give and receive information.

nonverbal communication: the sending and receiving of messages without the use of words.

active listening: being focused on the communication process.

feedback: a response that lets the speaker know you received and understood the message.

bully: a person who uses strength or power to persuade or pressure others (force or fear) to do something.

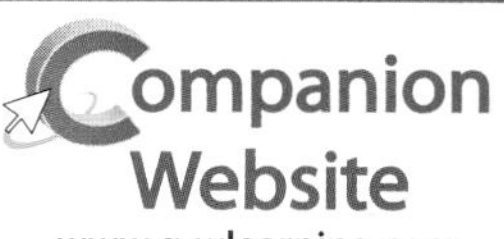

Study the Key Terms by completing crossword puzzles, matching activities, and e-flash cards at the website.

Main Ideas

- Relationships depend on good communication.
- Communication is both verbal and nonverbal.
- You can communicate effectively.
- Healthy communication helps you get along with others.

Communication is sending or receiving information, signals, or messages. See **1-16**. Developing good communication skills is important. These skills can help you enjoy life. You can better resolve conflicts. You can also communicate in healthy ways. This will help you be an effective listener and speaker. As a result, your self-concept will improve.

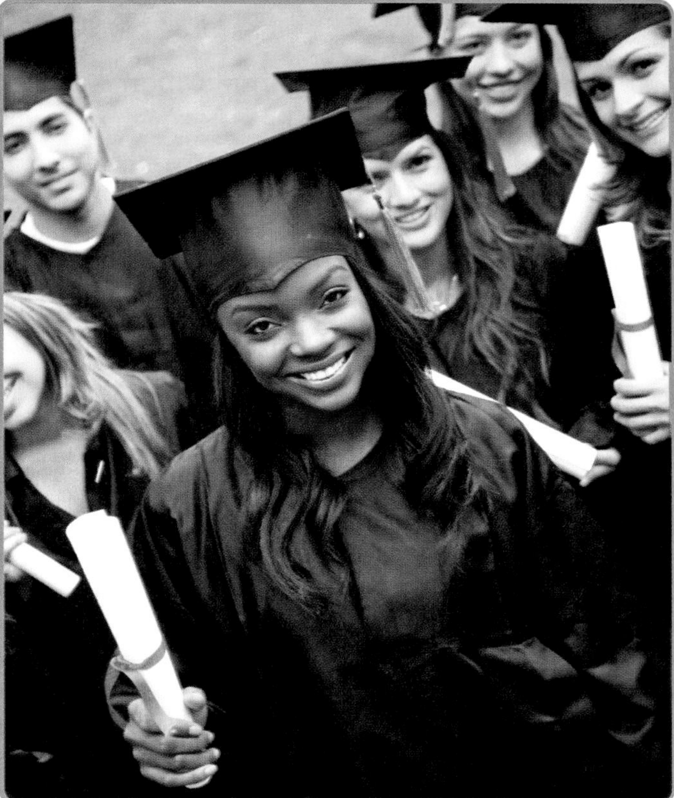

1-16 Graduating students communicate happiness and achievement.

How You Communicate

Relationships depend on communication. People use both verbal and nonverbal communication to share their feelings and ideas.

Verbal communication is the use of words to give and receive information. This includes both speaking and writing.

Nonverbal communication is the sending and receiving of messages without the use of words. *Body language* is a type of nonverbal communication, such as facial expressions and gestures. Sometimes, frowns or hand motions can say more than words. A light touch on an arm or shoulder sends a message. Your appearance is another example of nonverbal communication. The clothes you wear communicate a message about you.

You are always communicating how you feel. What you say and do lets people know how you are feeling. For instance, sometimes you tell people you are happy or sad. Other times, they can tell by your facial expressions or actions how you are feeling. You do not always need words to communicate.

As a child, you learned how to communicate. What you learned then affects how you communicate as you grow older. The way you communicate with friends and coworkers may be similar to the way you communicate with brothers or sisters. If you marry, communication with your partner may be based on how your parents communicate.

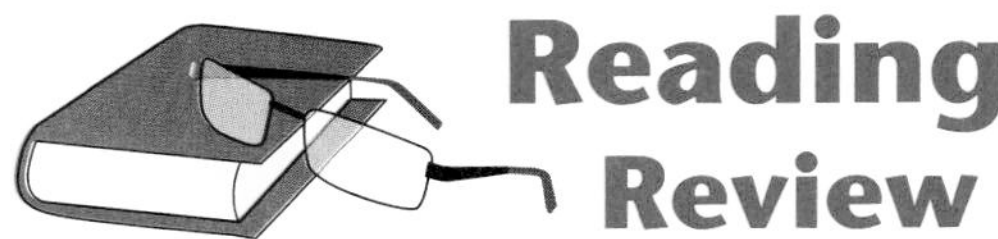

Reading Review

1. What is the difference between verbal and nonverbal communication? Give examples.
2. How can the ways you learned to communicate as a child affect you as an adult?

Communicating Effectively

Communication is a two-way process. To communicate well, you need to be able to speak and write clearly. This helps you send your message correctly. Being a careful listener is also important. When people listen carefully, they understand the message. When people communicate effectively, they can better understand one another. They get along better with others.

Writing is a second form of verbal communication. Written words are used to send messages and provide information. Think about how much you learn from books, magazines, and the Internet. Your schoolwork includes many written assignments. You write personal notes and letters to family members and friends. You can also use the Internet to keep in touch with them.

You need effective writing skills throughout your school years. Writing skills are also required for most jobs. Clear writing makes your messages easier to understand.

Another part of communicating effectively is listening. Listening is different from just hearing what is being said. **Active listening** is being focused on what is said and providing feedback. Active listeners give feedback. **Feedback** is a response that lets the speaker know you received and understood the message. To communicate effectively, you should follow the tips shown in Figure **1-17**.

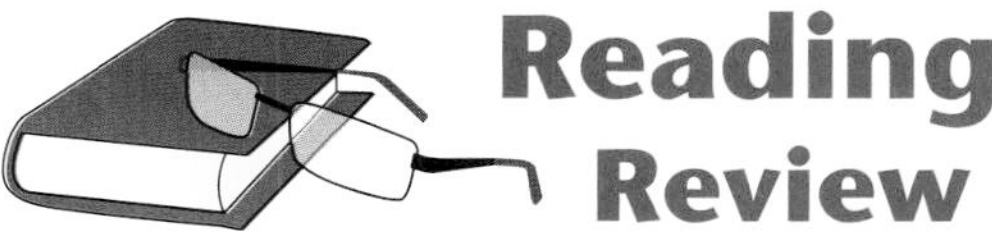

Reading Review

1. Why should you think before you speak with other people?
2. What writing skills do you need to write clearly?
3. What are the qualities of a good listener? Give examples.

Positive Behavior

Behavior is another form of communication. You can behave in a positive manner that communicates you care about others. You should always be polite and never hurt other people.

Also, show that you care about yourself and have a positive self-concept. Stand up for what you believe. People will respect you if you do. You will not always agree with everybody. You can disagree, however, without being afraid of making others angry. Using manners is a form of communication. Speaking respectfully to another, or standing patiently in line, sends a positive message you care about others.

Some people behave in a negative manner. They are more concerned with themselves than others. They are rude, hurt others, or put them down. If you treat people like this, they may not like you and try to avoid you. Some people do not stand up for themselves. They allow others to hurt them and treat them without respect. They may have a negative self-concept.

Tips for Effective Communication

To Speak Clearly

- *Pronounce words carefully.* Fast, mumbled speech is hard to understand. Do not drop the endings of words.
- *Keep your comments brief and to the point.* Do not make long, wordy statements. People may lose interest in what you are saying.
- *Pause before you speak.* This gives you time to know what you are going to say, and your voice will be stronger.
- *Think before you speak.* Always choose your words carefully to avoid hurting others. If people ask you for your opinion, tell them the truth. Do not, however, tell them in a way that may hurt their feelings or discourage them. Instead, tell them what you think in a positive manner. Try to be honest yet sensitive to their feelings.

To Write Clearly

- *Write neatly.* Practice your handwriting skills so people can read your writing.
- *Use correct grammar and spell words correctly.* If using a computer to write a message, use the grammar and spell check feature to check your message.
- *Think about what you want to write before you begin.* For instance, when writing a school paper, first make a few notes. Then prepare an outline before you start writing.
- *Have someone else read what you have written to make sure it is clear.* For instance, after you have completed a paper, ask a family member to read the assignment to check if it is understandable.

To Listen Actively and Provide Feedback

- *Pay attention to the speaker.* Keep your mind on what he or she is saying. Do not become distracted by your own thoughts.
- *Let the speaker know you are listening.* Smile or nod as he or she talks.
- *Ask questions if something is unclear.* Do not interrupt the speaker. Instead, ask questions when the speaker has finished.
- *Repeat what you think the speaker said.* This lets him or her know if you understood correctly.

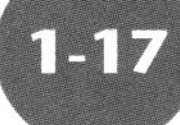

Developing effective communication skills will help you at home, school, and work.

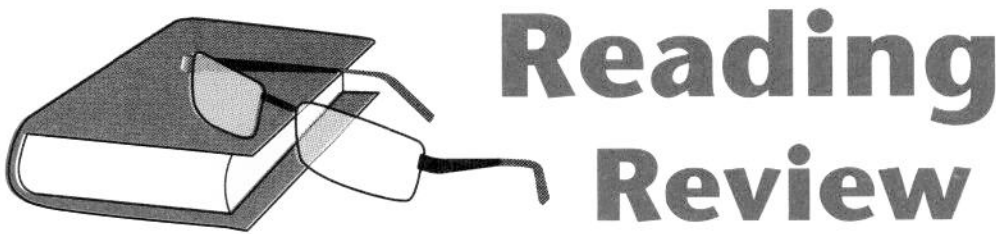

1. Think of three examples of positive behavior that communicates you care about yourself.
2. How can people who do not stand up for themselves get hurt?

Healthy Communication

Living successfully with others depends on effective communication skills. This is true in your daily life with your family and friends. This will also be true in your career when you have a job and work with others.

Having good communication skills increases your self-esteem and self-confidence. When you communicate well, you feel like a valued person.

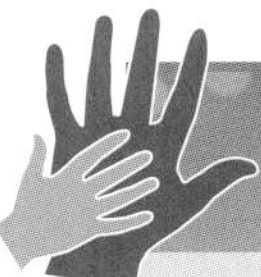

Safety Link

Prevent Bullying

Acting like a bully is an unhealthy form of communication. Bullying can be the use of written, verbal, or electronic expression, or a physical act or gesture. Some schools have guidelines to prevent bullying. If you experience bullying, share the details with an adult, such as a parent or teacher. Always use healthy communication.

You enjoy being with other people. Healthy communication means letting people know how you really feel. When you do, they can better understand you.

Try to express positive thoughts and feelings about other people. Do not assume people know you care about them. There are many ways to let them know. You can tell them in person. Write a letter or poem. Show how you feel by using nonverbal communication. You can make a drawing or give someone a hug or a smile.

Healthy communication often occurs when you feel good about yourself, and then you share that with others. There are times, however, when you do not feel good about yourself. You may take this out on other people. You may use harsh words to hurt them or ignore them. You may act like a bully. A **bully** is a person who uses strength or power to persuade or pressure others (using force or fear) to do something. These are unhealthy forms of communication that can hurt people.

When people feel hurt, healthy communication can still be present. If people are aware of others' moods, they can help. For instance, your mother may sense when you feel hurt, and respond lovingly. Your teacher may know you work hard in class, and offer praise.

Talk about your negative feelings. For instance, when your parents buy you new clothes, thank them. If you do not like the clothes, let them know. Explain why you do not like the clothes. Ask your parents if you can return them and choose what you like. Your parents should try to understand. When they tell you why they chose the clothes, you will better understand them.

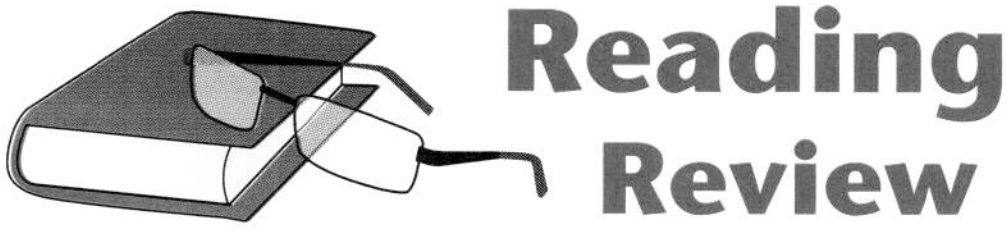

Reading Review

1. What are some benefits of healthy communication?
2. How can you let people know you care about them?
3. What are some signs of unhealthy communication?

Section Summary

- Relationships depend on communication.
- People communicate to share feelings and thoughts.
- You can use verbal and nonverbal communication to send messages.
- Communicating well includes speaking and writing clearly. Being an active listener is also an important part of communicating.
- Your behavior sends messages about you to others.
- Having good communication skills is healthy.

Section 1-6
Strengthening Families

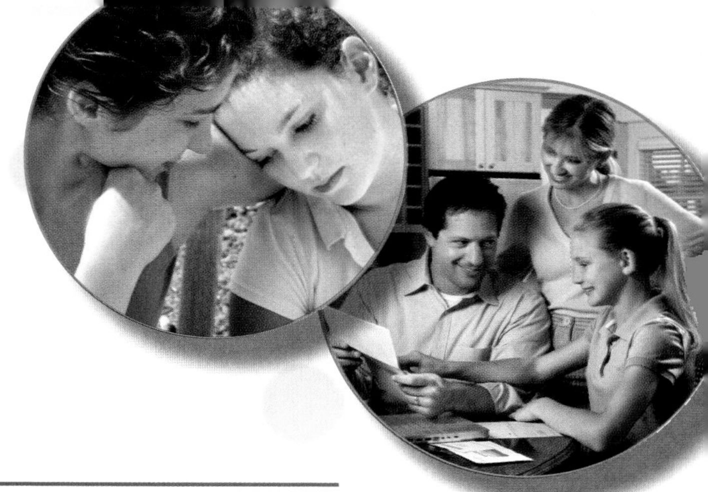

Objectives

After studying this lesson, you will be able to

- **define** *challenge*, *crisis*, *unity*, *solution*, *family council*, *conflict*, *conflict resolution*, *mediator*, *compromise*, *family counseling agency*, *shelter*, *hot line*, and *support group*.
- **list** some challenges of families.
- **describe** how challenges affect family members differently.
- **explain** the conflict resolution process.
- **apply** communication skills in finding solutions to disagreements.
- **identify** sources of help for family challenges.

Key Terms

challenge: a demanding or difficult task or situation that can be a source of distress.

crisis: affects the functioning of a family.

unity: a state of being in agreement, not being divided.

solution: an answer to a problem.

family council: an informal meeting to talk about issues concerning family members.

conflict: a disagreement between two or more people.

conflict resolution: the process of finding a solution to a disagreement.

mediator: a person not involved in the conflict, but helps settle the conflict.

compromise: an agreement in a conflict in which both sides are willing to give up a little of what they wanted.

family counseling agency: a group that works with family members to help them deal with changes and challenges.

shelter: a place that offers housing and food to people who have nowhere else to go.

hot line: a telephone service that offers immediate information to people who need help.

support group: a group of people with a similar challenge who provide support and help each other cope.

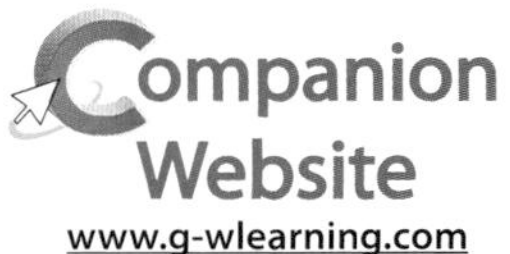

Study the Key Terms by completing crossword puzzles, matching activities, and e-flash cards at the website.

Main Ideas

- Every family has challenges.
- Challenges affect each family member in a different way.
- Families can solve many challenges together.
- Communication skills help resolve conflicts.
- Conflict resolution is the process of finding a solution to a conflict.
- Help from outside the family is sometimes needed to resolve challenges.

A **challenge** is a demanding or difficult task or situation that can be a source of distress. All individuals and families face challenges. Sometimes, they are small tasks like arguing about keeping your room clean and orderly. Other situations are large family challenges, such as illness, unemployment, drug abuse, or death. A bigger challenge is often called a crisis. A **crisis** affects the functioning of a family in negative or positive ways.

Positive effects of a crisis might be when a family member takes a new job with higher salary that requires moving to another city. This is positive for the family because of increased income, but could be difficult for children. For each family member, such challenges are real and must be faced. See **1-18**.

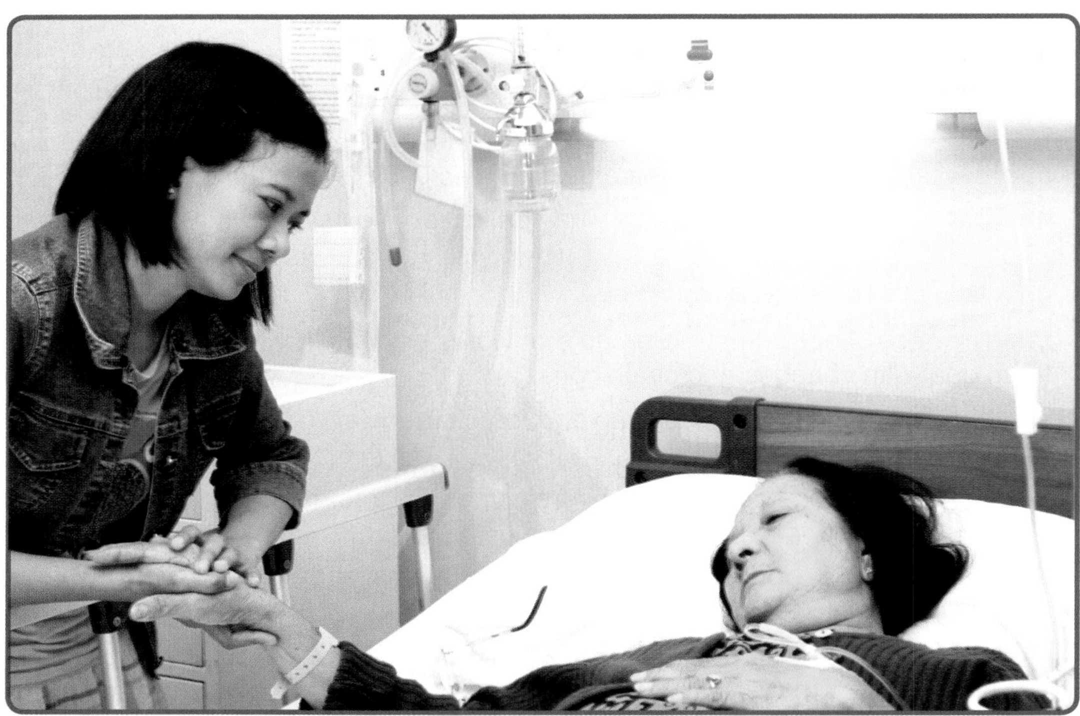

1-18 Illness or an accident requires adjustments for family members.

Different Points of View

When situations are difficult at home, each person may be affected differently. Young children, teens, and adults may each see the same problem from a different point of view.

For instance, young children have little understanding of money problems. Unless they lack food, shelter, and clothing, they may not even know a problem exists. Teens, on the other hand, need more than food, clothing, and shelter. They need supplies for school. They also want to have some of the items their friends have. They may feel angry if there is not enough money to buy these items. Adults are responsible for providing for the needs of their entire families. Money problems can cause adults to feel worried.

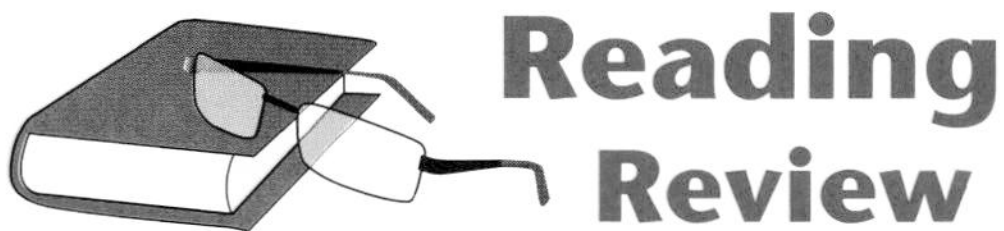

Reading Review

1. Why do similar challenges affect young children, teens, and adults differently?
2. How can you become more aware of the challenges your parents have? What can you do about it?

Addressing Challenges

Families can use several methods to deal with challenges. These methods include working together and talking openly. Sometimes families may have to seek outside help to deal with serious challenges or a crisis.

Unity means to agree, without being divided. When challenges occur at home, family unity makes them easier to face. Family members can agree to work together.

When family members share their feelings, challenges do not seem so bad. To young people, challenges sometimes seem bigger than they really are. Talking with parents may help young people see challenges in a more realistic way. Parents may be afraid to show their fear about family challenges. Sharing their concerns with their children can help the children understand the issues and give emotional support.

Some family challenges may have a very simple **solution**, or answer. It may just be a matter of talking about the challenge and deciding what to do. Other challenges, or a crisis, are harder to solve. Finding the answer may not be so easy. Family members may have to think and talk about the issues for hours, days, or even weeks before a decision can be reached.

When this happens, a family council can be helpful. A **family council** is an informal meeting to talk about issues concerning family members. Every member should be included, even younger children. They may not understand all that is said. They are, however, still a part of the family. See **1-19**.

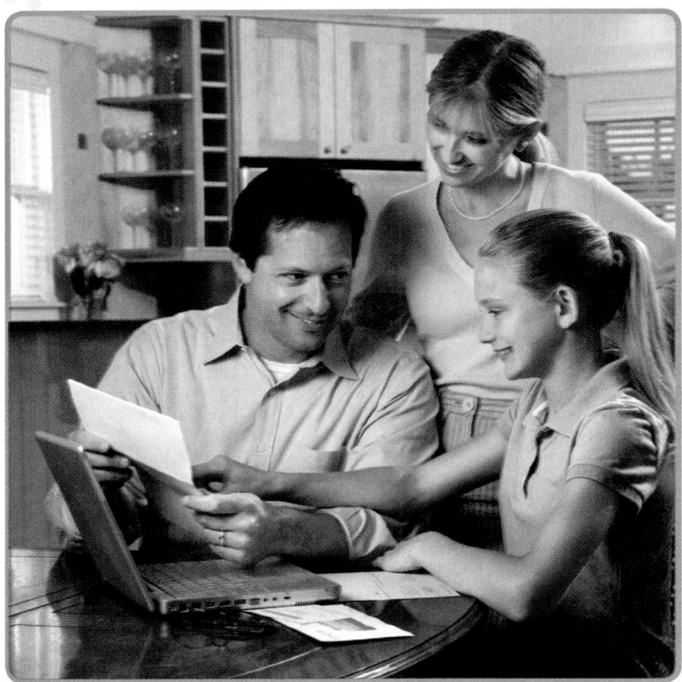

1-19 Family members should be given a chance to express themselves.

Discussing family issues gives members a chance to express their views. Talking about feelings helps increase understanding and trust. Sometimes, families may discuss serious issues, such as money challenges. Other times, they may talk about simple issues, such as which movie to see. Many families find that if all family members share a challenge, they can more easily reach a solution.

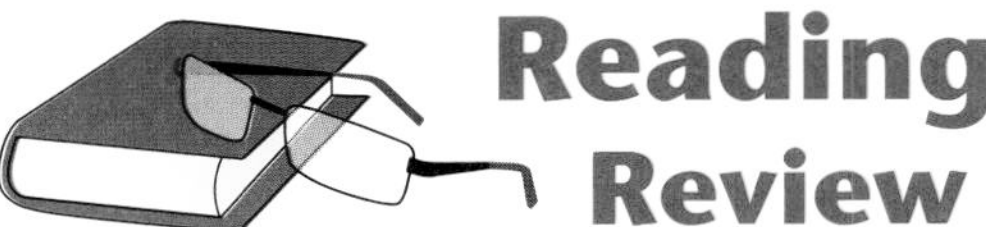

Reading Review

1. What can help make family challenges easier to face?
2. How can sharing feelings help when dealing with challenges?
3. How can family councils help solve family challenges?

Conflict Resolution

Sometimes, a challenge cannot be easily solved. It may turn into a conflict. A **conflict** is a disagreement between two or more people.

Conflicts often occur with family members and friends. This is partly because you spend so much time together. When conflicts are not resolved, relationships can be damaged by hurt feelings. **Conflict resolution** is the process of finding a solution to a disagreement.

First, make sure you find the right time to settle a disagreement. Choose a time when other people are not around. Allow sufficient time for everyone to talk, listen, and explore solutions.

Use good communication skills to help resolve conflicts. Express your feelings clearly. Be polite and avoid yelling or arguing. Attack the challenge, not the person. For example, you may say, "I feel frustrated when my ideas are not considered." This is more effective than saying, "You never pay attention to my ideas."

Good communication also involves talking *with* other people, not *to* them. Be an active listener. This helps you understand others' points of view. Family members need to share ideas, opinions, and feelings. This helps them find solutions to their challenges.

When a solution is still not found, a mediator may be needed. A **mediator** is a person who is not involved in the conflict, but who helps settle the conflict. This person will not be affected by the challenge. He or she can give a neutral viewpoint.

For instance, imagine you are having a conflict with a close friend. You may talk to your guidance counselor. He or she can act as a mediator to help find a solution. The mediator listens to both sides and asks questions. The mediator may suggest you and your friend try a compromise. A **compromise** is an agreement in which both sides are willing to give up a little of what they wanted.

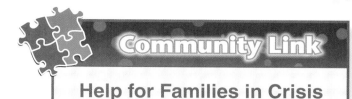

Help for Families in Crisis

Make a list of the organizations in your community that offer help to families dealing with serious challenges. Include in the list information on how families can best use these organizations.

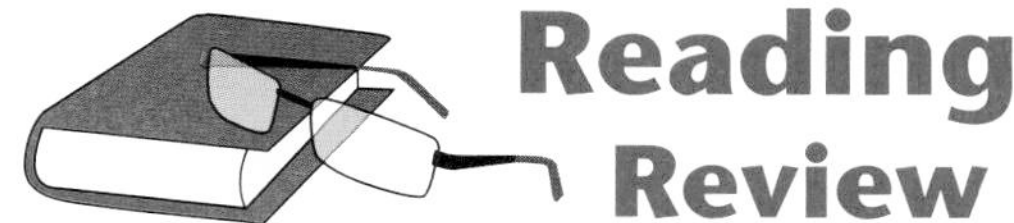

Reading Review

1. Why are communication skills helpful in resolving conflicts?
2. Describe a mediator.
3. What is a compromise? Give an example.

Seeking Help

For many young people, serious challenges or a crisis are difficult to understand. Divorce and death are two examples. They change the basic structure of the family. These changes may be hard to accept. People need to adjust without hurting themselves or others. It takes time and effort to understand and adapt to the situation.

When family troubles arise, it can be hard to think clearly. Some families share their challenges with one another. They work together to find solutions. Relatives, friends, and neighbors may provide support. See **1-20**. Other families sometimes need more help. They may talk with someone outside the family.

Discuss family challenges with someone who will understand. There are many people who can help. Family doctors and religious leaders are some examples. Teachers, school nurses, or counselors may also be able to help.

Community resources are other sources of help. Community resources include family counseling agencies and shelters. Hot lines and support groups also provide help for troubled families.

A **family counseling agency** is a group that provides families help as they adjust to changes and challenges in their lives.

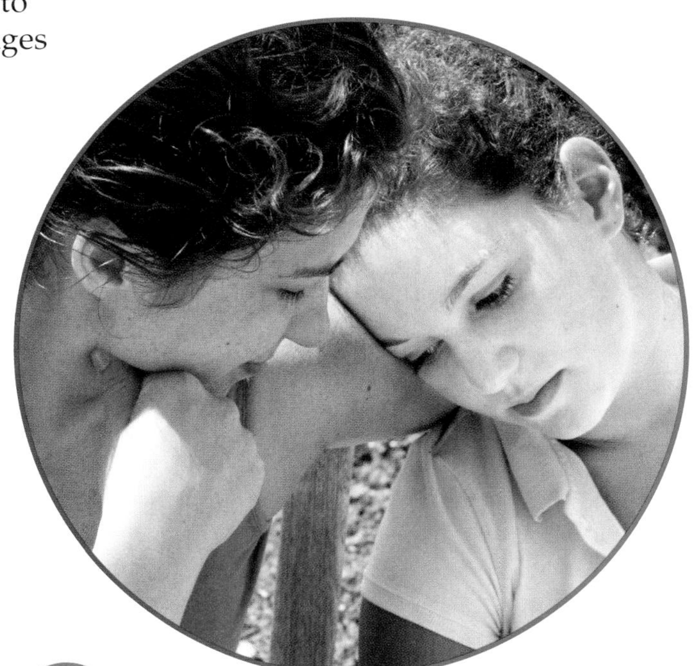

1-20 Support from others can help you get through family challenges.

A **shelter** is a place that offers housing and food to people who have nowhere else to go. Some shelters provide protection for people who are victims of abuse or violence.

A **hot line** is a telephone service that offers immediate information to people who need help. Hot lines often help people who are facing a crisis such as drug or child abuse. Most hot lines have toll-free numbers.

A **support group** is a group of people with a similar challenge who help each other cope. Some communities have a wide range of support groups. The groups may help people cope with drug or alcohol abuse, physical and mental illness, obesity, or grief. Some groups are for adults; others are for teens.

When a challenge or crisis occurs at home, the greatest source of strength for each family member should be the family itself. Family members should not waste time and energy finding fault and placing blame. Often, this does not help or make people feel better. Instead, they should try to find the best solution for the challenge or crisis. They need to be patient and understanding and help one another.

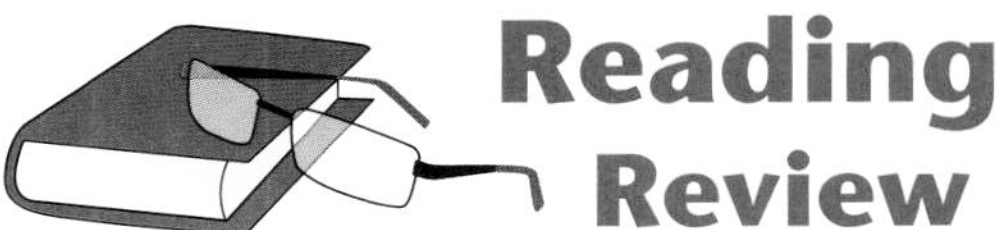

1. Why should you discuss a challenge or crisis with someone who will understand?
2. Whom could you turn to for help if you needed someone to talk with about a challenge or crisis?
3. How can a positive outlook help when trying to solve a family challenge or crisis?

Section Summary

- All families have problems.
- Family members often see the same challenge differently. They need to talk so they understand one another. This can help them solve the challenge together.
- A family council is useful in resolving issues.
- Conflict resolution is the process of finding a solution to a disagreement.
- A mediator may suggest a solution through compromise.
- Sometimes a family is faced with a crisis. The family can seek help from community resources. These include family counseling agencies, shelters, hot lines, and support groups.

Chapter Summary

No one else is exactly like you. Your personality and physical traits make you unique. As you grow from a child into an adult, your personality develops and changes. You grow physically, intellectually, socially, and emotionally. This time is called *adolescence*. During this time, you also learn to become more independent from adults.

As you grow and develop, your family supports you. Family members need to talk with one another about their feelings. Families can be of many different sizes and include many different members. Family types describe the makeup of a family.

Friends are also part of your support system. You can laugh and have fun with your friends. You can care about, trust, and respect your friends. Your peers can make you feel like you belong. Being open and friendly helps you make new friends and get along with your peers.

Your relationships with your family and friends depend on how well you communicate. Communication can be verbal and nonverbal.

Having good communication skills means letting people know how you really feel. This is both important and healthy.

Conflict resolution is the process of finding a solution to a disagreement. Conflicts often occur with family members and friends. Communication skills help resolve conflicts. A mediator may propose a compromise. A family council meeting may help resolve issues concerning family members.

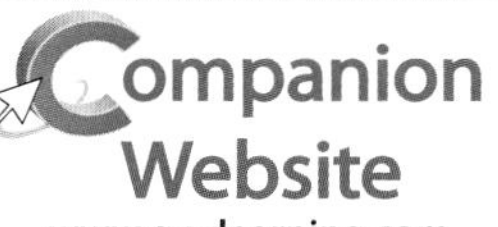

Review Key Terms and Main Ideas for Chapter 1 at the website.

Chapter Review

Write your answers on a separate sheet of paper.

1. List four personality traits that you have.
2. The way a person feels about his or her self-concept is called ______-______.
3. Being able to understand a science formula represents which type of growth and development?
4. List three developmental needs of young adolescents.
5. List three ways brothers and sisters can get along.
6. How can you show respect for older adults?
7. When your friends are in the same age group, they are considered ______.
8. When your friends influence you to make decisions that are not good for you, this influence is called ______ ______ ______.
9. Why is communication important in relationships?
10. Why is it sometimes helpful for families to have a family council meeting?
11. Explain how a mediator can help solve a conflict.

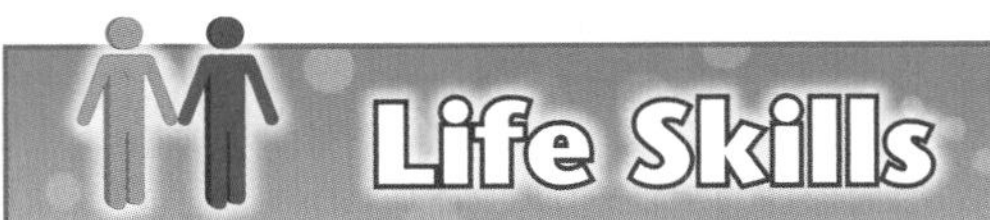

Life Skills

12. Prepare a five-minute oral presentation titled *The Importance of Character to Teens*. Your presentation should include your ideas about character. For instance, you may want to discuss what character is, how it is developed, and why it matters. Find positive examples to share. Practice your presentation before you share it with the class.

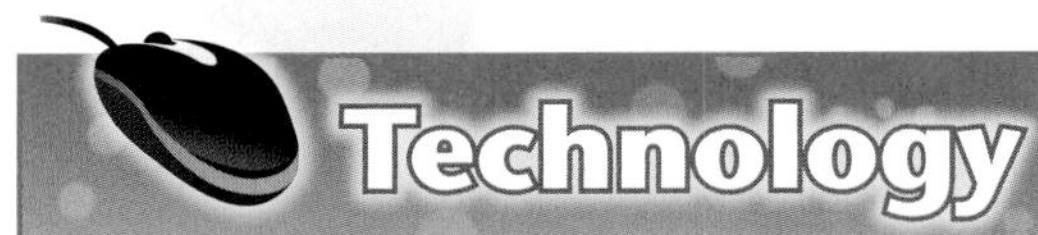

Technology

13. Using presentation software, create a presentation showing how you can say *no* to peer pressure. Include ways to stand up for yourself and make your own decisions. Share your presentations with the class.

Journal Writing

14. Begin a diary or a record that will show your growth and development during the adolescent years. It is helpful to review what you have written and see how you have grown toward adulthood. Write a brief summary every three months. Then discuss how you feel about your progress with a parent or trusted adult.

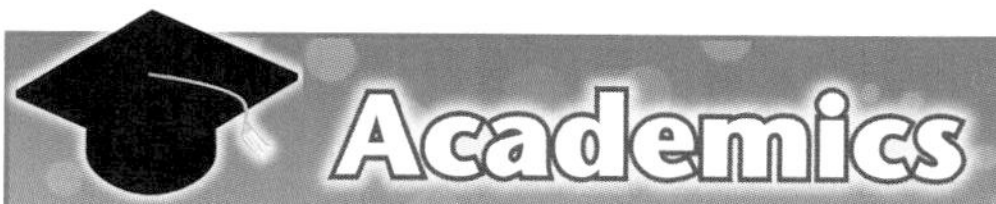

15. **Science.** Divide a sheet of paper into three columns. In the first column, list the four areas of growth and development. In the second column, write examples of how you have changed during the past year in each area of growth. In the third column, write examples of how you would like to change in each area during the year ahead. Think about how the changes listed in the second and third columns will help you grow toward adulthood.
16. **Social Studies.** Role-play a situation in which you are visiting a friend's home and do not behave properly. Discuss how you can change your behavior. Role-play the situation again showing the correct behavior.
17. **Speech.** Play the *telephone game*. As a class, sit in a circle. Your teacher will give a student a phrase. This student will whisper it to the next student. Continue until it has been passed around the circle. The last student will repeat the phrase aloud. Have the first student read the original phrase aloud. Compare the two versions. Discuss the importance of feedback and communicating effectively.

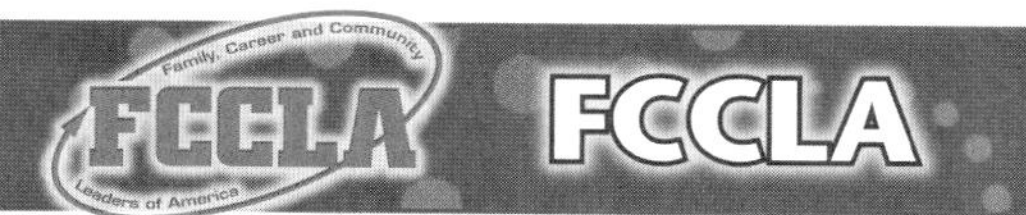

18. Think of a family situation that might cause challenges. Write how you would react to the challenge. Ask a parent and a brother or sister how they would react. Take notes and compare the answers. Share your findings with your family. Discuss how you can learn to understand one another better when family challenges occur. Then develop an FCCLA *Family Ties* project for the *Power of One* program. Obtain further information about this program from your FCCLA advisor.

Chapter 2
Learning About Children

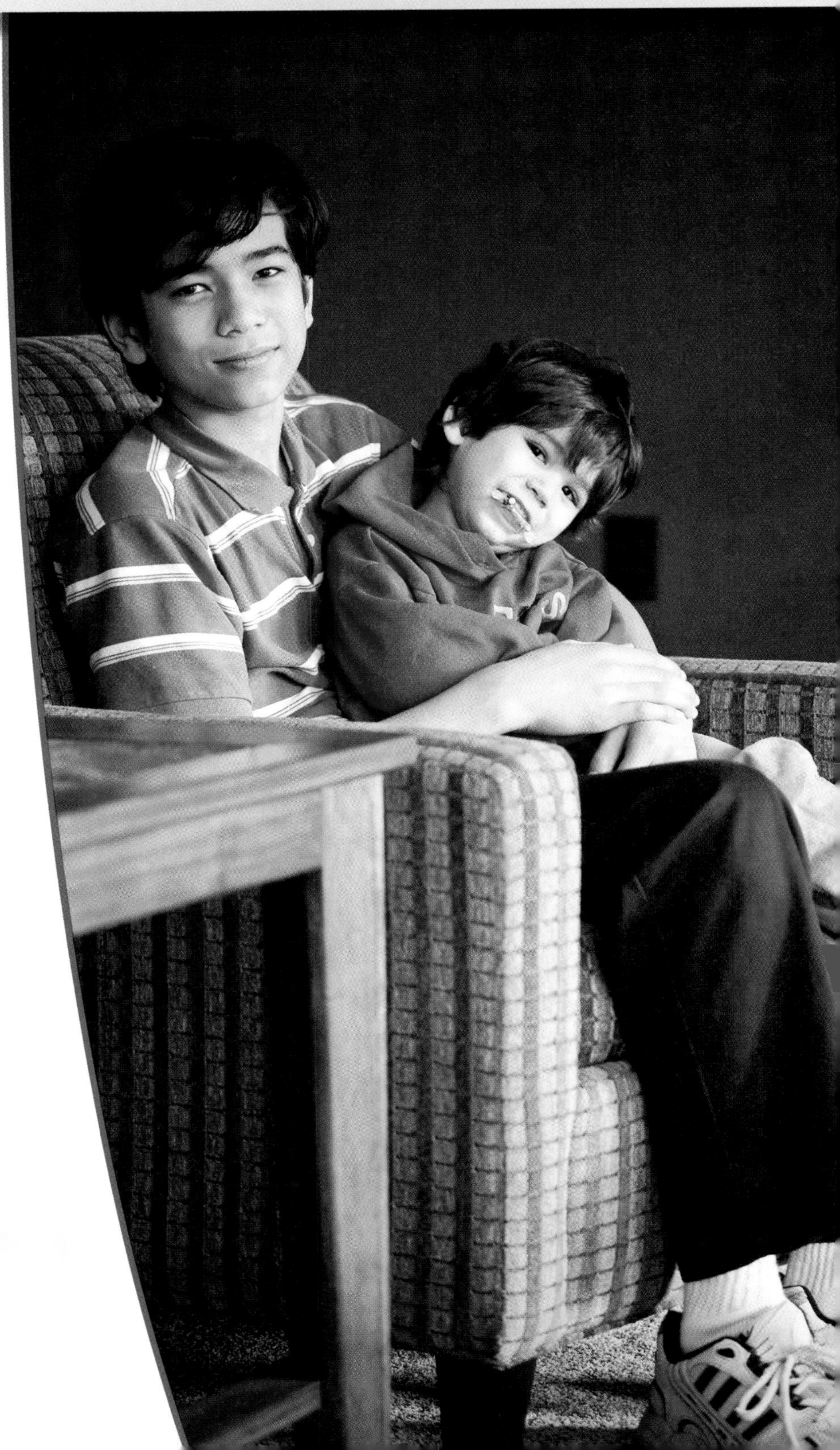

Sections

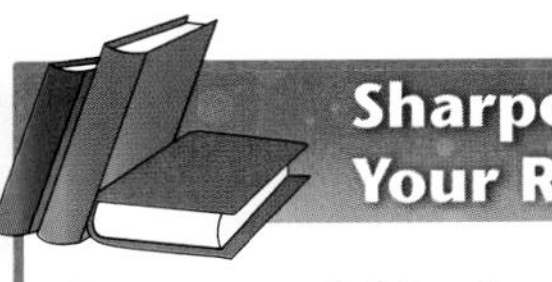

Sharpen Your Reading

As you read this chapter, write a *top ten* list of important concepts.

Concept Organizer

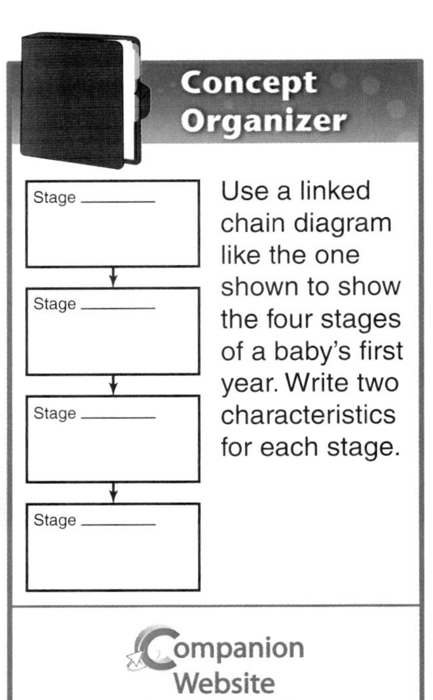

Use a linked chain diagram like the one shown to show the four stages of a baby's first year. Write two characteristics for each stage.

Companion Website
www.g-wlearning.com

Print out the concept organizer at the website.

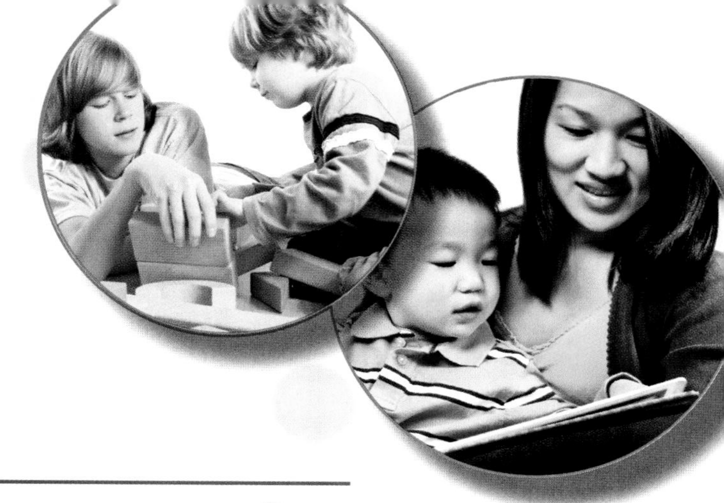

Section 2-1
Babysitting

Objectives

After studying this section, you will be able to
- **define** *babysitting*, *caregiver*, *limits*, *guidance*, *discipline*, *physical disability*, *intellectual disability*, and *gifted*.
- **list** some of the responsibilities of babysitters.
- **explain** how you can prepare to be a reliable babysitter.
- **describe** the tasks you need to perform when babysitting.
- **identify** special needs children may have.

Key Terms

babysitting: caring for children, usually during a short absence of the parents.

caregiver: a person who cares for children.

limits: boundaries or restrictions.

guidance: everything parents do and say to affect their children's behavior.

discipline: the use of various methods to help children learn to behave in acceptable ways.

physical disability: a condition that limits a person's ability to use part of his or her body.

intellectual disability: a condition that limits a person's ability to use his or her mind.

gifted: a child who has developed more quickly than other children the same age.

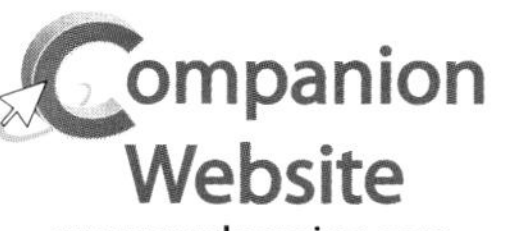

Study the Key Terms by completing crossword puzzles, matching activities, and e-flash cards at the website.

Main Ideas

- Babysitters are expected to treat children as their parents treat them.
- Keeping children safe and happy should be the main concern of a babysitter.
- Being a reliable babysitter takes a lot of preparation.
- Children with special needs should be treated like other children as much as possible.

Caring for children when their parents are absent for a brief time is called **babysitting**. When you babysit, you may care for younger brothers and sisters, cousins, or neighborhood children. Babysitting gives you a chance to learn about children. Sometimes, you may assist a parent or caregiver who is at home to care for a child. To be a responsible babysitter, you need to know how children grow and develop.

Responsibilities of Babysitting

The most important people in a child's life are the caregivers. A **caregiver** is a person who cares for children. See **2-1**. When you babysit, you are responsible for the children. You are a substitute for the parents. You are expected to treat children as their parents treat them.

Provide Guidance

Parents show their love by setting **limits**, which are boundaries or restrictions. Parents set limits to help children learn acceptable behavior and to keep them safe. For instance, parents may tell children they must complete their homework before going outside to play. This helps children learn to be responsible.

Limits are more effective when stated in positive ways. For instance, parents may say "Put your toys away" rather than "Don't leave your toys on the floor." By setting guidelines, parents can teach children to control their behavior.

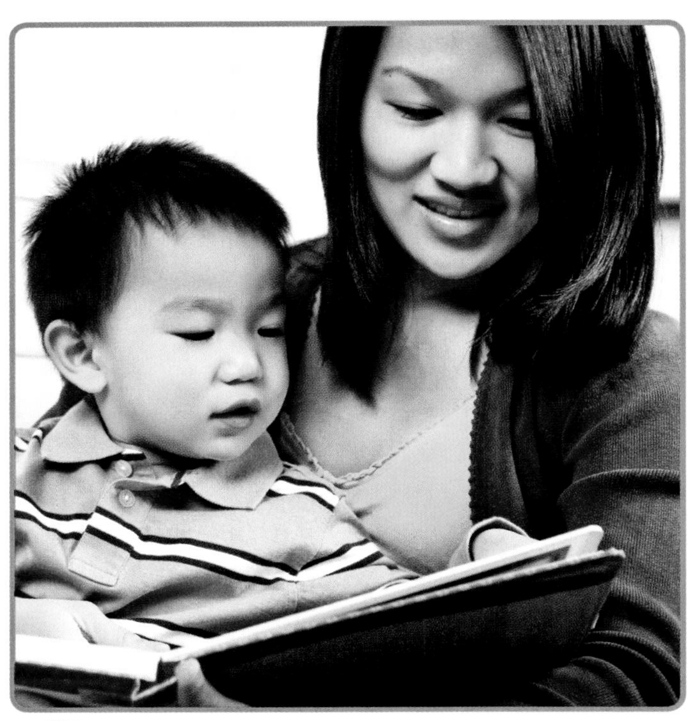

2-1 Caregivers can be parents, siblings, relatives, or babysitters.

Guidance and discipline may be needed to enforce some limits. **Guidance** includes everything parents do and say to affect their children's behavior. For instance, parents might model positive behavior by not becoming upset when they are frustrated. By modeling acceptable behavior, parents can help their children learn to control their own anger.

Discipline is the use of various methods to help children learn to behave in acceptable ways. Parents may use various styles of discipline to enforce limits. For instance, parents may teach their children to follow limits by setting a positive example. They may discuss reasons for limits. Parents may also praise their children when they follow the limits.

At times, children will ignore the limits parents set for them. When this occurs, parents must always be consistent when responding to the behavior. Parents are more likely to confuse children if they respond to an unacceptable behavior in a different way each time it occurs. Treating children consistently helps teach them to behave in acceptable ways.

In relationships with children, limits, guidance, and discipline are used with love. As a babysitter, find out what the limits are. Also, find out what kind of guidance and discipline the parents want you to use to enforce them.

Keep Children Safe and Happy

You are expected to keep children safe and happy when you babysit. Keeping them safe is a serious responsibility. Keeping children happy is sometimes as hard as keeping them safe. Following parents' instructions will help you reach these goals.

Never leave babies and young children alone, unless they are asleep in their beds. As they explore the world around them, accidents may occur. Stay with children and watch them. Play games and talk with them.

When an accident or illness occurs, you may need help. Call the parents or the doctor. Reliable babysitters are not afraid to ask for help. Keep the emergency phone numbers beside the phone for easy reference.

Do not give children medicine without a parent's or doctor's consent. If you think children may have taken medication on their own, call the parents at once to tell them.

Keeping children happy may require extra patience. They may become upset after their parents leave. Try to distract them. They will want to be talked to and held. Playing games and reading stories can help, too. Ask them to show you their favorite toys. Most children will become calm within a short period of time.

Succeed in Life

Keeping Children Safe

To keep children safe, you should follow these tips:

- Continuously watch over the infant or toddler in situations that pose any risk of injury.
- Never leave infants alone on a changing table or bed.
- Never leave infants or toddlers alone in the bathtub.
- Keep medicines, cleaning products, poisons, and matches locked up and out of the reach of children.
- Keep dangerous and breakable items, such as plastic bags and glass decorations, out of the reach of children.
- Keep small children away from touching stovetops, radiators, space heaters, sharp objects, or electric cords.
- Inspect all toys for small parts that children could swallow or sharp edges that can cut them. Place them out of reach of the child.
- Use safety gates to keep children from climbing up and down stairs.
- Never leave children alone in the house, even for a short time.
- Check children often while they are sleeping and playing.
- Keep first aid supplies and a flashlight handy in case of emergencies.

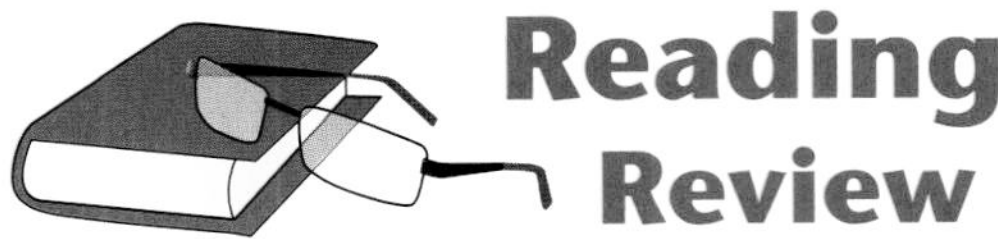

Reading Review

1. How can parents help their children learn acceptable behaviors?
2. What are two responsibilities you may have as a babysitter?
3. What can babysitters do to keep babies and young children from hurting themselves?

Preparing to Babysit

To be a reliable babysitter, you need to be prepared. Knowledge of how children grow and develop is important. You need to be patient and confident. You also need to be able to handle emergencies and act responsibly. A successful babysitter is caring and fond of children. A sense of humor helps, too.

Learn how children behave at each age. Read books about children. Observe children around you. Think about what you read and how it relates to what you observe. Remember this when babysitting.

Research community resources that are age appropriate for the child or children who will be in your care. Discuss these with a parent or caregiver. Suggest how you and the parent or caregiver could use such resources for learning experiences. You must have permission from the parent or caregiver to take a child away from home at any time, such as on a walk or to the park.

Before babysitting children for the first time, visit their homes to meet them and their parents. Tell the parents about your babysitting skills. Find out what duties they expect you to perform. Decide how much you will charge to babysit. Be sure the parents agree this is a fair amount.

Ask for any special instructions about caring for the children. What are their eating and sleeping habits? Do you need to feed them? If so, what foods should they eat? What time should they go to bed? What are their favorite toys? When you know and respect the rules, children cannot talk you into breaking them. Talk with the parents about the ways you try to guide children's behavior. See **2-2**.

Before the parents leave, ask for a phone number where you can reach them. Also, ask for phone numbers for the doctor, police, fire department, and local poison control center. Find out when you should call the doctor before calling the parents. Certain emergencies must be taken care of quickly.

Financial Literacy Link

Babysitting Rates

Before you decide how much to charge for babysitting services, you will want to consider several factors. Experience is one of the most important factors. For instance, a person with no babysitting experience may often receive several dollars less than a person who has years of experience. The number and age of children may also impact babysitting rates. For instance, caring for a baby or several children at one time often increases the hourly wage. Another factor to consider is the amount of additional work. When the job includes housework, cooking, or running errands, you may want to consider asking for more money.

Guiding Children's Behavior

- Give children time to change from one activity to another. Play is important. Children do not like to be interrupted. Warn a child five or ten minutes ahead of time.
- Use distraction to focus a child's attention on something else. If a child wants a book that he or she cannot have, offer another toy or book the child likes and can have.
- Smile when a child's behavior is good. Also, tell the child you approve of his or her behavior. Smiles and words help a child feel good about pleasing you.
- Use questions to help a child know what you expect. If you expect a child to pick up the toys when playtime is over, ask the child, "What are you supposed to do when you are finished playing with your toys?"
- Plan enough activities to keep a child busy. Try to have activities that will interest the child. A child may misbehave if he or she is bored. Remember that a child's attention span varies with different activities.

2-2 Follow these tips to reduce behavior problems.

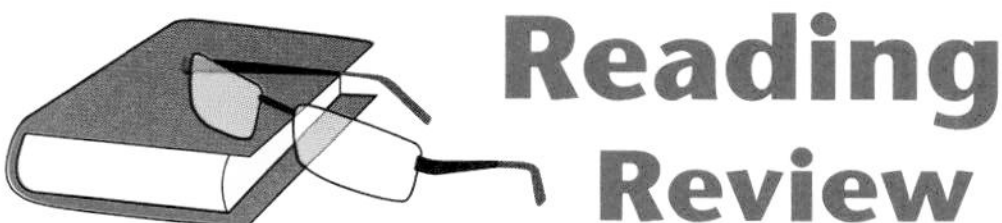

Reading Review

1. Why should babysitters visit the family before they babysit children for the first time?
2. What information should babysitters gather before the parents leave?
3. What kind of an emergency might require a babysitter to call the doctor before the parents?

On the Job

Following a few simple guidelines can help you be a successful, reliable babysitter. When you babysit, bring a notebook and pencil to write instructions. Wear comfortable clothes so you can play with the children. See **2-3**.

Bring reading material or homework to keep you busy after the children are asleep. Do not get so involved in your reading or homework, however, that you forget to check on the children. Only use the phone when necessary. This is not the time to be chatting with friends, even when the children are in bed. If you think you might want a snack, bring one with you. Do not eat the family's food unless they invite you to do so.

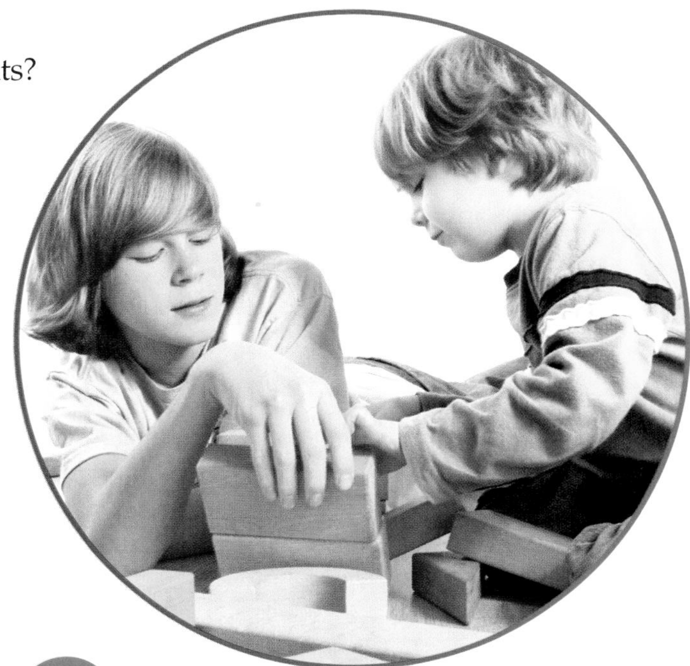

2-3 When you babysit, plan some activities you think the child might enjoy.

Make sure you respect the family's home. Handle dishes, decorations, and other breakable items carefully. Take care of furnishings. Fix or replace any objects that get broken or damaged. Leave the house as clean as when you arrived. Help the children pick up their toys before they go to bed or their parents arrive home.

Respect the family's privacy. Do not look through rooms, closets, or personal belongings unless the parents ask you to do so. Do not repeat anything the children say about the family. This is private information. If you find out about an action that may endanger the health or safety of the children, however, tell an adult whom you trust. The adult will aid you in getting help for the family, if needed.

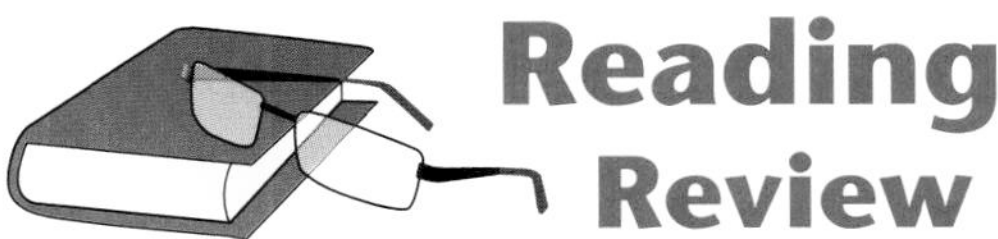

Reading Review

1. What reasons are there for not using the phone while you are babysitting?
2. How can you show respect for a family's privacy when babysitting?

Children with Special Needs

All children share certain basic needs. They all need food, clothing, and shelter. They need to feel safe and secure. Love and support are other basic needs.

Some children have special needs that go beyond basic needs. These children may have physical or intellectual disabilities. They may have special gifts or talents. Treat children with special needs like other children as much as possible.

Someday, you may babysit or work with children with special needs. The more you learn about these children, the better you will be able to care for them.

Some children have physical disabilities. A **physical disability** is a condition that limits a person's ability to use part of his or her body. Children with physical disabilities may need special tools to help them meet their needs. For instance, children who are blind may use guide dogs. Children who are hard of hearing may use hearing aids. Children with limited mobility may use wheelchairs or crutches. These tools help children with physical disabilities be more independent in their daily lives.

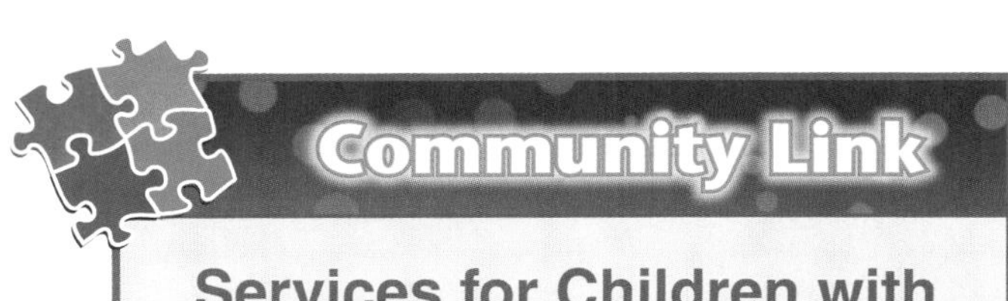

Services for Children with Intellectual Disabilities

Children with intellectual disabilities may benefit from special community programs that address their specific needs. For instance, some children may need special help to learn how to talk or read. Other children may need extra help to learn how to dress or feed themselves. With this help, children with intellectual disabilities are able to learn how to better meet their daily needs. Find out what resources are available in your community for children with intellectual disabilities. Share your findings with the class.

Children with intellectual disabilities also have special needs. An **intellectual disability** is a condition that limits a person's ability to use his or her mind. Intellectual disabilities can be caused by problems during pregnancy or birth. They can also be caused by injuries to the brain.

Children who are **gifted** have developed more quickly than other children of the same age. These children have different special needs. Children who are gifted may be skilled in English, math, art, music, or sports. Special programs help children who are gifted receive the extra attention they need to fully develop their skills.

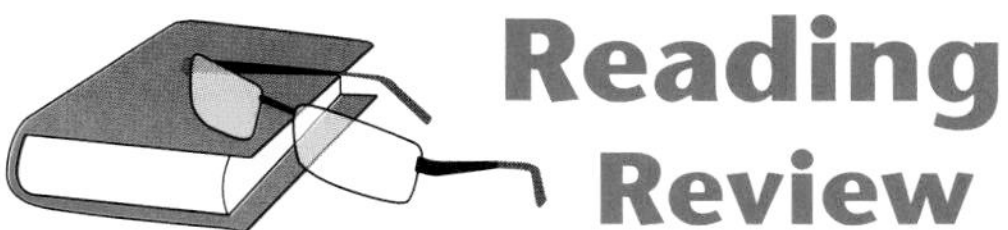

Reading Review

1. What are three needs all children share?
2. How can you learn to care for children with special needs?

Section Summary

- To be a responsible babysitter, learn how children grow and develop.
- Babysitters keep children safe and happy.
- Babysitters should prepare for their job by visiting the home and talking with the parents.
- Before you babysit, ask the parents for their instructions and follow them.
- Reliable babysitters can learn to help and care for children with special needs.

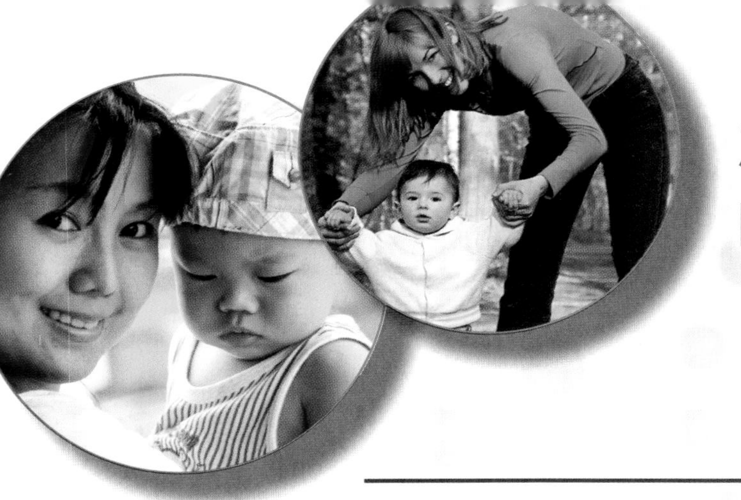

Section 2-2
Baby's First Year

Objectives

After studying this section, you will be able to

- **define** *newborn*, *dependent*, *reflex*, *infant*, *separation anxiety*, *childproof*, and *Sudden Infant Death Syndrome (SIDS)*.
- **state** why each child develops at a different rate.
- **explain** why babies are completely dependent at birth.
- **describe** how babies grow and develop during the first year of life.

Key Terms

newborn: a term used to describe a baby from birth to one month of age.

dependent: relying on another for support.

reflex: a natural, unlearned behavior.

infant: a term used to describe a baby from one month of age to one year of age.

separation anxiety: a fear that if parents leave, they will not return.

childproof: to make an area safe for children by keeping potential dangers away from them.

Sudden Infant Death Syndrome (SIDS): the sudden, unexpected death of a baby who seems healthy.

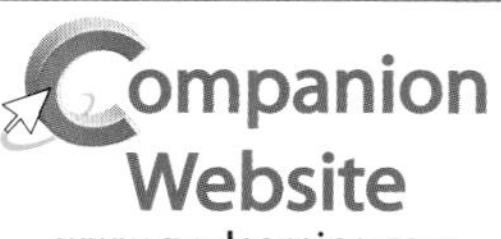

Study the Key Terms by completing crossword puzzles, matching activities, and e-flash cards at the website.

Main Ideas

- Babies grow and develop at different rates.
- Babies need a lot of love and care.
- Infants are constantly growing and changing.
- Dependent babies rapidly grow into active one-year-olds.

To care for children, you must understand how they grow and develop. Children differ in their physical, intellectual, social, and emotional growth. In this section, you will learn about babies during their first year of life. Children grow and develop rapidly during the first year.

Each Child Is Special

Every child is unique. Each develops at a different rate. Some start to walk, talk, and teethe earlier or later than others their age. Even brothers and sisters develop at different rates. See **2-4**. A younger brother may be able to put a puzzle together at an earlier age than his brothers or sisters. These differences are normal. They result from the influence of heredity and environment.

Although children grow and learn at different rates, they achieve developmental tasks in a certain order. The development of one skill leads to the development of the next. For instance, babies first learn to hold their heads up, then roll over. Soon they sit, crawl, stand, and walk. One skill builds on another.

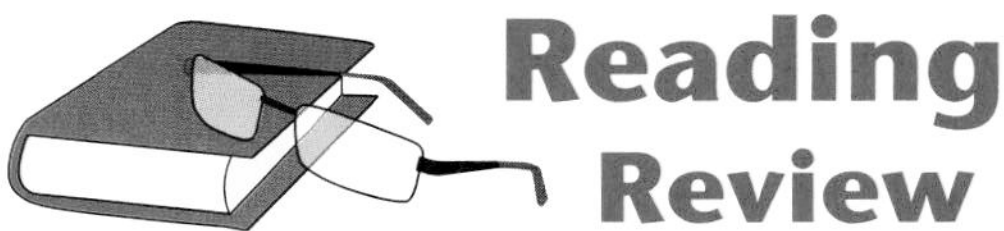

Reading Review

1. Think of two young children you know. Give examples of how their personalities are different.
2. Why do children achieve developmental tasks at different rates?

The First Month

From birth to age one month, a baby is called a **newborn**. Caring for a newborn is one of the greatest challenges a parent or caregiver faces. When babies are born, they are completely dependent. **Dependent** means they rely on others for support. For instance, newborns need someone to feed them and cover their bodies to keep them warm. They cannot perform these simple tasks for themselves.

At birth, a baby's body has a narrow chest and large abdomen. The average weight is 7½ pounds, and the average length is 20 inches. Babies grow rapidly, however, during the first year. Within a few months, the arms and legs fill out. The eyes may change color.

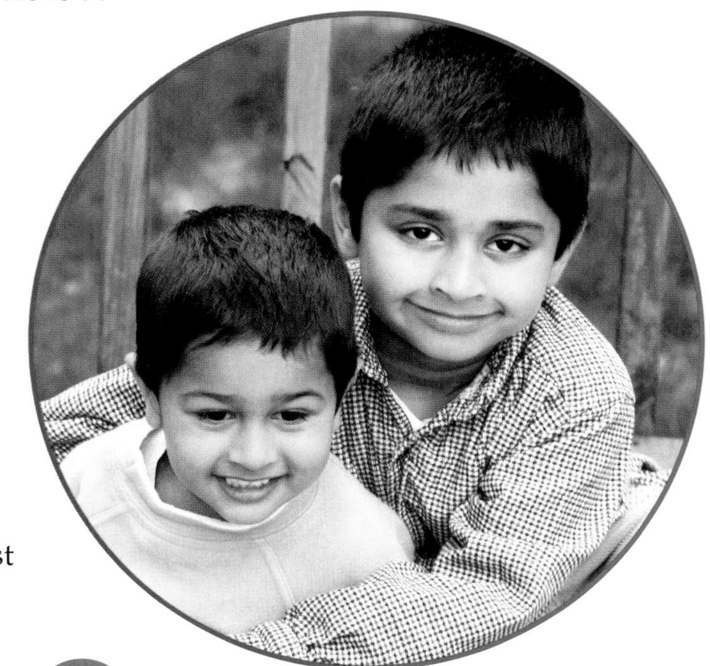

2-4 Parents with more than one child must remember children grow and develop at different rates.

Newborns do not have strong muscles. They have trouble controlling their actions. They cannot hold up their heads by themselves. Their heads, therefore, should be supported at all times. Babies' bodies need to be held firmly and securely for many months. Figure **2-5** shows how to support a baby's body.

Although their muscles are not strong, newborns are still able to perform some tasks. They use reflex movements. A **reflex** is a natural, unlearned behavior. Some reflexes are grasping, sucking, and rooting. The *Palmar (grasping) reflex* occurs when babies grasp any object placed in their hands. The *rooting reflex* occurs when you touch babies around their mouths, their heads turn, and their mouths search for food. The *sucking reflex* begins after newborns find objects with their mouths. The rooting and sucking reflexes help babies survive. These reflexes disappear within three to four months, when the muscles become stronger.

Newborns are aware of their surroundings. They can see, hear, feel, smell, and taste at birth. Their senses, however, are immature. A baby's senses develop and become stronger as the baby matures. Keep this in mind as you care for babies. Appropriate activities and toys help babies develop in all ways.

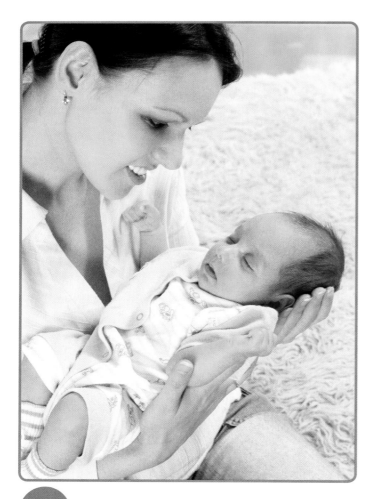

2-5 Infants' bodies need to be supported along the back and neck until their muscles become stronger.

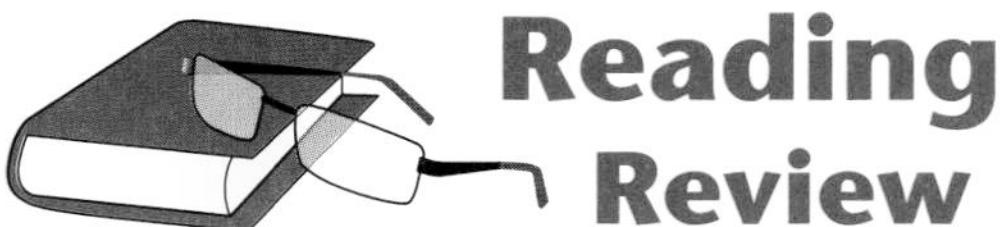

Reading Review

1. How are babies dependent on others at birth? Give examples.
2. How do the rooting and sucking reflexes help babies survive?
3. When caring for babies, why should you be aware of the development of their senses?

Two to Three Months

Infant is the term used to describe a child from one month of age to one year of age. As infants grow, they spend more hours awake. They have different ways of letting adults know what they want. When babies are awake, they may let adults know they want to play by smiling, cooing, and gently waving their arms and legs. When they get tired of playing, they may frown or look away.

Crying is one way infants communicate. They cannot tell you with words what they want or need. They have different cries when they are hungry, wet, sick, cold, or scared. They also cry when they want to be held or loved. When adults respond to a crying baby right away, the infant learns there is someone who will care for him or her. This helps the baby learn to trust adults.

If the needs of infants are not met during their first few months, they may quit trying to communicate their needs and become withdrawn. Their emotional and physical health may suffer.

Babies need a lot of love to grow and develop well. Love helps them learn to trust other people. They should be soothed when they are upset. They should also be held and touched when they are happy. Babies like to hear a calming voice. This is not spoiling them. This makes them feel warm and secure. See **2-6**.

Babies of this age learn to do many different tasks. They like to watch their hands and play with their fingers and toes. They smile. If they hear sounds, they look up for a few seconds or move their heads to follow sound. Babies kick their legs when lying down. If objects attract their attention, they reach for them. Infants also learn to roll from their sides to their backs.

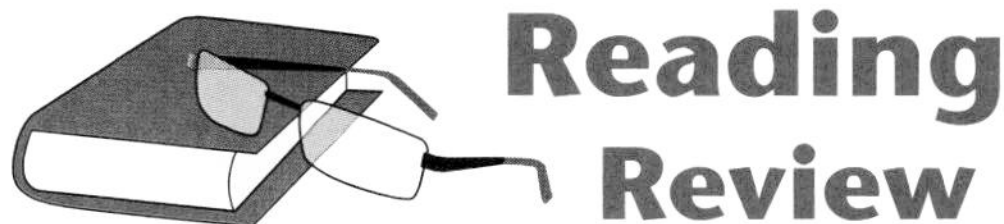

Reading Review

1. What are some reasons babies cry? Give examples.
2. What happens if babies' needs are not met during the first few months?
3. What are some tasks that three-month-olds can perform?

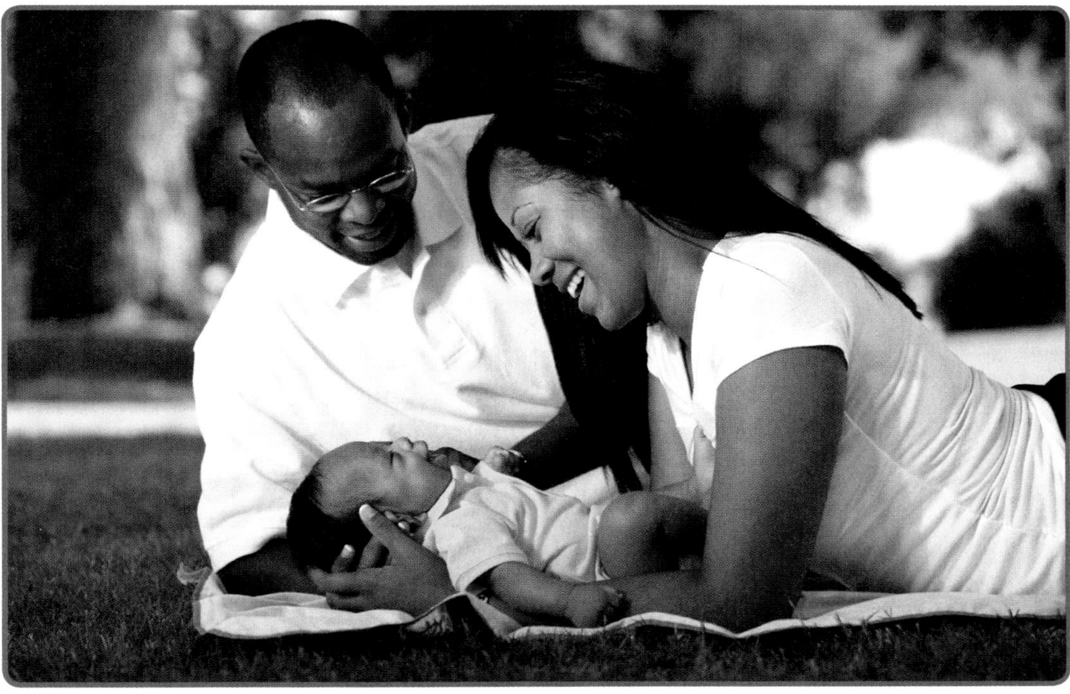

2-6 During the first few months of life, babies need a lot of love.

Four to Eight Months

Infants' muscles become stronger at four or five months of age. They may hold their heads up for a few minutes without support. They may begin rolling over by themselves. If they have trouble rolling back over, help them. They are still dependent on other people.

At this age, babies also start reacting more to people and their environment. They enjoy being held in a sitting position so they can look around. They smile more and may laugh out loud. See **2-7**. Between seven and ten months of age, they begin to babble. Most babies enjoy lying down for a while, playing with their hands or reaching for their toes. They also begin exploring their clothes, blankets, and other objects they can reach.

When placed in a sitting position, six-month-olds may sit alone. At this age, they learn to tell the difference between familiar and strange faces. Around six to eight months of age, infants often experience their first anxiety. **Separation anxiety** is a fear that parents will leave and not return. Infants like to be near their parents. They may become upset around strangers. Infants may even become upset when separated from parents for a short amount of time. This anxiety often fades by two years of age.

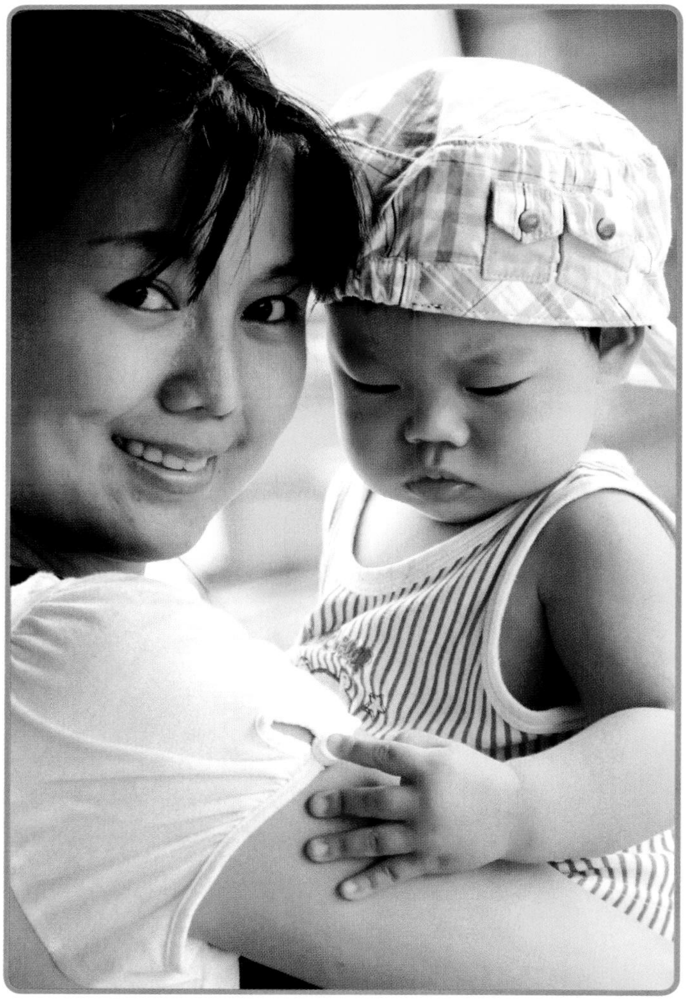

It should not take infants too long, however, to become familiar with new people. If people smile and talk to babies, they may smile or respond by babbling. Responding to babies' babbling in a consistent manner will encourage brain development.

Around seven or eight months of age, babies seem to be in constant motion. This is how they strengthen their muscles and learn to control their actions. When placed on the floor, they may kick their legs and wave their arms. They may also begin to move about and explore. They may kick and push themselves on their stomachs to get to objects beyond their reach. They may also roll over to get to objects. They can no longer be counted on to stay in one place.

Babies are curious at this age. They enjoy seeing, holding, and touching colorful objects. Toys of various sizes, shapes, and textures interest them. They like to bang objects together to make noise. They may drop their toys on the floor to see what happens. If their toys are hidden, they will look for them.

2-7 Babies four to eight months of age start interacting more with other people.

Place infants in safe, childproof places. To **childproof** means to make an area safe for children by keeping potential dangers away from them. For instance, a baby should not be left near stairs. A baby could be badly hurt from a fall.

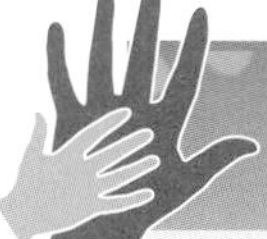

Safety Link

Keeping Infants Safe

Infants like to touch many objects. They learn how certain objects feel and taste. They want to put everything in their mouths. This is why you must keep small and sharp objects out of their reach. Otherwise, they could swallow something or hurt themselves. Do not allow infants to go near electric sockets, plants, or garbage.

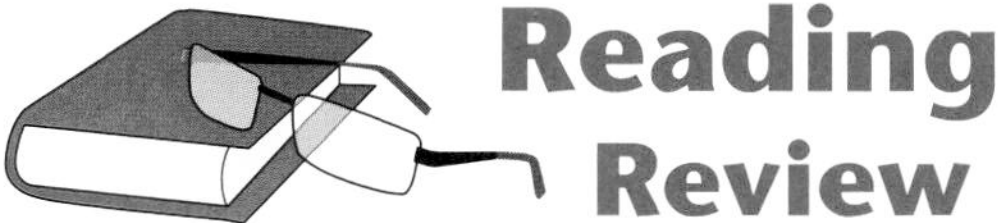

Reading Review

1. What tasks can four-month-olds perform that newborns cannot?
2. Why may six-month-olds become upset around strangers?
3. How do eight-month-olds strengthen their muscles? Give examples.

Nine to Twelve Months

From nine to twelve months, infants develop in many ways all at once. At this age, many babies go from crawling to walking. They may also begin talking. Some babies learn to walk and talk at the same time. Others may not develop either skill until later. Each baby learns at a different rate. See **2-8**.

By nine or ten months of age, most babies can move by themselves. They can sit up without help. They are no longer content to lie down and play. Most begin crawling from one place to another. Each baby has his or her own special way of crawling. For instance, Lena pulls herself along on her stomach. Tyler crawls on his hands and knees. Ella keeps her legs fairly straight and walks on her hands and feet. Each way is normal.

Also during this time, babies start learning the difference between right and wrong. They can tell when their parents approve or disapprove. They are learning how to act when someone says *no*.

By eleven months of age, babies begin to move around more. They may learn how to roll a ball to you. Infants this age may take a few steps while holding onto someone. They may even learn to stand, stoop, and stand again.

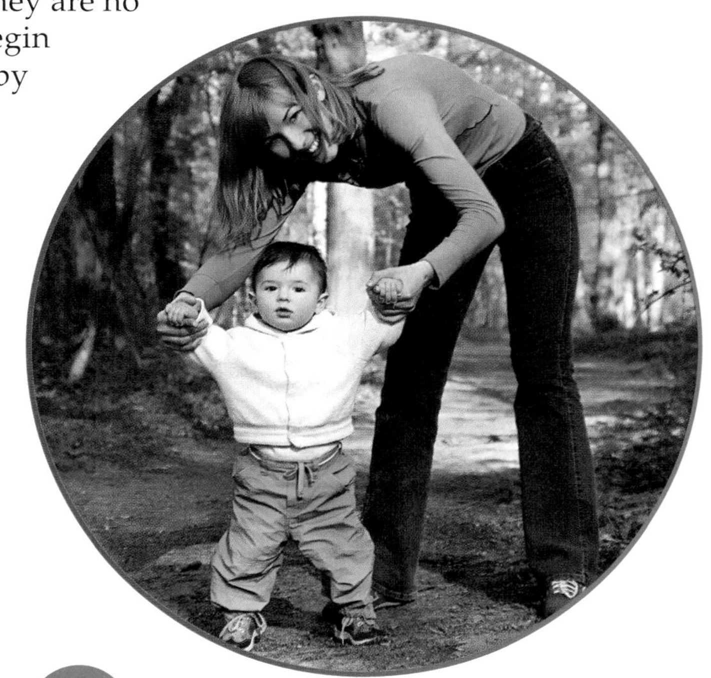

2-8 Each baby learns to walk at a different age.

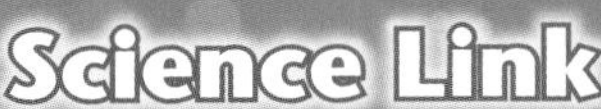

Infant Brain Development

If an infant is not stimulated, or is neglected, brain development is affected. The opportunities for new connections are lost. The baby does not learn as many skills. This can have lifelong effects on a baby's learning potential. This is why it is important to encourage development in babies through activities. For instance, babies like to be touched gently and spoken or sung to softly. Responding to infant babbles and coos is a form of conversation with the child. Infants learn by seeing and touching objects around them. They like to look at brightly colored objects and touch soft, fuzzy toys. They do not like strong smells or tastes.

At this age, babies learn to drink from a cup. They also feed themselves with their fingers. (They have not learned to use flatware yet.) Many times, as much food gets in their mouths as on themselves and the floor. Meals can become very messy.

At one year of age, babies may weigh three times as much as they did at birth. Most babies also grow one and one-half times in length during this first year. This is usually 9 to 10 inches.

One-year-olds seem to be busy all the time. They like to watch objects move. They watch cars, people, animals, and anything else they see. Other children fascinate them. Children of this age like to play and be held. Simple games such as pat-a-cake and peekaboo are enjoyed. One-year-olds like to put blocks in a cup and dump them out. They enjoy music, rhymes, and simple songs. They laugh and throw toys. They like to explore their surroundings.

One-year-olds usually sleep through the night and take morning and afternoon naps. Babies need a lot of rest to grow and develop properly.

During this time, babies may become shy with people outside the family. They may cry at the sight of friends or relatives. This is typical. It is a phase most children go through. It passes in a few months.

Early Brain Development

In recent years, early brain development has become an important topic of research. A person's ability to learn throughout life is tied to how well the brain develops. Parents and others who care for the baby can assist in early brain development. They do this by cuddling, playing with, and talking to the baby in a consistent manner. When these activities occur, messages are sent through the baby's brain. As the messages are sent, connections are made in the brain. These connections cause the baby's brain to become stronger and more active. This makes it possible for the baby to accomplish new skills. The more a baby is stimulated, the more active his or her brain becomes. Then, more and more connections are made.

Sudden Infant Death Syndrome (SIDS)

Sudden Infant Death Syndrome (SIDS) is the sudden, unexpected death of a baby who seems healthy. The true cause of SIDS is unknown. SIDS seems to occur, however, when a baby does not get enough air and stops breathing.

To reduce the risk of SIDS, infants should always sleep on their backs. See **2-9**. If babies sleep on their stomachs, they could press their faces into the mattress. Be sure to keep fluffy blankets or pillows away from infants. If babies place these items over their mouths, they could suffocate. Instead, place infants on a firm mattress with only a sheet or light blanket covering the mattress. No stuffed animals or other items should be in the crib.

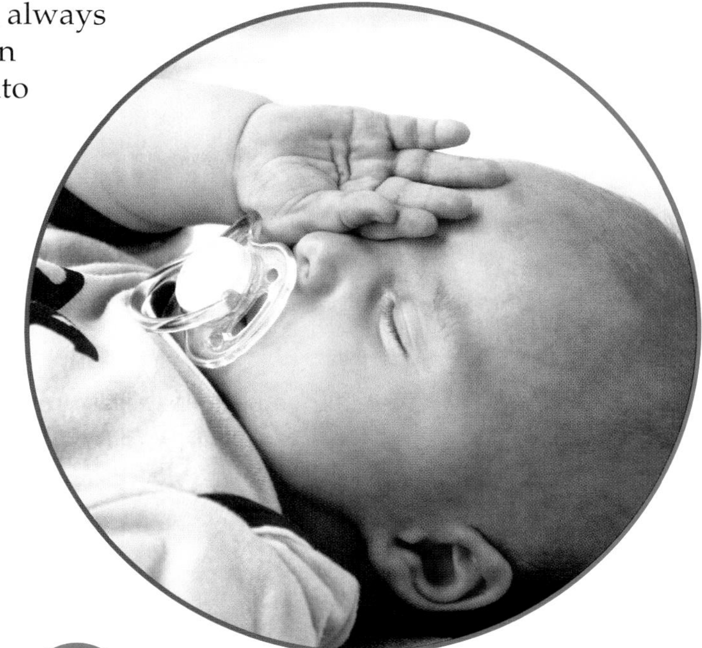

2-9 To reduce the risk of SIDS, babies should sleep on their backs.

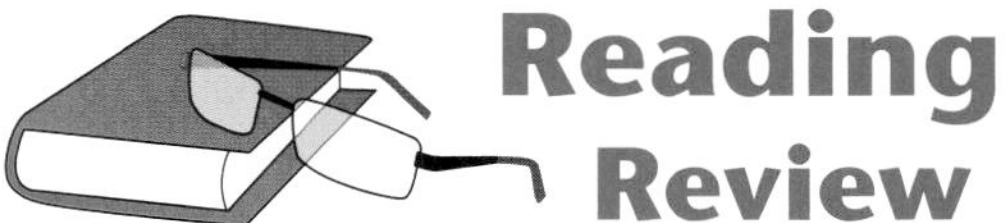

Reading Review

1. Why should you keep objects, such as buttons and safety pins, out of the reach of nine- to twelve-month-olds?
2. At what age do babies start to learn the difference between right and wrong?
3. What activities do one-year-olds enjoy? Give examples.

Section Summary

- To care for children, you must understand how they grow and develop.
- Growth is rapid during the first year of life. Each child grows at a different rate.
- Newborns are dependent on others to meet all their needs.
- As babies grow physically, they can roll over, sit, crawl, stand, and walk. They respond to the environment through smiling, cooing, movement, and play.
- By their first birthday, children often weigh three times as much as they did at birth. They may have grown 10 inches in length.
- One-year-olds are active and require attention to be safe.
- Talking with children in a consistent manner nurtures brain development.
- Childproofing areas to remove potential dangers is necessary to keep children safe.

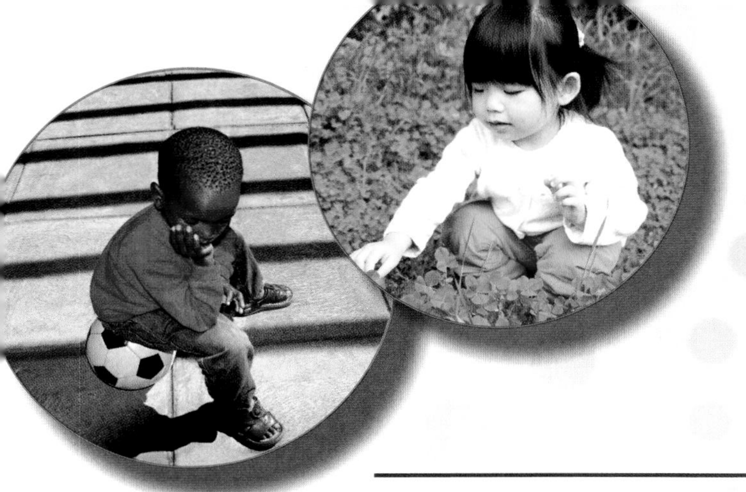

Section 2-3
The Toddler Stage

Objectives

After studying this section, you will be able to
- **define** *toddler*, *parallel play*, and *confident*.
- **describe** how children grow and develop during the toddler stage.
- **explain** how people can help toddlers gain confidence in themselves.

Key Terms

toddler: a child between the ages of one and three years.

parallel play: type of play in which toddlers play near, but not with, one another.

confident: being sure of yourself.

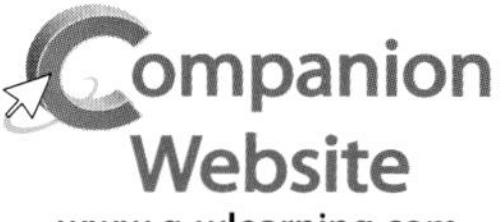

Study the Key Terms by completing crossword puzzles, matching activities, and e-flash cards at the website.

Main Ideas

- Toddlers grow and develop in many ways.
- Toddlers need love and support as they discover and explore the world around them.
- People who care for toddlers should create a safe environment for them.

A **toddler** is a child between the ages of one and three years. Toddlers often learn to walk between the ages of twelve and eighteen months. As they learn to walk, they begin exploring their environments. They start communicating more. They express more emotions and behave in new ways. You can support their freedom to grow and develop. You must also, however, protect them from injuries or harm. Caring for toddlers can be fun, but it is also a responsibility.

Physical Development

Toddlers' physical development is slower than that of infants. They do not gain weight as quickly as infants. Their bodies become longer and straighter. Toddlers often grow about two to three inches, and gain about six pounds per year. Body shape changes to more adult-like proportions, but toddlers still seem top-heavy.

Toddlers are always in motion. They spend a lot of time and energy moving. See **2-10**. This helps their bodies develop and lets them explore. They touch, feel, and taste objects. They may empty toy boxes, drawers, and kitchen cupboards to find objects. They rarely, however, put objects away. They move quickly from one activity to another.

As their muscles develop, toddlers are able to do more for themselves. They learn to use their fingers for tasks, such as using flatware to feed themselves. They place big pegs in pegboards and stack building blocks. Toddlers can turn the pages of books made from heavy paper. They dance to music. Toddlers also like to kick and throw balls. To reach objects they want, toddlers may even move furniture. They are becoming more independent.

As toddlers become more active, you need to reduce the chances for accidents. Remove any items toddlers should not touch. Use caution around pets. Toddlers may grab pets and hurt them. Always watch where toddlers go and what they do. This lets them explore safely and independently.

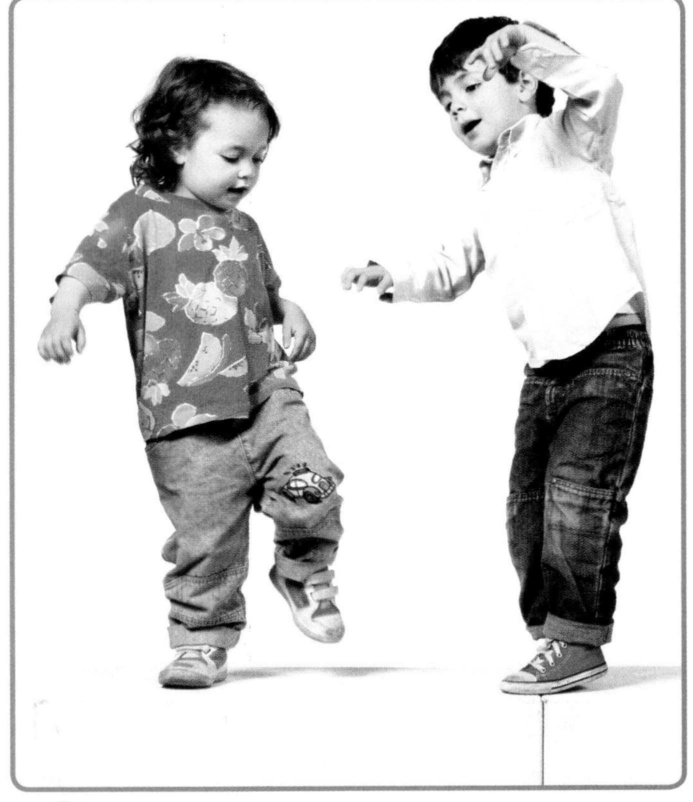

2-10 Toddlers find many ways to move about and play.

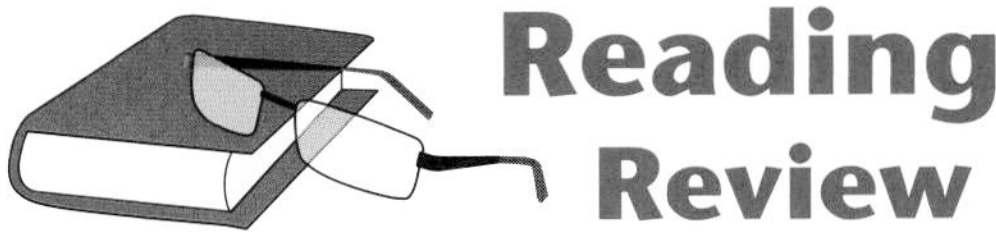

Reading Review

1. Why are toddlers able to do more for themselves than infants?
2. Why do you need to be concerned about the safety of a toddler?

Intellectual Development

Learning language and thought skills are part of the intellectual development of toddlers. As children grow, they develop the abilities to think and reason. They begin to form ideas and use language. Toddlers have experiences daily with people and their surroundings. These experiences help advance their brain development.

Speech begins as toddlers put sounds together. They begin speaking by repeating one-syllable words, such as *da-da* and *ma-ma*. Then they say these words repeatedly. Soon, their vocabularies grow to include names of objects with which they are familiar. They may be able to name parts of their bodies, such as *hand*, *foot*, *nose*, and *ear*. They may begin to tell others what they want, such as *juice*, *cup*, *up*, and *down*.

Remember that toddlers learn new words by listening to others. You should always speak correctly when talking with children. Never use baby talk or profane language.

Toddlers learn they can make their wants and needs known by talking. You may find toddlers easier to care for when they begin to talk. At times, you may still have to guess what children want. Toddlers often confuse the meanings of words. They may also mispronounce words. Being able to walk, however, adds to toddlers' ability to communicate. They can walk to objects they want.

Toddlers also understand what others say to them. They can follow short directions. "Roll the ball" and "Let's go out" are some examples.

Play is also important for toddlers' intellectual development. See **2-11**. Toddlers learn how objects work through play. They place items in a container and then dump them. They can complete simple puzzles. Looking at picture books and imitating songs are other play activities toddlers enjoy.

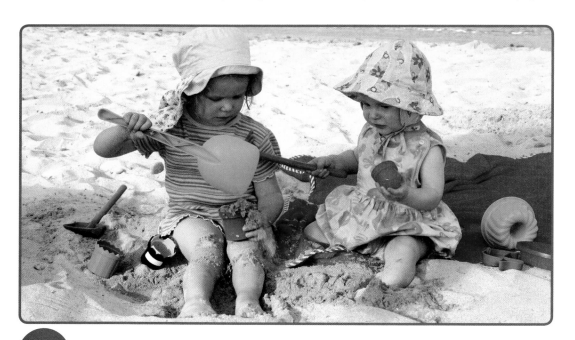

2-11 Hands-on play is important for intellectual development.

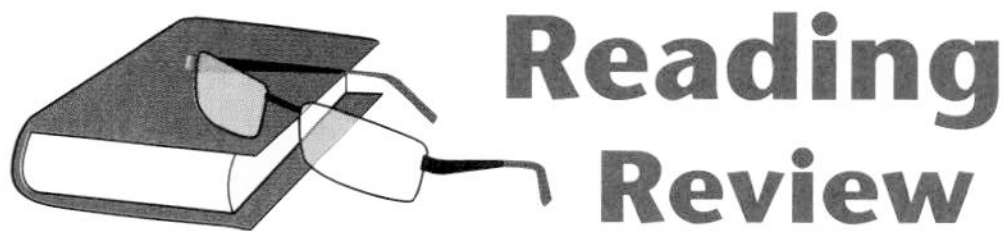

1. Why should you speak correctly when talking with a toddler?
2. Why are toddlers easier to care for when they begin to talk?

Social Development

As toddlers grow, they begin interacting more with others. They become more aware of their environments. They know they have abilities. As a result, they respond to situations differently from the way they did as infants.

Toddlers do not like to hurry. They do not understand the concept of time. They like to perform tasks by themselves, such as dressing and eating. This may take time. Be patient. When toddlers are forced to dress or eat more quickly, they may become discouraged and quit trying. Let toddlers do as much for themselves as possible. This helps them learn to be independent.

Toddlers do not always act the same from day to day. For instance, Chen may fasten all the buttons on his sweater today. Tomorrow, he may not be able to fasten any buttons. Emily may easily feed herself without a lot of mess one day. The next day, she may squeeze her food, mash it with her fingers, or drop it on the floor. Miguel may dress himself each day, then suddenly demand you do it for him. Changes in behavior can be caused by tiredness or desire for attention. This is typical behavior. It is part of the growth process.

The way toddlers play reflects their social development. One-year-olds mainly play by themselves. After two years of age, toddlers enjoy **parallel play**, or playing near other children, but not with them. They also have not learned how to share. They may take what they want from

Succeed in Life

Handling the Toddlers' *No Stage*

When toddlers are going through their *no stage*, they are testing adults. Allowing toddlers choices gives them fewer chances to say *no*. For instance, Ayana needs to wear a sweater. Ask her whether she wants to wear the blue sweater or the red sweater. This gives her a choice. If you ask her whether she wants to wear a sweater, she may say *no*. Then you will still have to convince her to wear a sweater.

Use a pleasant tone of voice when talking with toddlers. Explain the rules and your expectations for acceptable behavior. Keep the rules simple and state them clearly. Explain what will happen when the rules are broken. Repeat this information several times to help toddlers understand what you say and mean. Be consistent and follow through with what you say will happen when rules are broken. This guidance will help toddlers know what to expect.

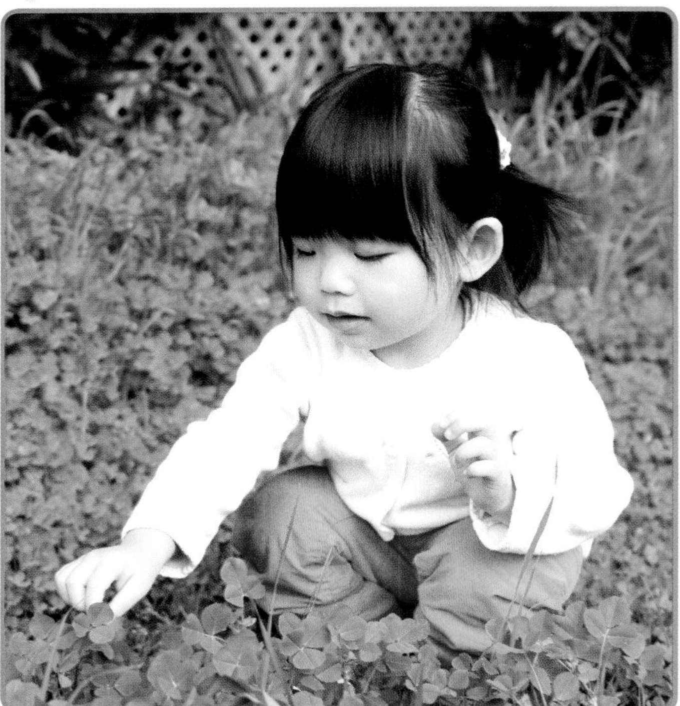

2-12 Toddlers are curious and enjoy exploring their surroundings.

other children. Show toddlers other toys to divert their interest. Explain that toys should be returned to their owners.

Toddlers are curious. They like to inspect toys or books. Toddlers like to taste, throw, and pull apart objects. This type of play helps them explore their surroundings. See **2-12**.

Toddlers often have a hard time choosing a favorite toy. You may need to offer only one or two playthings at a time. Choose toys carefully with children's safety in mind.

Toddlers like books, and they enjoy having others read to them. Another favorite play activity is imitating adults. Toddlers enjoy dressing up in adults' old clothes. They also like to act out adult experiences. They may use props such as toy dishes, cars and trucks, and stuffed animals.

The toddler stage is often called the *no stage*. Toddlers answer *no* to almost everything. They may say *no* because they hear it a lot. They may say *no* because people react when they say it.

Tell toddlers what they can do instead of what they cannot do. This will let toddlers know what you expect from them. For instance, Nathan keeps standing on a chair. You could say, "No, Nathan! Don't stand on the chair." A better response, however, would be, "Nathan, you need to sit when you are on the chair."

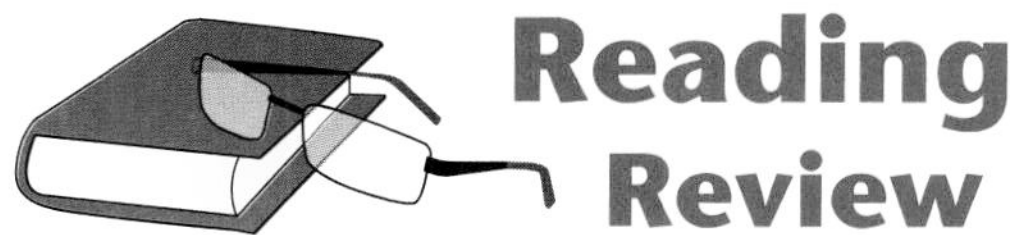

Reading Review

1. What can happen if you encourage toddlers to hurry?
2. What can cause toddlers to act differently from day to day?
3. Describe parallel play. Give two examples of the behavior of toddlers during parallel play.

Emotional Development

Toddlers are still developing emotionally. They easily become excited or upset. They may be excited about doing something new. Sometimes they are frightened. They may be afraid of strange people or places. To feel **confident**, or sure of themselves, they need love and support.

Toddlers can act upset in many ways. For instance, when their parents leave, toddlers may cry, act angry toward their babysitters, or refuse to eat. Often toddlers can be distracted if they are involved in activities they enjoy. This may help them feel less lonely. Separation anxiety is typical in toddlers.

Toddlers can become easily frustrated. They may not be able to perform certain tasks. They may want objects they cannot have. Often toddlers do not know how to act when they feel frustrated. They may become angry. See **2-13**. A temper tantrum may result. They may fall to the floor, kick, and scream. This is the only way they know how to express their feelings.

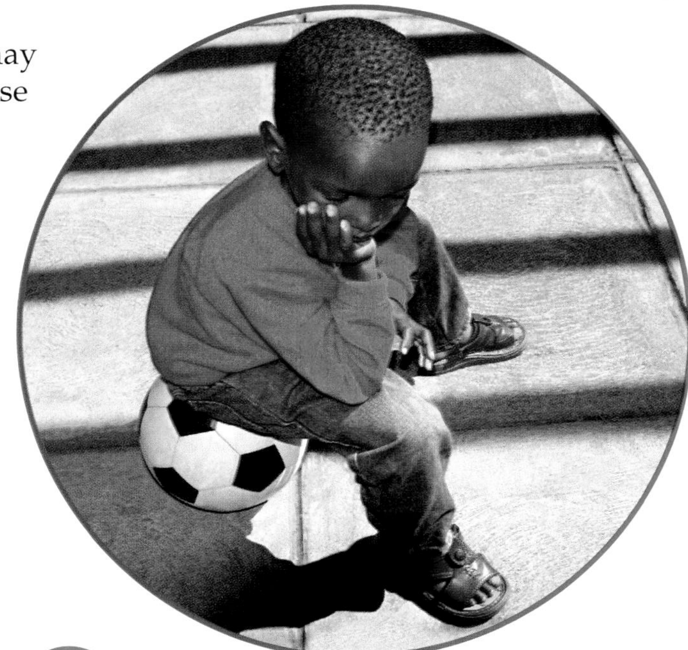

2-13 Toddlers may become difficult when they do not get what they want.

If this happens, treat toddlers calmly and gently. Scolding them does not help. Do not, however, let them hurt themselves or others. Show toddlers good ways to express their anger. Talk with them to help them express what is happening. You might say, "You are angry because Billy took your toy." You may suggest playing with other toys or reading a story.

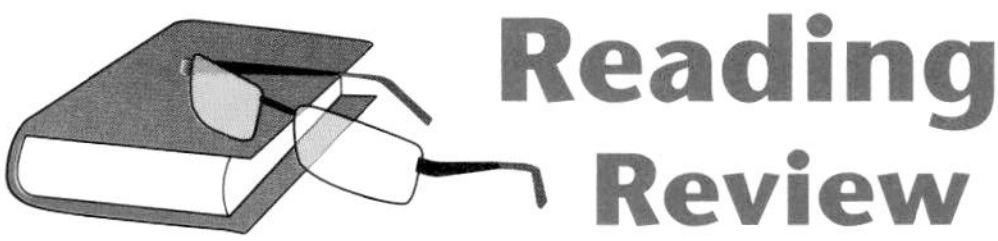

Reading Review

1. What should you do if children start crying after their parents leave?
2. How can you help toddlers express anger without hurting themselves or others?

Section Summary

- The toddler stage is a time of growth and exploration.
- A toddler's world grows as he or she learns to walk. Toddlers can move about and perform more tasks. They become more independent.
- Talking to toddlers helps them to communicate more easily.
- Toddlers' behavior may change from day to day.
- Sometimes, toddlers become frightened. Give them love and support to help them gain confidence in themselves and calm their fears.

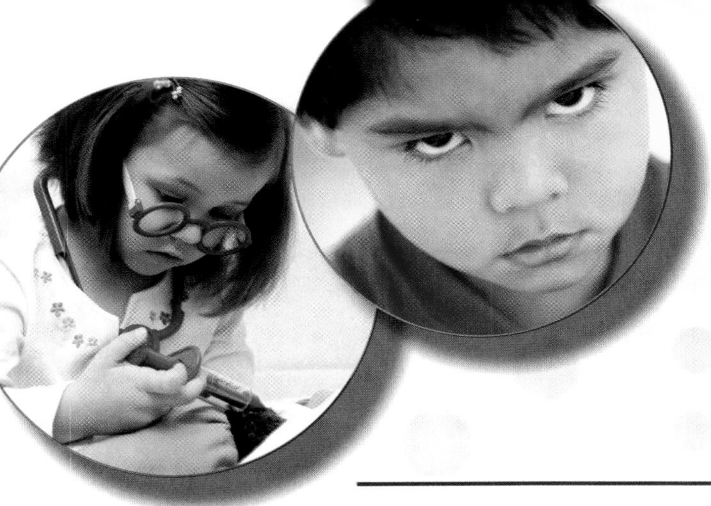

Section 2-4
Preschoolers

Objectives

After studying this section, you will be able to

- **define** *preschooler* and *cooperate*.
- **describe** how preschoolers grow and develop.
- **explain** how people can help preschoolers develop their independence.

Key Terms

preschooler: a child between the ages of three and five years.

cooperate: to act or work together with others.

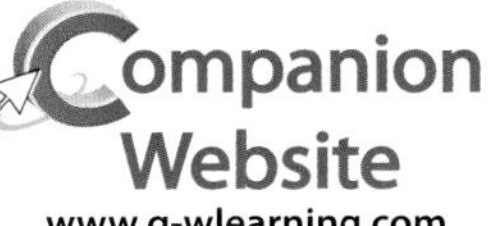

Study the Key Terms by completing crossword puzzles, matching activities, and e-flash cards at the website.

Main Ideas

- Preschoolers continue to grow and develop with the help of other people.
- Preschoolers are more independent than infants and toddlers.
- Preschoolers learn skills that prepare them for going to school.

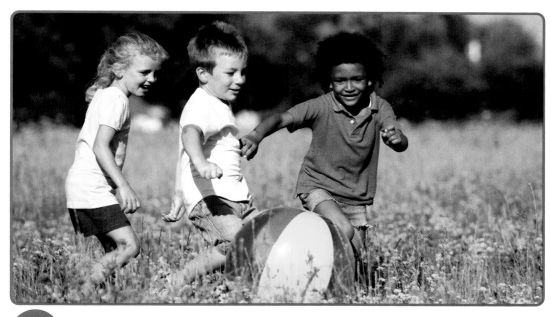

2-14 During the preschooler stage, children grow taller.

Preschoolers are children between the ages of three and five years. During this time, preschoolers are gaining greater independence moving about, talking, playing with others, and expressing emotions. Their bodies grow and develop in many different ways. See **2-14**. They gain greater ability to think, reason, and use language. Preschoolers tend to be more social and agreeable than toddlers. They are better able to express their emotions.

Physical Development

Preschoolers do not grow as fast as infants and toddlers. They gain weight slowly while growing taller. This makes them look slimmer.

The larger muscles of the arms and legs grow stronger during the preschool years. This allows preschoolers to enjoy active play. Preschoolers can climb trees or run up and down sidewalks. They can ride tricycles and use swings. These activities help preschoolers learn to control use of their large muscles.

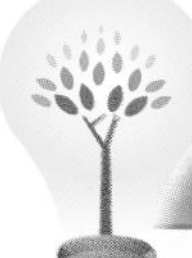

Think Green

Eco-friendly Play Dough

Making homemade play dough is not only a fun activity for young children, but it saves money, contains nothing toxic, and is biodegradable.

Ingredients
1 cup flour
1 cup warm water
½ cup salt
1 tablespoon vegetable oil
2 tablespoons cream of tartar
a few drops of food coloring

Mix all ingredients together, and stir over low heat. The dough will begin to thicken and look like mashed potatoes. Remove the pan from heat when dough pulls away from the sides and clumps. Allow it to cool enough to handle. Knead the dough on waxed paper until smooth and add food coloring. Always wash your hands before working with the dough. Store in airtight container in refrigerator.

After they learn to control their large muscles, preschoolers learn to use and control the smaller muscles of their hands and fingers. These muscles allow them to thread beads on a string and play with pegboards. Doing simple puzzles, cutting with scissors, and drawing with crayons also helps develop small muscle skills.

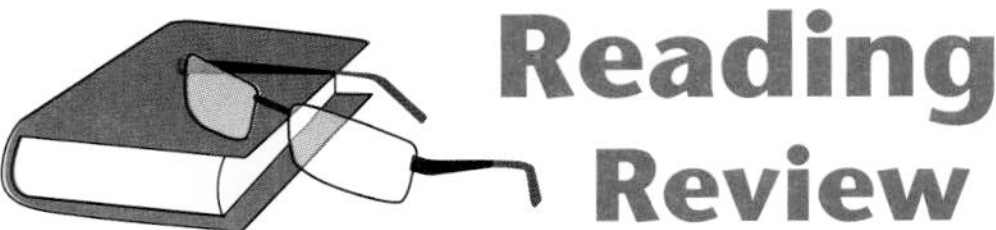

Reading Review

1. Why do preschoolers appear slimmer than toddlers?
2. What activities help preschoolers develop their smaller muscles?

Intellectual Development

Preschoolers have more developed thinking skills than toddlers. Preschoolers learn language and math skills. They learn to count and solve simple problems. Preschoolers can match and sort objects and name colors and shapes. They begin to discover cause and effect. Pretend play is a favorite activity. See **2-15**.

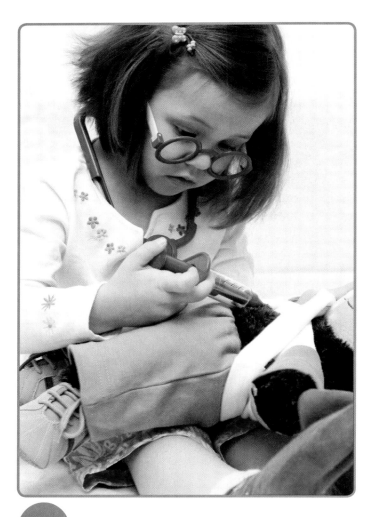

2-15 This preschooler enjoys pretending to be a doctor.

Preschoolers learn new words quickly. They practice by talking a lot. They talk about objects, events, people, and their actions. Preschoolers can answer simple questions and follow directions. They begin to use different parts of speech in their language. At first, you may not be able to understand preschoolers. As they grow, however, they begin to speak more clearly. You can help by speaking clearly to them. Always use proper language around preschoolers.

Some preschoolers have difficulty talking. They may repeat words or parts of words several times. This is often because their minds work faster than their tongues. Children usually outgrow this. You can help by listening patiently to preschoolers. Give them time to finish talking. Do not point out their speech pattern or criticize it. This will not help children correct the way they talk. Act as a model by pronouncing words correctly.

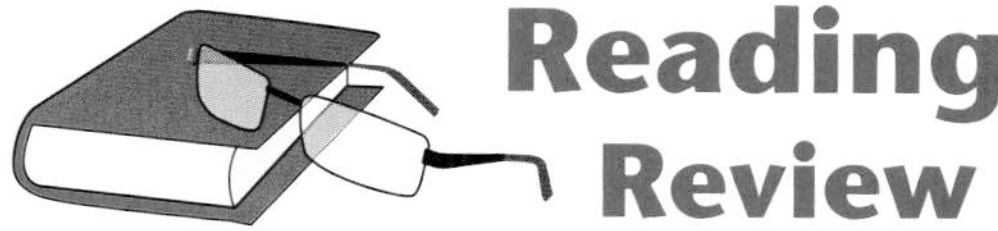

Reading Review

1. Why should you use proper language around preschoolers?
2. How can you help preschoolers who repeat words several times?

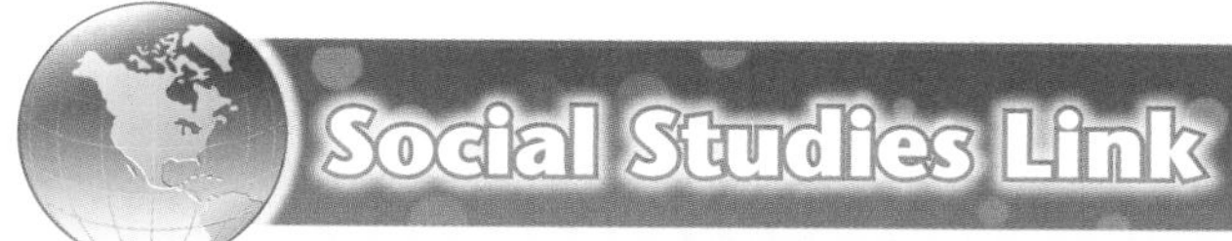

Social Studies Link

Providing Guidance

Children need to know how they are expected to behave. They also need to know what will happen if they do not meet those expectations. For instance, you could say to Liam, "The blocks are for building. If you throw the blocks, you will lose your turn to play with them."

Follow through on warnings you give to children. In the previous example, you must take the toys away from Liam when he throws them. If you do not, he will not learn what will happen as a result of his actions. He will also not learn to believe what you say.

Social Development

Preschoolers are more independent than toddlers. They still, however, need love and support. As preschoolers learn new skills, praise them. This helps them gain confidence in themselves and their actions.

Preschoolers like to perform tasks by themselves. "I want to do it" is a common request. They want to dress and feed themselves. They want to help adults. They may ask to help set the table, feed the dog, or empty the garbage. Preschoolers should be allowed to help with tasks. This is how they learn to perform bigger tasks and develop independence.

Often, it is hard for preschoolers to switch from one task to another. For instance, Nilay does not like to stop playing when it is time for a bath. He agrees, however, after a while. Soon he is having fun playing in the water. Then, he refuses to get out of the tub because he is enjoying his bath. Be patient when caring for preschoolers. They are still learning.

Preschoolers do not say *no* as often as toddlers. They sometimes have difficulty, however, making up their minds. Help them by using simple directions. When you ask Kaya if she wants to go to the store, she may quickly decide. Other times, she may take a long time to decide. If this happens, tell her, "Let's go to the store." Be sure to still let preschoolers make decisions when they do not affect other people.

When you correct children's behaviors, they may become upset. If this happens, try removing them from the activity. Watch them until they are calm. Do not yell. This will only upset the children more. Try to remain patient and calm.

Preschoolers play and share with other children. They learn to **cooperate**, or act or work together with others. Sometimes, they may fight. They often, however, make up quickly. They may need help learning how to be a friend. Set positive examples for them. Let them know how they should or should not act.

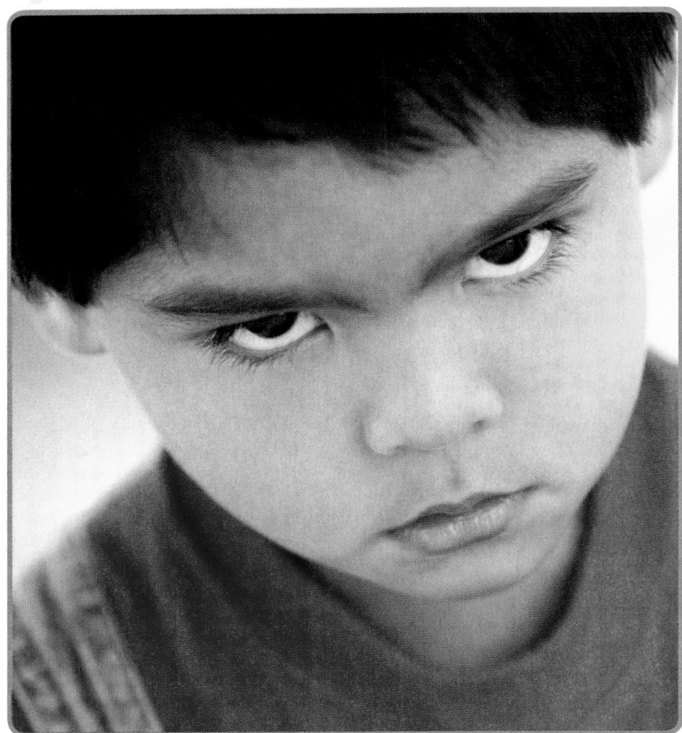

2-16 Guidance can help prevent preschoolers from hurting themselves or others.

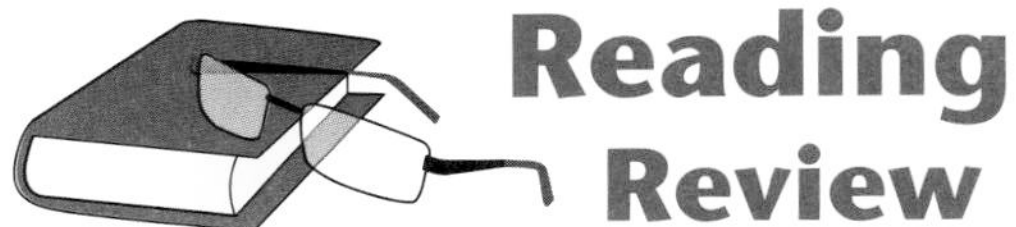

1. How can praise help preschoolers become more independent?
2. When should you let preschoolers make decisions?
3. Why should you always follow through on warnings you give children?

Emotional Development

As preschoolers grow, they learn how to better express their emotions. They still, however, need people to guide and support them. Tell and show preschoolers how you expect them to express themselves. Make them feel loved and wanted. This helps them develop positive self-concepts.

Preschoolers' moods may change quickly. See **2-16**. One minute, they may be playing happily. The next, they may start throwing toys or hitting people. Tell them right away this is wrong. Explain to them what they can and cannot do. You may say, "Blocks are for stacking. You do not throw them." Tell them, "You must not hit people. It hurts." You may want to give them a pillow to hit or a foam ball to throw. This way, they cannot hurt anyone or break anything.

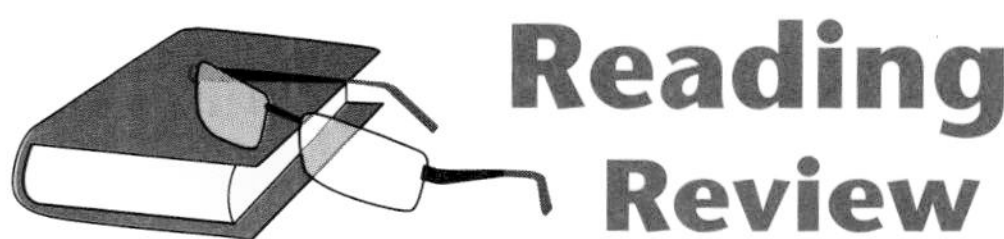

1. What helps preschoolers develop positive self-concepts? Give examples.
2. What should you do when preschoolers' moods change?

Section Summary

- The preschool years extend from age three to five years.
- Preschool children learn many new physical, intellectual, social, and emotional skills. This helps them develop their independence.
- Preschoolers need a lot of love and support during this time.

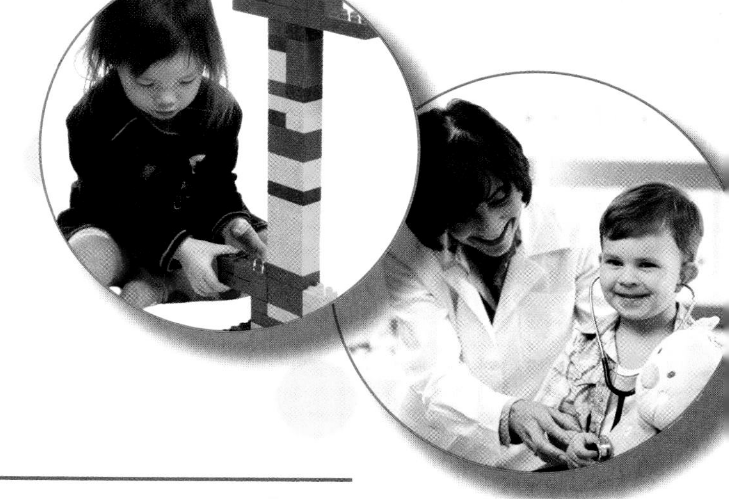

Section 2-5
How Children Learn

Objectives

After studying this section, you will be able to
- **define** *learning* and *time-out*.
- **give examples** of activities that help infants learn.
- **explain** how toddlers and preschoolers learn.
- **describe** how communicating with children helps them learn.

Key Terms

learning: gaining information or skills through engaging in play that provides hands-on materials.

time-out: a guidance technique in which a caregiver instructs a child to move away from others to a place where he or she must sit quietly.

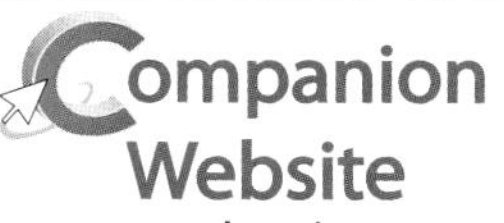

Study the Key Terms by completing crossword puzzles, matching activities, and e-flash cards at the website.

Main Ideas

- Children need learning experiences.
- Communication between children and adults helps children learn.
- Children can learn how to behave in ways acceptable to themselves and others.

Children learn an almost endless amount of information during their first five years of life. **Learning** is gaining information or skills through engaging in play that provides hands-on materials. Learning through play is important, especially during the early years. Children learn by exploring the world around them. All children need praise and encouragement to learn.

Infants

Infants learn by using their senses. They learn when they touch, see, hear, smell, and taste. For instance, Aria's parents have given her a rattle as her first toy. Aria grasps the rattle and learns what it feels like. She learns what it tastes like as she puts it in her mouth. When she shakes it, she learns what it sounds like.

Playing helps infants learn new concepts. They can also learn how to control their bodies. Peekaboo teaches them that objects or people can disappear and return. Waving good-bye and playing pat-a-cake helps them control their hands and arms.

Infants learn to speak by making sounds. Let them know you enjoy the sounds they make. This encourages them to make more sounds. You can also help infants learn to speak by talking to them. They imitate how people talk. The more words they hear people use, the more they learn. They can also learn that people express their thoughts and feelings by using words. See **2-17**.

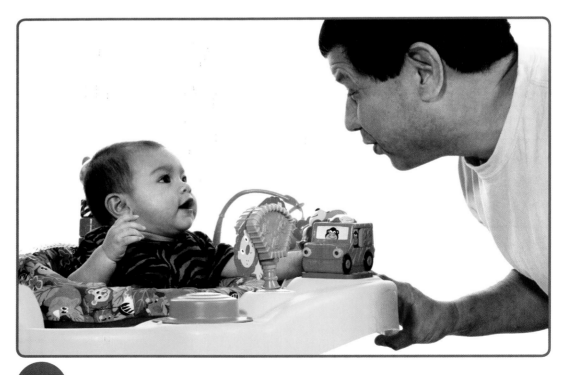

2-17 Encouraging infants to make sounds helps them learn about speech.

Infants need love and attention in order to learn. As people around infants love and care for them, the infants respond by wanting to learn more. For instance, Mark's parents hold him close and talk to him. They stroke his cheek and rub his body. They feed and bathe him. As a result, Mark feels loved and secure. He feels free to learn by exploring the world around him.

As adults hold, feed, bathe, and play with infants, they communicate emotions. For instance, when an adult is nervous about holding a baby, the infant can sense the adult's fear. The infant may respond by crying more than usual. On the other hand, when an adult holds a baby securely, the baby senses love. This helps the infant develop trust in the adult.

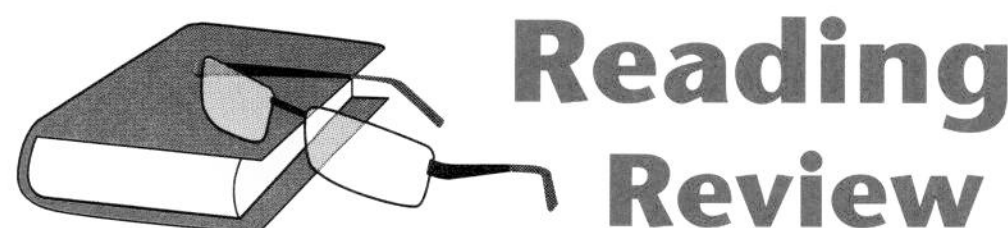

Reading Review

1. How can infants learn through play? Give examples.
2. How can talking to infants help them learn to speak?

Toddlers and Preschoolers

As toddlers and preschoolers learn new skills, their behavior may swing from independence to dependence. Amir may try jumping from a step, but hold on to his father's hand. Madison may run after a pigeon in the park. Then she may return suddenly and want a hug from her mother. Understanding the growth and development of children can help you be sensitive to these swings of behavior.

When you help children learn, they enjoy childhood more. This also makes it easier for them to learn when they start school. Give toddlers and preschoolers the chance to explore their surroundings and try new tasks. Let them see and talk about new events and objects. Let them feel objects that are safe to touch. See **2-18**.

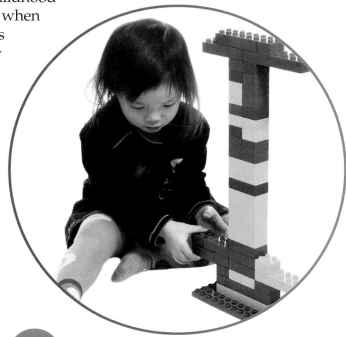

2-18 Children are often fascinated by objects like building blocks.

Young children learn many skills and concepts. They learn how to count. They can identify shapes and colors. They learn how words and sounds are used. Children learn skills and concepts best when they are allowed to play.

Children can learn about numbers through many daily activities. You can play counting games with children, such as counting toes, fingers, or blocks and other toys. You can use numbers when talking. You may hold an apple and say, "Here is one apple." You may offer crackers and say, "You may have two crackers." Let

Children's Books

Reading to children can help them learn how words and sounds are used. Nursery rhymes help them learn about sounds and rhythms. Identifying pictures in books helps them learn the meaning of words. They can also learn to match words with real objects. For instance, they learn from a picture book what an orange looks like. When you ask them to choose an orange from a fruit bowl, they can identify which piece of fruit to choose. Visit your local library and select a book you think would interest children the most. Arrange to read the book to a local preschool class.

the children count and decide how many to choose. Letting children use measuring cups or spoons to prepare simple recipes can also help them learn number skills.

You can help children learn about concepts such as size, shape, and texture. Use descriptive terms when talking with children about objects they see and use daily. You might say, "That building is tall," "Your cookie is round," or "Sandpaper is rough."

You can also help children learn about colors. Talk about the red sweater, the blue ball, the yellow sun, and the green grass. Show children these objects as you talk about them.

Learning to care for themselves is another skill children need to learn. For instance, they should learn how to dress themselves and decide what colors to wear. This may not be easy for them at first. They may need your help. Children may have to practice these tasks many times. Be patient. When children succeed, they feel good about themselves.

Children like to help adults. For them, learning to pour milk and sweep floors are often fun tasks, not work. Adults and children can have fun together doing laundry or setting the table. Children can also have fun and learn by caring for plants or pets. Doing household tasks helps children learn responsibility. If children enjoy doing these tasks, their positive feelings toward work later in life may be greater.

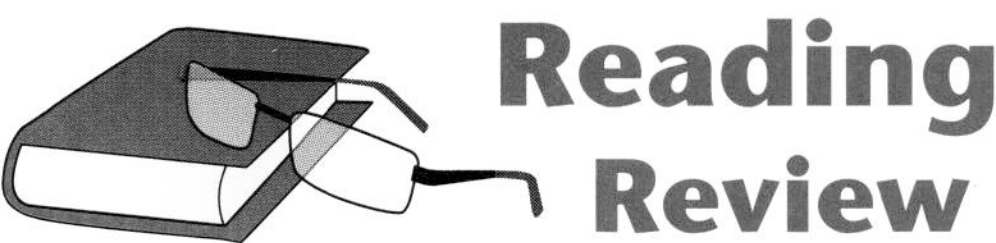

Reading Review

1. How can you help children learn about concepts such as size, shape, and texture?
2. How can reading to young children help them learn?
3. Why may children need your help learning to care for themselves?

Communicating with Children

When you talk to children, speak correctly. In order for them to learn to use the correct words to describe objects, you must set an example. This will help them when they start school. If you use incorrect words to describe objects, children will also use the incorrect words. When they start school, they will have to learn to use the correct words. This can cause children to become discouraged.

Children need to feel you care for and understand them as they are learning. They like to receive praise when they learn to behave correctly or perform tasks for themselves. See **2-19**. For instance, when children tie their shoelaces for the first time, praise them. Say, "You tied your shoelaces correctly!" Smile and encourage them to do it again. Such rewards are important for children as they are learning.

When you care for children, encourage them to try new tasks. Show interest in what they do. This encourages them to keep learning and trying. When children make mistakes or do not succeed, they become discouraged. Do not criticize them. This does not help them learn. When they are discouraged, they need patience and understanding. They need to know you love and accept them. Be an active listener when they share their feelings.

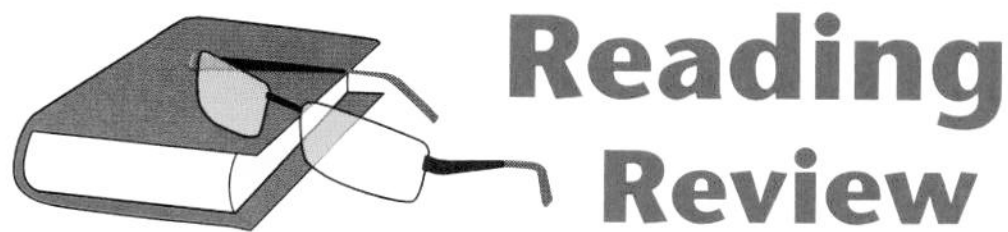

Reading Review

1. Why do you need to speak correctly to children?
2. How can you let children know you care for and understand them?

Behavior

Children need to act in ways that are acceptable to themselves and others. They need to learn right from wrong. They need to know how to behave in different situations. See **2-20**. Acceptable behavior helps children get along with others. It gives them confidence.

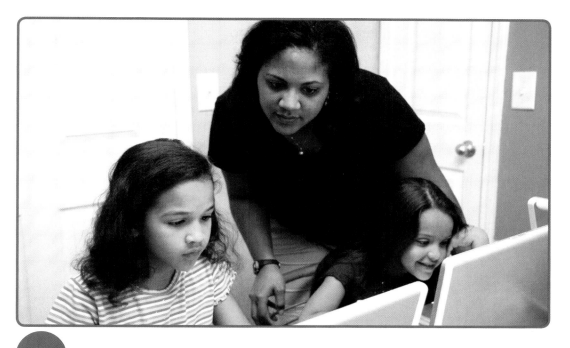

2-19 Children should receive a lot of encouragement when learning new tasks.

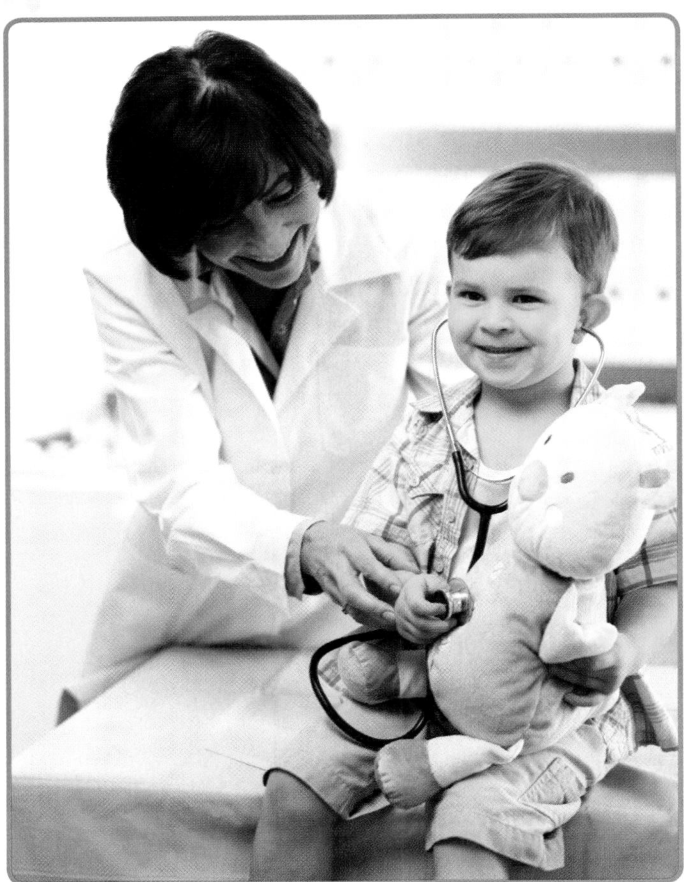

2-20 Children can learn how to behave during physical exams.

Telling children what they can do is a positive way to teach acceptable behavior. This lets children learn what they can do instead of what they cannot do. This also lets them decide how they want to behave. Children need encouragement. Too many no's and not enough praise may make them afraid to try new tasks.

Sometimes, you need to say *no* to children. They may be doing something that is harmful or unacceptable to others. If you show them how to behave correctly and praise them, they will learn acceptable behavior. Also, when children learn that some types of behavior are unacceptable, they can say *no* to other people. This can help them avoid being taken advantage of or hurt.

Sometimes, caregivers may use a time-out to help correct a child's conduct. In a **time-out**, a caregiver instructs the child to move away from others to a place where he or she must sit quietly. Let children know what behaviors will result in time-out. Also, explain the length of the time-out. The length of time should be reasonable, such as one minute per year of age. When you find a child misbehaving, say firmly, "time-out." Then move the child to a place to sit quietly for the brief time you have stated.

Every child should know what behavior you expect. During the time-out, explain to the child why you are not happy with his or her conduct. Be positive and patient. For instance, you may say, "When I see you hitting John, I am unhappy because you are hurting him." Time alone gives the child a chance to calm down and reflect on his or her behavior. If the child does not sit quietly, restart the time. You must make sure the child obeys the time-out rules. Otherwise, the child will not take you seriously.

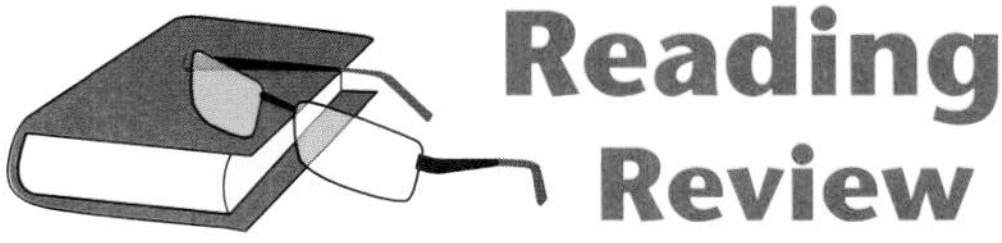

Reading Review

1. Why should you tell children what they could do instead of what they cannot do?
2. How can you help children learn acceptable behavior?
3. How do you use a time-out? Why do some people feel it is effective?

Section Summary

- Learning during the first five years helps children grow and change.
- Children learn by using their senses. They also learn by playing.
- Communicating with children helps them learn.
- Praise children and encourage them to try new tasks. This helps children learn acceptable behavior.
- Children learn acceptable behavior by being told what to do, rather than what *not* to do.
- Time-out is a technique used to help correct a child's conduct.

Chapter Summary

Learning about children can help you when you babysit. You will know how to keep children safe and happy. You will also be able to help them grow and develop. During the first five years of their lives, children grow and develop in different ways and at different rates. At birth, they are dependent on others to take care of all their needs. By the time they reach five years of age, children are ready to attend school all day on their own.

Each year, children become more independent and learn new skills. They learn by using their senses and playing. They also learn from other children, teens, and adults.

During this time, children need a lot of love and support so they gain confidence. Communicating with children helps them learn. Praise them and encourage them to try new tasks. This helps children learn acceptable behavior. Time-outs can be used as a guidance technique to help correct a child's conduct.

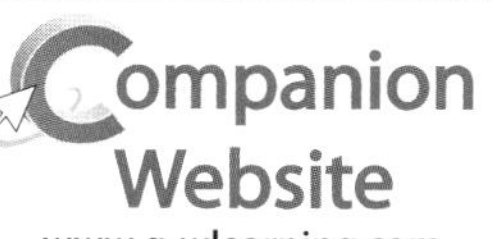

Review Key Terms and Main Ideas for Chapter 2 at the website.

Chapter Review

Write your answers on a separate sheet of paper.

1. What are three ways you can prepare to babysit a child for the first time?
2. How can you help a gifted child when you are babysitting?
3. Use + to identify the traits that describe infants at birth. Use – to identify the traits that do not describe infants at birth.
   A. Is completely dependent.
   B. Has strong muscles.
   C. Needs support for head.
   D. Can control actions.
   E. Uses reflex movements.
4. How do babies communicate their needs?
5. What do toddlers need to feel confident?
6. What are two reasons toddlers may say *no* a lot?
7. List three ways you can calm preschoolers who become upset when you correct their behavior.
8. How do infants learn to speak?
9. Give an example of how you can help a child learn about numbers.
10. What should you do if a child does not sit quietly during a time-out?

Life Skills

11. You will be working as a babysitter three mornings a week during the summer months. Maria is four years old. Her mother has a home office and needs the time to take care of her real estate business. When you met with Maria's mother, she asked you to plan activities that would promote a preschool child's development. Create a list of activities you could do with Maria to aid in her physical, intellectual, emotional, and social growth and development. Present your ideas to the class.

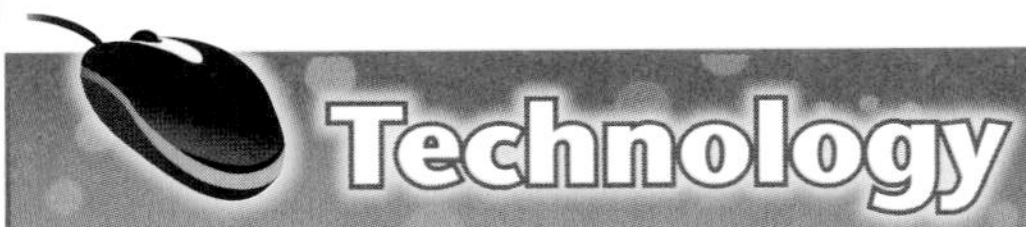

Technology

12. Visit the website for the American Association of Poison Control Centers, www.aapcc.org, to locate the Poison Control Center in your area. Find the telephone number and list the tips to protect children from poisons in the home.
13. Research the Internet for information about infant brain development. Enter the key words *infant brain development* to begin your search. Record the websites you found most helpful. Write a short report about your findings to share with the class.

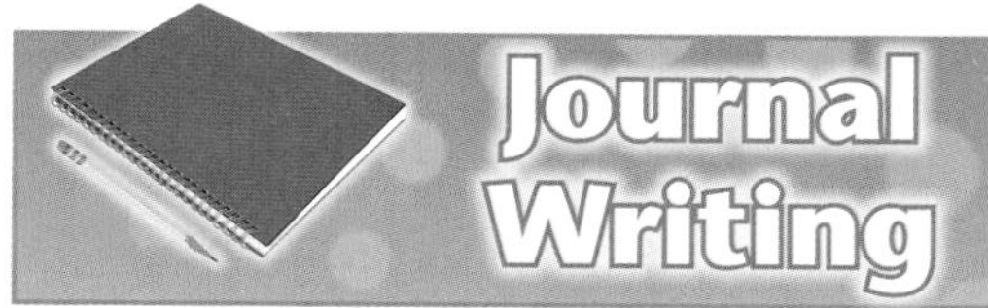

14. Interview your parents about some of the unusual or interesting things you did as an infant, toddler, and preschooler. What are your earliest memories? Are they positive ones? Start a section of your journal about your experiences and feelings during that time of your life. This may help you relate to babies and young children you babysit.

Academics

15. **Writing.** Write a short story about a situation between a toddler and a babysitter in which the toddler keeps saying *no*. Explain in your story how the babysitter deals with this situation.
16. **Science.** Choose a developmental task you would like to help preschoolers learn. Select several games designed to teach this task. Give a demonstration to the class showing how you would use these games to help teach the child the task.
17. **Speech.** Observe a group of preschoolers. Take notes on how they practice saying new words. Notice the similarities and differences in how their language skills develop. Discuss your findings with the class.
18. **Social Studies.** Plan a *dramatic play corner* for a toddler. List the play items and dress-up clothes you would choose for the child to use for different activities. Make notes about precautions you should take to keep the child safe during dramatic play.

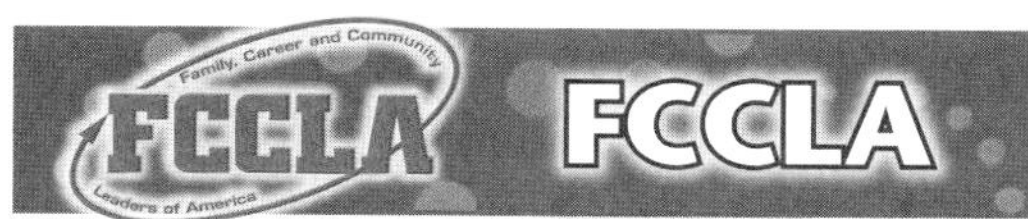

19. Many families have a hard time balancing the need to work with the costs of good childcare. Think about the childcare needs in your community, especially for families with babies and young children. Brainstorm to find some lower-cost options for families who must use childcare, but cannot afford the traditional higher-cost care centers. This activity can be done in a small group. Develop an FCCLA *Focus on Children* project for the *STAR Events* competition based on your ideas. Obtain further information about this program from your FCCLA advisor.

Unit 2

You—A Manager

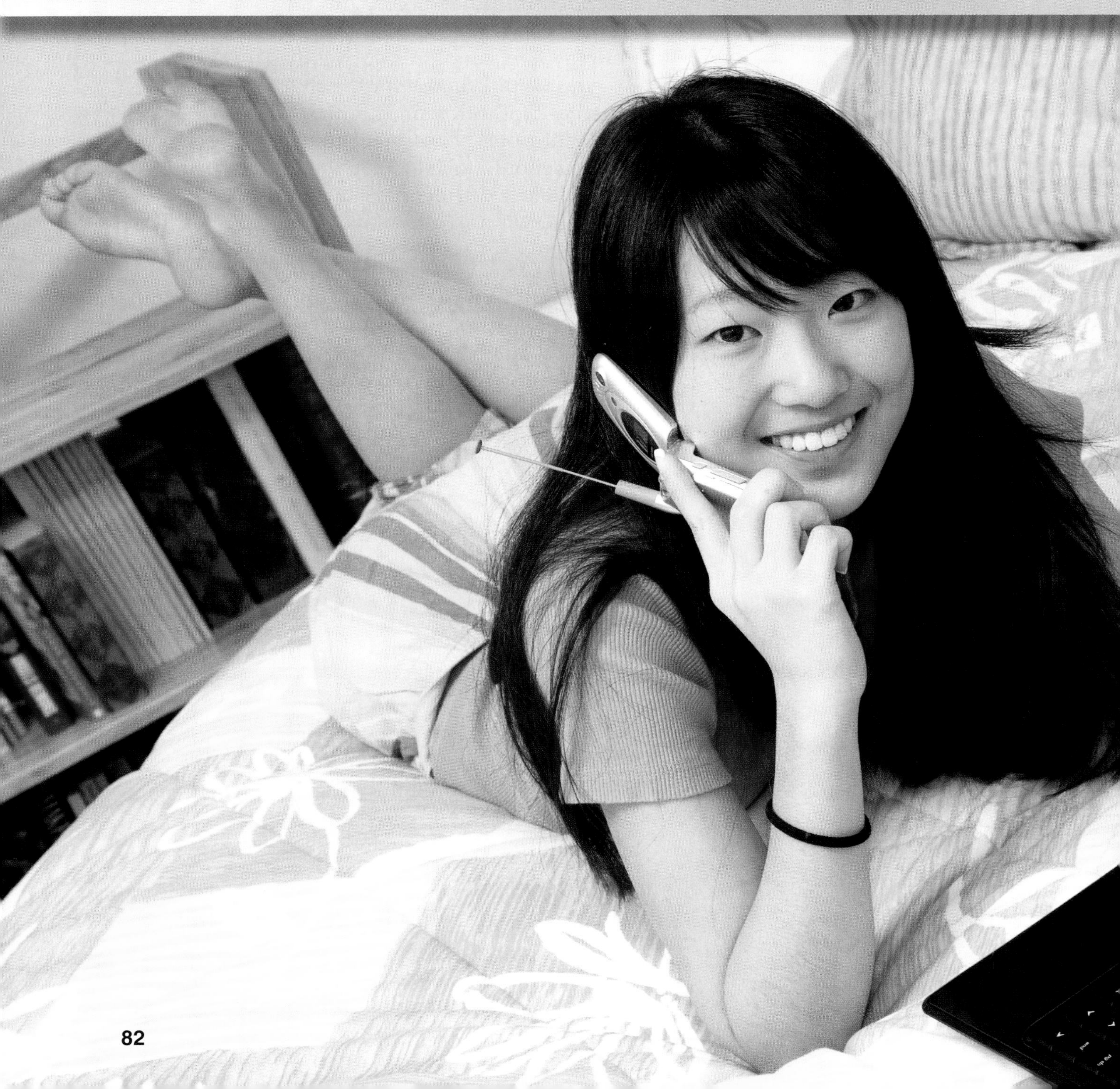

Chapter 3	Making Decisions
Chapter 4	Managing Daily Living
Chapter 5	Managing Your Living Space
Chapter 6	Managing Your Environment

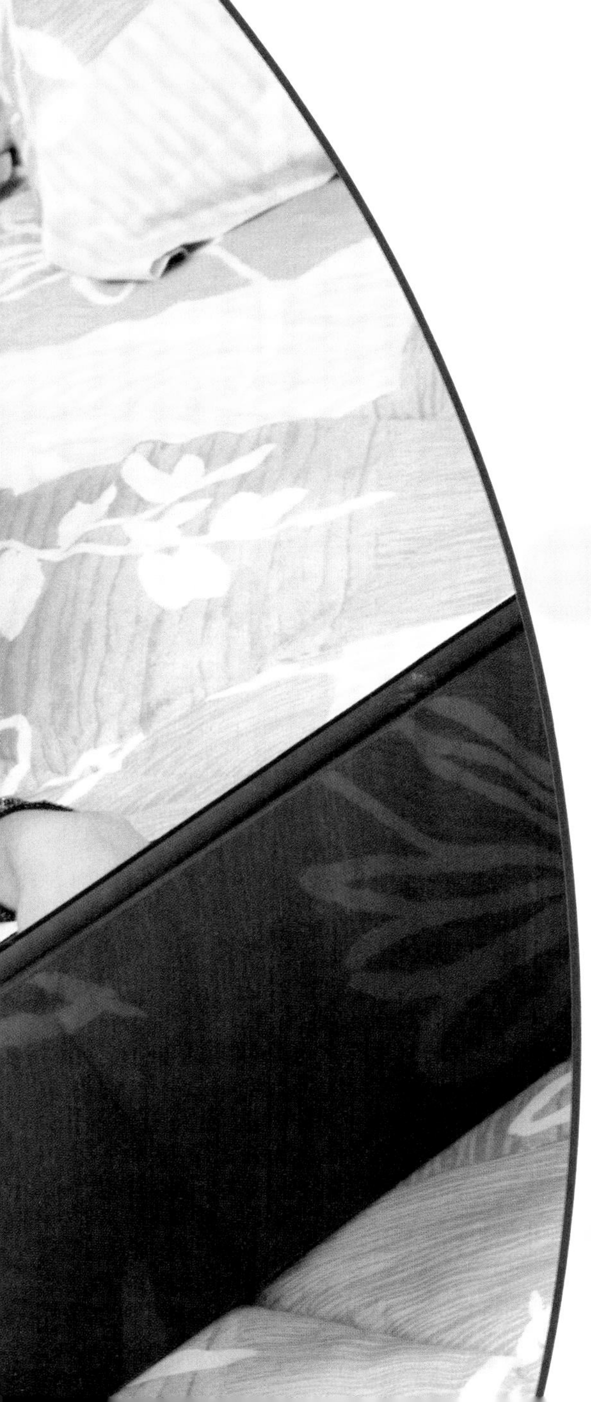

Exploring Careers

The following careers relate to the information you will study in Unit 2. Read the descriptions and then complete the activity to learn more about the careers that might interest you.

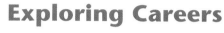

Career	Description
Customer service representative	Works to maintain a good relationship between a business and its customers
Interior designer	Plans and designs interior spaces for every type of building and residence
Personal trainer	Works with clients to attain and/or maintain physical fitness
Environmental engineer	Develops solutions to environmental problems
Financial planner	Advises clients about investments and helps them to manage their assets
Real estate agent	Guides clients through the buying and selling of real estate property
Quality-control inspector	Monitors quality standards for various manufactured products
Administrative assistant	Helps an office run smoothly through performing and coordinating clerical activities

Activity: Pick three careers you find interesting. Conduct online research to find the salary ranges of people just starting in those careers. In which industries might each career be found?

Chapter 3
Making Decisions

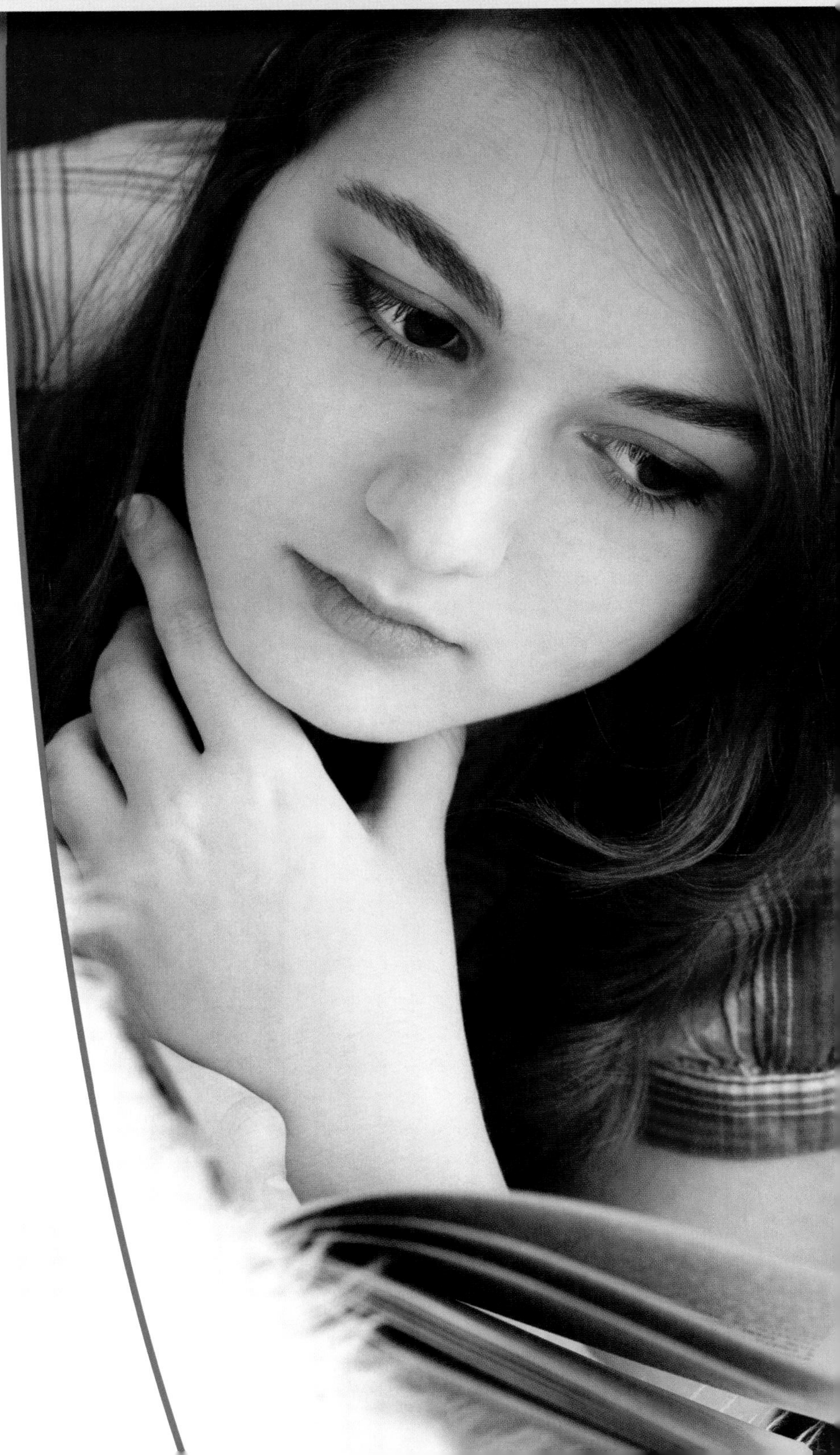

Sections

3-1 Your Needs and Wants
3-2 Your Resources
3-3 Your Values and Goals
3-4 Your Decisions
3-5 Making a Difference in Your Community

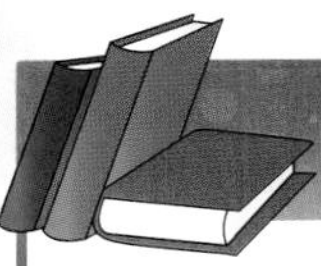

Sharpen Your Reading

After reading each section (separated by main headings) write a three- to four-sentence summary of what you just read. Be sure to paraphrase and use your own words.

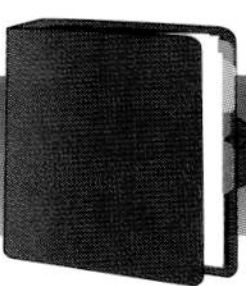

Concept Organizer

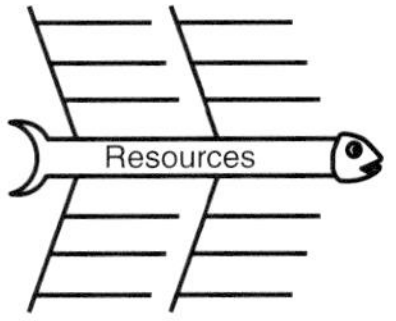

Use a fishbone diagram like the one shown to list the four ways resources can be grouped. List two resources found in each of the four groups. Which of those resources do you have direct control over?

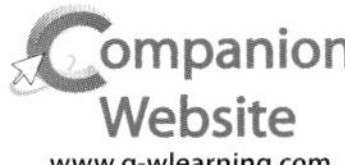

Print out the concept organizer at the website.

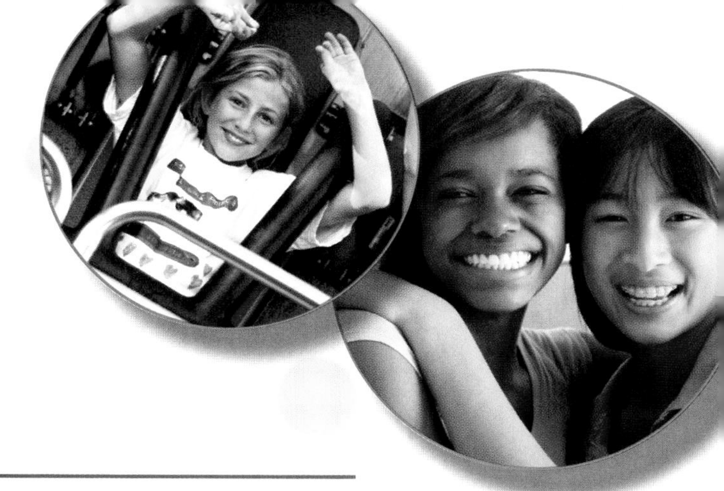

Section 3-1
Your Needs and Wants

Objectives

After studying this section, you will be able to
- **define** *needs* and *wants.*
- **list** basic physical and emotional needs.
- **explain** how wants are different from needs.

Key Terms

needs: the basic items you must have to live.

wants: the extra items you would like to have, but are not necessary to live.

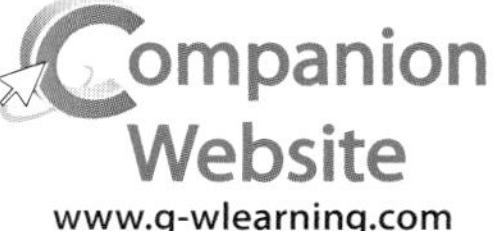

Study the Key Terms by completing crossword puzzles, matching activities, and e-flash cards at the website.

Main Ideas

- You have basic physical and emotional needs.
- Wants can make your life more satisfying.

Your needs and wants affect your life. **Needs** are the basic items you must have to live. **Wants** are the extra items you would like to have, but are not necessary to live. Needs and wants affect how you use your time, skills, and talents. They affect your feelings. They even affect how you get along with others.

Physical Needs

Abraham Maslow, a famous psychologist, developed a theory of human needs. He believed that each person has the same basic *physical needs*. These needs include food, clothing, and shelter. Maslow also believed that people must first meet their physical needs before they fulfill any other needs and wants. See **3-1**.

Most adults are able to meet their own basic physical needs. They earn money to pay for food, clothes, and shelter. Other people, such as babies and children, or those who are sick, must depend on others to help them meet their needs. People who are victims of disasters, such as floods and tornadoes, also depend on others for help. They need to have clean food and water, dry clothes, and safe places to sleep.

Helping those who are not able to meet their basic physical needs is everyone's responsibility. For instance, giving canned goods to a food bank will help people provide meals for their families. Donating money to a charity can help others meet their basic needs. Volunteering your time is a way you can help people without spending any money.

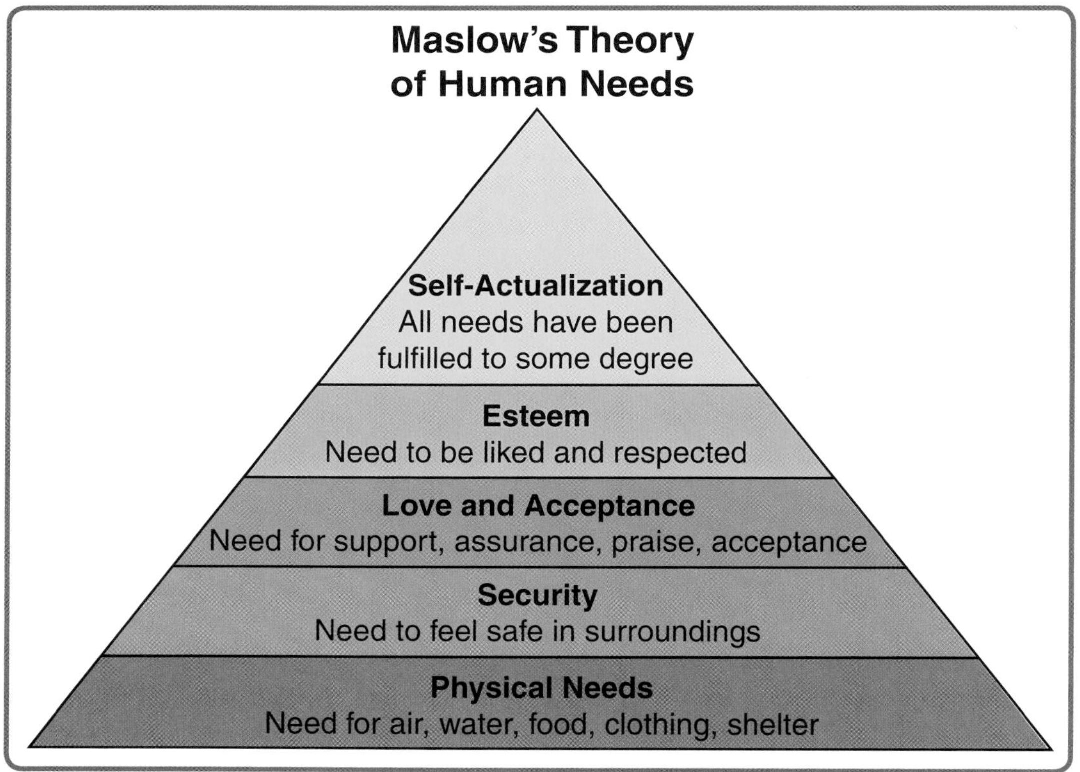

3-1 According to Abraham Maslow, you must meet your basic needs before you can fulfill other needs.

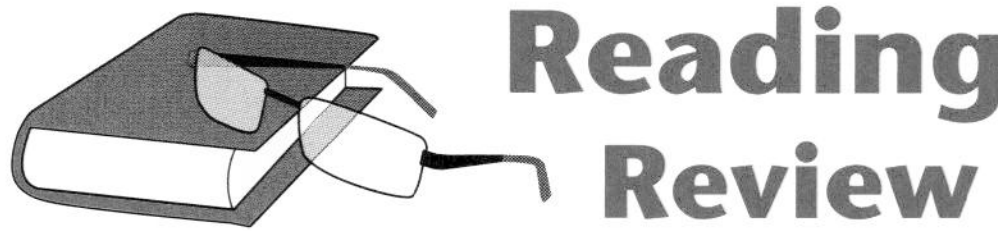

1. Why must people first meet their basic physical needs?
2. How can you help other people meet their basic physical needs?

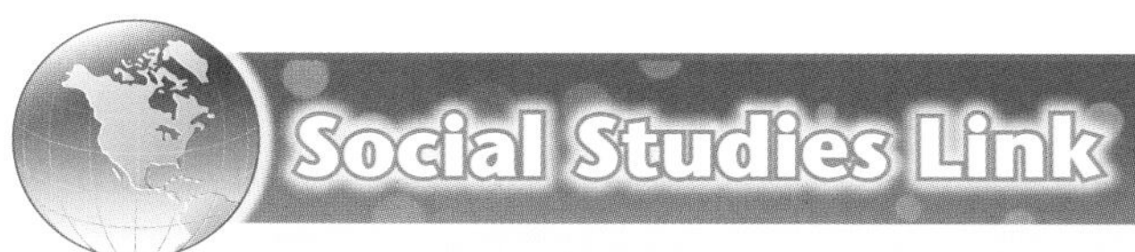

Meeting Emotional Needs

There are both healthful and unhealthful ways to meet basic emotional needs. Healthful ways allow you to meet your needs without preventing you from meeting other needs. Unhealthful ways may allow you to meet one need, but prevent you from meeting another need. For instance, being president of an after-school club is a healthful way to gain recognition and help others. On the other hand, if you gossip to gain recognition, you may lose friends in the process. This would be an unhealthful way to meet your need for recognition. Think about healthful ways in which you can meet your emotional needs for love and acceptance.

Emotional Needs

In addition to physical needs, people have basic *emotional needs*. According to Maslow's theory, these emotional needs include feeling secure and safe and being liked by others. Gaining recognition, feeling good about yourself, and reaching your potential are also emotional needs. Others believe that having new experiences is an important emotional need.

Everyone needs to feel safe from harm. They need to feel secure in their daily routines. Knowing their belongings are safe can also make people feel secure. When individuals feel secure, they are often more relaxed and happy.

People need to feel that others like them and want to spend time with them. To meet this need, people will often develop and maintain friendships. See **3-2**.

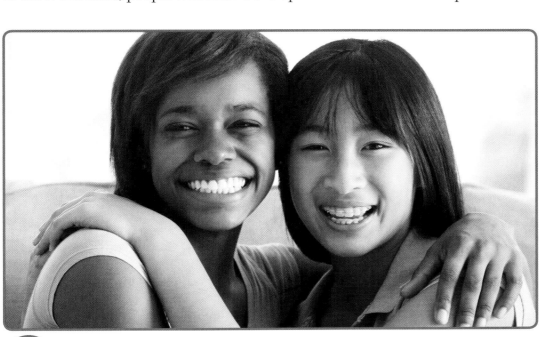

3-2 Being friends with someone can help meet your emotional need to be liked by others.

Some teens may join a dance group or a book club to meet new people. Feeling love and acceptance from others often helps people feel more secure in their relationships.

Individuals also need others to notice them and to make them feel special. You may like to have others pay special attention to you. Some people may gain recognition by trying to excel in certain areas, such as sports, academics, or the arts. They want to earn the respect of others. Receiving praise and support from others can also make people feel more special.

If you are like most people, you enjoy some changes in your life. You have an emotional need to have different experiences. These experiences can be fun and help you learn more about the world around you. Joining a volunteer program or a youth group are just a few examples of ways to try different experiences.

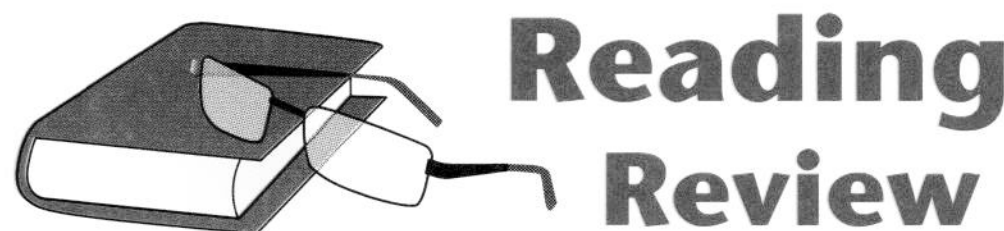

Reading Review

1. How do you meet your need for recognition?
2. How do you meet your need for new experiences?

Wants

Wants are different from basic needs. Basic needs are limited. Wants, however, can be unlimited. Most people are not able to fulfill all their wants.

When you fulfill your wants, your life may be more satisfying. For instance, you may want a musical instrument so you can join a band. You

Succeed in Life

Needs versus Wants

How are needs different from wants? Foods are one example of the difference between needs and wants. People can meet their basic need for food with a few low-cost, healthful items. For many people, however, these foods may not fulfill their wants. Some may want a variety of foods they enjoy eating. Others may want to try different foods away from their homes.

Clothes are another example of the difference between needs and wants. People can often fulfill their basic need for clothing by having a few simple items. Most people, however, want more clothes than they need. Some want clothes that show their status. They want to gain recognition by having clothes in the latest fashions.

You will not always fulfill your wants with material items. Think of what you want in your life. You might want to be healthier. You may want to have an understanding friend or a better relationship with a family member. These wants can influence the dreams you have for your future.

may believe that when you are a member of the band, your life will be more fun. You may think about the new friendships you can develop.

You need to think about how your wants affect others. It can be harmful when your wants cause others to not meet their needs. For instance, you may want to spend all your free time in your room listening to music or reading. When you do this, however, then your family does not get to spend quality time together. Your family may feel you do not enjoy spending time with them. It is important for you to think about the consequences of your wants.

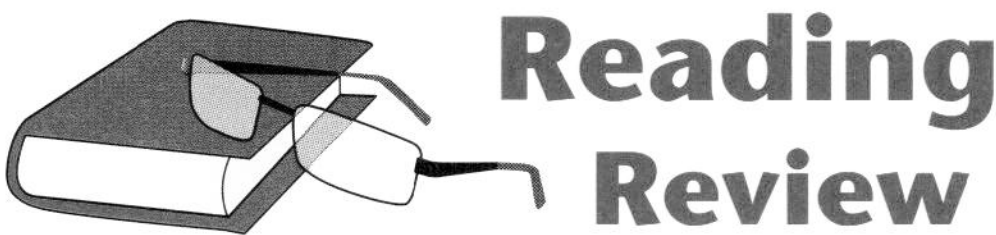

Reading Review

1. How are wants different from needs? Give examples.
2. What is something you may *want*, but do not *need*?

Section Summary

- Everyone has needs and wants.
- Basic physical needs are those needs you must meet before any other needs and wants.
- Emotional needs relate to a person's peace of mind and happiness.
- Wants are items you would like to have, but are not necessary to live. You must meet your needs before you can fulfill your wants.

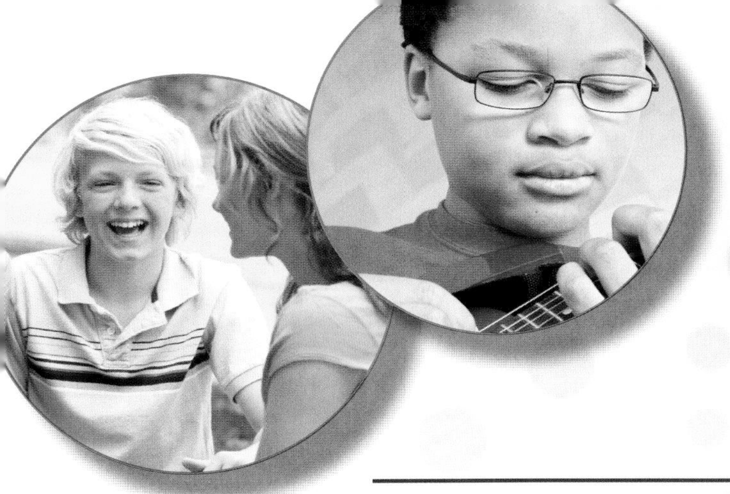

Section 3-2
Your Resources

Objectives

After studying this section, you will be able to
- **define** *resources*, *human resources*, *nonhuman resources*, *private resources*, *community resources*, and *scarce*.
- **list** the different types of resources.
- **explain** how resources can be developed.
- **describe** ways in which resources can be used.

Key Terms

resources: assets that can be used to meet needs and fulfill wants.

human resources: the qualities and traits people have within themselves to get what they need or want.

nonhuman resources: objects and conditions available to people to help them meet needs and fulfill wants.

private resources: resources owned and controlled by a person or a family.

community resources: resources shared by everyone and paid for through taxes.

scarce: a resource that is limited in supply.

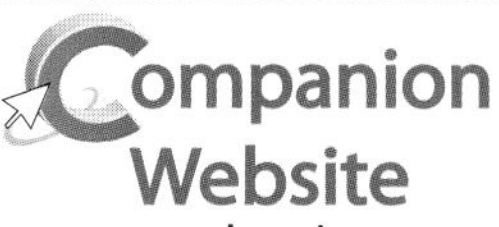

Study the Key Terms by completing crossword puzzles, matching activities, and e-flash cards at the website.

Main Ideas

- Resources help you meet needs and fulfill wants.
- Resources can be identified as human, nonhuman, private, or community.
- You have the ability to develop your resources.

Resources are assets that can be used to meet needs and fulfill wants. Without resources, you cannot accomplish what you want to do. You need resources to reach your goals now and in the future. There are many types of resources available to you.

Human Resources

As a student, you use your human resources daily. For instance, your ability to learn and how you learn are human resources. Knowing how you learn best can help you be a better student. Make a list of your five most important human resources. Write a brief summary describing how each resource can help others such as your family, friends, and community.

Types of Resources

Resources can be grouped as human and nonhuman. **Human resources** are the qualities and traits people have within themselves to get what they need or want. Your human resources are yours alone. They are like no one else's resources. They are part of you. Human resources include knowledge, skills, and talents. Health, energy, time, personality, creativity, and work habits are other human resources. See **3-3**. Human resources are also called *personal resources*. Your human resources make you special.

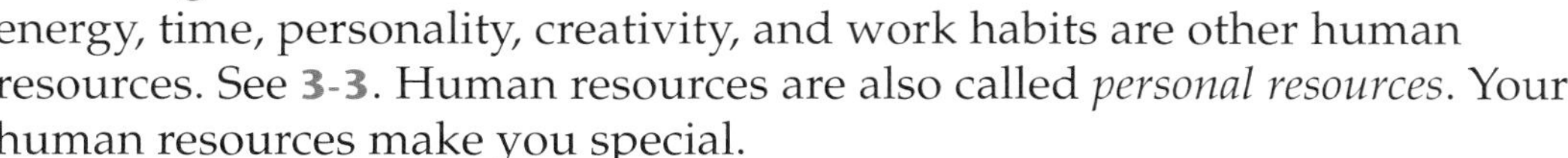

Nonhuman resources are objects and conditions available to people to help them meet needs and fulfill wants. Nonhuman resources include material and environmental resources. *Material resources* are the objects

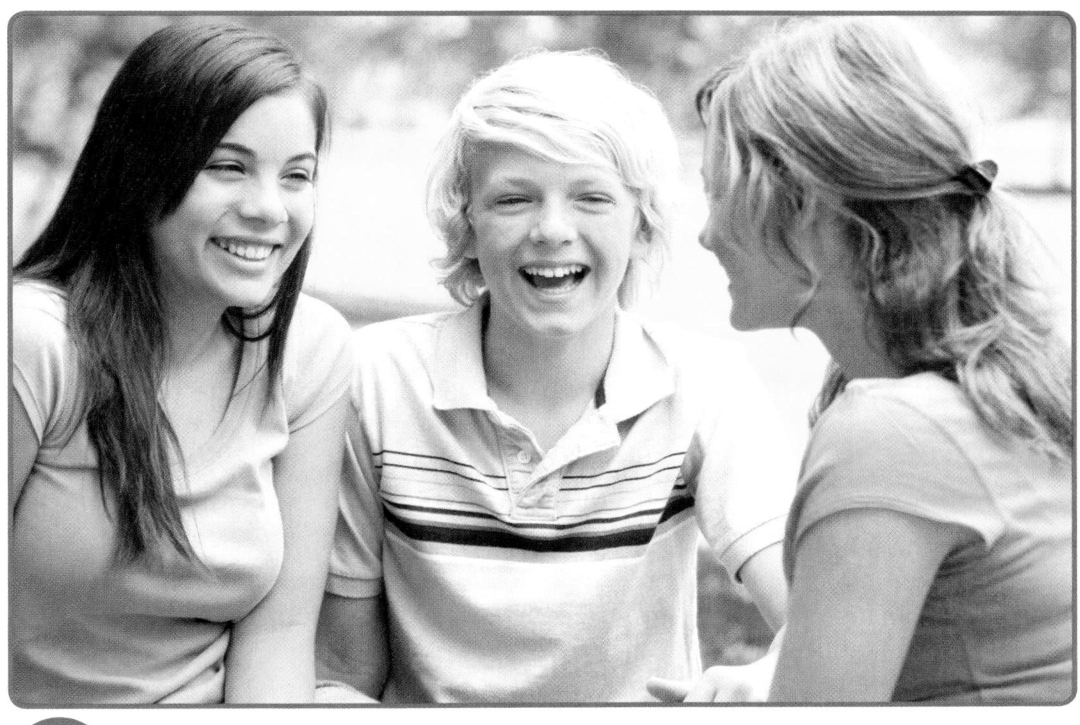

3-3 Your personality and ability to make friends are human resources.

you own. Examples are money, DVDs, and clothes. *Environmental resources* are assets found in nature. They include air, water, and soil. All material resources come from environmental resources.

Resources can also be grouped as either private or community resources. **Private resources** are owned and controlled by a person or a family. One example of a private resource is income. Others are houses or cars owned by a family. Human resources are also private resources.

Community resources are shared by everyone and are paid for through taxes. They are also called *public resources*. These resources are available through the local, state, and federal levels of government. If you are in a public school reading this book, then you are using a community resource. Other examples of community resources include roads, parks, libraries, and fire and police protection. Community resources are nonhuman resources.

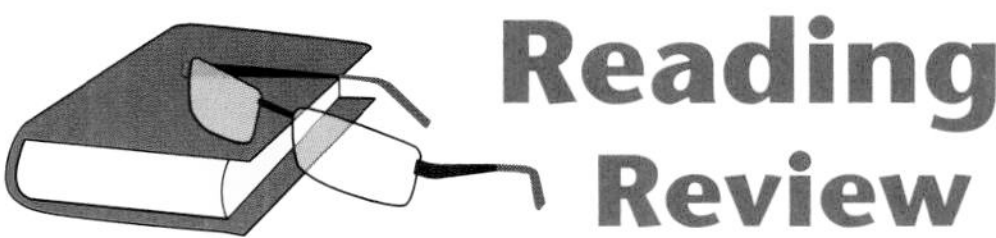

Reading Review

1. How do you use your human resources as a family member? Give examples.
2. What community resources do you use?

Financial Literacy Link

Your Resources Affect Future Earnings

Developing your human resources will help you make better use of your nonhuman resources. For instance, you may enjoy working with computers. These skills may help you earn an income in your future career. Therefore, your skills and knowledge, or human resources, will provide the ability to earn money, which is a nonhuman resource. What skills can you develop now to help you earn an income in the future? Start with activities you like. For instance, if you love to draw or play an instrument, you can plan to take advanced lessons. This can help you to become good enough to turn your skill into a career.

Using Resources

You can use resources in a variety of ways. You can trade one resource for another resource. For instance, Tracy's neighbor is paying Tracy to walk his dog while he is on vacation. Tracy is trading her time and skills for money. When you walk to the store instead of riding in a car, you are trading your energy for gas.

It is important to use resources without wasting them. Some resources are **scarce**, which means they are limited in supply. Scarce resources can run out. For instance, many communities experience water shortages when the supply of clean water becomes scarce. People can cope by reducing their use of water. They can turn off the water when brushing their teeth. They can take showers instead of baths.

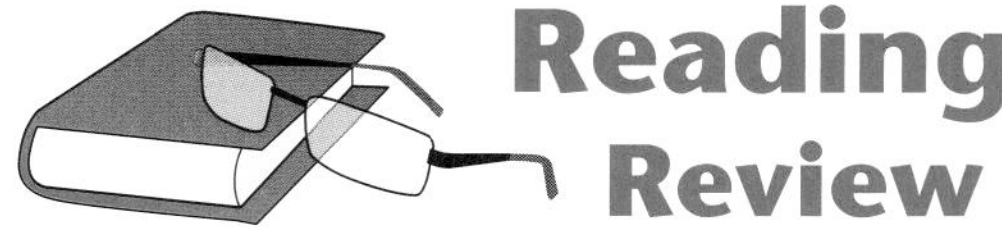

Reading Review

1. How can one resource be traded for another resource?
2. Why is it important to avoid wasting resources?

Developing Your Resources

Developing your resources is important. The more resources you develop, the more goals you can reach. There are many ways to develop your resources, especially your human resources. Increase your knowledge and learn new skills. Work on improving the skills you already have. You can also develop new interests, learn more about yourself, and improve your health. See **3-4**.

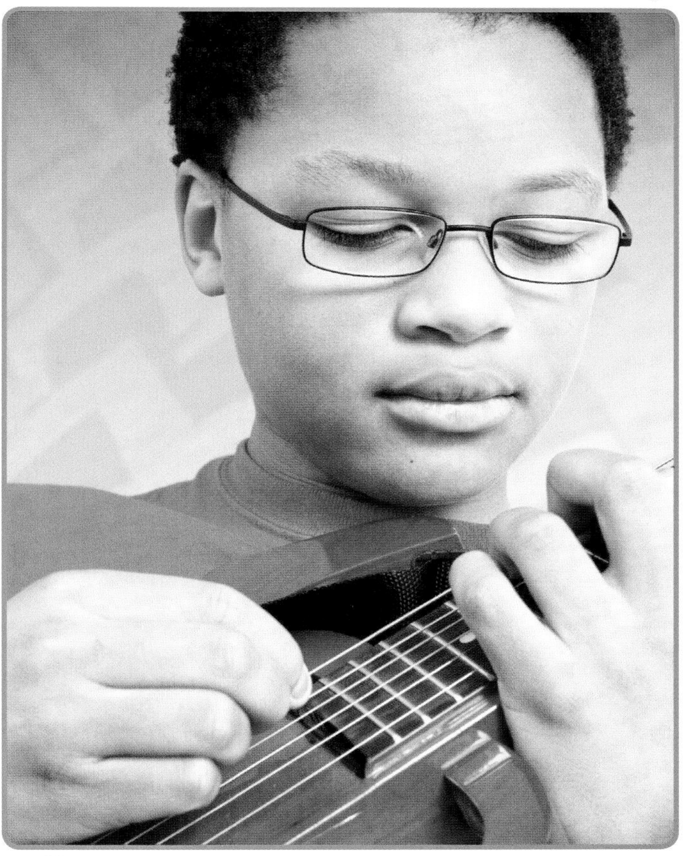

3-4 Learning to play a musical instrument can help you develop your human resources.

Families are the main influence in helping young children develop their human resources. As you grow older, you begin taking responsibility for your own development. You become the only person who can choose how to develop your human resources. As a student, you can develop your intelligence by reading, going to school, and meeting new people. You can develop your skills through practice. You can improve your health by being physically active and eating right.

How you choose to develop your resources is an important decision. You must make this decision for yourself. All people develop their resources differently. It depends on their needs and wants. Also, some people are born with more resources than others. They may be wealthy. They could live in an area where there are many chances to explore new interests and develop skills. No matter what, all people should work toward improving themselves.

Everyone has special skills that can be developed as resources. See **3-5**. You may excel at swimming, writing, or dancing. You may be artistic or get along well with other people. You may not yet have discovered your special skills. Many famous people did not discover their special skills until they were older.

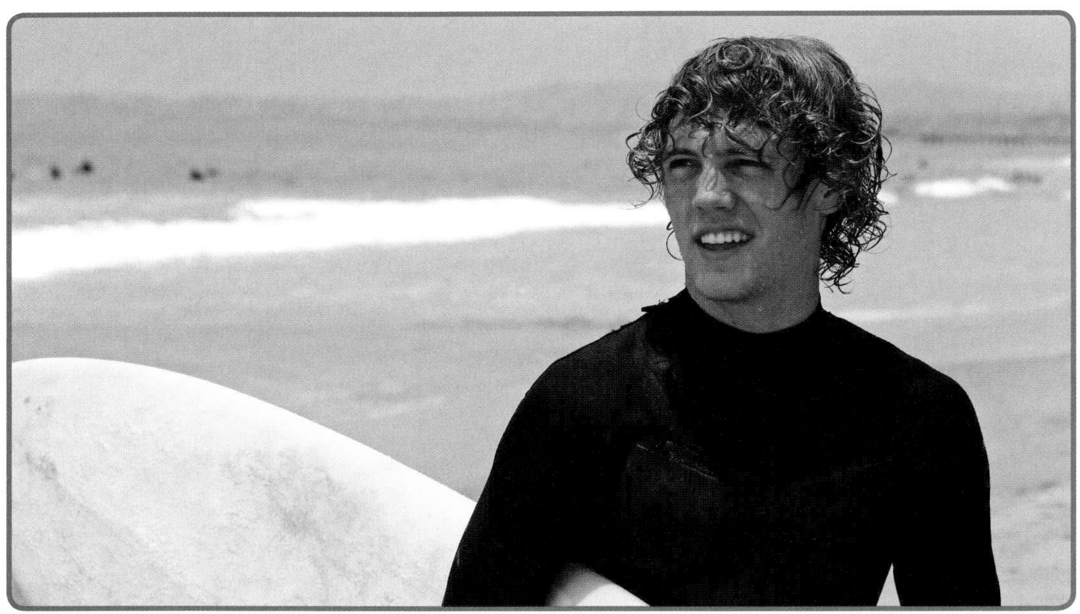

3-5 Some skills need practice to be developed. Others occur naturally.

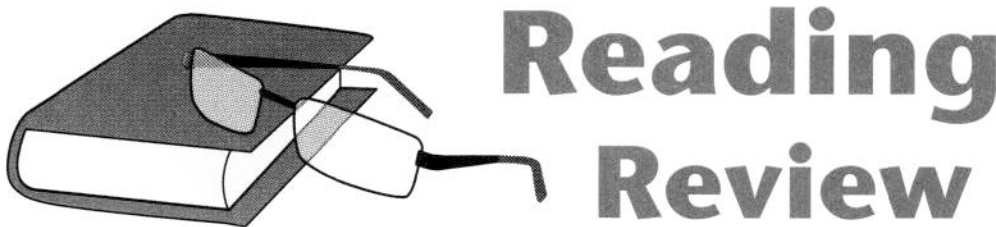

Reading Review

1. How can you develop your human resources? Give examples.
2. How can developing your human resources now help you develop your nonhuman resources in the future?

Section Summary

- You use your resources to meet needs and fulfill wants.
- Resources can be human or nonhuman, and private or community.
- You can choose how to develop your resources.
- Developing your human resources helps you to better use your nonhuman resources.

Section 3-3
Your Values and Goals

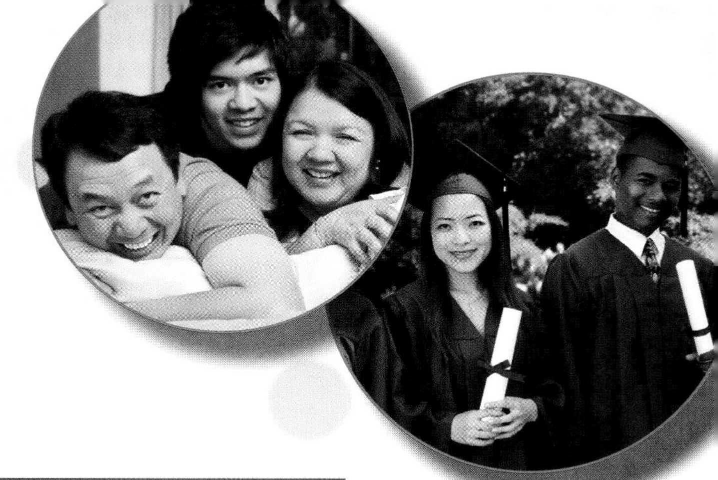

Objectives

After studying this section, you will be able to
- **define** *values*, *goals*, *short-term goals*, *long-term goals*, *priorities*, and *standards*.
- **give examples** of values and goals.
- **state** how values and goals are related.
- **give examples** of how values affect priorities.

Key Terms

values: strong beliefs or ideas about what is important.

goals: what you want to achieve.

short-term goals: what you plan to get done soon.

long-term goals: what you hope to accomplish at a later date.

priorities: goals that are more important to you.

standards: a means of measuring how well you achieve your goals.

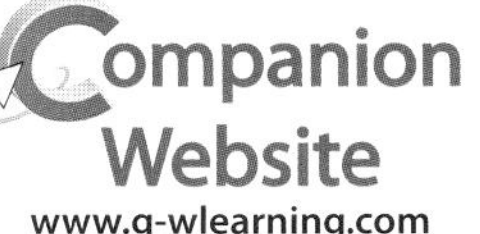

Study the Key Terms by completing crossword puzzles, matching activities, and e-flash cards at the website.

Main Ideas

- Values and goals affect your wants, how you make decisions, and how you use your resources.
- Values affect the goals you try to achieve.
- Priorities are important goals that must be met first.
- Standards help you judge how well you have met your goals.

Community Link

Learning Values from Others

You learn values from what others say and do. For instance, young children are strongly affected by their parents' values. They notice how their parents act and what they say. For instance, when parents volunteer to help with a food drive, children often learn to value community involvement. Some children are also influenced by the values of their religious training.

As children get older, they have more experiences outside the home. Their friends and teachers may have values different from their parents. Children may consider these values. They may then accept some of the values, and reject others.

What is most important to you in life? What do you hope to do today and in the future? The answers to these questions are determined by your values and goals. **Values** are strong beliefs and ideas about what is important. **Goals** are what you want to achieve. Your values and goals affect the life you lead.

Values

Your values are part of you. See **3-6**. They serve as guides for how you live your life. They provide direction for your actions. Knowing your values can help you make satisfying decisions.

You can have many different values. A few examples are freedom, service to others, and strong family ties. You and your family's views on religion, education, health, and security are also values. Your values affect what you want and how you act. They also affect how you use your resources and the decisions you make, or choose not to make. For instance, you may value being healthy. To maintain a healthful lifestyle, you choose to be physically active and eat healthful foods.

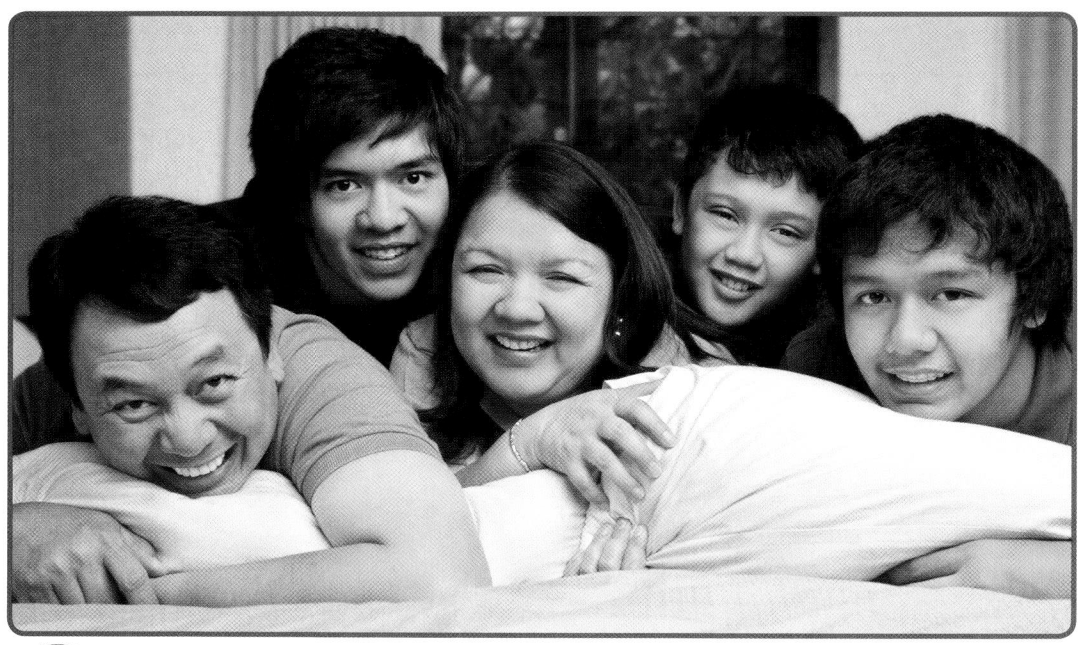

3-6 You learn many of your values from your family.

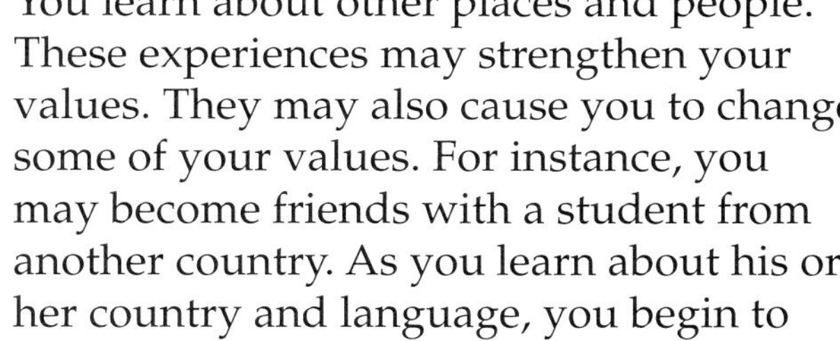

You also learn some values from your experiences. Throughout your life, you continue to have new experiences. You learn about other places and people. These experiences may strengthen your values. They may also cause you to change some of your values. For instance, you may become friends with a student from another country. As you learn about his or her country and language, you begin to value learning about different cultures.

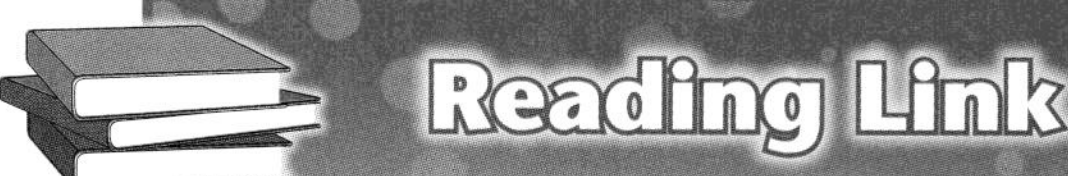

Goals and Priorities

Choose a famous historical figure you admire. Then visit your local library and select a book you can read to learn more about this person's lifetime goals and achievements. What were the goals this person was striving to achieve? How did this person's values affect his or her goals? What were the most important goals, or top priorities? Present an oral report of your findings to the class.

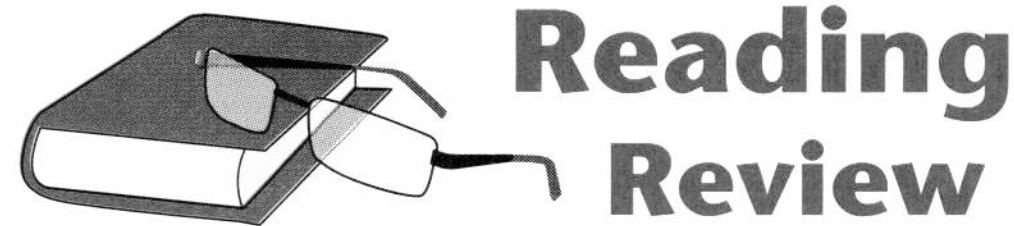

Reading Review

1. What are some of your values? How do they affect the decisions you make?
2. How can other people affect your values? Give examples.

Goals

Goals are what you are striving to achieve. Your values affect the goals you decide to set for yourself. If you value a good education, you may set a goal to complete additional homework for extra credit. If you value having a nice bike, you may set a goal to save enough money to buy the one you want.

Goals can be short- or long-term. **Short-term goals** are what you plan to get done soon. They may take a day or week to achieve. For instance, you may want to earn money to go to a movie this weekend.

Long-term goals are what you hope to accomplish at a later date. They may take a year or several years to achieve. A long-term goal may be saving money to buy a car. Long-term goals often take time to plan and are reached one step at a time.

Short-term goals are related to long-term goals. You may not reach your long-term goal if you do not reach your short-term goals first. For instance, your long-term goal may be to go to college. Your short-term goals should include getting good grades and saving money. Otherwise, it may be hard to reach your long-term goal.

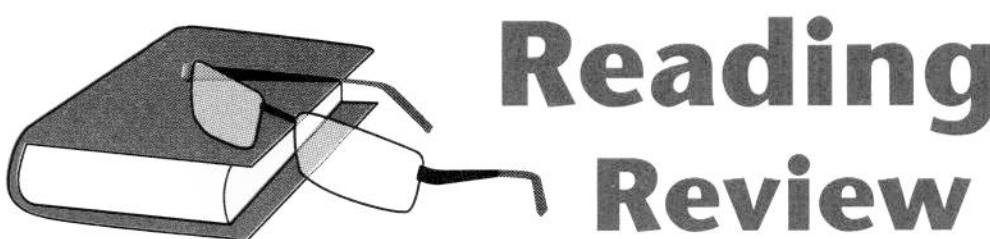

Reading Review

1. How do your values affect your goals? Give an example.
2. How are short-term goals related to long-term goals?

Priorities

Priorities are the goals that are more important to you. See **3-7**. Your *top priorities* are the most important goals. You must meet your priority goals before you meet other goals. For instance, Mackenzie has to write a paper for English class and complete a science project. She wants to learn how to play a new song on the piano. She also wants to learn how to play her new video game. Mackenzie needs to choose the goals that are most important to her. She should then complete these goals first. The goals Mackenzie chooses are her priorities.

Your values may affect the way you prioritize your goals. *Prioritize* means to list or rate in order of importance. The more values you have that relate to a goal, the better your chances are of reaching that goal. For instance, you may value having good friends and being well liked. Therefore, you will make getting along well with others a priority.

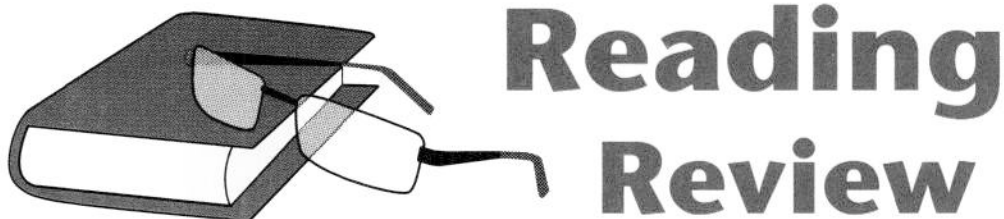

1. What are top priorities?
2. How do values affect your priorities?

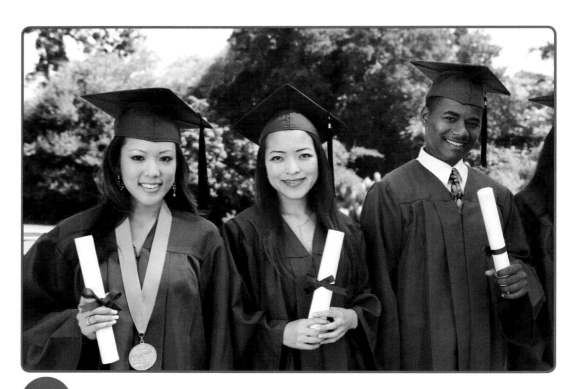

3-7 Graduating from college is a priority for many people.

Standards

Standards are a means of measuring how well you achieve your goals. Each person has a different set of standards.

Many standards come from your family. For instance, Jordan's family has high standards for maintaining good grades. To meet those standards, Jordan set a goal to get an *A* in math. If he does poorly on a math test, Jordan feels he has not met his standards.

Some standards are based on scientific knowledge. For instance, research shows that food choices affect health. Therefore, you may set a goal to follow healthful eating guidelines. Reviewing your daily food choices can help you find out if you have met your standard for eating right.

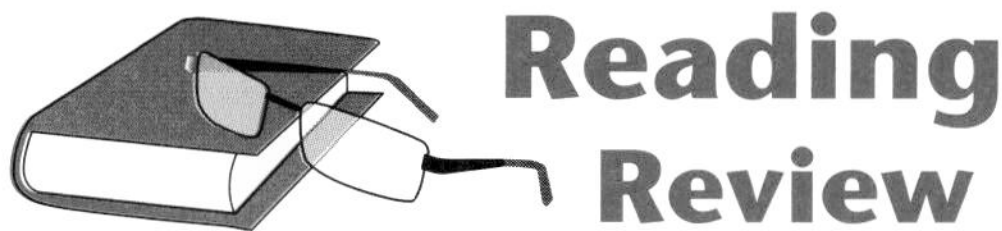

Reading Review

1. What are two factors that affect standards?
2. What are some of your standards?

Section Summary

- Values are beliefs and ideas about what is important.
- Your values affect your decisions, goals, actions, and priorities. They are learned from people and events that affect you.
- Values may change as you grow and develop.
- Goals are what you hope to achieve. Goals can be both short- and long-term.
- Priorities are the important goals you must meet first.
- Your standards can help you judge how well you have met your goals.

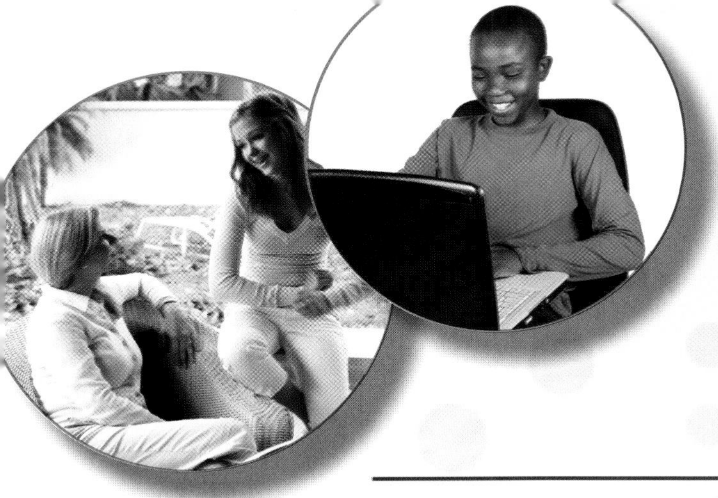

Section 3-4
Your Decisions

Objectives

After studying this section, you will be able to
- **define** *decision*, *ethics*, *ethical decision making*, *decision-making process*, *alternatives*, and *trade-off*.
- **describe** how to make an ethical decision.
- **apply** the decision-making process.

Key Terms

decision: a choice you make about what to do or say in a given situation.

ethics: thinking about why something is right or wrong.

ethical decision making: applying ideas of right or wrong to specific situations.

decision-making process: a set of six basic steps to help you make decisions, solve problems, or reach goals.

alternatives: options available to choose from when making a decision.

trade-off: the giving up of one thing for another.

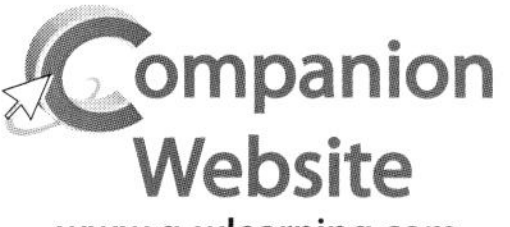

Study the Key Terms by completing crossword puzzles, matching activities, and e-flash cards at the website.

Main Ideas

- You are responsible for the decisions you make.
- It is important to make ethical decisions.
- There are six steps in the decision-making process.
- The planning process can help groups function more effectively.

To make the best use of your resources to meet your goals, you must be able to make wise decisions. A **decision** is a choice you make about what to do or say in a given situation. Some decisions require much thought and consideration. There are steps you can follow to help you make wise decisions. You can also reach group goals using a planning process.

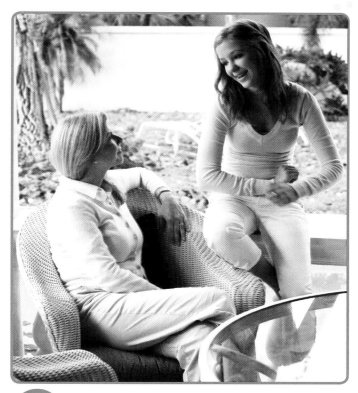

3-8 Ask for advice from family members when learning to make important decisions.

Decisions

You often have to make many decisions every day. Some of your decisions may be easy to make. For instance, you decide what clothes you will wear to school. You also decide what to eat for breakfast. You may make these decisions without a lot of thought. They are almost habit.

At times, smaller decisions may affect your daily routine. Major decisions, such as going to college, getting married, and having children, can affect you for the rest of your life. These decisions are harder to make and should involve much thought and reflection.

You will make many decisions throughout your life. See **3-8**. As a teen, you are already making some decisions. You must accept the *consequences*, or what happens as a result of your decisions. You are responsible for your decisions, whether they are unwise or wise. This is called *personal responsibility*. You need to learn to make decisions carefully.

Adults can help you learn how to make wise decisions. They can guide you and let you know from their own experiences which decisions are wise. Adults, however, cannot always be with you. You will need to practice making your own decisions.

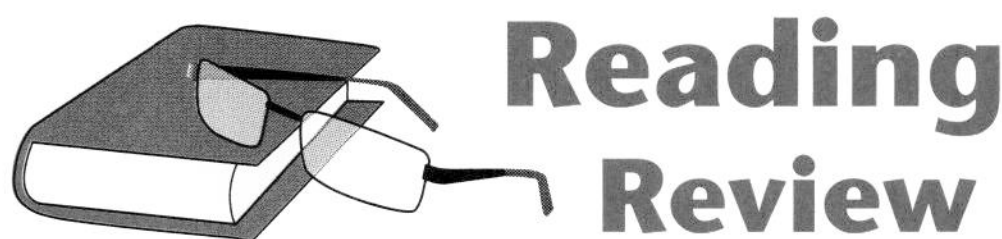

Reading Review

1. Why do you need to learn to make decisions carefully?
2. Why should you practice making your own decisions?

Ethics

There are times when you have to think about making the right decision. **Ethics** is thinking about why something is right or wrong, or good or bad. You practice **ethical decision making** when you apply ideas of right or wrong to specific situations. To determine if a decision is right or wrong, consider the following questions:

- Will your decision help or hurt others?
- What would a responsible person do?
- Is your decision consistent with your values?
- Would you want others to know about your decision?

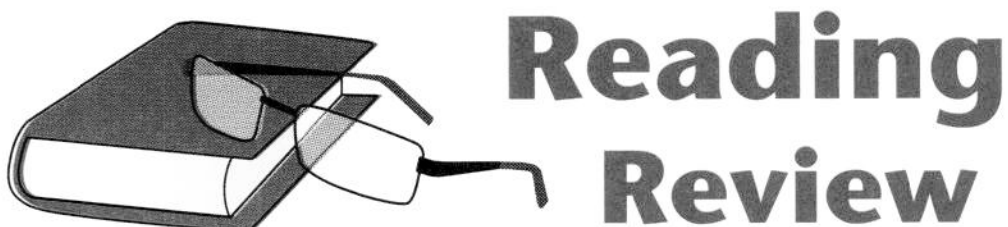

Reading Review

1. Give an example of an ethical decision.
2. Why is it important for your decisions to be consistent with your values?

The Decision-Making Process

You can use the decision-making process to help you make decisions. The **decision-making process** is a set of six basic steps to help you make decisions, solve problems, or reach goals. See **3-9**. The decision-making process includes the following steps:

1. **Define the problem.** The first step is to clearly define the problem you need to solve. A problem may include a decision you need to make or a goal you need to reach. For instance, Miguel is now a member of his school's soccer team. Practice takes a lot of after-school time. Before joining the soccer team, Miguel would use the time after school to study. He also takes part in other activities during the evenings, such as scouts and a local youth group. Miguel identifies his problem by asking, "When can I complete my homework?"

Succeed in Life

Ethical Decision Making

If you learn that what you are planning to do is wrong, it is important to think about your choices. For instance, Arah found a paper on the Internet that matched her term paper assignment. At first, she thought it could save her time and assure her a good grade on the paper.

When thinking through the consequences, however, Arah determined that it would hurt her if she cheated on the assignment. She would not learn the skills needed to write the paper. *Plagiarizing*, or passing off work that was not hers, would hurt her self-confidence. She reflected that a responsible person would not steal another person's work. Her values of honesty and fairness were not consistent with copying the paper. Arah also knew that she would not want her parents, teachers, or friends to know she plagiarized a paper. Arah decided it was not the right thing for her to do.

Steps in the Decision-Making Process

Step 1. Define the problem.
Step 2. Examine alternatives.
Step 3. Consider how choices relate to goals.
Step 4. Identify acceptable choices.
Step 5. Decide on one choice.
Step 6. Evaluate results.

3-9 Following these six steps can help you make decisions.

2. **Examine alternatives.** **Alternatives** are the options available to choose from when making a decision. When you make major decisions, list the advantages and disadvantages of your alternatives. *Advantages* are the positive points. *Disadvantages* are the negative points. Miguel thinks about his alternatives. Playing on the soccer team takes a lot of time during the week and on the weekends. He really enjoys playing soccer, however, and being a member of the team. He knows the physical activity is good for him. Miguel also enjoys his evening activities, which take time. He has been a member of scouts and the youth group for several years. He likes to spend time with his friends and do worthwhile projects.
3. **Consider how choices relate to goals.** No one else has the same values, wants, needs, resources, goals, standards, and priorities as you. Miguel wants to go to a good college. To do this, he needs to study and get good grades.
4. **Identify acceptable choices.** Once you examine your alternatives and consider your choices, you are ready to identify acceptable choices. Be sure to carefully consider all your choices. Miguel identifies his acceptable choices. They include (a) quitting the soccer team or (b) giving up some evening activities.
5. **Decide on one choice.** You need to take responsibility for the decision you make. Miguel decided to make a trade-off. A **trade-off** is the giving up of one thing for another. Miguel chose to give up some of his evening activities for soccer. He told his scout troop that he had to take time off during soccer season. When he made his decision, Miguel knew he would miss being with his friends from the troop. He decided to accept this as a result of making his decision.
6. **Evaluate results.** The last step of the process is to evaluate the results of your decision. People often make the same decisions over and over again without thinking. By evaluating your decision, you may avoid repeating an unwise decision. After the soccer season ended, Miguel evaluated his decision. His grades were good because he was able to do homework in the evening. He also ended the season with some new friends and improved soccer skills. In addition, he was still in touch with his friends from his scout troop. Miguel became active in this group again. He concluded that he made a wise decision.

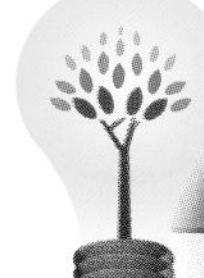

Think Green

Build an Organic Garden

Organic gardens are becoming more common and they are good for both the environment and the community. Organic means no chemicals or pesticides are used. Many people believe an organic garden is safer for the people working in the garden and eating the food. You can work with a group of students or neighbors to create a community garden. Use the FCCLA five-step planning process to help you identify concerns and set a goal. Then form a plan to create the garden. Be sure to evaluate your actions and make any necessary improvements. Your garden might even become a model for others in the community to follow.

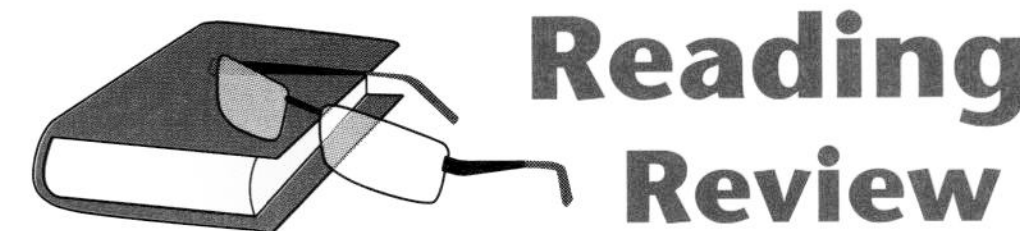

Reading Review

1. What are the six steps of the decision-making process?
2. Why do you need to be able to make your own decisions?

Contributing to Group Decisions

You are part of a group in each of your classes. Class discussions give you and your classmates a chance to talk about different topics and make decisions. By taking part in class discussions, you can find out what your classmates are thinking and feeling. You can also express your thoughts and feelings. Discussing current events, school policies, and important social issues with your classmates can help you understand your decisions about these issues.

You may also belong to an after-school group such as a sports team, band, youth group, or scout troop. Each of these groups makes decisions, too. Some groups elect leaders to make decisions.

You may be a member of a student organization such as Family, Career and Community Leaders of America (FCCLA). FCCLA is a group offered through a school's family and consumer sciences department. FCCLA helps teens develop leadership skills for life through projects that address family issues, career exploration, and community involvement. Members of this group use a five-step planning process to reach group decisions and goals. **See 3-10**. The steps in the planning process are as follows:

1. Identify concerns.
2. Set your goal.
3. Form a plan.
4. Act.
5. Follow up.

You can use tools such as the decision-making and planning processes when you are part of any group. Sometimes, group decisions can be harder to make than personal decisions. This is because group members may have many different ideas based on their needs, wants, values, goals, priorities, and standards. They may have a conflict about what is the best decision.

When making group decisions, you need to gather and examine information carefully. It is better to discuss topics or subjects when you know the facts. That is why reading and doing research are part of your schoolwork.

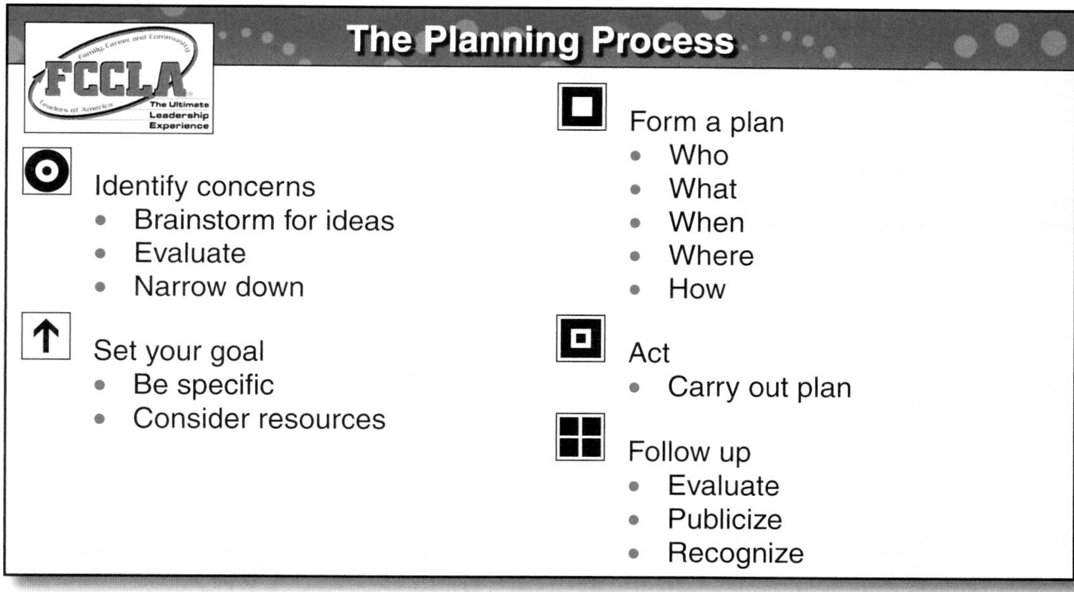

The Planning Process
FCCLA
Family, Career and Community Leaders of America
The Ultimate Leadership Experience
Identify concerns
• Brainstorm for ideas
• Evaluate
• Narrow down
Set your goal
• Be specific
• Consider resources
Form a plan
• Who
• What
• When
• Where
• How
Act
• Carry out plan
Follow up
• Evaluate
• Publicize
• Recognize

FCCLA

3-10 The FCCLA Planning Process can help you reach your individual as well as group goals.

Although your ideas are important, you need to be able to support them with facts.

The group decision-making skills you learn now will help you in the future. In your community, you will be able to help make group decisions. On the job, you will be better able to help solve group problems. Decision making can help you as a member of any group.

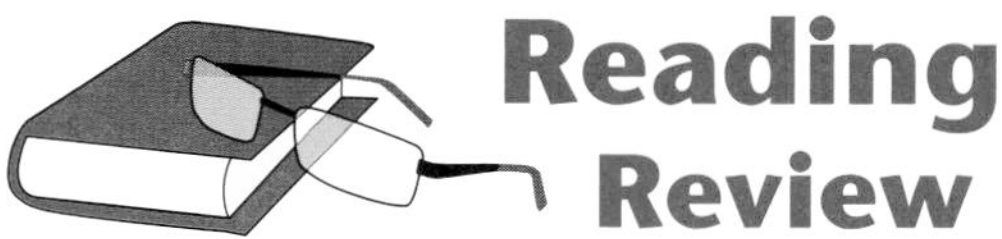

Reading Review

1. How can you benefit by taking part in group decisions?
2. Why do you need to gather and examine information when making group decisions?

Section Summary

- It is important for you to learn to make decisions carefully.
- Ethical decision making means that you apply ideas of right or wrong to a given situation.
- Following the six steps in the decision-making process will help you make decisions.
- The planning process can help you make decisions in groups.

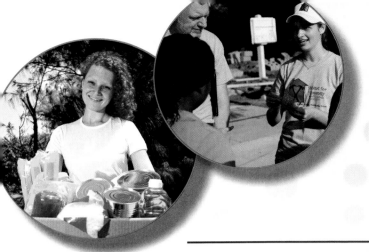

Section 3-5
Making a Difference in Your Community

Objectives

After studying this section, you will be able to

- **define** *leadership*, *integrity*, *teamwork*, *citizenship*, *civic engagement*, *service learning*, and *social entrepreneur*.
- **explain** qualities of effective leaders and strong team members.
- **describe** ways to contribute to your community through civic engagement, service learning, and social entrepreneurship.

Key Terms

leadership: the ability to inspire others to meet goals.

integrity: a commitment to do what is right.

teamwork: work done by a group in a cooperative manner.

citizen: a member of a community.

citizenship: the ways in which citizens handle their responsibilities.

civic engagement: actions that individuals and groups take to identify and solve the problems of their communities.

service learning: a strategy where students use their academic skills to provide services for their community.

social entrepreneurs: individuals who identify the problems of societies and develop plans to change the world in positive ways.

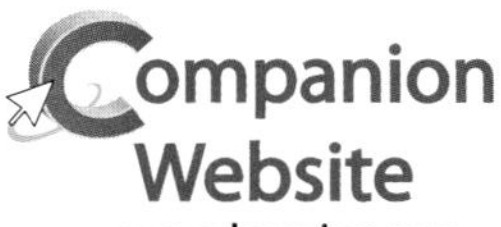

Study the Key Terms by completing crossword puzzles, matching activities, and e-flash cards at the website.

Main Ideas

- You can develop teamwork and leadership skills.
- Responsible citizens identify and solve the problems of their communities.
- Civic engagement, service learning, and social entrepreneurship are ways people can make a difference in their local and global communities.

There are many ways to make improvements in your community. As individuals and as group members, you can take actions to make positive changes locally and globally. Many schools encourage students to use their academic skills to help others by volunteering in their communities. Some individuals are able to use their skills to solve a large, worldwide problem affecting many people.

Being a Leader and a Team Member

Working with groups, such as FCCLA, can help you develop leadership and teamwork skills. See **3-11**. **Leadership** is the ability to inspire others to meet goals. Leaders value the needs and interests of others. They set examples for others to follow. They guide group decisions.

Effective leaders have certain qualities that help them influence group members. They are knowledgeable about group issues, which helps them make wise decisions. Leaders must have courage to do what needs to be done. Effective leaders should have friendly, caring personalities. They must be organized and have good time management skills to meet goals. Effective leaders also have **integrity**, which means they are committed to doing what is right. Leaders need enthusiasm to motivate group members so they are excited about achieving goals.

Teamwork is work done by a group in a cooperative manner. Effective team members listen to others in the group. They respect different points of view. Others will want to work with you if you demonstrate a positive attitude, honesty, fairness, and tact. Encouraging all team members to work and contribute will make a stronger team.

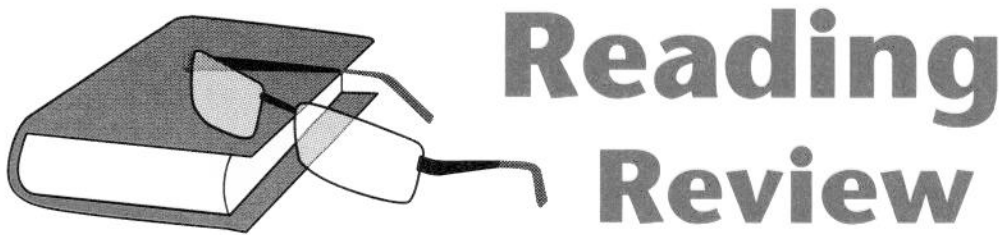

Reading Review

1. Which traits of an effective leader would you like to develop?
2. How can you be a leader in your school?
3. List four traits of a strong team member.

Giving to the Community

There are many ways to make a difference in your community. You are a **citizen**, or a member of a community. The way you handle the responsibilities of being a citizen is called **citizenship**. Responsible citizens search for ways to make improvements in their communities.

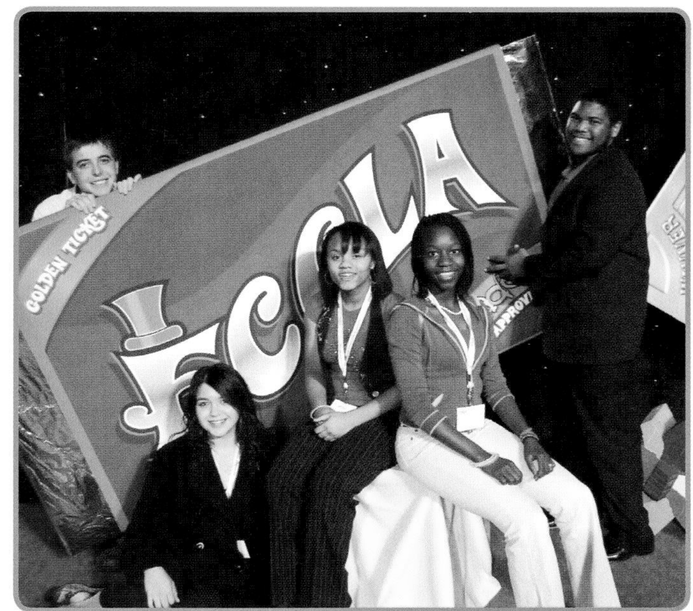

FCCLA

3-11 Groups such as FCCLA can help you develop skills to be a better leader and team member.

Civic engagement includes the actions that individuals and groups take to identify and solve the problems of their communities. It can include volunteering on an individual basis as well as taking action as a group.

For instance, Dion was concerned about the amount of litter he was noticing in his neighborhood. He first decided to meet with a few of his friends to explain his concerns. They developed a plan to take turns picking up the litter. Then they decided to present their plan to members of the neighborhood association. This resulted in more people becoming involved to keep the neighborhood clean. Dion acted both as an individual and as a group member.

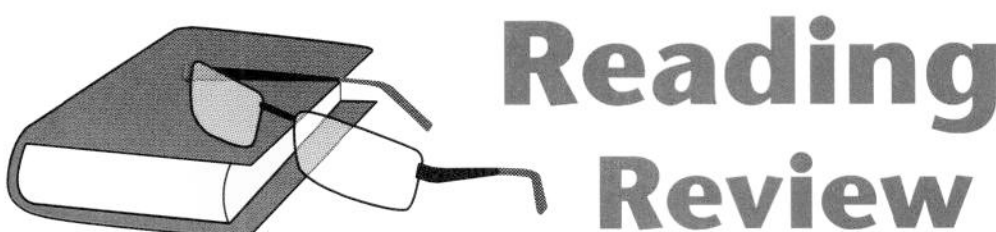

Reading Review

1. What does it mean to be a responsible citizen? Find examples in your local newspaper of good citizenship.
2. Give an example of civic engagement.

Service Learning

Service learning is a strategy where students use their academic skills to provide services for their community. After students volunteer, they reflect or think about what they learned. Doing meaningful, real projects can be positive experiences for the students and their communities. See **3-12**.

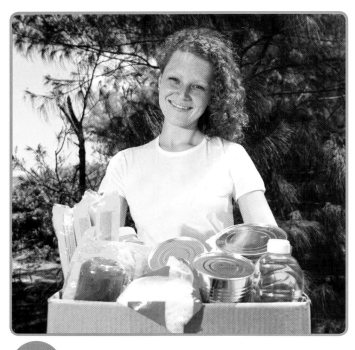

3-12 This girl enjoys working as a volunteer to collect donations for the community food bank.

For instance, one middle school class decided to apply what they learned in nutrition class to improve the lives of children. They were concerned about the number of overweight children at the nearby elementary school. Some students volunteered to teach nutrition classes after school for the children. Others volunteered in the after school program to encourage the children to be more physically active. At the end of the nine-week project, students reflected on the experience. They noticed improvements in the children's health habits. The middle school students also learned more about nutrition. The students wanted to continue the project and identified ways to make further improvements.

In another class, students conducted a service learning project for a children's hospital. They learned the hospital needed simple cloth dolls for children undergoing surgery. The doctors could draw on the dolls to explain surgical processes to the children. The children could also draw on the dolls so they looked like them. Students were able to use their sewing skills to make the dolls. They delivered the dolls and saw how they would be used. The students thought about all they had learned in the process.

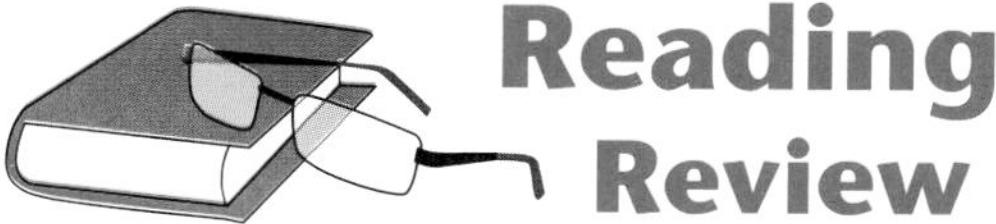

Reading Review

1. Give an example of a service learning project.
2. Consider what you have learned in your classes. How can you use this knowledge to help your community?

Social Entrepreneur

There are special talented individuals who sometimes go beyond giving service to their communities. **Social entrepreneurs** identify the problems of societies and develop plans to change the world in positive ways. They use their skills to organize, create, and manage projects that will address the problems.

There are many examples of social entrepreneurs. In 1976, Professor Muhammad Yunus developed a research project where small loans, or microcredit, could be given to the rural poor in Bangladesh. Today, microcredit agencies help people all over the world with the principles he established. In 2006, Yunus was awarded the Nobel Peace Prize for his work with microcredit. Another example is TOMS Shoes, which was founded in 2006 by Blake Mycoskie. With every pair of shoes sold, TOMS donates a new pair of shoes to a child in need. See **3-13**.

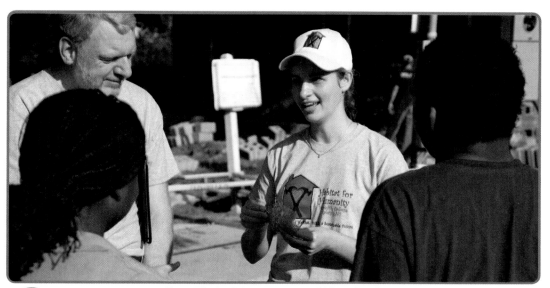

Dave Timberlake, courtesy of Meredith College Marketing Department

3-13 Habitat for Humanity is an example of an organization that was started by a social entrepreneur.

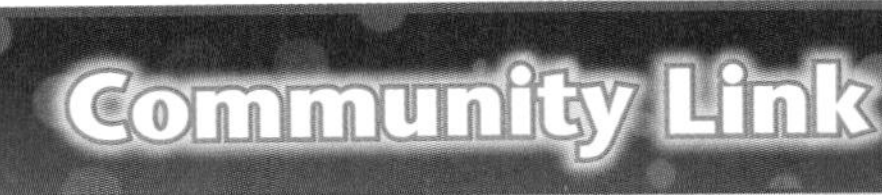

Social Entrepreneurs

Throughout history, individuals have seen a need and developed a plan that makes the world better. For instance, Florence Nightingale from the United Kingdom was concerned about the conditions in hospitals. She established the first school for nurses. As a result, hospitals all over the world improved. In the early 1900s, Ellen Swallow Richards from the United States was disturbed that school children were not getting nutritious lunches. She founded the *penny lunch program* in Boston, which became the first school lunch program. List some other examples of social entrepreneurs.

A growing number of young social entrepreneurs are making a difference in the world. In Canada, Craig Keilburger was twelve years old when he first learned of child labor. *Child labor* occurs when children under a legal age are forced to work long hours in harmful conditions. These children are often denied education.

Craig read an article about a young boy who was killed in Pakistan for speaking out against child labor. He began to research this problem and with his friends formed an organization called *Free the Children*. The organization now builds schools as better options for children in many developing countries that use child labor.

When Zach Hunter was twelve years old, he became concerned with the number of people enslaved through human trafficking. He founded Loose Change to Loosen Chains (LC2LC), to raise awareness and funds to end modern-day slavery. Now, people and student groups of all ages collect change and contribute to the organization.

Responsible citizens can make a difference in the world. Schools that focus on civic engagement and service learning are teaching good citizenship skills. Social entrepreneurs are those special individuals who use their skills to solve major problems in the world.

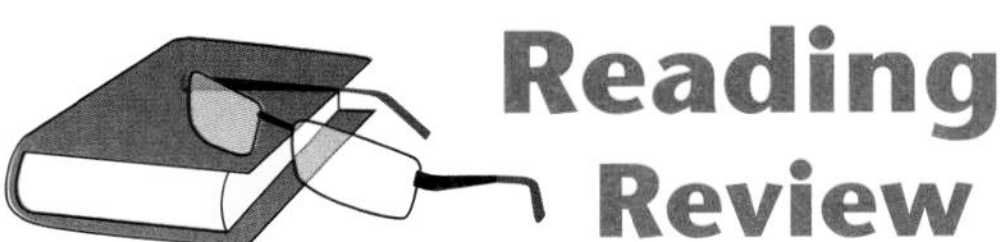

1. What is the difference between a volunteer and a social entrepreneur?
2. Give an example of a social entrepreneur from the past and one from today.

Section Summary

- School groups can help you develop the qualities of an effective leader and team member.
- Schools can also help you make a difference in the community through civic engagement and service learning.
- Social entrepreneurs are solving problems of societies through creative problem solving and action.

Chapter Summary

As a teen, you learn to make decisions. To make wise decisions, you need to know about needs, wants, resources, values, goals, priorities, and standards. These factors play an important part in the decision-making process.

Your needs and wants affect your life in many ways. They affect your feelings, how you get along with others, and how you use your time and skills. You often make decisions based on your needs or wants.

Resources are what you use to meet needs and fulfill wants. The types of resources that are available to you often determine how you will make a decision.

When you make a decision, you are often trying to reach a goal. Your goals are based on your values or what you believe is important.

There are six basic steps to follow in the decision-making process. The first step is to define the problem. The second step is to examine alternatives. The third step is to consider how choices relate to goals. The fourth step is to identify acceptable choices. The fifth step is to decide on one choice. The sixth step is to evaluate results. Thinking about whether the decision is right or wrong leads to ethical decision making.

While you are a student, joining school groups or student organizations, such as FCCLA, can help you learn how to be part of a group. This will help you develop leadership and teamwork skills.

Responsible citizens find ways to improve their communities. Schools promote good citizenship through civic engagement and service learning. Social entrepreneurs use their skills and talents to improve societies by identifying and addressing major problems.

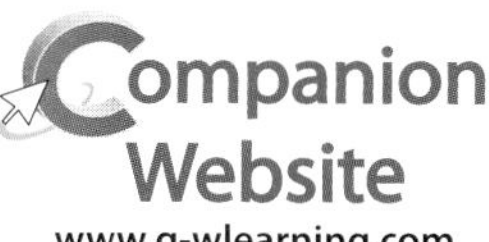

Review Key Terms and Main Ideas for Chapter 3 at the website.

Chapter Review

Write your answers on a separate sheet of paper.

1. Give examples of three physical needs and three emotional needs.
2. Give an example of a healthful way to meet an emotional need. Give an example of an unhealthful way to meet an emotional need. Explain your answers.
3. True or false. Most people dislike new experiences.
4. How are needs different from wants? List two examples.
5. Give examples of three human resources and three nonhuman resources you have.
6. Planning to go to a baseball game this weekend is a ______-term goal.
7. Jim wants to teach small children. He believes education is very important. He thinks he could make a difference as a teacher. What is Jim's goal? What does Jim value?
8. What happens as a result of your decisions?
9. List the six steps of the decision-making process. Next to each step, give an example of an action that could be taken to help make a specific decision.
10. What are three characteristics of a good team member?
11. Give two examples each of service learning and social entrepreneurs.

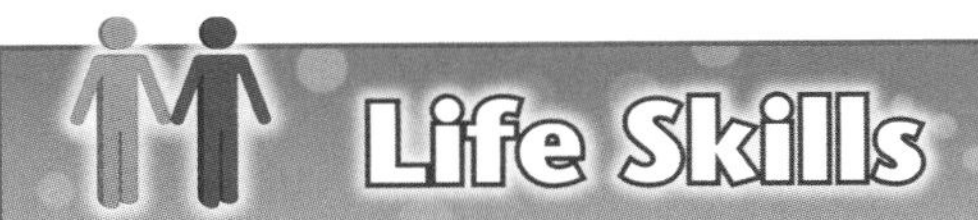

12. When Vicky Jones was in the third grade, her father died. Her mother works to support Vicky and her younger brother and sister. Mrs. Jones makes just enough money to support the family. Vicky is now in the eighth grade. She wants to go to college when she graduates from high school. She knows her mother will not be able to afford college tuition. Help Vicky make a plan to reach her goal of attending college. Be sure to consider short- and long-term goals, resources, and any trade-offs Vicky might have to make.

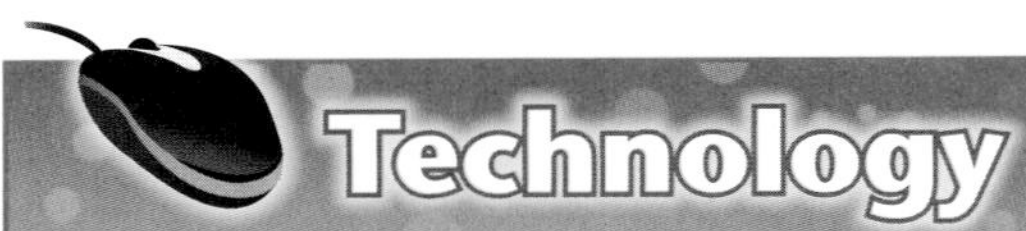

13. Use the Internet to research a current public figure whom you admire. Identify the values, standards, and priorities that have directed this person's life. Why do you admire this person? How has he or she contributed to a community, country, or the world? How can you follow this person's example?

14. In your journal, write three goals you would like to achieve by this date next year. Make a list of the resources you will need and the steps you will take to achieve your goals. How do your needs, wants, and values affect the goals you choose? Which standards will you use to measure how well you achieve your goals?

Academics

15. **History.** Look in the library or online for books or articles about a famous person who did not develop his or her talents until he or she was older. Write a one-page report about this person.
16. **Social Studies.** Look in your local telephone book for five public resources your city or town offers. Make a poster illustrating these resources. Your title might be *Look What (name of your city or town) Has to Offer!*
17. **Writing.** Survey students at your school about the qualities they think describe an effective leader. Who are the leaders they admire most? Write an article for the school newspaper reporting the results of your survey.
18. **Speech.** In small groups, brainstorm ways to successfully make group decisions at school. Then, as a class, use the suggestions to make a group decision. Discuss how this activity can help you throughout life.
19. **Writing.** Think of ways in which people you know have made a difference in the community. Write a letter to one person and thank them for their contributions in your community.

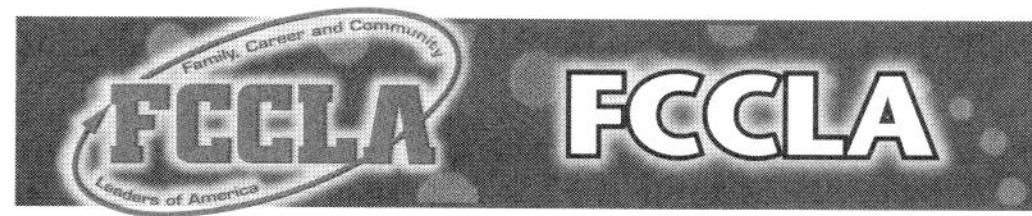

20. Identify and analyze all of the groups you are involved with in your school, family, work, or community. Which of these groups function as teams? How do the teams compare with one another? What are the different roles in any given team? Pick one team and determine ways to improve teamwork among team members. Complete an FCCLA *Take the Lead* project for the *Power of One* program. Obtain further information about this program from your FCCLA advisor.

Chapter 4
Managing Daily Living

Sections

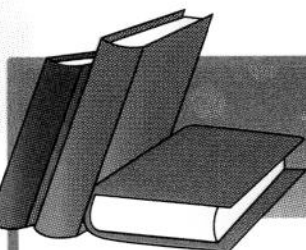

Sharpen Your Reading

As you read the chapter, put sticky notes next to the sections where you have questions. Write your questions on the sticky notes. Discuss the questions with your classmates or teacher.

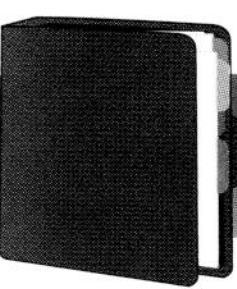

Concept Organizer

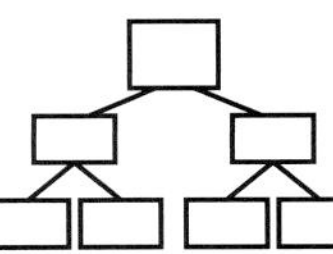

Use a tree diagram like the one shown to determine the major expense categories in your budget. List two examples of each one that are part of your personal budget.

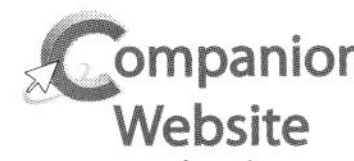

Print out the concept organizer at the website.

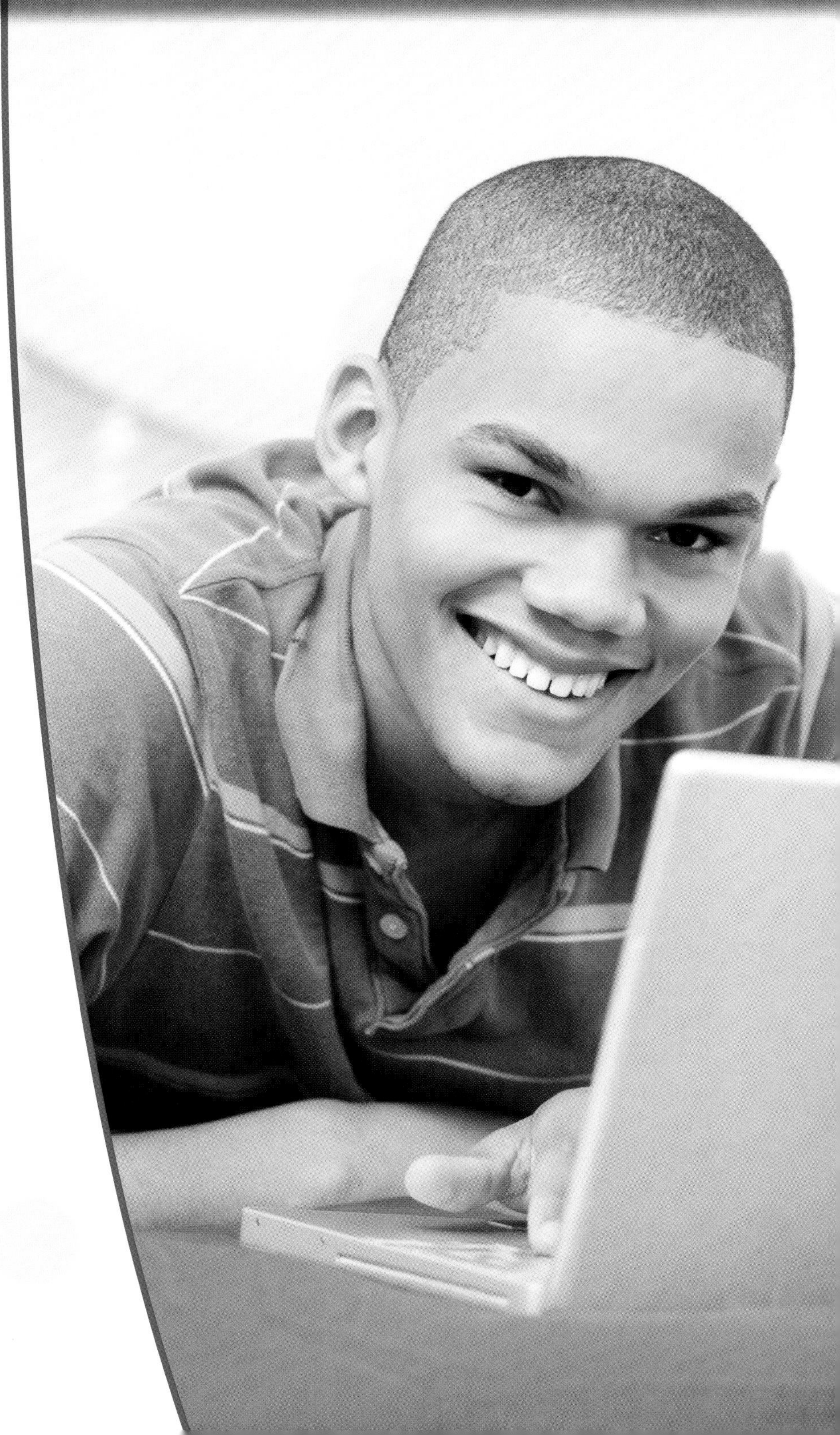

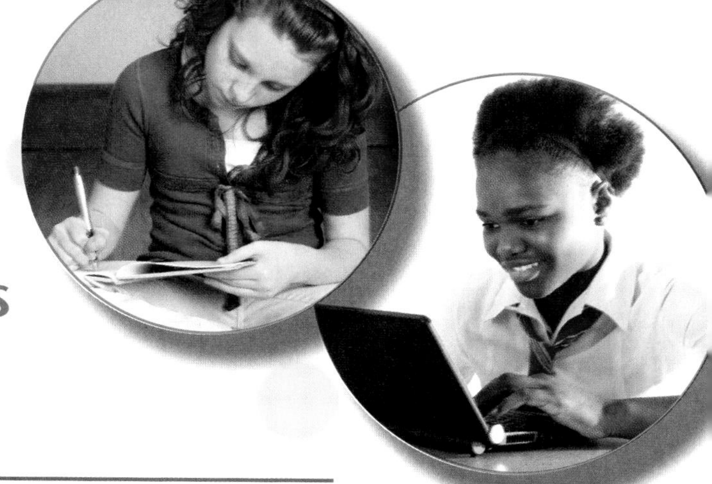

Section 4-1
The Management Process

Objectives

After studying this section, you will be able to
- **define** *management*, *management process*, *schedule*, *implement*, *evaluate*, *time management*, *habit*, *procrastinate*, and *learning style*.
- **identify** the steps in the management process.
- **explain** how you can manage your time.
- **determine** how you can improve your study skills.

Key Terms

management: using resources to reach goals.

management process: a series of steps for reaching a goal. The steps include setting a goal, planning, implementing, and evaluating.

schedule: a written plan for reaching a goal within a certain period of time.

implement: to carry out a plan of action.

evaluate: to judge an entire plan of action.

time management: the skill of organizing your time so you can accomplish tasks.

habit: a repeated pattern of behavior.

procrastinate: to put off difficult or unpleasant tasks until later.

learning style: the conditions under which you learn best.

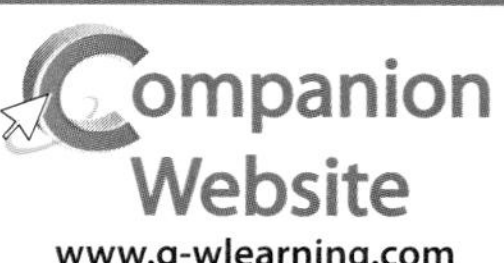

Study the Key Terms by completing crossword puzzles, matching activities, and e-flash cards at the website.

Main Ideas

- The management process helps you set and reach goals.
- You can learn to manage your time.

Do you ever feel you are not in control of your life? Are you unable to finish tasks because time passes too quickly? If so, you need to learn more about the *management process*. Understanding the management process and how it works can help you get the most from your resources.

The Management Process

Management is using resources to reach goals. You can reach your goals by following the management process. The **management process** is a series of steps for reaching a goal. The steps include

- setting a goal
- planning
- implementing
- evaluating

Setting a Goal

The first step in the management process is setting a goal. Sometimes, people set unrealistic goals. These goals are often impossible to reach. Learn to set realistic goals, which are goals you can achieve. Reaching goals is easier if you set priorities and focus on one goal at a time. See **4-1**.

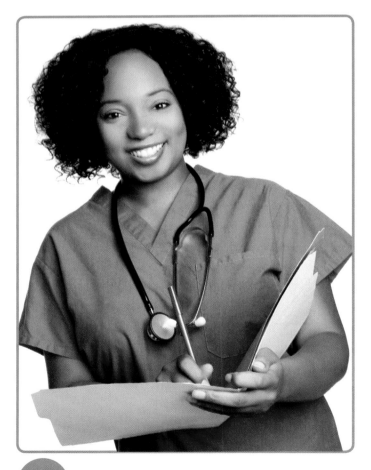

4-1 The management process can help you reach your career goals.

For instance, Tiago is an overweight teen who wants to lose 20 pounds. He set a goal to lose the weight before the school dance. The dance, however, is in two weeks. Tiago decided to ask his family and consumer sciences and health teachers for advice. After doing so, he realized he set an unrealistic goal. His teachers told him that losing more than one or two pounds a week is unhealthful. They also told him it is very unlikely he could lose 10 pounds in one week.

Therefore, Tiago changed his goal. He decided to gradually lose 20 pounds by following a healthful diet. This way, he would be able to keep the weight off by eating sensibly.

Planning

After you set a goal, you must make plans. Begin by asking yourself, "What do I need to do to reach this goal?" Look at the resources you have and decide which actions to take. Then, make a schedule for meeting your goal. A **schedule** is a written plan for reaching a goal within a certain period of time. It should show when you will perform your actions and in what order. See **4-2**.

Tiago made a list of the resources he could use to reach his goal. These resources included his family and consumer sciences teacher, family doctor, and health teacher. He asked his family and consumer sciences teacher for information on nutrition. He talked to his family doctor about planning a healthful diet. He also talked to his health teacher about ways he could become more physically active. All this information helped Tiago develop a sensible meal plan. He also made a schedule of when he could fit more physical activity into his daily routine.

Implementing

Once you make your plans, you must implement them. **Implement** means to carry out your plan of action. During this step, check your progress. Make sure you are following your plan. After checking, you may need to make changes in your plan.

In order to follow his plan, Tiago made some changes. Instead of buying lunch at school every day, he started making his own lunch. This way he would be sure to follow his personal meal plan. Tiago also avoided playing a computer game right after school. Instead, he would work out in the school's gym and weight room before going home. At first, this was hard for Tiago. He had to get used to waking up earlier in the morning to make his lunch. He also had to get used to coming home later from school. He was, however, able to quickly adjust to his new routine.

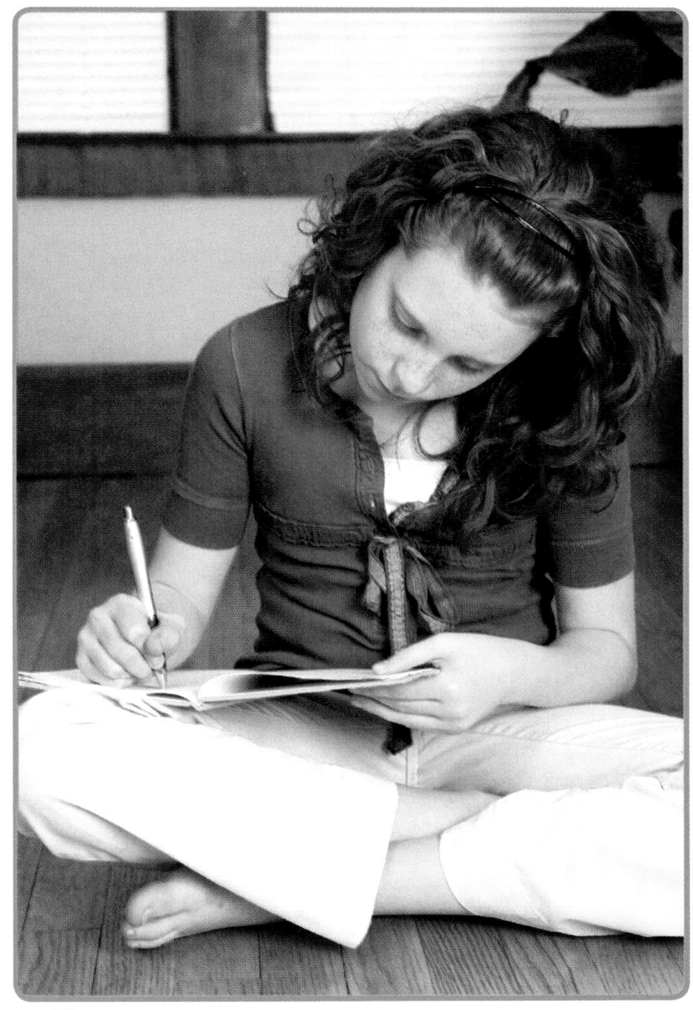

4-2 Use a calendar or planner to check the progress of your plan and make needed changes.

Evaluating

The last step of the management process is to evaluate. **Evaluate** means to judge the entire plan of action. After you complete your plan, evaluate whether it was a good plan. You also need to evaluate your goals. Evaluating plans and goals can help you improve your management skills. If you find that your plans were weak or your goals were unrealistic, you can make changes in the future.

After Tiago lost 20 pounds, he evaluated his weight loss plan. Although it had taken a long time to lose the weight, he felt good about his plan. It taught him to eat sensibly and get enough physical activity. Now that he has lost the weight, he knows he will be able to stay at the weight he wants.

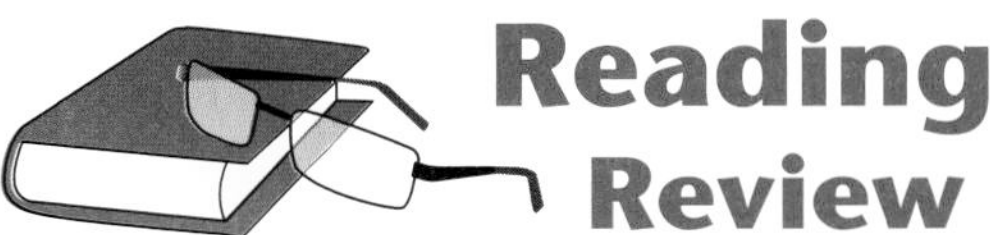

Reading Review

1. What are the steps of the management process?
2. Why do you need to set realistic goals? How do you go about doing this?
3. Why do you need to check the progress of your plan?

Time Management

Time is a limited resource. There are only 24 hours in each day for you to use. Sometimes, you may not have enough time to do the tasks you want. Some people may be able to accomplish more than you do in a day. You may wonder how you can better use your time. Using the management process can help. **Time management** is the skill of organizing your time so you can accomplish tasks.

Time	Activity
6:00 am	wake and shower
7:00 am	eat breakfast
8:00 am	school
9:00 am	↓
10:00 am	↓
11:00 am	↓
12:00 pm	lunch
1:00 pm	school
2:00 pm	↓
3:00 pm	↓
4:00 pm	soccer practice
5:00 pm	↓
6:00 pm	eat dinner
7:00 pm	homework
8:00 pm	TV
9:00 pm	go to bed

4-3 Keeping an hourly record of your activities can help you better manage your time.

Making a daily to-do list can also help you manage your time. The list reminds you of what you want to do each day. As you complete each item, cross it off the list. This can make you feel good about yourself.

Be sure to evaluate whether your to-do list has helped you better manage your time. If it has not, analyze what you have done. See what improvements you can make, and then try again.

You can identify ways in which you waste time. To do this, keep track of how you spend your day. See **4-3**. Some common time wasters include habit, clutter, and procrastination. A **habit** is a repeated pattern of behavior. Watching TV for long periods of time can be a habit. Other habits that can hurt your time management include talking on the phone and playing a video game. Habits can also be helpful. For instance, Kyle does his homework every afternoon

Succeed in Life

Improving Time Management Skills

To improve your time management, start by analyzing how you spend your time. For one day, keep a record of everything you do each hour. Your record may include sleeping, going to school, reading, listening to music, visiting with friends, or watching TV. By keeping a record of how you spend your time, you will be able to see where you waste time.

Next, plan how you want to spend your time. Set goals for what you want to do each day. Goals that are the most important should be your top priorities. Try to meet these goals first.

To implement your plan, create a schedule. Write everything you want to do that day and plan a time to do it. Following your schedule will help you do what you want to do. Write important appointments on a calendar so you remember them. Some people keep their schedules on their phones or on computers.

when he gets home from school. When he is finished, he plays video games. This habit allows him to finish his work before playing.

Clutter occurs when your personal belongings are unorganized. If your closet is cluttered, it may take you more time to get dressed in the morning. If your locker is messy, it may take you a long time to find your books and important papers. Organizing your belongings can help you save time.

Sometimes you may procrastinate. To **procrastinate** is to put off difficult or unpleasant tasks until later. Instead of doing your weekly chores, you watch TV or talk on the phone. People often procrastinate if they are scared of doing a task. For instance, Zahra wants a good grade on her book report, but she is afraid she will not do well. Therefore, she procrastinates until there is not enough time to do a good job on the project.

It is important to tackle areas in which you are procrastinating. If you have two projects to do, then do the one you dislike first. For instance, you may have both math and English homework. Start with the one you dislike the most. Once you finish, you will feel good about your accomplishment. Then do your other homework. This will help you avoid wasting time.

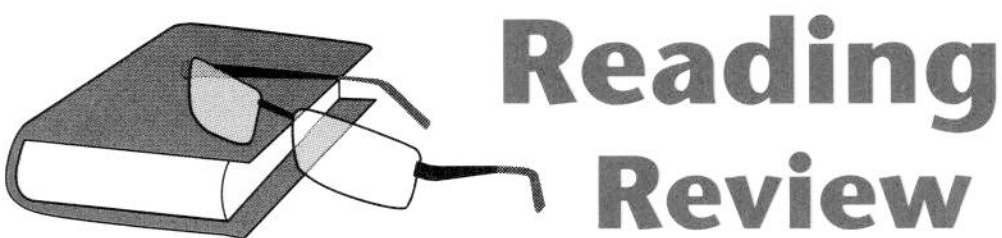

Reading Review

1. Why do you need to analyze how you use your time?
2. How does making a schedule help you manage your time?
3. What are three common time wasters?
4. Why do you need to respect other people's time?

Study Skills

Time management is an important study skill. Scheduling can help you better use your study time. Set aside a certain time and place to study each day. See **4-4**. Plan to study during the time of day you work best. Some people work better in the morning, while others work better at night. Make sure you allow enough time to complete your assignments. Some projects may take days or even weeks to complete. Do not try to finish a big project all at once. Instead, plan to work on it for an hour or two each night. This will make it seem easier, and you will often do a better job.

Your **learning style** describes the conditions under which you learn best. Think about the ways you learn best. Do you benefit most from seeing the material? If so, you may like to study by copying notes, using highlighters, and having written instructions. Do you learn best when you listen? You may remember more if you hear a lecture. To study, you can read out loud or listen to a recording. You may prefer to work with your hands. In this case, you may learn from doing a project.

Different people learn best under different conditions. Some like to work in a quiet room, while others prefer background noise. Some teens learn best when they study by themselves. Some need to work with others. By identifying your preferred learning style, you can use this information to be a better student. You can make the most of your study time.

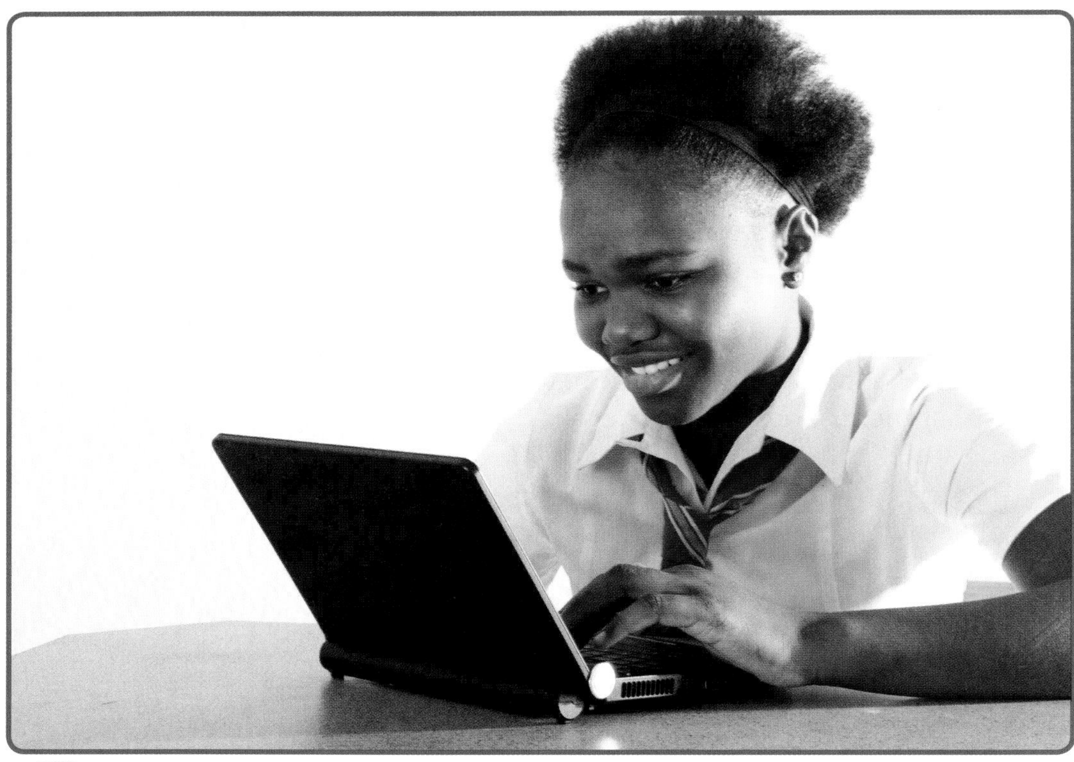

4-4 Scheduling a quiet place to study is important.

Succeed in Life

Improving Your Study Skills

Having time management skills is important to develop good study skills. If you do not set aside a certain time each day to study, you may have difficulty completing assignments. Pick a place that will provide the least amount of distractions. Avoid talking or texting with friends while you are trying to study. Also, avoid Internet surfing or other personal time-consuming activities online.

Create a list of everything you need to accomplish before you begin studying. Also, make a list of any supplies you need. This will help avoid interruptions.

Think about your current study habits. Do you study at a certain time each day? What is your study area like? Is it quiet or full of distractions? Do you make a list of everything you need before you begin? Do you take time to gather the supplies you need? Think about your answers to these questions and create a plan that will help you improve your study skills.

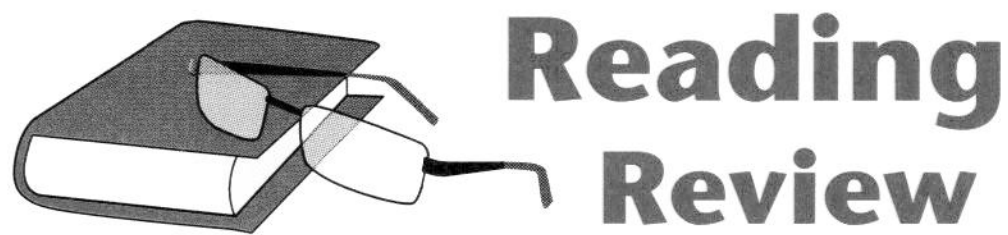

1. Explain how time management is an important study skill.
2. What are the three examples of learning styles?

Section Summary

- The management process steps include setting a goal, planning, implementing, and evaluating.
- Following these steps will help you reach your goals and get the most from your resources.
- You can also learn to manage your time better by following the steps of the management process.
- Using time management skills can help you be a better student.

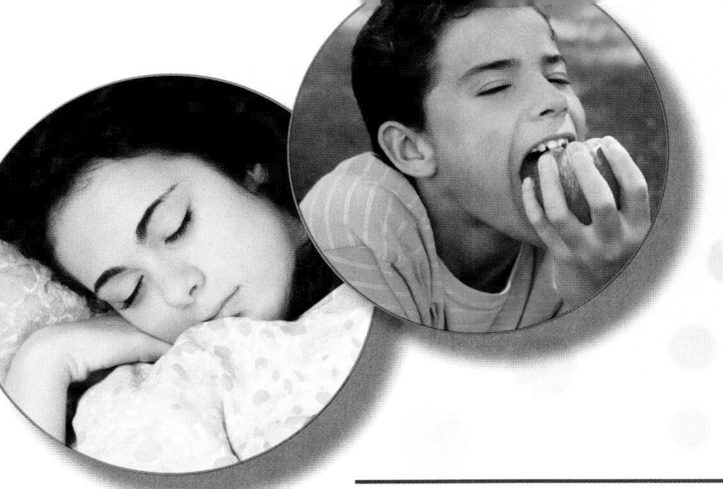

Section 4-2
Managing Your Health and Appearance

Objectives

After studying this section, you will be able to
- **define** *lifestyle*, *appearance*, *wellness*, *addiction*, *image*, *posture*, and *stress*.
- **give examples** of ways to promote wellness.
- **explain** why physical activity and rest are important to appearance.
- **show** how to use good posture when standing, walking, and sitting.
- **explain** how to manage stress.

Key Terms

lifestyle: the continuing way in which a person lives.

appearance: the way you look.

wellness: state of physical, emotional, and mental well-being.

addiction: a physical dependency to a substance.

image: the mental picture others have of a person.

posture: the way you hold your body when standing, walking, or sitting.

stress: emotional, mental, or physical tension felt when faced with change.

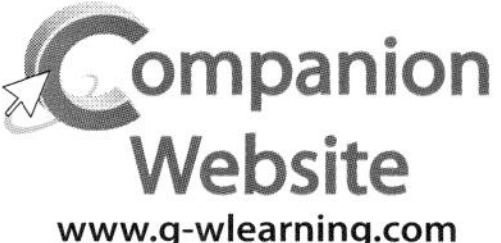

Study the Key Terms by completing crossword puzzles, matching activities, and e-flash cards at the website.

Main Ideas

- Health habits can affect the way you look.
- Eating right and getting plenty of rest and physical activity are important to your health and appearance.
- Good posture makes you look and feel better.
- Stress can be both positive and negative.

When you feel good about yourself, you are better able to manage your life. You have an improved lifestyle. A **lifestyle** is the continuing way in which a person lives. Managing your health can make you feel better and give you energy. It can improve your **appearance**, or the way you look. You need to care for your body on the inside as well as on the outside.

A healthful lifestyle promotes wellness. **Wellness** is a state of physical, emotional, and mental well-being. Eating foods that are good for you can improve your health. Also, avoid unhealthful habits. Being physically active and resting can contribute to wellness. Having a positive image and managing stress are other factors.

Eating Right

Eating the right foods in the proper amounts while you are young will help you build a healthy body. Certain foods can help you be healthy and prevent disease. These are fruits, vegetables, low-fat or fat-free milk, and whole grains.

Many snack foods do not provide any health benefits. Foods such as chips, soft drinks, candy, cakes, and pastries usually contain high amounts of sugar, fat, and salt. Eating too many foods that are not good for you may lead to weight, skin, and health problems.

Selecting healthful snacks can contribute to your health and appearance. It is a good idea to eat more vegetables and fruits and to drink more milk and fewer sugary beverages. See **4-5**.

Most people care about their appearance. You probably care about how you look. The food you eat can make a difference in your appearance. Eating the right foods in the proper amounts will help you look and feel your best. You will be better able to maintain the best weight for you. Eating the right foods can also keep your hair shiny, your skin smooth, and your eyes bright.

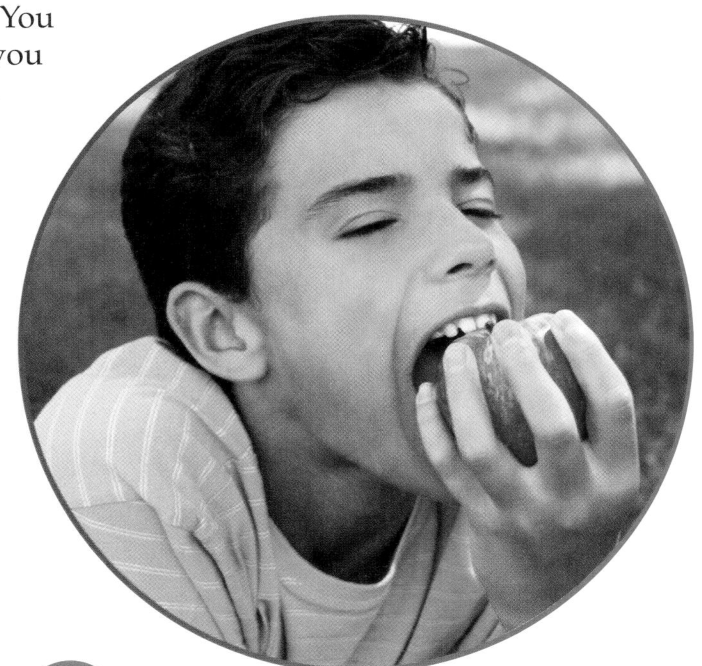

4-5 You will look and feel better when you select healthful snacks.

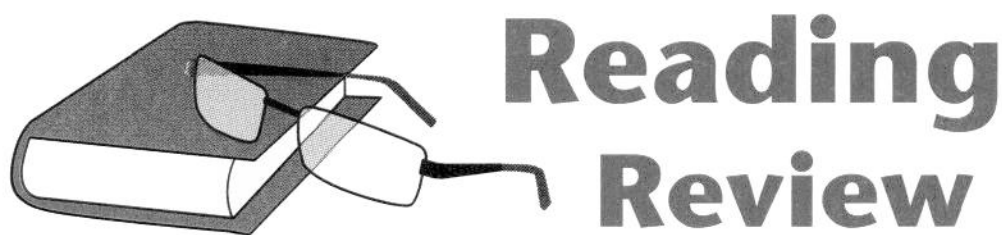

Reading Review

1. What foods can help you be healthy and prevent disease?
2. Why should you limit the amount of candy, chips, and soft drinks you consume?

Avoiding Drugs, Alcohol, and Tobacco

Many substances can be harmful to your health. Drugs can keep the body from functioning normally. Drugs can affect the mind. Alcohol is classified as a drug. It can slow reflexes and cause loss of muscle control. Alcohol can also cause lasting damage to the body if used too much. The liver, stomach, and heart may be harmed. People who do not eat because they drink too much may even starve themselves.

Cigarette smoking is the largest cause of preventable illness. Many people die each year because of tobacco use. As smoke is inhaled, the nose, throat, and lungs are irritated. The lungs and heart are damaged. Cigarettes can harm nonsmokers through secondhand smoke.

Drugs, alcohol, and tobacco can have lasting effects on health. They often cause **addiction**, which is a physical dependency to a substance. Addictions are very hard to overcome. People with addictions often need a lot of help and support to recover. Many adults developed unhealthful addictions during their teen years. To maintain a more healthful lifestyle, avoid using drugs, alcohol, and tobacco now and in the future.

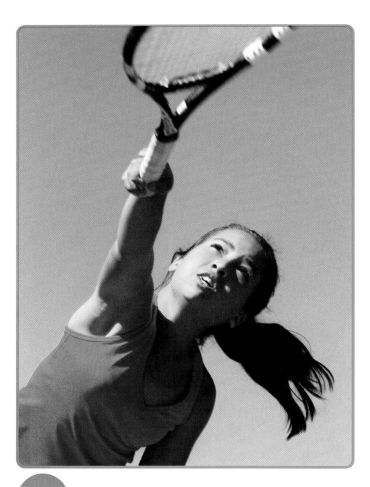

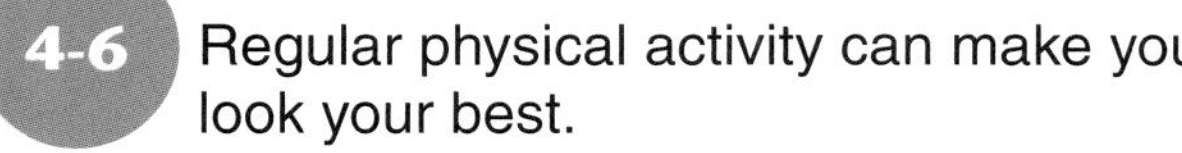

4-6 Regular physical activity can make you look your best.

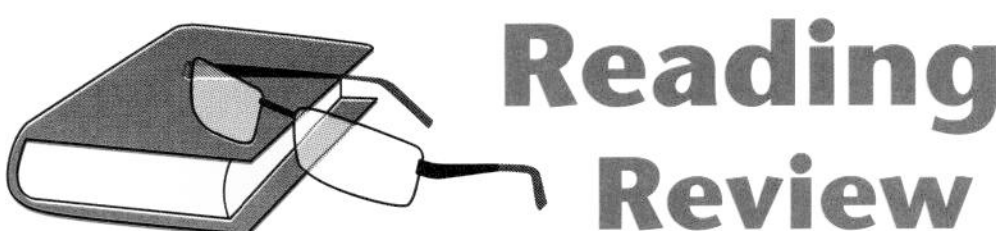

Reading Review

1. How can drugs, alcohol, and tobacco affect your health? Give examples.
2. What are the dangers of an addiction?

Being Physically Active

Being physically active is another way to improve your health and appearance. It can help you control your weight and feel more energetic. Physical activity can build your muscles and endurance. It also helps you resist diseases. You will feel more alert and learn better when you are physically fit.

Physical activity, such as walking, skating, and riding a bike helps keep you physically fit. You can take part in team sports such as football, soccer, basketball, and volleyball. See **4-6**. Getting regular physical activity with friends can be fun. Dancing, skiing, and aerobics provide good fitness opportunities. Doing errands or chores around the house also counts as physical activity. *Keep moving* is a golden rule for fitness.

When you do not get enough activity, you may feel tired. For instance, you may stay home all day and watch TV. Then you may feel tired from sitting all day. Being physically active will give you more energy. You will not feel as tired.

Physical activity can help you manage stress. Physical sports such as jogging and tennis are great ways to work off steam. Working out can make you sleep better at night. You will feel more relaxed. You can keep your muscles strong, healthy, and flexible. Your posture will improve. You will look better.

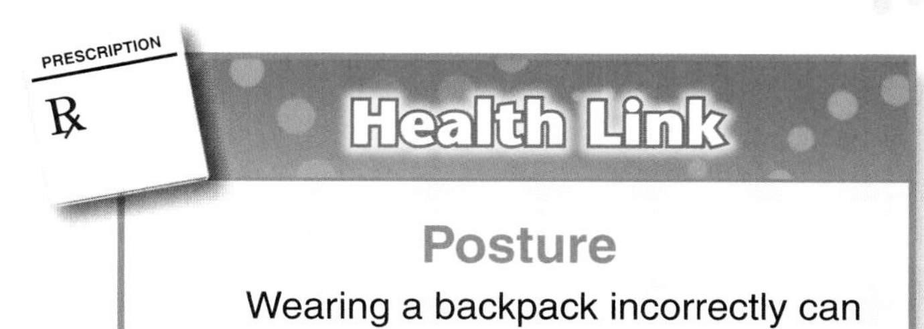

Posture

Wearing a backpack incorrectly can damage your posture. It is important to use both shoulder straps to evenly distribute the weight. Many students wear backpacks that are too heavy. This can cause permanent damage to the spine. You should not carry more than 15 percent of your body weight in a backpack. For instance, if you weigh 125 pounds, your backpack should weigh 19 pounds or less.

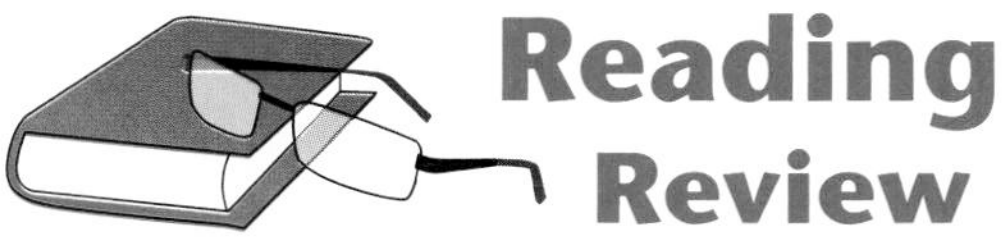

1. What are three benefits of being physically active?
2. What types of activities would you enjoy doing to be more physically active?

Establishing Your Image

Being physically fit can contribute to your appearance. You will project an image of health. **Image** is the mental picture others have of you. This can contribute to your self-concept. Your image can be influenced by your posture and your attitude.

Posture

Posture is the way you hold your body when standing, walking, or sitting. Your posture may reflect how you feel about yourself. Good posture can make you look and feel better.

Good posture when standing includes keeping your chin up and your head held high. Your legs, shoulders, and back should be straight. Always hold your body straight. If you round your shoulders and slump forward, you look sloppy. When you have good posture, your clothes will look better on you. Whether you are tall or short of stature, you appear self-confident.

Sitting straight will help you feel rested. You become tired when you slump. If you sit at a computer, it is important to support your back. Your muscles tire when you slip down in a chair.

Attitude

Your attitude can also affect your image and energy level. People who are positive reflect self-confidence. If you are self-confident, you can have the courage to deal with new experiences. Your attitude will often improve, too.

Positive feelings can make you feel energetic. Negative feelings can decrease your energy. For instance, you may not want to go out with your friends because you feel too tired. After you go, you may start to have a good time. Your attitude becomes more positive. Your energy level increases. When you are excited about something, you have more energy.

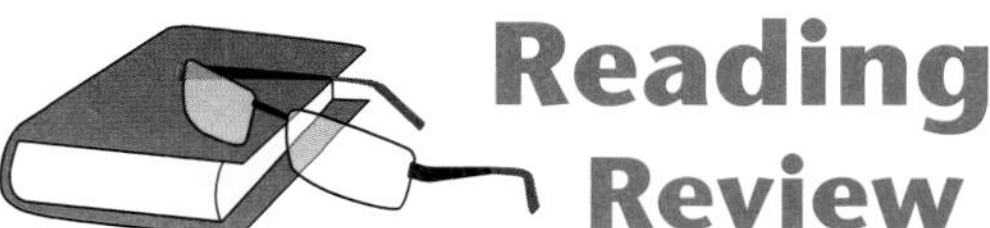

Reading Review

1. How can your posture reflect your self-confidence?
2. How can your attitude affect your image?

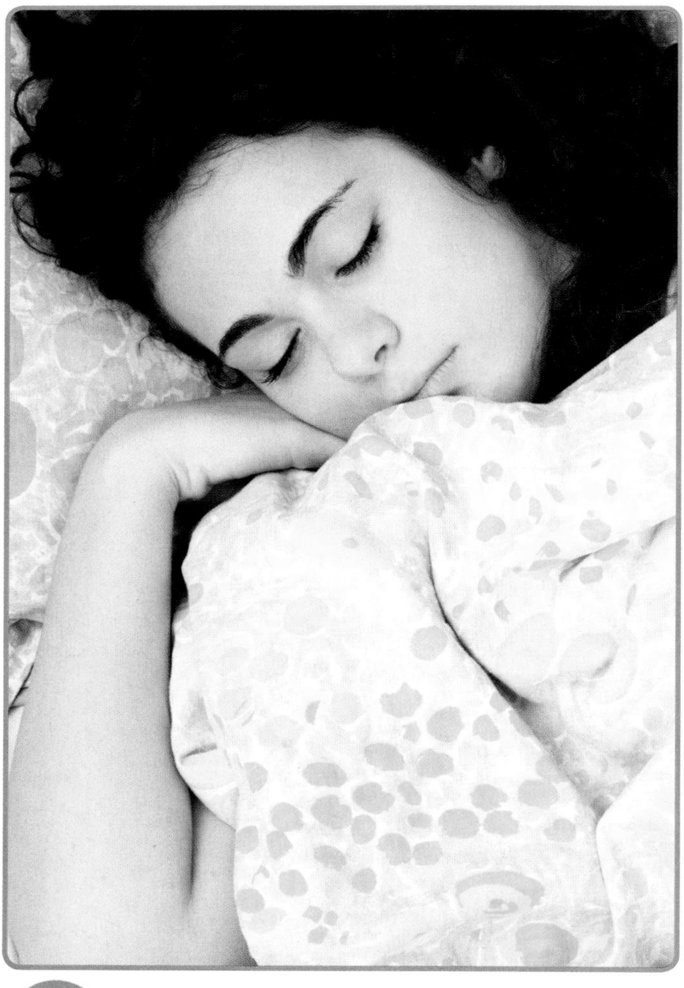

4-7 If you do not get enough sleep, you will not feel your best.

Getting Enough Rest

When you get enough rest, you look fresh and feel energetic. You add to your good health. When you are tired, your appearance, attitude, and health are affected. You may feel grouchy. Dark circles may appear under your eyes. You may not have enough energy. This can keep you from reaching your goals. See **4-7**.

Many teens need eight to ten hours of sleep each night. If you stay up late at night and get up early in the morning, you will not get enough sleep. You cannot make up lost sleep by sleeping late on the weekends. Try to get enough sleep every night.

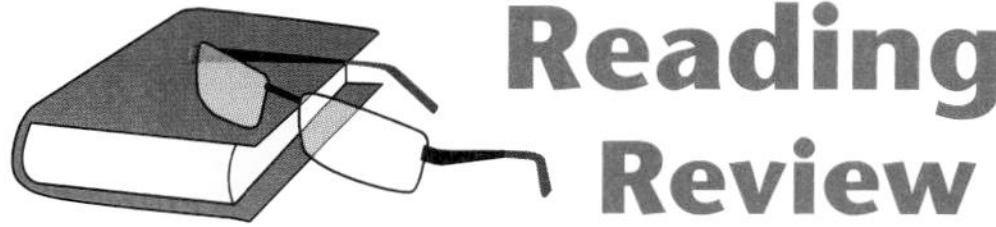

Reading Review

1. How can getting enough rest affect your appearance?
2. Why is it important to get enough sleep every night?

Handling Stress

Some people set too many goals. They do not have enough time and energy to meet their goals. This can cause stress. **Stress** is emotional, mental, or physical tension felt when faced with change. You can feel stress when you are in a new setting. Stress can also be caused by having too much to do.

When you are feeling stressed, your hands may become sweaty. Your heart may beat rapidly. You may even feel dizzy. These are all physical signs of stress. There are also emotional signs of stress. They include crying easily or acting bored, cranky, or depressed. People react differently to stress.

The leading cause of stress is change. When you are in a new setting, it is normal to feel uncomfortable. Moving to a new school or neighborhood is very stressful for many teens. Divorce, death, and illness can also cause stress. These events may cause changes in your family. A change in your family can be very hard to accept.

Following a healthful lifestyle can help reduce stress. You will be better able to cope with problems and changes if you feel your best. When you are tired, do not have enough energy, or do not eat right, situations may seem worse than they really are. Everyday problems may seem bigger. They may not be as easy for you to handle. For instance, if you are tired, you may think you do not have anything nice to wear to school. When you get enough sleep, you can be creative and put together new outfits.

Talking with someone can also help you feel less stressed. See **4-8**. Your family members and friends can often help you find ways to deal with your stress. Guidance counselors are trained to help teens learn to deal with stress. Listening to others can reduce your stress and help you deal with your problems.

Not all stress is negative. Without a certain amount of stress, you would not get up and go to school. Stress can make you study for a test. The stress of meeting new people can make you care more about how you look. The stress of a new job can make you work harder.

Stress in life cannot be avoided. The secret in handling stress is to learn how to recognize it in your life. Then, it is important to learn ways to cope with stress.

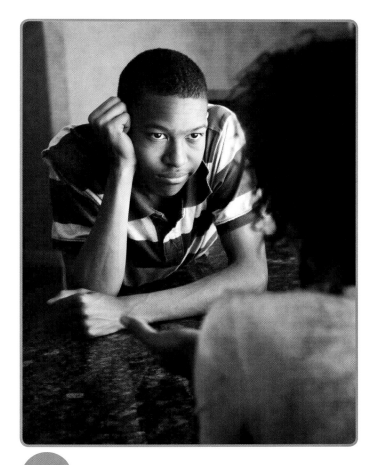

4-8 Talking with someone you trust can help you deal with stress.

Succeed in Life

Managing Your Stress

There are other actions you can take to manage your stress. You can practice good time management skills. You can prepare for events ahead of time. If getting ready for school is stressful, choose your clothes the night before. If you are worried about being in a new place, learn as much about it ahead of time as possible.

Take time to relax and have fun. Physical activity can help you cope with stress. Solving puzzles, playing games, and reading can take your mind off your stress. Many people tell their problems to their pets. Sometimes, just taking a walk will make you feel better. Many teens like listening to music when they are feeling stressed. Hobbies can be relaxing, too. What actions can you take to better manage your stress?

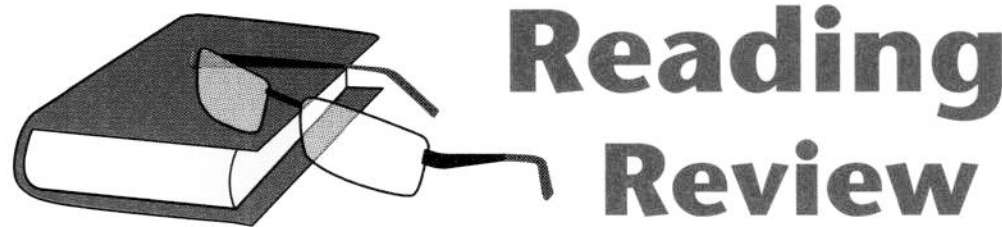

1. What are some signs that you are feeling stressed?
2. How can living a healthful lifestyle help you reduce stress?
3. How can you manage your stress? Give examples.

Section Summary

- Eat healthful foods and get plenty of physical activity to help you build a healthy body. These habits plus getting enough sleep and having correct posture can help you look and feel your best.
- Living a healthful lifestyle can help you better manage stress.

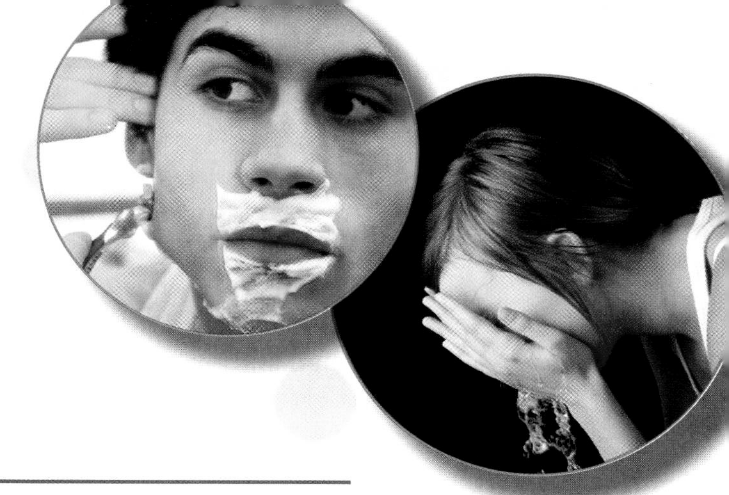

Section 4-3
Managing Your Looks

Objectives

After studying this section, you will be able to

- **define** *grooming*, *pores*, *deodorant*, *antiperspirant*, *dermatologist*, *manicure*, and *pedicure*.
- **explain** the importance of keeping your body clean.
- **list** the steps in keeping your hair and scalp clean.
- **explain** how to care for teeth.
- **state** how to care for hands and feet.

Key Terms

grooming: cleaning and caring for your body.

pores: tiny openings in the skin.

deodorant: a product that helps destroy or cover unpleasant body odors.

antiperspirant: a product that helps control wetness and covers unpleasant body odors.

dermatologist: a doctor who specializes in treating the skin.

manicure: a method of caring for hands and fingernails.

pedicure: a method of caring for feet and toenails.

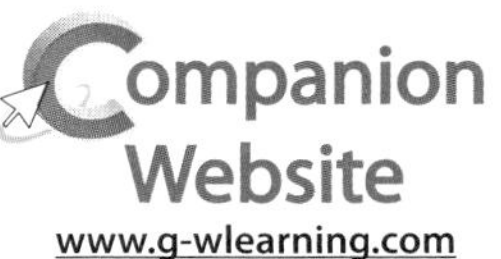

Study the Key Terms by completing crossword puzzles, matching activities, and e-flash cards at the website.

Main Ideas

- Good grooming adds to your health and appearance.
- There are steps you can follow to care for your body.

Grooming is cleaning and caring for your body. Good grooming habits help you look attractive and feel positive about yourself. These habits can add to your health by preventing illness. Being well-groomed is a factor in getting and keeping a job.

It is important to form good grooming habits while you are young. You will probably keep some of the habits you form now for the rest of your life. Part of managing your daily living includes making plans to care for your appearance.

Keeping Clean

Your skin has **pores**, or tiny openings. Pores give off oil and sweat that collect on your skin. Dirt and dust from the air also collect on your skin. You need to wash often to remove these substances. If you do not, your body may have an unpleasant odor. Blemishes may develop on your skin. See **4-9**.

When you shower, bathe, or wash your face or hands, be sure to rinse away all traces of soap. Soap left on your skin can cause it to become dry and irritated.

Bathing and showering regularly can help prevent body odor. These grooming habits, however, cannot do the job alone. You also need to use a deodorant or antiperspirant. A **deodorant** is a product that helps destroy or cover unpleasant body odors. An **antiperspirant** is a product that helps control wetness and covers unpleasant body odors. These products are applied to the underarm area. They work best when used right after a bath or shower.

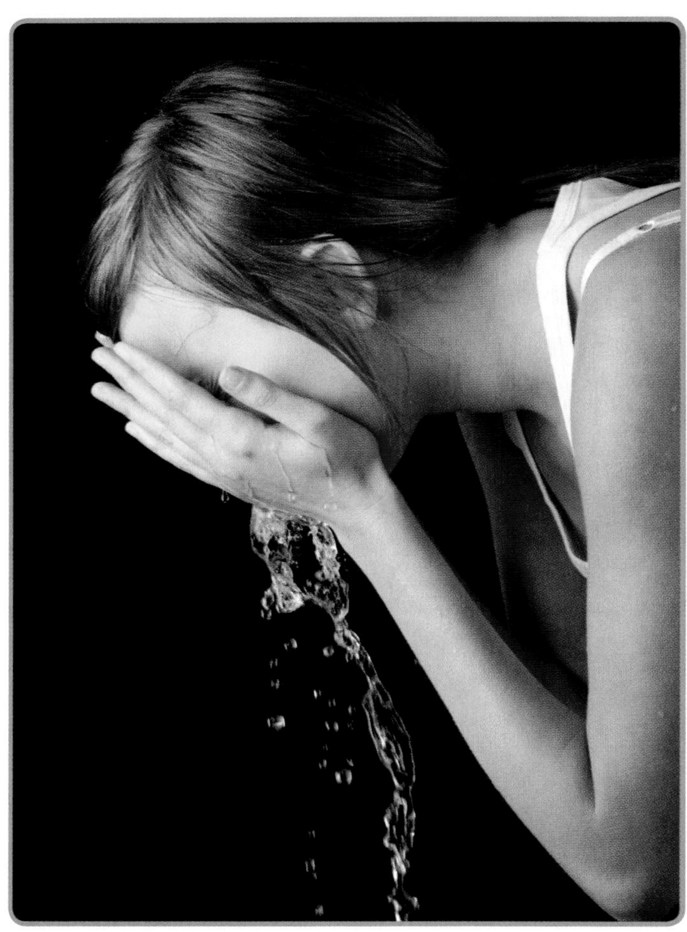

4-9 Wash your face thoroughly at least twice a day.

As a teen, you are growing in many ways. This growth causes chemical changes in your body. Some of these chemical changes may cause blemishes such as blackheads and pimples. These often occur around the nose and on the chin and forehead. They may also occur on the back and chest. When pimples develop, they should not be squeezed. This can cause infection and scarring.

If you have blackheads or pimples, wash the affected areas often with soap. Eating right, being physically active, and getting plenty of rest may also help clear up your skin. Doctors also suggest drinking at least eight glasses of water a day. For severe skin problems, see a dermatologist. A **dermatologist** is a doctor who specializes in treating the skin.

Succeed in Life

Proper Hair Care

When you wash your hair, use your fingertips to rub your scalp. This will help loosen any dirt or dandruff. Be sure to get your scalp clean. This is where the oil comes from that causes dirty hair. Be careful not to rub with your fingernails. If you scratch your scalp, you may get an infection. Also, if you rub too roughly, your hair may become tangled. This may cause strands of hair to break or split.

Rinse your hair thoroughly to remove all traces of shampoo. You may want to use a conditioner that adds moisture and body as well as removes tangles. If you have braids, you may want to use a deep-conditioning treatment once a month. After washing your hair, use a comb instead of a brush to gently comb out the tangles.

Remember that your hair is delicate. When brushing your hair, be careful. Brushing too hard can damage your scalp and hair.

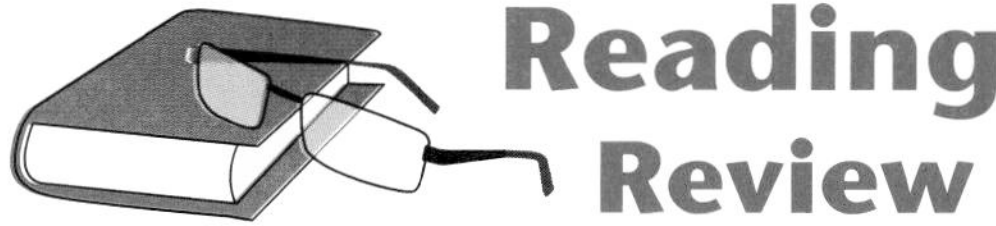

Reading Review

1. What is the difference between a deodorant and an antiperspirant?
2. What can happen if pimples are squeezed?

Hair Care

Your hairstyle is a frame for your face. A good hairstyle can help you look attractive by accenting your positive features. The shape of your face and your type of hair determines how a hairstyle will look. Have a friend, parent, barber, or hairstylist help you choose a flattering hairstyle.

When choosing a hairstyle, also consider the type of hair you have. Look at the texture. If it feels hard and wiry and looks thick, you may have coarse hair. If it feels smooth and soft and looks thin, you may have fine hair.

Is your hair straight, wavy, or curly? This will influence the best style for you. Also, think about your activities. Decide how much time you are willing to spend caring for your hair. For instance, you may be in sports and need a hairstyle you can care for easily.

Hairstylists can also change the appearance of your hair through various procedures. See **4-10**. Use caution when using chemicals with your hair. Many

Hairstyling Terms	
Relaxers	Chemicals applied to straighten hair.
Perms	Chemicals applied to add curls or waves to hair.
Color	Chemicals that will change the color of the hair.
Weaves	Weft of hair (natural or synthetic) bonded, sewn, or braided into hair.
Braids	Hair that is divided into small sections with three or more strands intertwined.
Locks	Strands of hair that are permanently intertwined. Hair that would normally shed is caught up with the rest to form a cordlike *lock*.

4-10 These procedures can help you create popular hairstyles. They can also damage your hair.

chemicals that relax, perm, or color the hair can cause damage. Braids that are too tight can cause hair loss or breakage.

After you have a good cut, be sure to get your hair trimmed on a regular basis. Trimming hair prevents split ends. This keeps your hair healthier. Many young men get their hair trimmed every four weeks. Young women may get their hair trimmed every six to ten weeks. Your hair grows approximately one-half inch per month.

To keep your hair and scalp clean and healthy, wash your hair regularly. How often people wash their hair varies. Wash your hair when it gets dirty. People with oily skin often have oily hair. Oily hair needs to be washed more often than dry hair. Select a shampoo based on your type of hair.

Some flaking of skin cells from your scalp is normal. Excessive flaking is a condition called *dandruff*. Some shampoos are made to treat dandruff. If you have an extreme case, you may need to see a doctor. Also, do not use other people's combs or brushes. This can transfer unhealthful scalp conditions.

After you wash your hair, you can let your hair dry naturally. You can also use a blow dryer. If you use a blow dryer, be careful. Heat can cause your hair to break and split. Keep the blow dryer at least six to eight inches from your hair. Keep it moving constantly so your hair does not get too hot.

Let your hair cool from the heat before brushing it. Make sure it is completely dry before using a curling iron or hot rollers. Hair that has been treated with chemicals is easily damaged by heat.

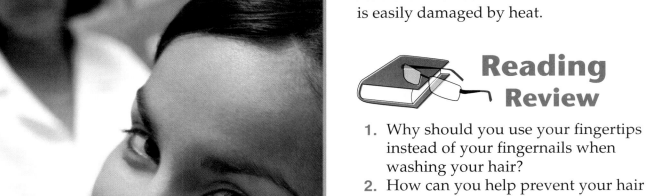

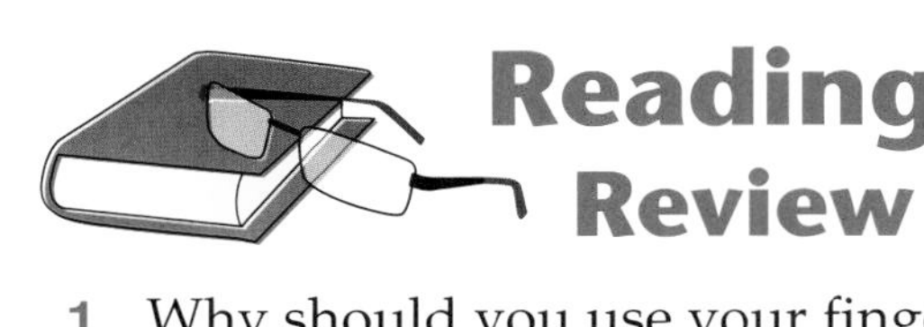

Reading Review

1. Why should you use your fingertips instead of your fingernails when washing your hair?
2. How can you help prevent your hair from being damaged by heat?

Caring for Your Teeth

Healthy teeth and gums are important to your health. It is important to care for your teeth properly. Visit your dentist every six months. See **4-11**. Your dentist will examine your teeth and give you advice on how to care for them.

Removing food from your teeth is important. Regular brushing will help your teeth stay clean and gums healthy.

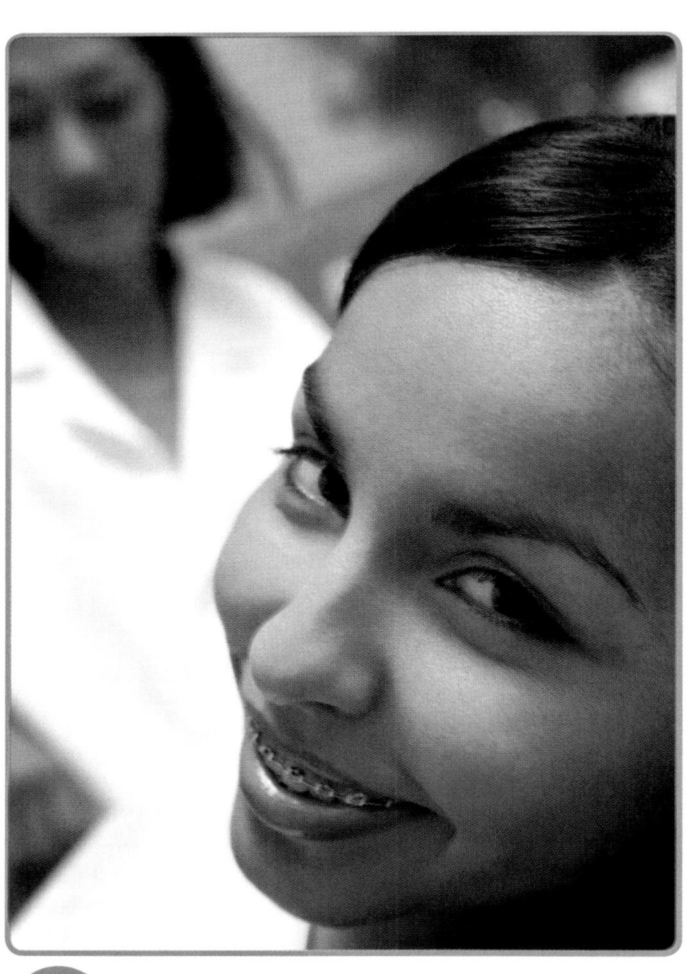

4-11 An orthodontist is a dentist who can help with straightening teeth.

You should brush your teeth after each meal. This helps remove food from around and between your teeth. If you are not able to brush, rinse your mouth out with water.

Also, use dental floss at least once a day. Dental floss is used to remove food from between the teeth and at the gums. Using dental floss is as important as brushing. Many cavities are caused by pieces of food that cannot be removed with a toothbrush. Your dentist can show you the correct way to brush and use dental floss.

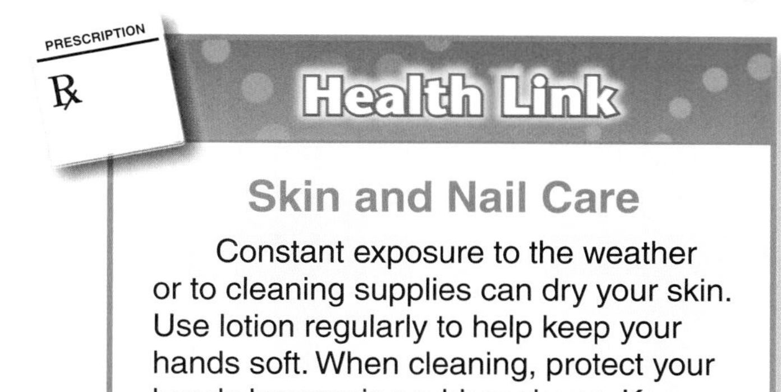

Skin and Nail Care

Constant exposure to the weather or to cleaning supplies can dry your skin. Use lotion regularly to help keep your hands soft. When cleaning, protect your hands by wearing rubber gloves. Keep your nails strong and healthy by avoiding the habit of biting your fingernails.

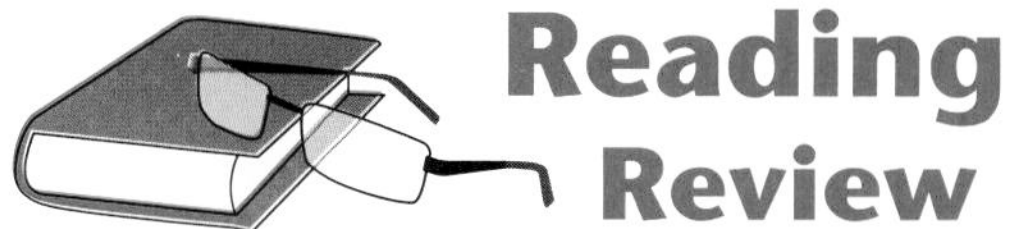

1. How often should you brush and floss your teeth?
2. What should you do if you cannot brush your teeth after a meal?

Caring for Your Hands and Feet

Wash your hands thoroughly several times a day. This will keep them looking good and prevent spreading germs. Always wash your hands before meals and after using the toilet.

When you wash your hands, use warm water and soap. Lather the soap on your hands and wrists. Use a nailbrush to remove dirt under your nails and around your cuticles. Remove all traces of soap with warm water. Dry your hands thoroughly. This helps prevent rough, chapped hands, which can be painful.

To keep your nails attractive and in good condition, you can give yourself a manicure and a pedicure. A **manicure** is a method of caring for hands and fingernails. A **pedicure** is a method of caring for feet and toenails. It is important for both males and females to take care of their hands and feet.

To give yourself a manicure or a pedicure, first file and shape or trim your nails. Then soak them in warm, soapy water to soften the cuticles. Finally, push back the softened cuticles. Some girls may want to apply nail polish to their nails.

Shoes and socks that do not fit properly may cause foot and back pain, blisters, and rough spots on your feet. Do not wear shoes and socks that can cause these problems. When you buy shoes, try on both shoes to check the fit. One of your feet may be larger than the other. Make sure both shoes are comfortable.

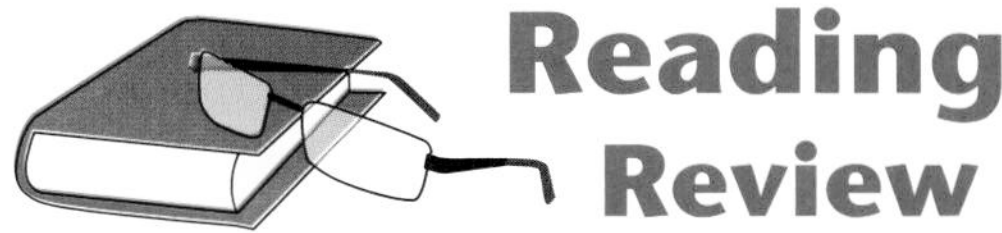

1. What are the steps to follow when washing your hands?
2. Why is it important to try on both shoes when buying a new pair?

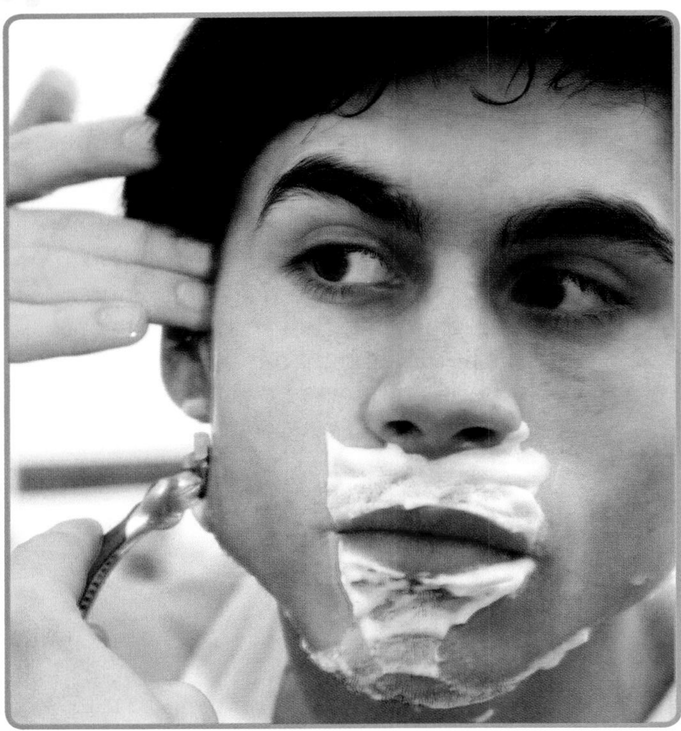

4-12 Shave carefully to keep from cutting yourself.

Personal Care

As girls begin to grow into adults, hair growth under their arms and on their legs becomes heavier. Guys start growing more hair on their faces, arms, legs, chests, and under their arms. Girls may shave their legs and underarms. Guys usually shave their faces.

When shaving, choose a razor that is comfortable to hold and easy to use. Wet the area to be shaved with warm water. Apply shaving cream or a rich lather of soap. This helps soften your hair. It also helps prevent the razor from cutting or irritating your skin. See **4-12**. Shave in the opposite direction from which your hair grows. Rinse off the soap or cream after shaving. Then apply lotion to your face or legs to prevent dryness.

Some teen girls wear makeup. Makeup includes eye shadow, powder, blush, mascara, and lipstick. There are special types of makeup for different skin types and problems. Read the labels on the makeup packages to make sure you have the right type for you. Salespeople at cosmetic counters can also help you.

Apply makeup lightly. This helps keep the look natural. Makeup should also be applied to clean skin. Always remove makeup before going to bed. Makeup applied to dirty skin or makeup left on overnight can lead to skin problems. This can result in blackheads and pimples.

Do not lend makeup or borrow it from other people. Germs can be spread through makeup.

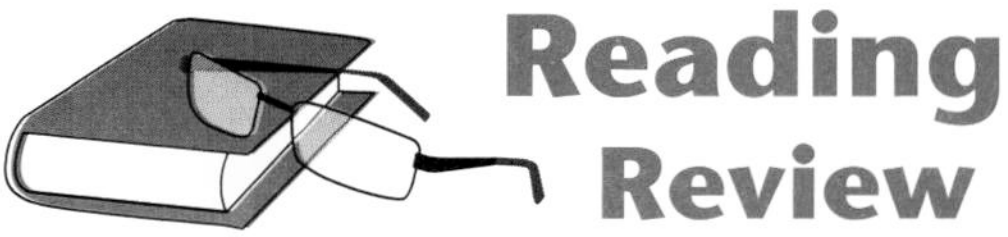

Reading Review

1. How does applying shaving cream or a rich lather of soap help when shaving?
2. What can happen if you leave makeup on overnight?

Section Summary

- Keeping your body clean will help you feel and look more attractive.
- To be well-groomed, take proper care of your skin, hair, teeth, and nails.
- Some of the grooming habits you form now will probably continue throughout your lifetime.

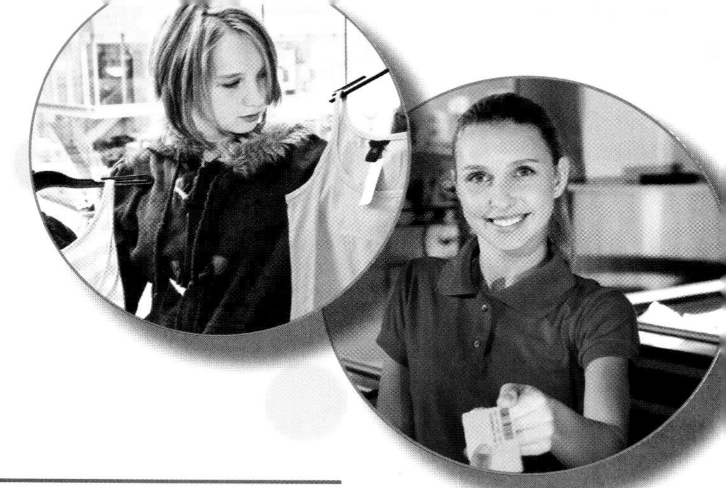

Section 4-4
Managing Your Money

Objectives

After studying this section, you will be able to
- **define** *income*, *money management*, *budget*, *fixed expenses*, *flexible expenses*, *credit*, *consumer*, and *warranty*.
- **tell** how to make a budget.
- **list** the different ways to pay for purchases.
- **give examples** of how you can shop wisely.

Key Terms

income: the money you earn.
money management: the process of planning and controlling the use of money.
budget: a plan for spending.
fixed expenses: costs that remain the same on a regular basis.
flexible expenses: costs that may change from month to month.
credit: a way to pay that lets you buy now and pay later.
consumer: a person who buys or uses goods and services.
warranty: a written guarantee for a product from the manufacturer.

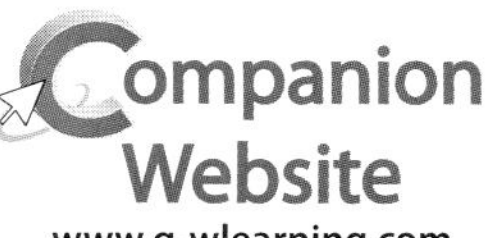

Study the Key Terms by completing crossword puzzles, matching activities, and e-flash cards at the website.

Main Ideas

- Making a budget can help you better control your money.
- You can pay for purchases in a variety of ways.
- Good consumer skills can help you save money.

You may get money as a gift or as an allowance. You may earn money babysitting or doing yard work. The money you earn is called your **income**. Your income may be small. You can, however, begin developing money management skills. **Money management** is planning and controlling the use of money. You can use these skills now and in the future as your income increases.

Making a Budget

An important part of money management is making a budget. A **budget** is a plan for spending. Before you make a budget, keep a record of all the money you spend in one week. This helps you better understand your spending habits.

The first step in writing a budget is to list all your income. Knowing how much money you earn can help you control your spending. You know how much you have to spend.

Next, list your expenses. Expenses can be both fixed and flexible. **Fixed expenses** are costs that remain the same on a regular basis. Examples may include music lessons or a car payment. See **4-13**. **Flexible expenses** are costs that may change from month to month. Examples may include movies, video games, books, clothes, or eating out.

The money you save should be listed as a fixed expense in your budget. When you save, you are setting aside money from your income for later and unexpected uses. You may also be saving for a special purchase. For instance, Zoe is saving money to buy a new bike. Each week, she puts the same amount of money in her savings account.

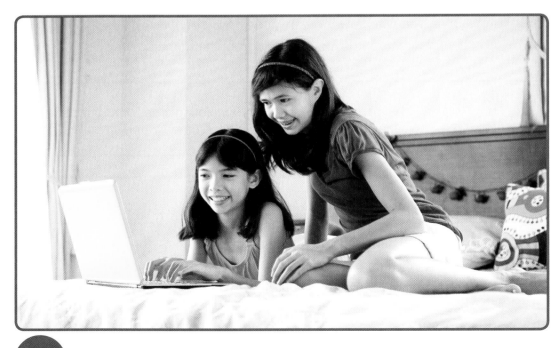

4-13 A monthly Internet fee is an example of a fixed expense.

To keep track of your budget, set up a record-keeping form. See **4-14**. This form will show you how well you are following your budget. First, add your income and then your expenses. Compare the two totals. They should be the same or very close. If your expenses are more than your income, reduce your flexible expenses or increase your income. You cannot spend money you do not have. If your income is greater than your expenses, you can spend more money. You may also decide to save more money.

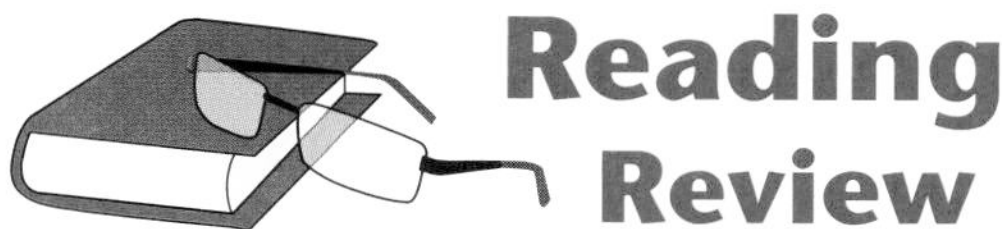

Reading Review

1. How can a budget help you manage your money?
2. How do record-keeping forms help you keep track of your budget?

Paying for Purchases

You can pay for items using cash or a layaway plan. You can also use checks and credit, debit, or gift cards. When you go shopping, decide in advance how much money you plan to spend. You should also decide which payment method you want to use. This will save you time when you are ready to make your purchase.

Monthly Budget			
Income		**Expenses**	
Allowance	$60.00	**Fixed Expenses**	
Babysitting	$75.00	Music lessons	$45.00
Gifts	$25.00	Savings	$20.00
		Flexible Expenses	
		Movies	$16.00
		Snacks	$15.00
		Music	$15.00
		Clothes and Accessories	$34.00
		Books and Magazines	$5.00
		School Supplies	$5.00
		Other Expenses	$5.00
Total	$160	**Total**	$160

4-14 Following a written budget can help you avoid overspending.

Financial Literacy Link

Use Credit Wisely

Using credit can add to the cost of an item when interest and finance charges are added. Many credit cards charge an annual fee for having a credit card. Credit cards also have a finance charge. This includes the interest, service and transaction fees, and other fees for the loan. There is usually a *grace period* of 25 days in which no interest fees are charged, if the bill is paid in full. Having a credit card can lead to overspending. If you do not pay your credit card bills on time, then it will be difficult to get credit in the future.

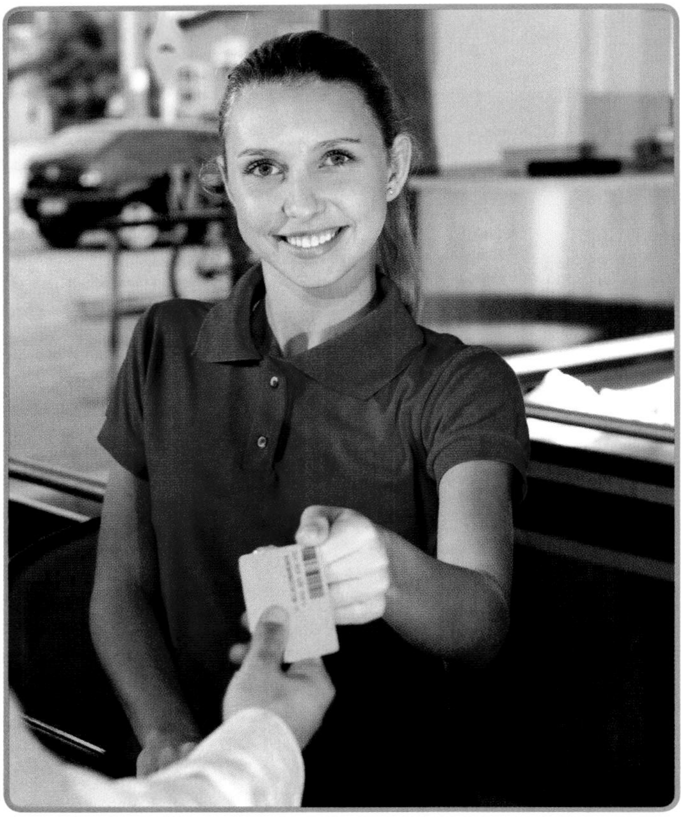

4-15 Before you use a debit card, ask your bank if there are additional fees for using it to make purchases.

Using cash is an easy way to pay. When you use cash, you know exactly how much money you are able to spend. Before you pay, make sure you have enough cash with you. As you pay, count the bills and change carefully. Also, be sure to count the change you receive.

If you do not have enough cash, you may want to use the store's layaway plan, if available. A *layaway plan* is an arrangement in which you pay a small deposit for the item so the store will hold it for you. Then, you must make payments each week or month for a certain amount of time. When you finish paying for the item, you can take it home.

Paying with checks is similar to using cash. When you write a check, however, the bank deducts the money from your checking account. The bank then adds the money to the account of the person or business receiving the check. Keep in mind you cannot write checks for more than the amount of money you have in your account. Some stores do not accept checks.

Your bank may also issue you a debit card. You can use a *debit card* to electronically deduct the amount of a purchase from your checking account. See **4-15**. You will be given a Personal Identification Number (PIN) to protect your debit card from being used by others. Do not share your PIN with anyone.

Another way to buy purchases is with credit. **Credit** is a way to pay that lets you buy now and pay later. Credit is often used if you do not have enough cash or are buying a costly item. People must apply for credit cards. Companies then issue the cards to people who earn enough money and can afford payments.

A *gift card* allows you to spend a designated amount on purchases. You may receive a gift card or a prepaid credit card for future purchases as a present. Remember to treat the cards as cash and keep them in a safe place.

Always handle cash, checks, and debit, gift, and credit cards carefully. Carry them in a wallet or purse. Keep your wallet or purse close to you. Do not lay it down when you are shopping. Do not share your debit or credit card security codes or other personal information, except to show proof of identification to the salesperson.

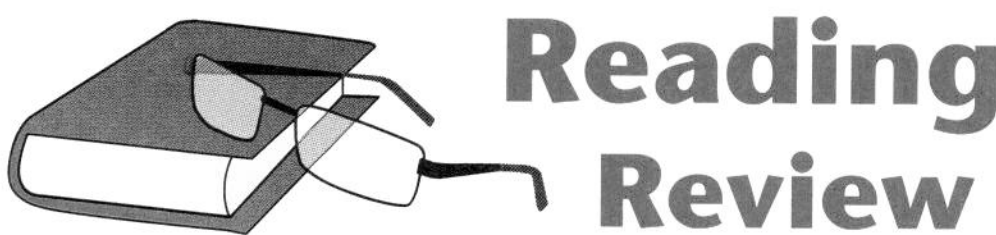

Reading Review

1. If you do not have enough cash on hand, what other forms of payment can you use?
2. Why should you always handle cash, checks, and debit, gift, and credit cards carefully?

Consumer Skills

A **consumer** is a person who buys or uses goods and services. You are a consumer when you shop. You are also a consumer when you use a service. For instance, when you get a haircut, you are being a consumer. As a consumer, you can learn skills to help you manage your money. You will learn to get the most for your money.

One important skill is *comparison shopping*. When you shop, you may notice the price of a product often varies from store to store. In order to get the most for your money, compare prices at several stores.

You should also learn how to figure the unit price of the product. The *unit price* is the cost for each unit of measure or weight. Usually, if you buy a large amount of a product, its unit price will be lower than the small amount. This may not, however, be the best size for you to buy. If you do not use the product quickly, it may spoil. Also, if you are trying a new product, you may want to buy the smallest size to test it.

Besides comparing price, you should also compare quality. *Quality* refers to how well a product is made. It also refers to how well a product performs and how long it lasts. A high price for a product does not always mean quality. Sometimes, a lower-priced product may be of better quality. See **4-16**.

You can gather information about the quality of products from many sources. For instance, you want to buy a new gaming system. Ask friends or family members

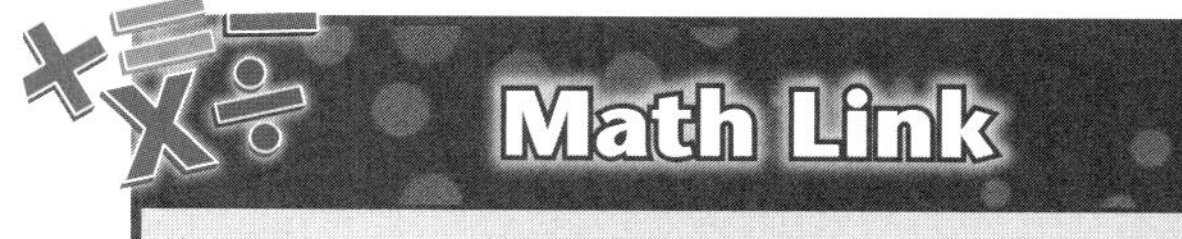

Math Link

Figuring Unit Price

To find the unit price of a product, divide the price of the product by the unit of measure or weight. After figuring the unit price, compare the products to see which is really less costly. For instance, one bottle of shampoo weighs 8 ounces and costs $6.40. The unit price is $.80 an ounce. Another bottle of shampoo weighs 10 ounces. It costs $10.00. The unit price is $1.00 an ounce. The first bottle of shampoo is less expensive than the second bottle. What would the unit price be for a bottle of shampoo that weighs 6 ounces and costs $5.25?

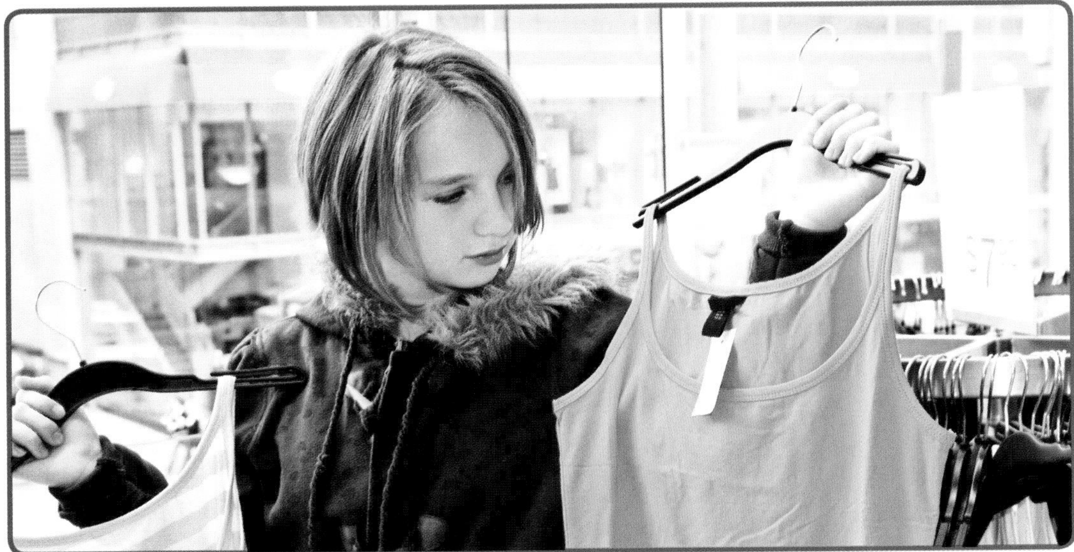

4-16 When you are shopping, compare both price and quality to get the most for your money.

who have bought the gaming system what they think. Talk to salespeople who sell gaming systems. Read about them in consumer magazines, such as *Consumer Reports*. Research various gaming systems online.

Be sure to read the labels on products when you are shopping. The government regulates what must be included on product labels. Labels can give you information about nutrition and package contents. Labels also include directions for use of the product and the warranty. A **warranty** is a written guarantee for a product from the manufacturer. Some information on labels is not as important. For instance, companies often put information on labels to help them sell their product.

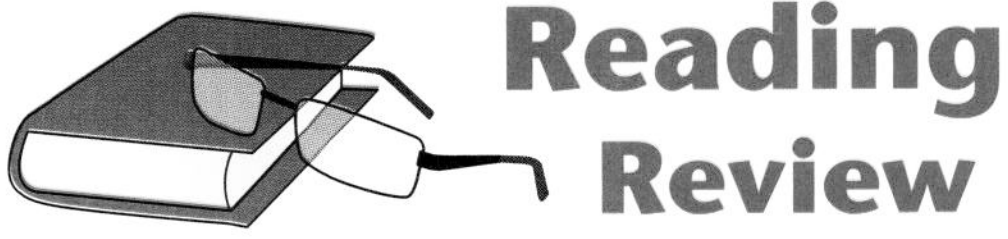

Reading Review

1. Should you always buy the lowest-priced product? Why or why not?
2. What helpful information should you look for on labels?

Section Summary

- As a consumer, you need skills in money management.
- Making a budget and following it can help you learn money management skills.
- There are various ways to purchase items.
- You can also learn to shop wisely. These skills will help you get the most for your money.

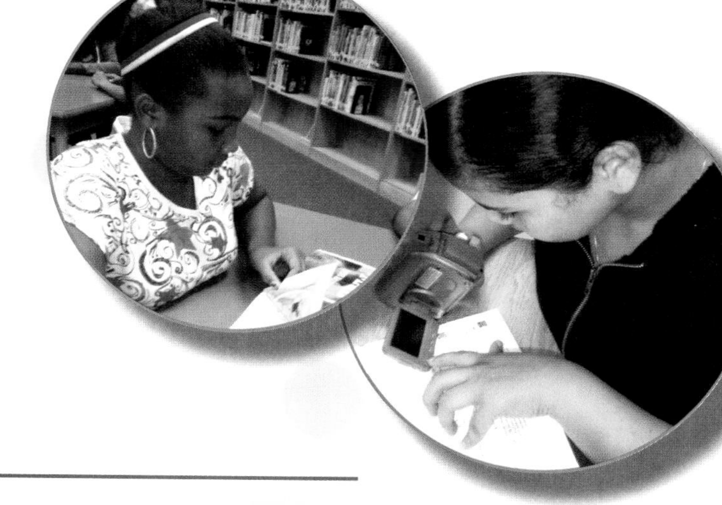

Section 4-5
Making Consumer Decisions

Objectives

After studying this section, you will be able to

- **define** *consumer decisions*, *mass media*, *advertising*, and *impulse buying*.
- **explain** how needs, wants, values, and goals affect consumer decisions.
- **give examples** of how peers, mass media, and advertising can affect what you buy.
- **list** the six basic consumer rights.
- **tell** how you can be a responsible consumer.

Key Terms

consumer decisions: choices you make about how to spend your money.

mass media: a means of communicating to large groups of people.

advertising: the process of calling attention to a product or a business through the mass media.

impulse buying: making an unplanned or spur-of-the-moment purchase.

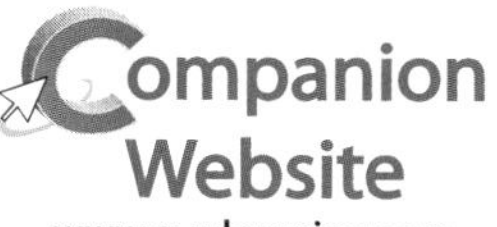

Study the Key Terms by completing crossword puzzles, matching activities, and e-flash cards at the website.

Main Ideas

- Your needs, wants, values, and goals affect your consumer decisions.
- Peers, mass media, and advertising affect consumer decisions.
- You have six basic consumer rights.
- You can be a responsible consumer.

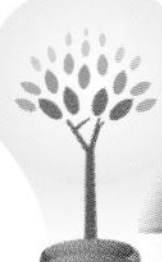

Think Green

Disposable or Reusable?

If you value the environment, you may choose a reusable product over one you cannot reuse. For instance, some people prefer to buy reusable sports bottles rather than bottled water. They are concerned with the number of disposable water bottles added to landfills daily.

Investigate how plastic bottles are disposed at your school. Are there recycling bins? Conduct a trash audit by looking at the number of plastic bottles in the general trash containers. Think about why people buy so many plastic water bottles. What makes this a good or bad consumer decision? What is the better choice for you?

You make decisions as a consumer every day. Someday, others may depend on you for financial support. Your money management skills may then be even more important. The way of life for you and your family will depend on your consumer decisions. Knowing your consumer rights and responsibilities can help you make good decisions.

Consumer Decisions

Consumer decisions are choices you make about how to spend your money. When you buy a product, you make decisions. You may not even be aware of some of these decisions. They are, however, important. Sometimes, outside pressures may affect your decisions.

When you shop, you should think about your needs, wants, values, and goals. They affect how you earn money and how you manage it. Many needs and wants can be met by spending money. For instance, people meet their need for shelter by buying or renting a home. Learn to make consumer decisions that will let you meet as many needs and fulfill as many wants as possible. See **4-17**.

Your values and goals also affect your consumer decisions. Your values help you decide which products to buy. If you value the environment, you may

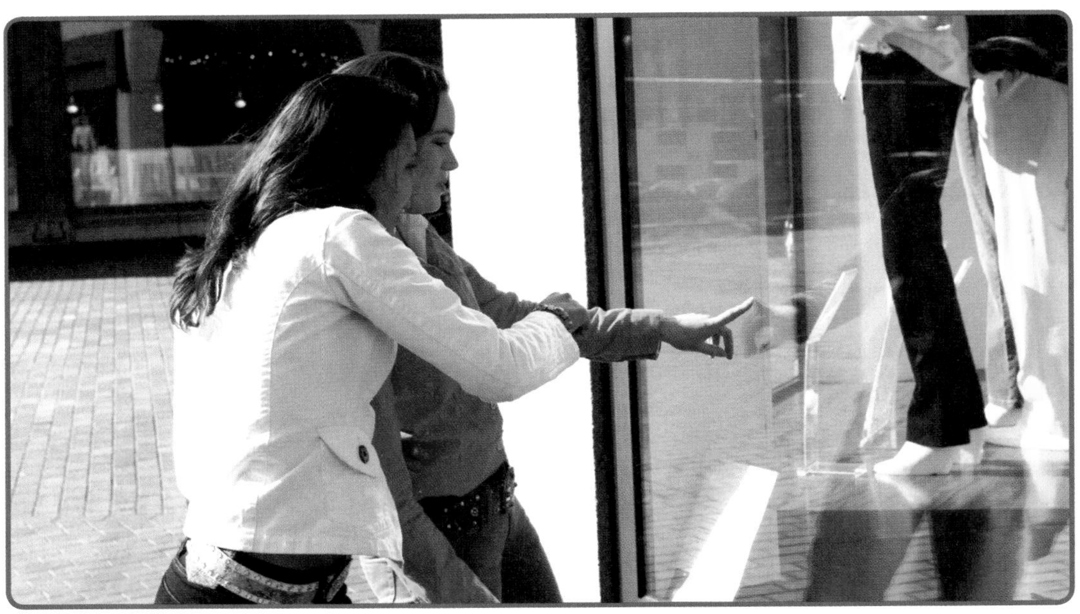

4-17 You cannot always afford to buy what you want.

choose a reusable product over one you cannot reuse. Your goals affect how you use your money. For instance, your goal may be to buy a new pair of skis. While you are saving money for the skis, you may spend less on other products.

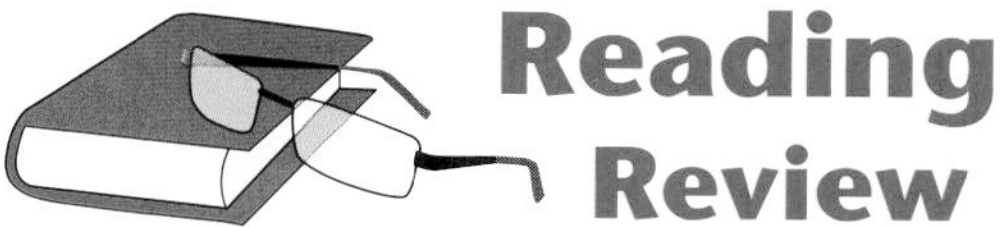

Reading Review

1. How can your consumer decisions affect your family?
2. How do your values help you decide which products to buy?

Outside Pressures

Your consumer decisions are affected by a number of outside pressures. These pressures include peers, mass media, and advertising.

Your peer group can affect your consumer decisions. As a teen, it is normal for you to want to fit in with your peers. You want to look and act like them. You may decide to buy products because your peers have them. This can give you a feeling of belonging. It may also help you fit in with the group. Be careful, however, not to give in to peer pressure when you know it is wrong.

Mass media is a means of communicating to large groups of people. It includes TV, radio, movies, billboards, magazines, Internet, and newspapers. Mass media can affect your consumer decisions. You may buy clothes or copy hairstyles you see on TV or in magazines. You may buy music you hear on the radio. Magazines and newspaper articles show people what is popular and trendy.

The most powerful pressure from mass media comes from advertising. **Advertising** is the process of calling attention to a product or business through the mass media. Companies pay the media to use their advertisements. They hope the advertisements will sway consumers to buy their products. See **4-18**. The price of products includes the cost of advertising. As a result, consumers really pay for advertising.

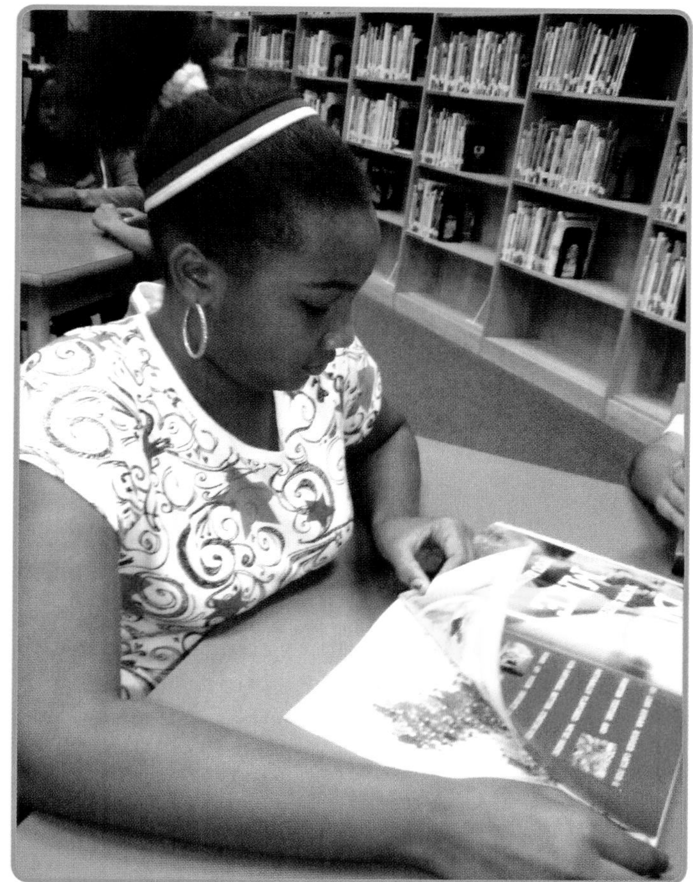

Deborah Tippett

4-18 Magazine advertisements influence many consumer decisions.

Many ads can be found on the Internet. Banners and pop-ups can appear while you are online. Most companies have websites to advertise their products. Consumers are encouraged to visit the websites to gain information. Some sites have contests and games. The contests are often used to collect e-mail addresses and other information about the shoppers.

Advertisements can be useful when they provide information about a product or service. Useful information includes facts about the size and color of the product. The uses of the product and its price are important. Knowing what care the product needs is also helpful. Advertisements give you information to compare products and services. This helps you make informed decisions.

Advertising can also influence you to buy products you do not need and may not want. These advertisements only want you to buy. Few or no facts are given about the product. Attention is given to emotions or feelings connected to the product. Advertisements use appeals to make you think you need the product. They may say you will be happier with their product. Some ads promise you will be popular. Others say you will look better if you use their service.

Advertising appeals can lead to impulse buying. **Impulse buying** is making an unplanned or spur-of-the-moment purchase. Impulse buying is unwise because you may not be sure what you want to buy. You also may not have enough information to be ready to make a good decision. Take time to get the facts about what you want to buy. Do not be rushed into a quick decision by advertisements.

As a responsible consumer, view advertising carefully. Use it to help you gather information about products. Do not be pressured to buy something you do not need or want.

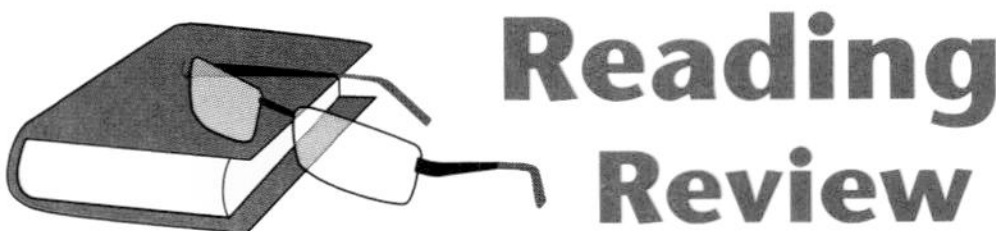

Reading Review

1. How can peers influence you to buy certain products?
2. How can the mass media affect your consumer decisions?
3. How can you use advertising to make informed decisions?

Consumer Rights

In 1962, the Consumer Bill of Rights was created. It stated that consumers have four basic rights. They are the right to choose, the right to be heard, the right to safety, and the right to be informed. Two other basic rights were added later. They are the right to redress and the right to consumer education. These rights protect you from unsafe products and services. They also give you power as a consumer. See **4-19**.

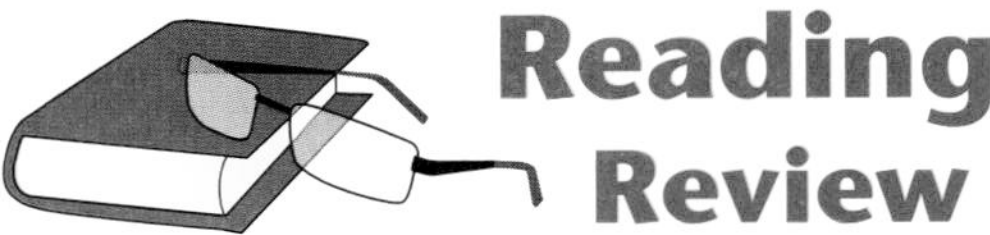

Reading Review

1. How do you benefit from your consumer rights?
2. How do government agencies help protect your consumer rights?

Consumer Rights	
The Right to Choose	You have the right to choose among products and services. When you shop for a product, you can choose from more than one brand. You have a choice about where to buy products and services. You can choose to buy the products and services that are the best for you.
The Right to Be Heard	You have the right to speak out when you have a complaint about a product or service. You can express your point of view about laws that affect consumers.
The Right to Safety	You have the right to know the goods and services you buy are safe. Government agencies test products to make sure they are safe. The agencies keep unsafe products from being sold. These agencies also listen to your complaints about unsafe products.
The Right to Be Informed	You have the right to the facts you need to make informed consumer decisions. This means having the correct information about credit costs, and how to use and care for products.
The Right to Redress	The right to *redress* means that wrongs done to you will be corrected. If you buy a flawed product, you have the right to return it to the store. The store should listen to your complaint and act upon it. Government and consumer agencies can help you with this.
The Right to Consumer Education	You have the right to information about your consumer rights. The government provides ways for you to learn about your rights. It publishes pamphlets and offers programs to inform you of your rights and the laws concerning them. They also use websites to educate the consumer.

4-19 These are some of the rights you have as a consumer.

Consumer Responsibilities

With rights come responsibilities. To keep your consumer rights and have them be meaningful, you must behave responsibly. Take action to make these rights work for you. Think about your responsibilities when you use products and services. The following are tips on how to be a responsible consumer:

- When you shop, comparison shop. Refuse to buy poor quality products. Choose only the services that best meet your needs. Refuse to buy goods and services that are harmful or cause pollution.
- Write to manufacturers and the government to express your concerns and complaints. Share your compliments with them, too.
- Use products safely if you expect them to remain safe. See **4-20**. If a product is unsafe, report it to the seller, the manufacturer, and the government.

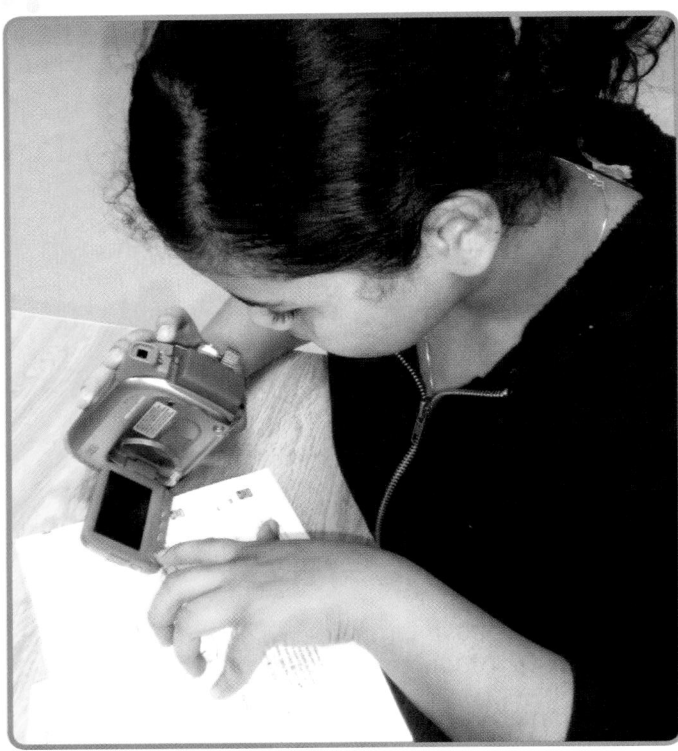

Deborah Tippett

4-20 Read use-and-care manuals to learn how to correctly use products.

- If you have a problem with a product, talk to the seller. If you are fair and polite, most sellers will listen. Sometimes, however, you may need to write the manufacturer about the problem. Most product labels include the address of the company. You may also be able to find the company's address online or at your local library.
- Keep informed of new consumer laws. Read government pamphlets explaining your rights. Read findings published by agencies that test new products.

You also have other responsibilities as a consumer. You can help control store losses by handling goods carefully so they do not break or become damaged. Do not shoplift. Take good care of what you buy. Avoid wasting products. Do not overbuy during shortages. Instead, share limited supplies.

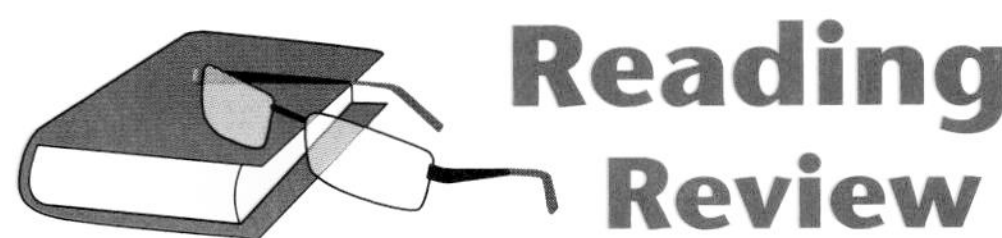

Reading Review

1. How can you show responsibility as a consumer?
2. What can you do to help control store losses? Give examples.

Section Summary

- Your needs, wants, values, and goals affect your consumer decisions.
- Your peers, the mass media, and advertising also affect some of your consumer decisions.
- There are six basic consumer rights.
- As a consumer, you also have responsibilities.

Chapter Summary

The management process helps you set and reach goals. There are four steps in the management process. First, set a goal. Then work out a plan or schedule to meet that goal. The third step is to implement or carry out a plan of action. The fourth step is to evaluate the goal and plan. Was it a good plan? Was the goal realistic?

The four-step management process can help you succeed as you begin making more decisions about your life. You will use the management process over and over again. It will help you make decisions about how to manage your health and appearance. It will also help you manage money.

Your consumer decisions are more important as you become more responsible for spending money. Your needs, wants, values, and goals affect your consumer decisions. Your peer group affects what you decide to buy and when. Mass media and advertising also influence what you buy.

There are six basic consumer rights that protect you as a consumer. Along with these rights come responsibilities. Understanding these can help you make good consumer decisions.

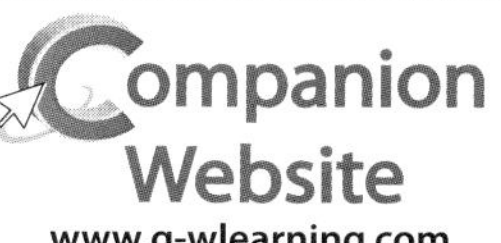

Review Key Terms and Main Ideas for Chapter 4 at the website.

Chapter Review

Write your answers on a separate sheet of paper.

1. List the four steps of the management process.
2. A written plan for reaching goals within a certain period of time is a(n) _____.
3. _____ is a physical dependency on a substance.
4. How can drugs and alcohol affect your health?
5. How can physical activity affect the way you feel?
6. What does your posture tell others about you?
7. True or false. Most teens need no more than six or seven hours of sleep each night.
8. True or false. Change is the leading cause of stress.
9. How can you benefit from having good grooming habits?
10. The tiny openings of the skin are _____.
11. What can you do to prevent body odor?
12. True or false. Blow dryers should be kept six to eight inches from your hair.
13. You should use dental floss at least _____ a day.
14. Why is comparison shopping a good skill to have?
15. Give examples of how advertising can influence your consumer decisions.

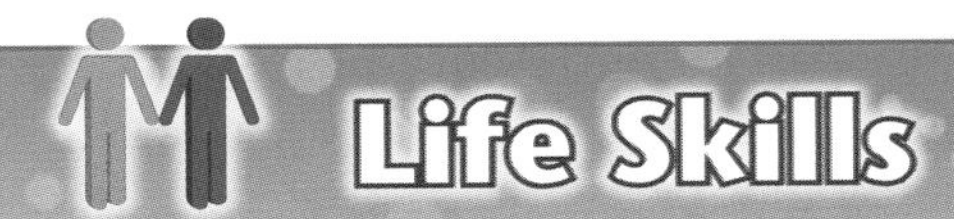

16. Your next-door neighbor, Kevin, has asked for your advice. He is having trouble staying awake in school. He feels tired and sluggish during the day. He often procrastinates in turning in his work at school. His grades are falling and his parents are upset with him. This is causing him to feel stress. You know he comes home from school and gets on the computer in his room to play games for hours. He is not physically active, and he eats a lot of junk food. Think about advice you could give Kevin to improve his lifestyle. Use the management process to help Kevin develop a plan to improve his life. How could this plan relieve some stress? What time management hints could you share with him? What strategies for improving his health could you suggest?

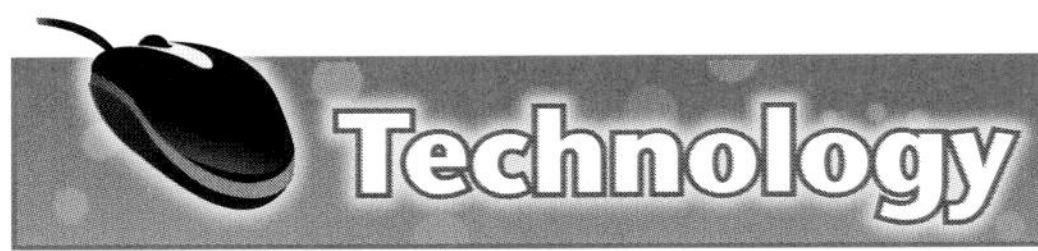

17. On the Internet, research current information and guidelines on the use of backpacks. Create a presentation of your findings using presentation software. In your presentation, include information on injuries caused by not wearing the backpack correctly and carrying too

much weight. Also, list ways to cut down on the weight in a backpack. Share your presentations with the class.

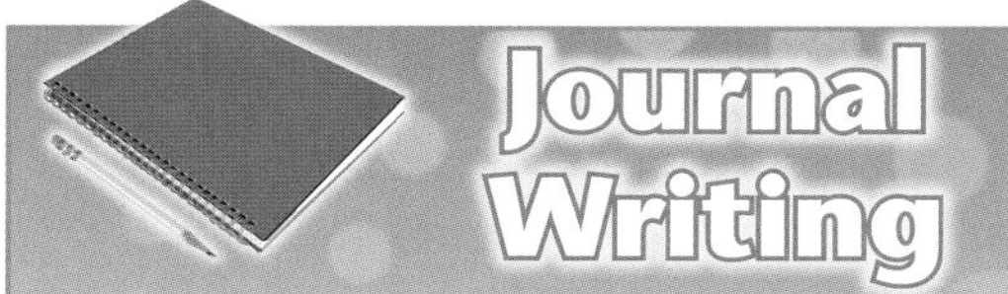

18. For one day, keep a record of all your activities in your journal. Then analyze how you spent your time. Look at how much time you spent sleeping, eating, attending school, doing homework, and relaxing. Based on this record, make a schedule for yourself to follow the next day. Allow time for your priorities. Also, allow time to relax. Try following your schedule. How did following your schedule help you to better manage your time?

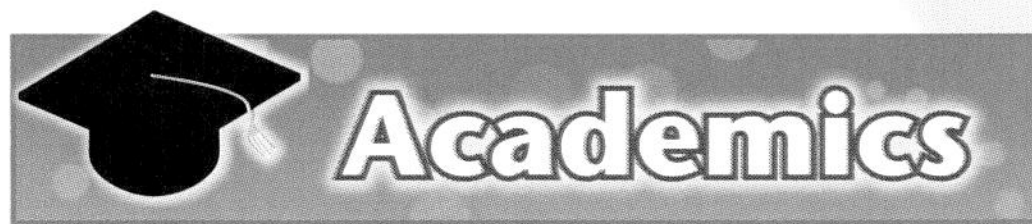

19. **Financial Literacy.** You received $50 from your grandparents for your birthday. Make a budget for how you will spend this money. Keep in mind the many different ways you can use your money.
20. **Writing.** Write a short story about a teen who has a goal to reach. Show how this teen uses the steps in the management process to reach this goal.
21. **Math.** Go to a store and find a product that comes in several sizes. Write the price for each size of the product. When you return to class, figure the unit price for each size of this product. Discuss whether the product with the lowest unit price would be the best buy for you.
22. **Speech.** Role-play a situation in which you are returning a defective product to a store. Show right and wrong ways to do this. As a class, discuss the consumer rights and responsibilities involved in this situation.

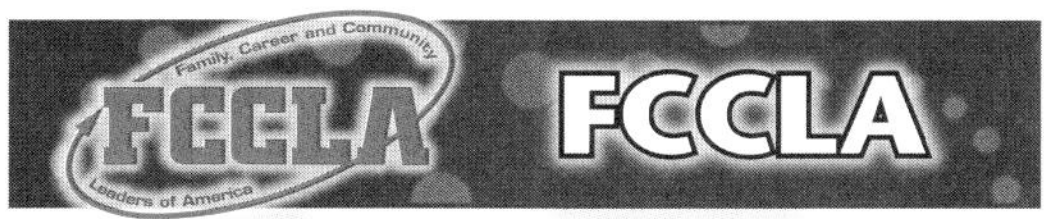

23. Track and plan your personal spending over the next three months so it stays within your income. Think of creative ways to make the most of the nonhuman resources you have access to now. Are there ways you and your friends can help each other save money? What activities and purchases could become part of a group effort? What are some new and different ways to acquire things you may want that do not require cash? Develop an FCCLA *Cash Control* project for the *Financial Fitness* program. Obtain further information about this program from your FCCLA advisor.

Chapter 5
Managing Your Living Space

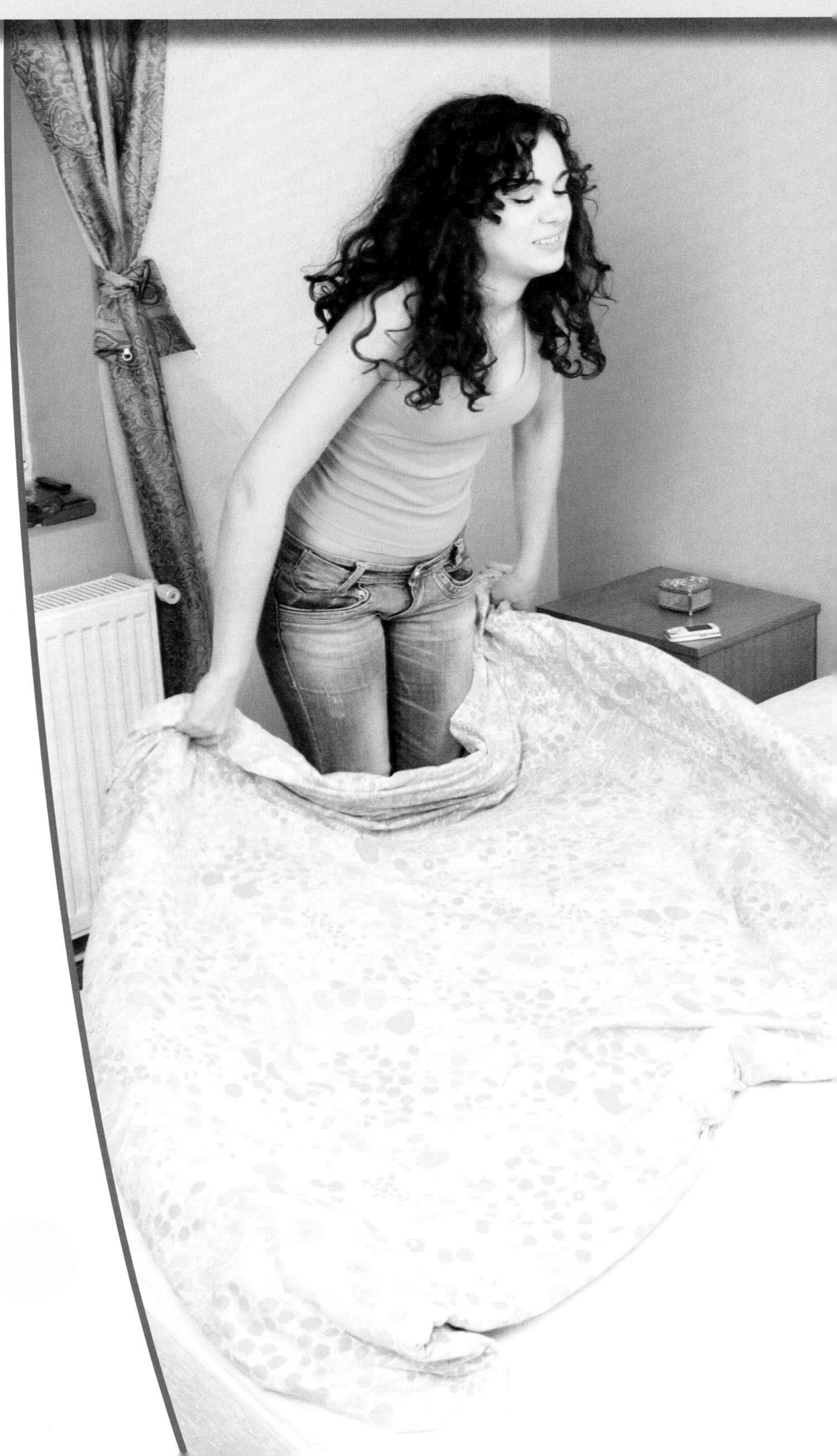

Sections

5-1 Your Living Space
5-2 Home Safe Home
5-3 Caring for Your Home

Sharpen Your Reading

Take time to reread sentences or paragraphs that cause confusion or raise questions. Rereading will clarify content and strengthen your understanding of key concepts.

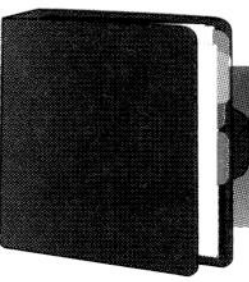

Concept Organizer

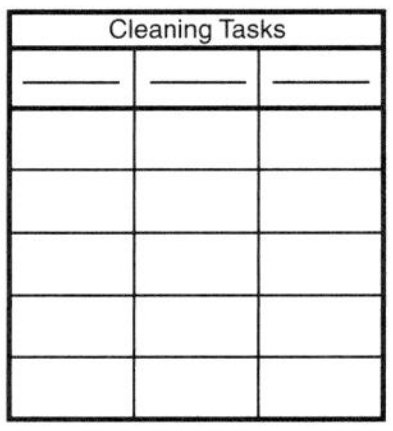

Cleaning Tasks		
____	____	____

Some cleaning tasks need to be done more often than others. Use a chart diagram like the one shown to list how often most cleaning tasks should be done. Show the three time periods; then write the recommended tasks under each one.

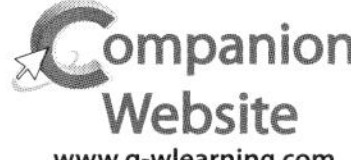

Print out the concept organizer at the website.

Section 5-1
Your Living Space

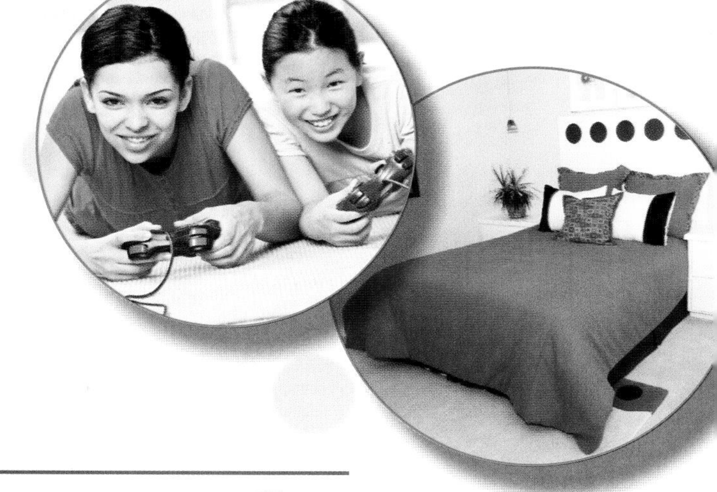

Objectives

After studying this section, you will be able to
- **define** *home*, *house*, *universal design*, *scale floor plan*, and *traffic patterns*.
- **describe** ways homes meet needs.
- **give** some tips for sharing space in a home.
- **show** how to use a scale floor plan.
- **explain** how the elements and principles of design and your values, goals, and resources can affect the way you decorate your space.
- **list** some tasks you can perform when moving to a new home.

Key Terms

home: any place people live.

house: a freestanding, single-family dwelling.

universal design: the concept of designing homes and environments to be flexible and functional for all residents, including those with disabilities.

scale floor plan: a drawing that shows the size and shape of a room.

traffic patterns: paths people follow as they move within a room.

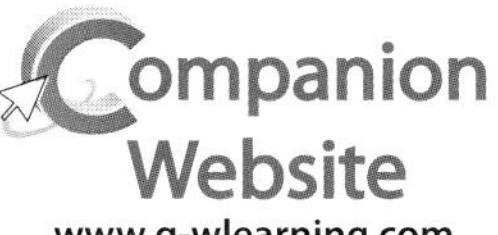

Study the Key Terms by completing crossword puzzles, matching activities, and e-flash cards at the website.

Main Ideas

- Homes meet physical, emotional, and social needs.
- Every home has shared space and private space.
- Carefully arranging your furniture and storage space can help you make the best use of your room.
- Your values, goals, and resources will affect how you decorate your space.
- Moving can be stressful, but there are tasks you can perform to make the transition easier.

Your living space is in your home. A **home** is any place people live. Apartments, mobile homes, and houses are all types of homes. A **house** is a freestanding, single-family dwelling.

Homes Meet Needs

Homes meet many needs for people. See **5-1**. Your home meets your physical needs for shelter and safety. Having a roof over your head protects you from bad weather. Having locks on your doors helps protect you from crime.

Homes help meet people's emotional needs. Your home is a place where you are free to express yourself. Having a home gives you a sense of belonging.

Your home can also meet some of your social needs. You can enjoy being with family members and friends in your home. You can treasure moments alone in your home, too.

A home should meet each family member's needs. **Universal design** is the concept of designing homes and environments to be flexible and functional for all residents, including those with disabilities.

For instance, if a family member has a physical disability, he or she needs to be protected from falling. Special features, such as ramps and wider hallways and doors, can be built. These design features allow those who use wheelchairs and crutches to move safely.

Kitchens and bathrooms can also be specifically designed for people with physical disabilities. The height and accessibility options of important areas, such as cooking surfaces and showers or bathtubs, can be adjusted. See **5-2**.

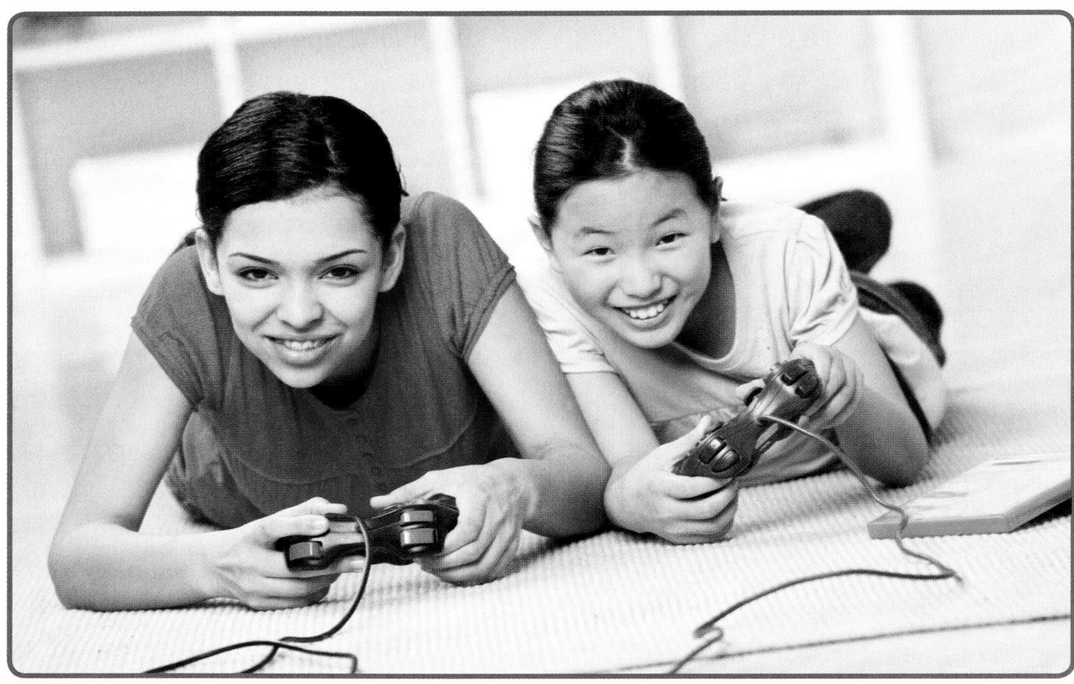

5-1 At home, you can relax and spend time playing with friends.

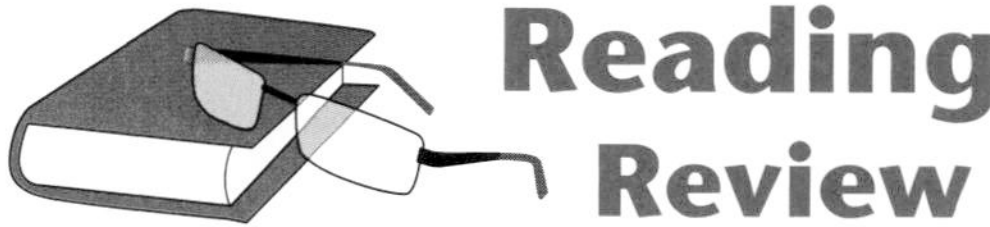

1. What physical needs can a home meet? How can a home meet these needs?
2. What are some of the emotional and social needs a home can help you meet?
3. What are some examples of universal design?

Sharing Space

In every home, there is shared space and private space. *Shared space* is the area you share with members of your family and guests. You need to make shared space comfortable for everyone. You can contribute by helping take care of the space.

Private space is an area that is only yours. It can be a bedroom or part of a room. You may read, study, or listen to music in your private space. You may just spend time thinking or relaxing with friends there.

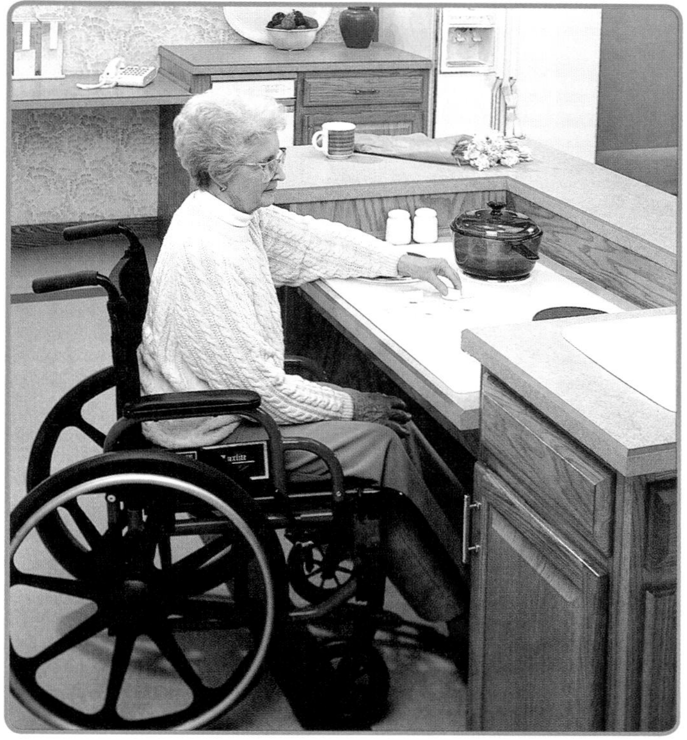

Whirlpool

5-2 Specially designed kitchens are safer for people with physical disabilities.

Even if you share a bedroom, you and your brother or sister can both have private space. To avoid problems when sharing a room, you must respect each other's rights. This means respecting your brother or sister's privacy when he or she wants to be alone. If the door is closed, knock before going into the room. Respect his or her belongings, too. If you want to borrow something from your brother or sister, ask first. Make it clear you would like him or her to show you the same respect.

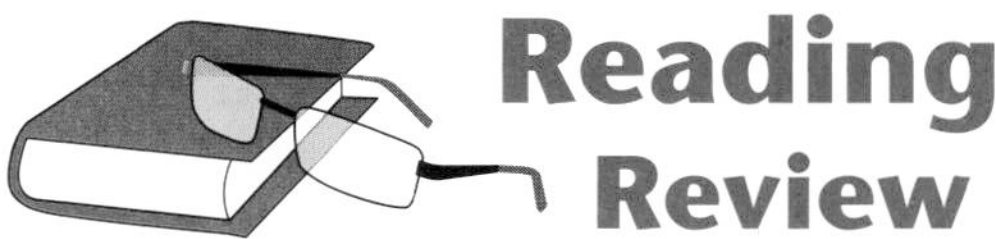

1. Name some shared spaces in your home. How can you help to keep these spaces comfortable for everyone?
2. What can you do to help avoid problems when sharing a bedroom?

Arranging Your Space

Even if you share a room, careful planning can help you get the most from your private space. Plan how to arrange your furniture and your storage space. If you share a room with your brother or sister, discuss these plans together.

Math Link

Drawing a Scale Floor Plan

You can draw a scale floor plan of your room on graph paper. First, measure the length and width of your room. Then, measure or locate the dimensions of each piece of furniture you want to use in the room. Finally, use colored paper to cut out scale-sized pieces to represent your furniture. Place the furniture pieces on your scale floor plan. Try different arrangements. When you find the best arrangement, glue the pieces on your floor plan. You can also use a computer graphics program to draw your room and furniture to scale.

A **scale floor plan** is a drawing that shows the size and shape of a room. Using a scale floor plan can help you arrange the space in your room for the best advantage. A certain number of inches on the scale floor plan equals a certain number of feet in the room. Special symbols are used to show doors, windows, and closets. The symbols for the room in Figure **5-3** are defined next to the scale floor plan.

Drawing a scale floor plan can save you time and energy. You can find a good arrangement before you move the furniture.

When arranging furniture, allow space for traffic patterns. **Traffic patterns** are the paths people follow as they move within a room. Leave at least two feet of space between pieces of furniture so people have room to walk. Also, leave space to use the furniture. For instance, you need room in front of a dresser to open the drawers.

Once you have arranged your furniture, decide how to arrange your belongings. You can use hidden or displayed storage space to store objects in your room. *Hidden storage* is space for storing items out of sight. Hidden storage spaces include closets, chests, or trunks. *Displayed storage* is space for storing items in view. Displayed storage spaces include shelves, desks, and tables. Some guidelines for arranging your storage space are listed in **5-4**.

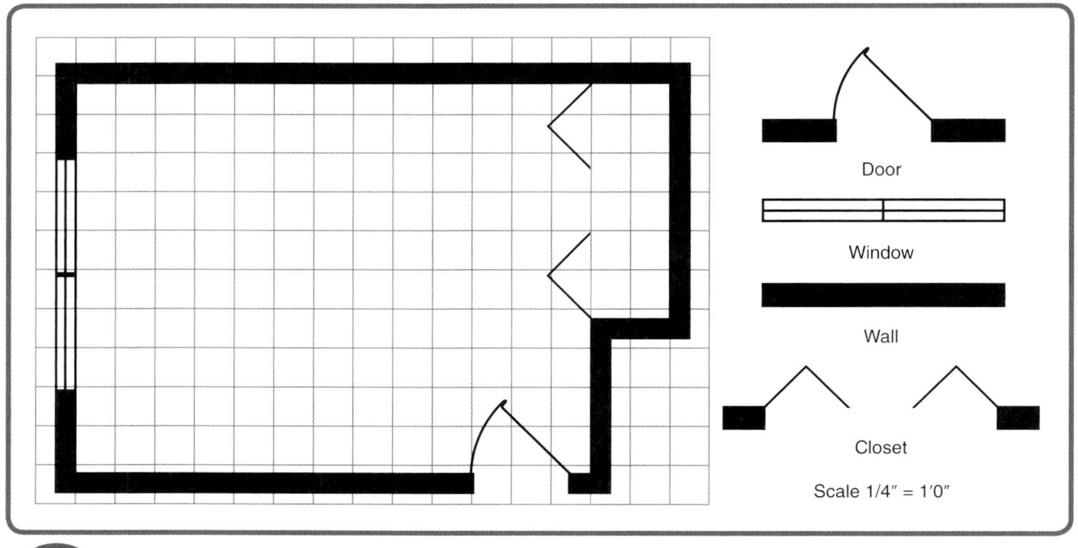

5-3 You can save time and energy by arranging furniture on a scale floor plan first.

Storage Guidelines

- Store items near the area where they are most often used. For instance, keep your alarm clock on your nightstand.
- Store items you use often, such as hairbrushes and combs, in easy-to-reach places. Items you only use once a year, such as holiday decorations, can be stored in places that are hard to reach, such as a high shelf.
- Use all available space. Look for space that is not being used. It is easy to put up nails or hooks in your closet. You can also add extra shelves and clothes rods.
- Be creative. Use hidden and displayed storage to your advantage. Any hollow object can be used for storage. For instance, baskets, crates, storage cubes, and pottery all make great storage containers and look good.

5-4 These guidelines can help you make the most of your storage space.

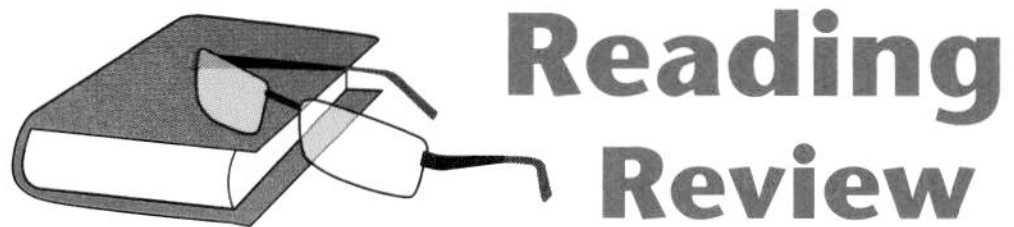

1. How can using a scale floor plan help you arrange furniture?
2. What kinds of items do you store in hidden storage? What kinds of items do you store in displayed storage?

Decorating Your Space

The way you decorate your space can say a lot about you. The elements and principles of design can help you make good design decisions for a visually pleasing room. Taking your values, goals, and resources into consideration is also important.

The Elements of Design

When deciding how to decorate your private space, think about using the five elements of design to express yourself. These include color, texture, line, shape, and spacing. Each of these elements is a building block of the final decorating scheme.

Color may be the most obvious element. Blues, greens, and purples are *cool colors*. Yellows, reds, and oranges are *warm colors*. Some colors go better together than others. See **5-5**.

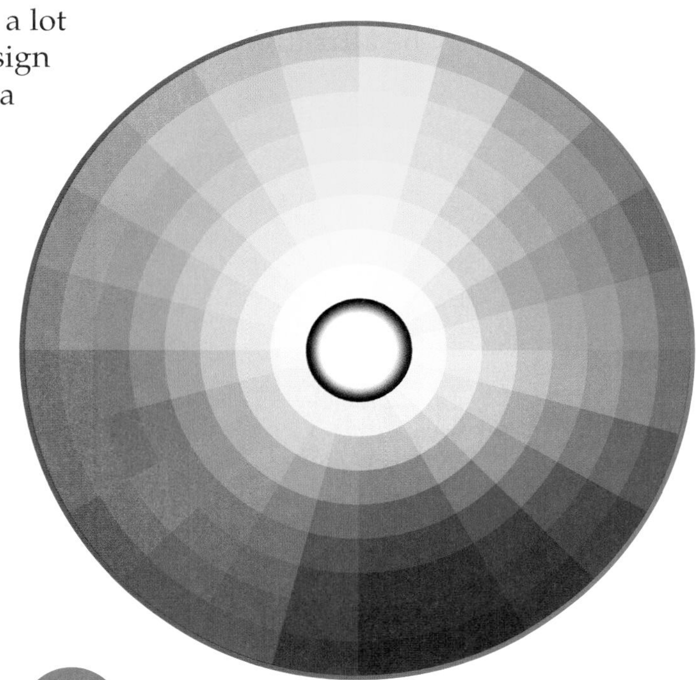

5-5 The color wheel is a commonly used tool that shows all color relationships.

The colors you choose can affect the feeling of your room. For instance, blues and greens tend to feel relaxing, while shades of red are more stimulating. If you live in a cold climate, using warmer colors can help your room seem warmer. While those living in hot climates may prefer shades of the cooler colors.

Texture means the look and feel of the objects, furniture, and décor in your room. For instance, you may have soft, fuzzy pillows or a hard, smooth metal desk. Texture adds dimension and also affects how a room feels.

Line refers to the overall directions of the objects in your room. Your furniture can have straight, curved, or diagonal lines. So can the designs on the fabrics in your room. Curved lines tend to look delicate and peaceful. Straight lines tend to look sturdy and forceful.

Shape is the overall geometric outline of your room's objects. Most beds and dressers are rectangles. You may have tables in the shapes of circles or ovals. Think about the number of different shapes in your room. Too many different ones can cause disharmony.

Spacing refers to the amount of space between objects. Too much space can cause a room to look bare and sterile. Too little space can make a room look cluttered and overwhelming.

The Principles of Design

The elements of design will help you to use the five principles of design and achieve the look you want. These include proportion, balance, emphasis, rhythm, and unity.

Proportion is the relation of objects' sizes in a room to the room itself. For instance, a small room would be overpowered by very large furniture. A large room, however, needs either more or larger furniture to be attractive.

Balance means that different items in a room occur in equal or proper amounts. You would not want most of the display items on your dresser on one side only. It would look off balance. This principle applies to everything in your room.

Emphasis is having a piece of the room as the visual center of attention. Emphasis is important and can be achieved in a number of ways. For instance, placing an unusual piece of painted furniture by a mirror creates a visual emphasis. So does using a very different color from the rest of the color scheme. See **5-6**.

Rhythm shows the patterns in a space. Placing a series of items somewhere or using patterned fabrics creates visual movement, or rhythm.

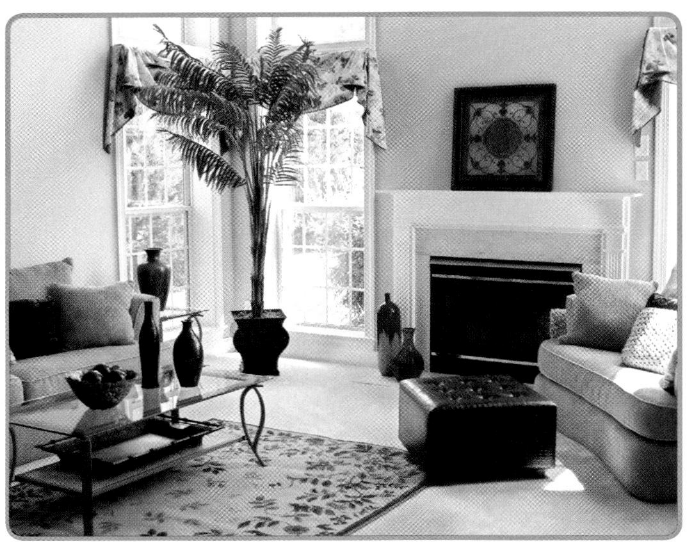

5-6 The large palm tree in front of the windows creates visual emphasis in this room.

Unity refers to the overall appearance of a room's contents. Everything in the room looks like it belongs together, and the space is visually pleasing.

Your Values, Goals, and Resources

Your values often affect your decorating decisions. For instance, suppose you value comfort. You may choose to have floor pillows and beanbag chairs in your room. On the other hand, you may value neatness. In this case, you may feel that floor pillows and beanbag chairs look messy.

Your goals for using your room may also affect your decorating decisions. See **5-7**. If your goal is to study in your room, you will probably want to create space for a desk. If your goal is to visit with friends, however, you may want to have several comfortable chairs in your room.

Your resources affect how you decorate your space, too. If you have time, you may decide to paint your room in your favorite color. If you have some money, you may decide to buy a new picture frame or desk lamp. If you have sewing skills, you may decide to make new curtains or decorative throws. If you are creative, you may think of unusual and inexpensive ideas for decorating.

You may not be the only one who will be affected by your decorating decisions. Make sure your parents approve your decisions before putting your plans into action. They may even contribute to your plans. If you share a room, consult your brother or sister first. He or she should also agree to your decorating decisions. You may even decide to decorate your room together.

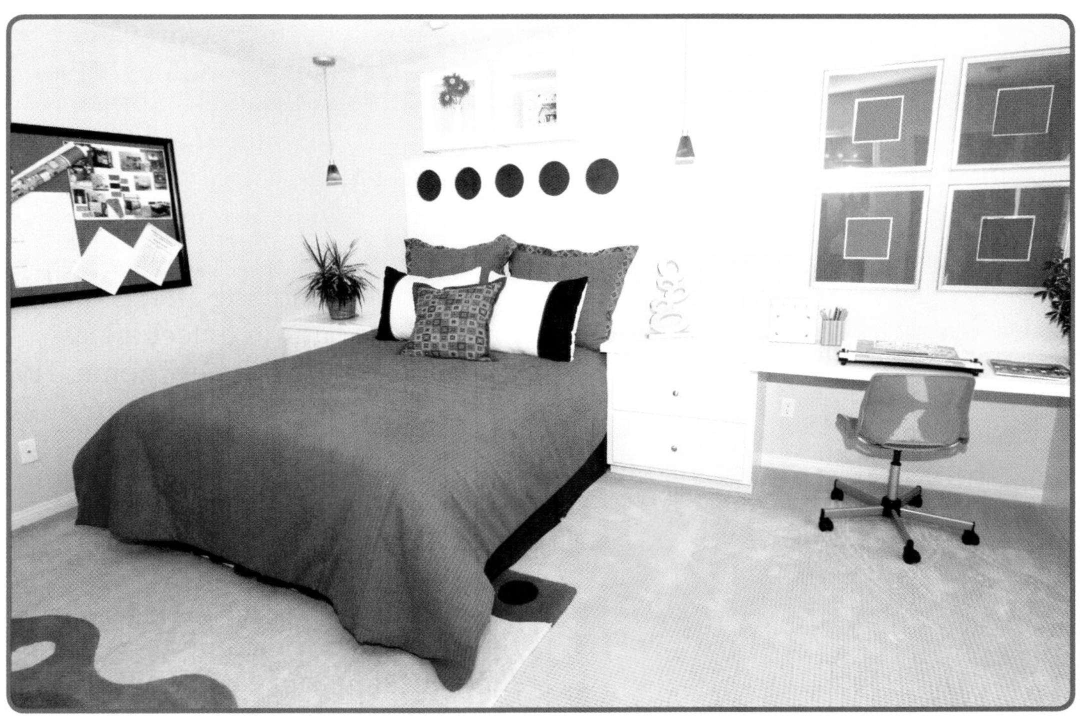

5-7 The decorations in your room can reflect your values and goals.

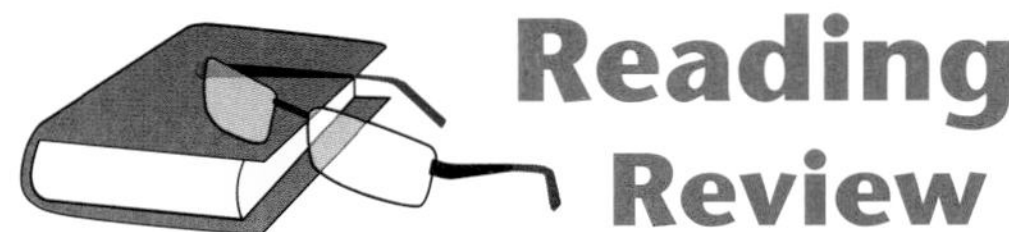

Reading Review

1. What are some ways you can use the elements and principles of design to decorate your room?
2. How can your values, goals, and resources affect your decorating decisions?

Moving

Approximately one in five families moves in a given year. Many of them move to new homes in their own towns. Some, however, need to move to a new state for a parent's job or another important reason. Moving is considered to be one of the more stressful events in a person's life. It is hard for everyone in the family, especially if you have lived in the same home for a long time.

If moving far away, it is hard to leave your friends, school, and your familiar neighborhood. Change is often difficult, but it can also be rewarding. You will be able to make new friends and have new experiences to share with your old friends. Social media and cell phones help to stay in touch with your old friends so they seem closer.

Moving involves the packing and physical transfer of all belongings. Plus, your home must be cleaned well for the new residents. On the other end, it involves unpacking, sorting, and putting those belongings away in your new home. See **5-8**.

Remember that moving affects the entire family. It is natural to feel uneasy until you get used to your new home. Try to look at moving as a new adventure.

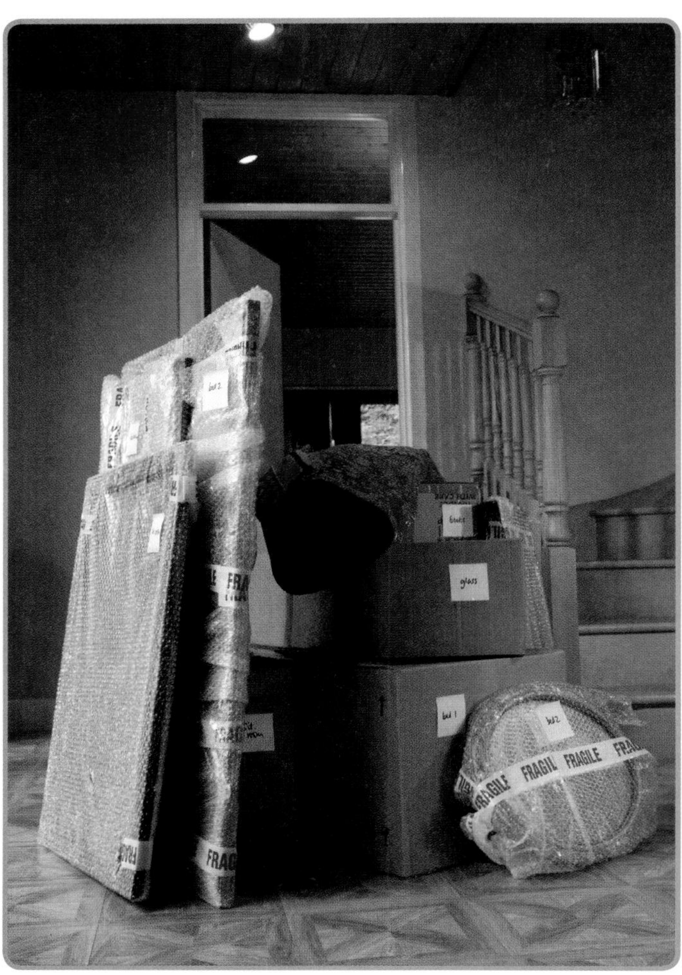

5-8 Labeling boxes when you move makes it easier to locate items later.

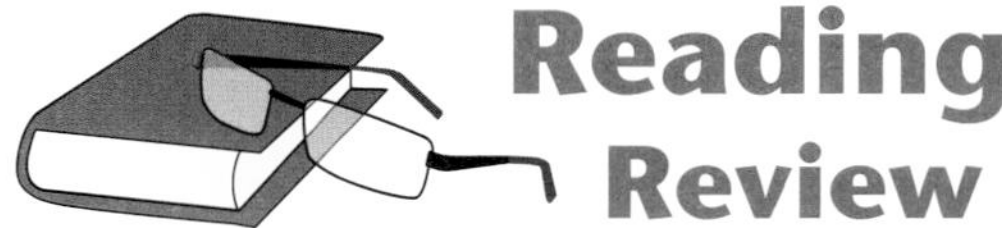

Reading Review

1. Why is moving considered stressful?
2. What are some tasks you can do that will help make moving easier?

Succeed in Life

Preparing to Move

There are some tasks you can perform to make moving easier. For instance, go through all your clothing and other items to determine what is worth taking with you. Moving is a good time to discard what you no longer need, does not fit, or is broken. You can donate items in good condition to charities.

Once you have the proper sizes of boxes for your personal property, start packing. Make sure you carefully wrap anything breakable. Use a heavy marker to indicate your name and the room on the outside of the boxes.

You can also help with any of the necessary cleaning duties when the house is empty. Once you reach your new home, it can be fun to help unpack and find new ways to arrange your furniture and belongings. You may also want to decorate your new room differently than your old one.

Section Summary

- Your living space, or your home, helps meet some of your physical, emotional, and social needs.
- Some of your living space is shared, and some is private.
- Using scale floor plans and your room's storage can help you arrange your space.
- The elements and principles of design can help you decorate your space to suit your unique personality.
- Thinking about your values, goals, and resources can also help you decorate your space to suit your lifestyle.
- Moving can be stressful for the entire family. You can make the transition easier by helping with the packing, cleaning, and unpacking.

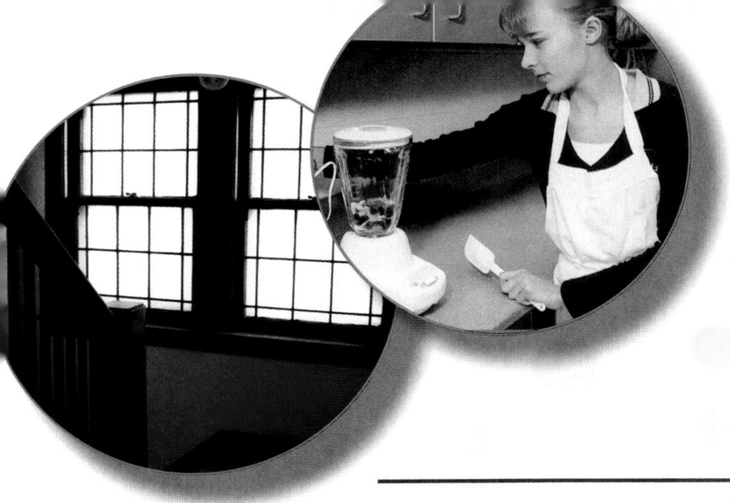

Section 5-2
Home Safe Home

Objectives

After studying this section, you will be able to
- **define** *accidents*, *fatal*, *toxic*, and *appliance*.
- **describe** some common household accidents.
- **list** steps that should be taken to prevent household accidents.
- **tell** how you can help keep your home secure.

Key Terms

accidents: unexpected events causing loss or injury.

fatal: deadly.

toxic: poisonous.

appliance: a tool run by electricity or gas.

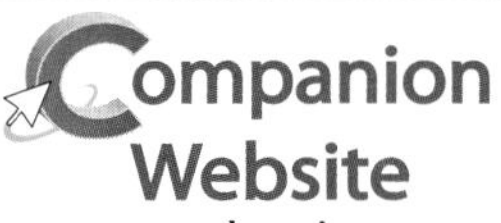

Study the Key Terms by completing crossword puzzles, matching activities, and e-flash cards at the website.

Main Ideas

- Falls, fires, poisonings, and electric shocks are common household accidents.
- Many household accidents can be prevented.
- You can protect your home from break-ins.

Homes can meet your need to live in a safe, secure place. Homes, however, can sometimes be unsafe. Accidents can happen. **Accidents** are unexpected events causing loss or injury. Common household accidents result from falls and fires. Other accidents are caused by poisoning or electricity. Most accidents can be avoided. As a family member, you are responsible for helping to make your home a safe place.

Preventing Falls

Falls are the most common accidents in the home. Children and older adults are the most likely people to fall. Children need safety gates to protect them from stairs. Older adults may need handrails in certain areas of their homes, such as in the bathroom.

Keep the floors clear of clutter. Make sure objects are stored when not being used. It is easy to trip on toys, shoes, and other items left on floors.

Clear sidewalks of ice and snow. Use sand or salt for extra traction on icy walks.

Bathrooms are common areas for falls to occur. To prevent falls, put nonskid mats or decals in showers and bathtubs. Clean up spilled water quickly. Otherwise, others could slip and get hurt. See **5-9**. Put nightlights in bathrooms and hallways.

In the kitchen, use sturdy step stools or ladders to reach high cabinets. Do not climb on the tops of counters. Clean up all spills right away.

If your home has stairs, make sure they are well lit and have solid handrails. Hold on to the handrails when you go up and down stairs. It is safer to walk up and down stairs instead of running. Otherwise, you could fall or trip.

You can also trip on rugs that are not securely tacked to the floor. Nonskid backing should be put under throw rugs and other rugs that cannot be tacked down. Do not store items on the stairs.

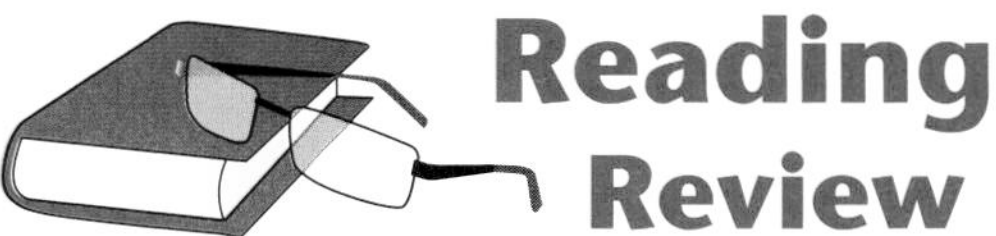

Reading Review

1. Who is most likely to fall in the home? What can cause falls?
2. How can you help prevent falls from happening in your home?

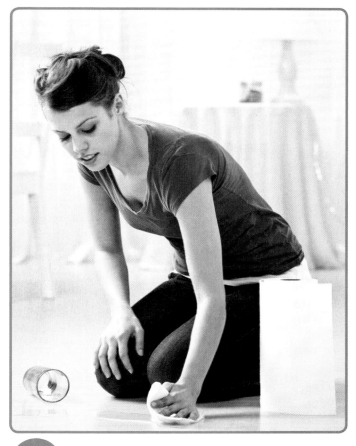

5-9 Clean up spills as soon as they occur to help prevent falls.

Preventing Fires

Fires are very dangerous accidents. They are often **fatal**, or deadly. Most fatal fires occur at night, while people are asleep. Inhaling large amounts of smoke from the fire is often more deadly than the actual flames. All homes should have smoke detectors located near or in the bedrooms, kitchen, and stairwells. See **5-10**. Keep a fire extinguisher in the kitchen, as well.

If possible, sleep with your bedroom door closed. If there is a fire, you will have more time to escape before the smoke reaches you. If you wake up and smell smoke, touch your door. If it feels warm, do not open it. Smoke and heat rise, so drop to the floor and crawl away from the door. If you can, wrap a wet towel around your mouth and nose so you can breathe without inhaling the smoke. All families should have day and night fire escape plans.

After you escape, call the fire department. In most areas, the emergency number for fire and police is 911. Learn and memorize the emergency number for your area. When you call, state your name, address, and the problem clearly. Do not hang up until you are sure you have given all the important information.

Home fires can start in a number of different ways. For instance, overloading the electrical circuits in your home can overheat the wiring and start a fire. Therefore, do not have too many plugs in one outlet.

Burning candles should never be left alone. Make sure they are out of the reach of young children. Keep the flames away from objects that could easily catch fire, such as curtains.

To help conserve fuel, many families use space heaters or wood stoves. You should read the instruction booklets for all your heat sources. Learn how to use them safely. Saving money on fuel bills will not be important if your home is destroyed by fire.

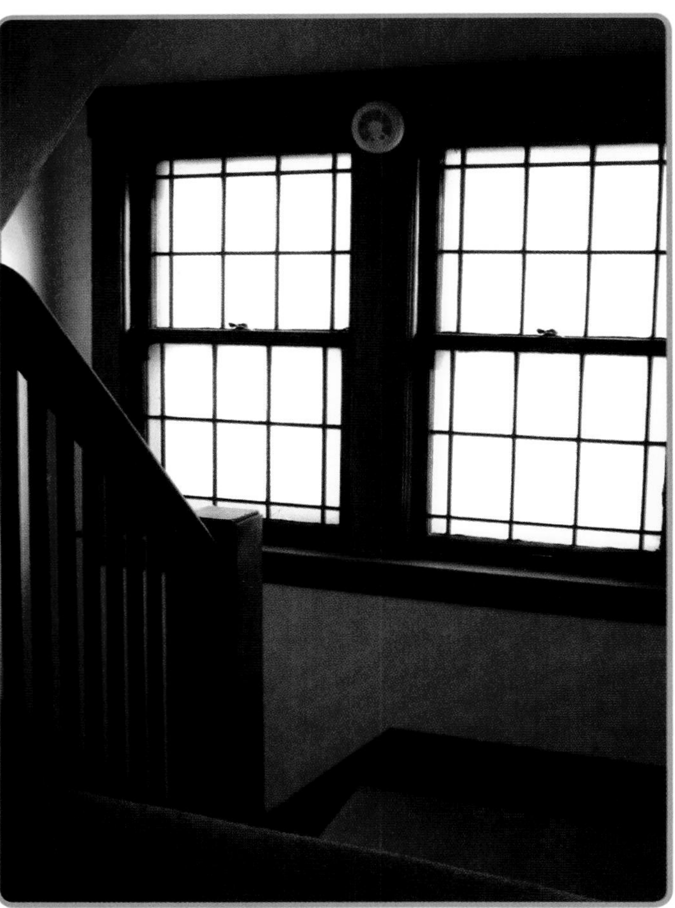

5-10 Check smoke detectors regularly to make sure they work properly.

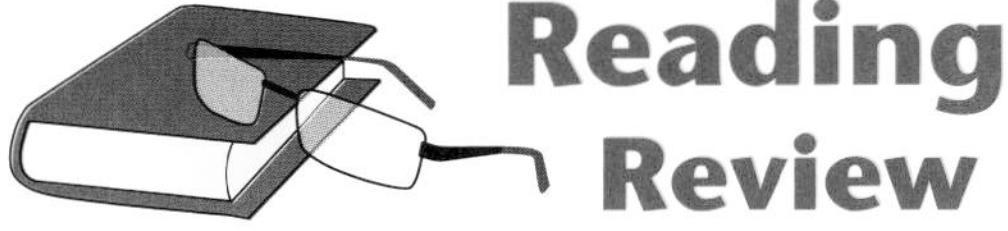

Reading Review

1. What should you do if you wake up and smell smoke?
2. What information should you give if you have to call the fire department?

Preventing Poisonings

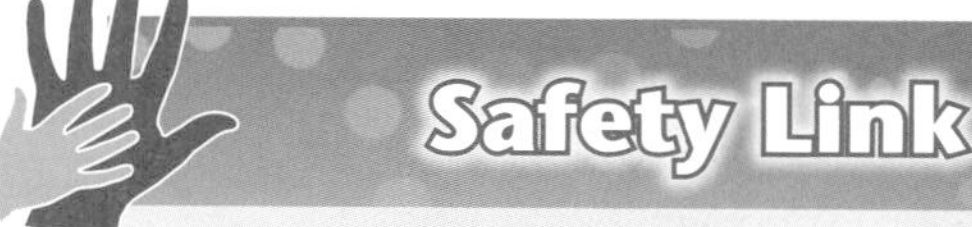

Cleaning Products

Never mix cleaning products containing chemicals. They can emit toxic fumes when mixed. These can make you sick or hurt your eyes. For instance, you should never mix a cleaner that contains bleach with one that contains ammonia. Read directions on all products carefully before using them.

Toxic, or poisonous, substances can be found in most homes. These substances are often in household cleaners, insecticides, and many medicines. Read the labels on all cleaners and insecticides. Follow the directions carefully. Most cleaners and insecticides are toxic. If you swallow or inhale them, they can poison or hurt you.

Store all toxic substances away from young children. Children are the most likely victims of accidental poisoning. They do not understand that poisons are dangerous. They like to explore and often swallow objects that attract their attention. You can buy special *childproof* latches to keep children out of cabinets and drawers.

Never tell children that medicine is candy. Do not let them see you taking medicine. They like to copy what you do. Many medicine bottles come with childproof caps to protect children.

Never store toxic substances in food containers. Someone could mistake the substances for food. Poisoning could result.

To determine if a product is toxic, check the label. It should also state what to do if an accidental poisoning occurs. Labels tell you how to safely use products. They may also tell you how to dispose of the container and any unused product when you have finished. Be sure to read and follow all label directions carefully.

If an accidental poisoning happens in your home, act quickly. Follow the directions on the product label. Then call the toll-free phone number on the label or the local poison control center. Calmly state the problem. Have the container with you so you will have complete information.

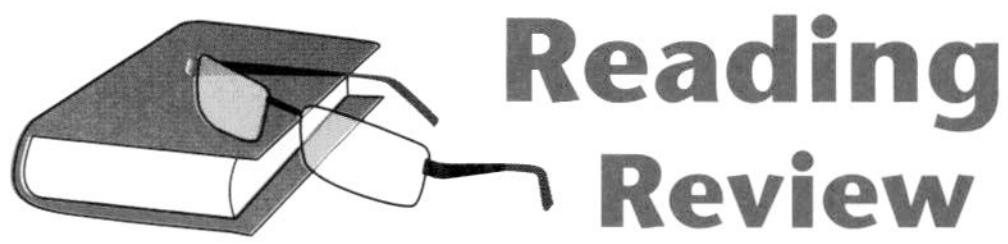

Reading Review

1. Why should you not tell children that medicine is candy?
2. What should you do if someone in your home has been poisoned?

Preventing Electrical Accidents

Electricity can cause two major problems in the home. The first is fire. The second is electric shock. A person can receive a shock when using electric appliances. An **appliance** is a tool run by electricity or gas. See **5-11**.

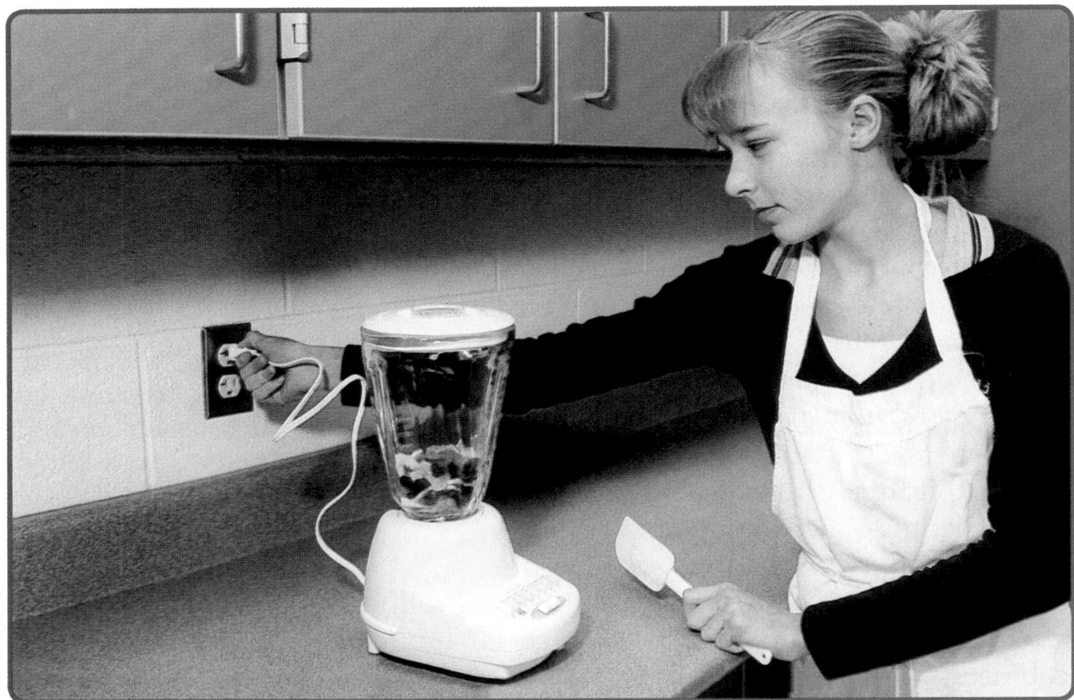

Steve A. Wilson

5-11 Always use electric appliances with care.

Wet skin attracts electricity far more than dry skin. Never touch an electric appliance or its cord if you are wet—or standing in or near water. This could cause an electric shock that can injure or kill you. Always unplug appliances before cleaning them. Keep appliances away from bathtubs, showers, and sinks.

When you buy electric appliances, look for the Underwriter's Laboratories (UL) label. Appliances with the UL label meet the latest safety requirements.

Use products safely to prevent electric shock. Pull electric cords from outlets by the plug rather than the cord. Never use appliances if they are broken, cracked, or have frayed cords. Have them repaired or discard them.

Protect young children from electric shock. They like to play with outlets, which are often located within their reach. If there are young children in your home, buy covers for your outlets. Also, never let children play with electric appliances.

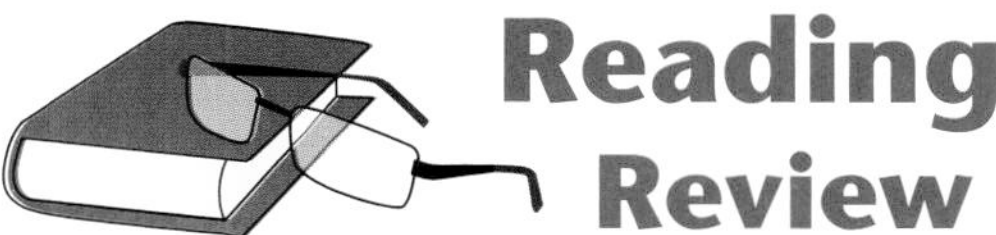

Reading Review

1. How can you prevent receiving an electric shock when using appliances?
2. Why should you not use an appliance that is broken or has a frayed cord?

Securing Your Home

In addition to preventing accidents, you should also know how to protect your home from break-ins. To keep your home safe, always lock your doors and windows. Make sure your locks are secure. Leave a light on when you are gone at night. Burglars do not like to enter occupied homes.

If a person you do not know calls, do not identify yourself. Never tell a caller you are home by yourself. You can always tell the person your parents are busy and cannot come to the phone. Do not let strangers in your home. Before you open the door, always ask, "Who is it?"

When your family leaves for a vacation, make your home look like you are still there. Ask a neighbor or friend to collect your newspapers. Have the post office hold your mail until you return. Use a light timer so your lights go off and on at certain times.

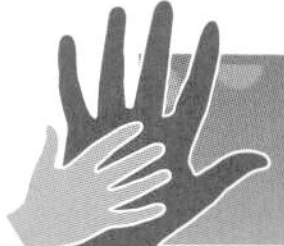

Safety Link

Home Security

Some homes have home security systems that alert the police if there are intruders. Inexpensive monitors can be installed. For instance, motion sensors will sound an alarm if someone opens a door or window. This can give you a chance to call 911. Also, sensors on outside lights turn them on when someone walks near the lights. Prepare a list of questions to ask a police officer about how to secure your home and prevent break-ins.

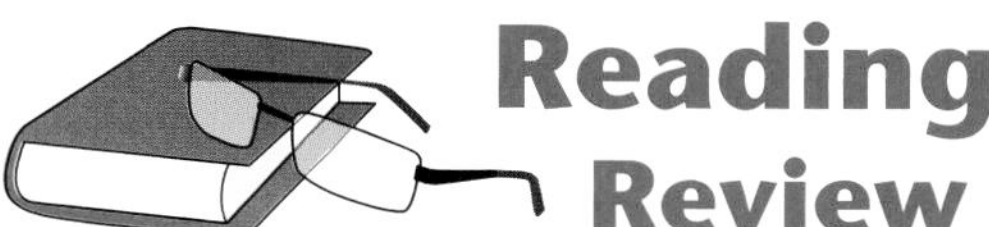

Reading Review

1. How can you protect your home from break-ins? Give examples.
2. Why should you not let people know you are home alone?

Section Summary

- It takes a lot of effort and care to make your home safe.
- Most household accidents result from falls, fires, poisons, and electricity.
- Everyone in your family is responsible for protecting your home from accidents and break-ins.

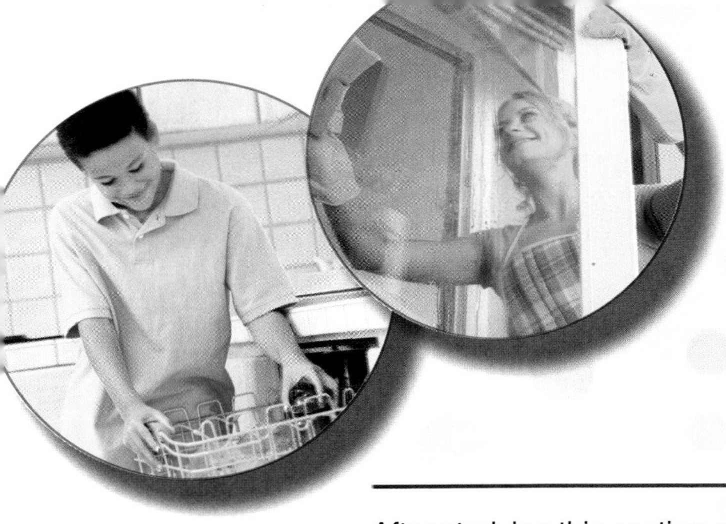

Section 5-3
Caring for Your Home

Objectives

After studying this section, you will be able to
- **define** *compost*, *environmentally friendly products*, and *biodegradable*.
- **list** household cleaning tasks that need to be done on a regular basis.
- **make** a family cleaning schedule.

Key Terms

compost: a mixture of decaying organic matter used to improve soil structure and provide nutrients.

environmentally friendly products: products that are effective and safe for the environment.

biodegradable: capable of decomposing under natural conditions.

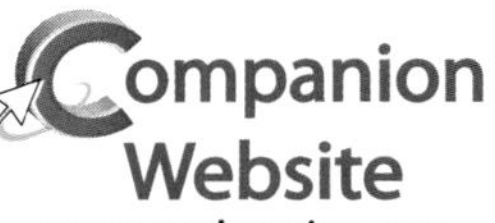

Study the Key Terms by completing crossword puzzles, matching activities, and e-flash cards at the website.

Main Ideas

- You should clean your home on a regular basis.
- A cleaning schedule is helpful in caring for a home.
- You can select cleaning products that are safe for you and the environment.

There are many benefits to having a clean home. When your home is clean, it is a more healthful place to live. When you clean a messy room, you can see your results. This can give you a sense of pride. You can also enjoy your home more when it is clean. You can relax. You can have friends over without being embarrassed.

Why Clean?

When you clean often, cleaning is easier and takes less time. Your furniture, carpets, and other belongings last longer when you take care of them. See **5-12**.

To keep your home clean, certain tasks need to be done. How well each task is done will depend on your family's needs and standards of cleanliness. Some people want very clean and neat homes. Others do not like to spend a lot of time cleaning. Their homes may be less clean and neat. As a family, you need to decide how clean you want your home to be.

There are daily, weekly, and occasional cleaning tasks that help to keep your home clean and comfortable. Having plants, pets, or a yard means you will have extra tasks to do.

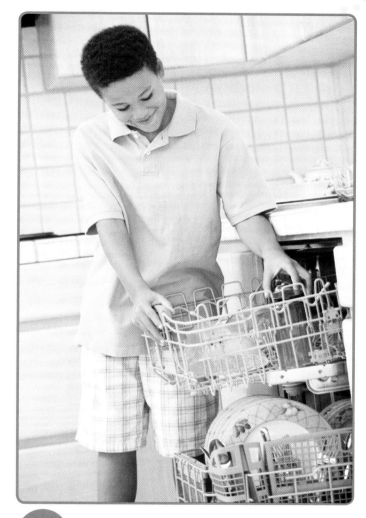

5-12 Doing tasks frequently will help keep your home clean.

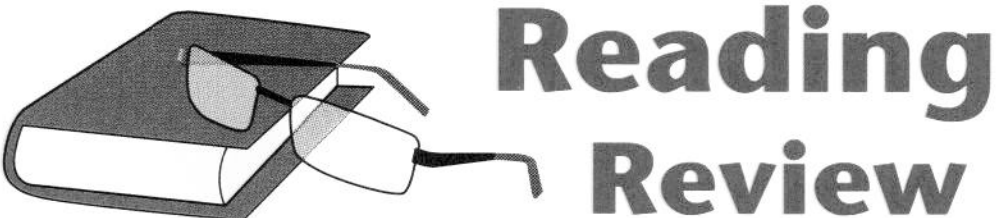

Reading Review

1. What are some benefits of cleaning your home often? Give examples.
2. Why do some families spend more time cleaning than other families?

Daily Tasks

Some household tasks should be done daily. Doing these tasks will help keep your home looking neat. Doing daily tasks will also make the weekly cleaning much easier.

Cleaning the Kitchen

Kitchens must be cleaned each day to prevent odors and germs. This means wiping tables and counters. You also need to wash the dishes and scour the sink.

Straightening the Home

Everybody should pick up his or her belongings. Some families put a basket in the hall for all belongings that are not put away. Some also have a tray or basket near the front door for keys, messages, and mail. This also includes keeping your bedroom tidy by making your bed and hanging up or putting away your clothes.

Emptying Trash, Recycling, and Composting

Remove trash easily by using trash can liners. Sort glass, paper, plastic, and cans for recycling. Follow the directions from your local recycling center. See **5-13**.

Compost is a mixture of decaying organic matter used to improve soil structure and provide nutrients. Some families put their yard and food waste in a compost bin outside. Doing so prevents that waste from going to the landfills. Composting is good for the environment. Compost improves the soil in a yard or in containers for planting. Some neighborhoods have community gardens with compost bins.

Cleaning the Bathroom

Keep clean sponges handy in the bathrooms. Use them to wipe the sink, bathtub, and shower after each use. This simple activity makes the weekly cleaning much easier.

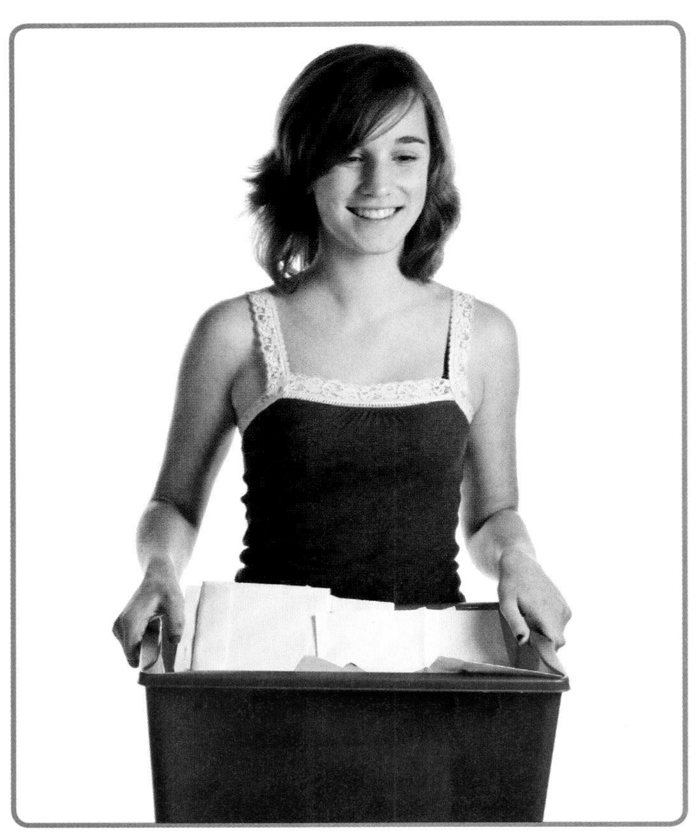

5-13 Recycling can cut down on waste in landfills.

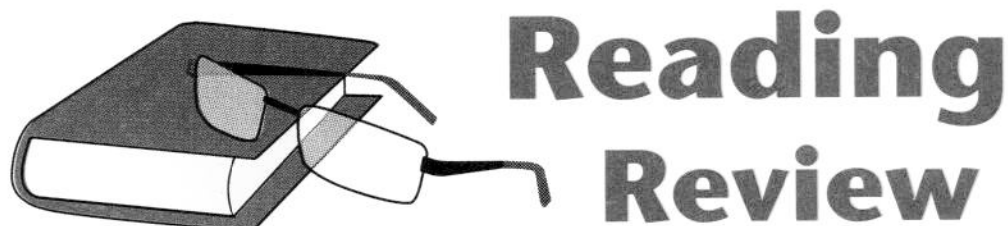

Reading Review

1. Why should everybody pick up his or her own belongings?
2. Why is composting good for the environment?

Weekly Tasks

Several household tasks need to be done weekly. Performing weekly tasks will help keep your home clean.

Changing Bed Linens

Changing your bed linens is easy. Put the fitted sheet on the mattress using alternate corners. Then put on the top sheet and smooth out all the wrinkles. Tuck it in, along with any blankets at the foot of the mattress. Lastly, put the pillowcases on the pillows.

Cleaning the Floors

Carpets need to be vacuumed. Floors need to be mopped or swept.

Dusting and Polishing the Furniture

Feather dusters are good for light dustings. Old socks you can slip over your hand or reusable rags are good for heavy dusting and polishing. You may want to use wax or dusting spray, too.

Cleaning the Bathroom

Clean the toilet, sink, bathtub, and shower with bathroom cleaners that will not scratch the surfaces. Thorough cleaning keeps germs and mildew from growing.

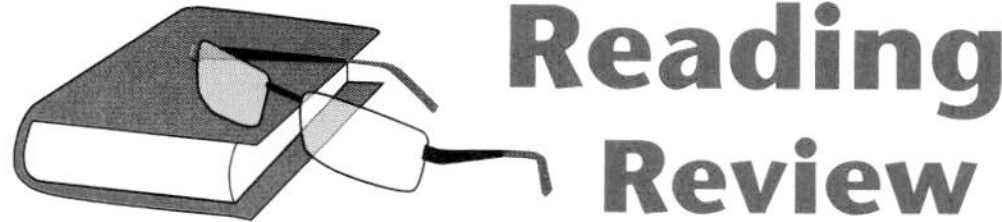

Reading Review

1. What is the order you should follow for changing your bed linens?
2. Why should the bathroom be cleaned thoroughly?

Occasional Tasks

Some household tasks need to be done occasionally. They may need to be done only once a month or once or twice a year.

Cleaning Windows

Use a window cleaner or water mixed with a small amount of ammonia. Also, use lint-free rags, such as old sheets. These can be washed and used again. See **5-14**.

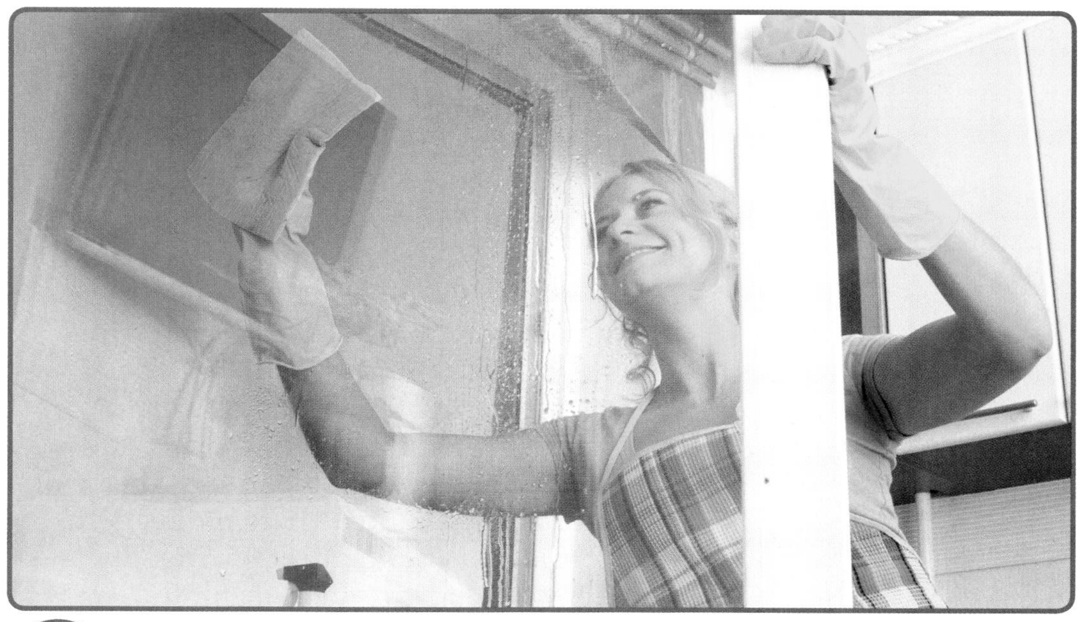

5-14 Windows are only cleaned occasionally. Make sure to do a good job when you clean them.

Cleaning Woodwork and Walls

Wipe woodwork and walls with fingerprints and other dirt on them. Remove hard-to-reach cobwebs found in corners and around ceilings with a pillowcase over a broom.

Cleaning the Oven and Refrigerator

Clean the oven and refrigerator once a month. Read the instruction booklets for both appliances. Your oven may be self cleaning. It may have special features, such as removable doors, to make manual cleaning easier. It is important to follow cleaning directions carefully and use the correct products.

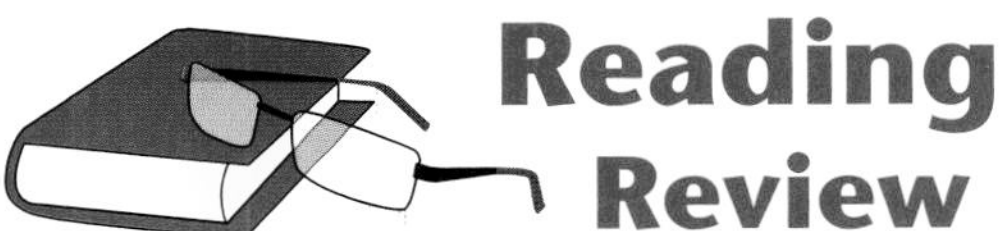

Reading Review

1. Why may some household tasks only need to be done occasionally?
2. How can you clean hard-to-reach areas of walls and woodwork?

Cleaning Supplies

Many of the cleaners used in the home can be harmful to the environment. They can be toxic or poisonous. Read labels on cleaning supplies to see if you have any that contain toxic ingredients. For instance, while bleach can kill germs and whiten surfaces, it is toxic to the environment and can harm you if swallowed.

Many products contain perfumes, which can pollute the air. Think of all the products in your house that have a fragrance. For instance, you will find perfumes in furniture polish, air fresheners, and dishwashing detergents.

Many people want to use **environmentally friendly products** that are effective and safe for the environment. Often these products are made from natural ingredients such as lemons and baking soda. **Biodegradable** products are capable of decomposing under natural conditions. These products break down quickly and go back to the soil. They will not cause pollution. These products are considered environmentally friendly. They are effective and safe for the air, the surfaces, the fabrics, the pets, and the people within your environment.

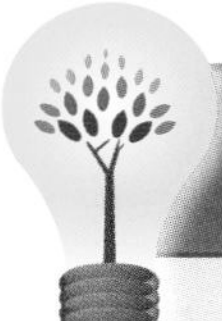

Think Green

Green Home Cleaning

You can substitute inexpensive nontoxic substances for hazardous cleaners. This will reduce the poisons in your home, pollution in the environment, and save money. For instance, you can use lemon as a disinfectant in the kitchen. You can use cornstarch to remove grease stains on carpeting. Vinegar is also an inexpensive nontoxic substance you can use for cleaning the home. Vinegar helps cut grease when washing windows and floors. Use 3 tablespoons of vinegar to 1 quart of water.

It is easy to reduce the amount of toxic materials you buy. Some general rules for managing toxic household products include the following:

- Select the least toxic products for your home.
- Buy only what you need.
- Read and follow instructions on the labels.
- Avoid aerosol spray cans.
- Dispose of toxic waste as recommended.

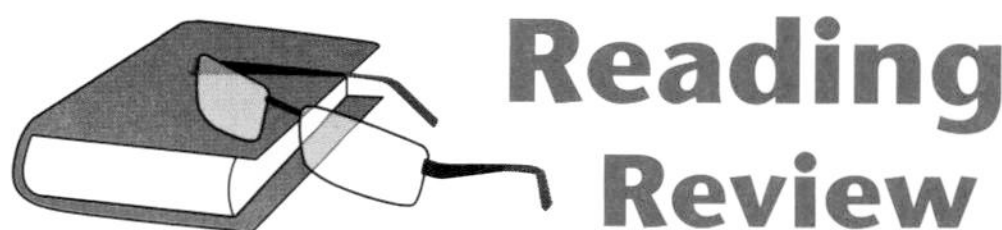

Reading Review

1. Give examples of household cleaners that can be harmful to the environment.
2. Why do many people prefer environmentally friendly products?

Working Together

To help share cleaning tasks, families can make a cleaning schedule. More work will get done when everybody helps. No one will feel like he or she is doing all the work.

To make a schedule, first list all the tasks that need to be done and when. Next, decide who is responsible for each task. Be sure to divide the tasks evenly among the family members. Rotate the tasks to be fair. See **5-15**. Keep in mind how long it takes to do each task.

When making a cleaning schedule, think about the amount of time each family member has available. Parents who work outside the home may have less time to clean on weekdays. They may want to do their cleaning on the weekend. When you are out of school for the summer, you may have more time for cleaning.

Cleaning Schedule

Task	Week One	Week Two	Week Three	Week Four
Set kitchen table	Mom	Dad	Suzanne	Izzy
Clean off kitchen table	Dad	Suzanne	Izzy	Joel
Clean and put away dishes	Suzanne	Izzy	Joel	Mom
Straighten living room	Izzy	Joel	Mom	Dad
Feed pets	Joel	Mom	Dad	Suzanne

5-15 A weekly family schedule lets everyone see his or her tasks.

You should also think about the tasks you like to do. You may like to work indoors instead of outside. You may prefer to clean the bathroom instead of doing laundry. Volunteer to do the tasks you like most.

Let everyone in the family help, especially young children. See **5-16**. Find tasks they can do well. For instance, Sofia is a five-year-old. She likes to help on cleaning days. Her task is to dust. This makes her feel needed. There are many cleaning tasks that are appropriate for children of all ages.

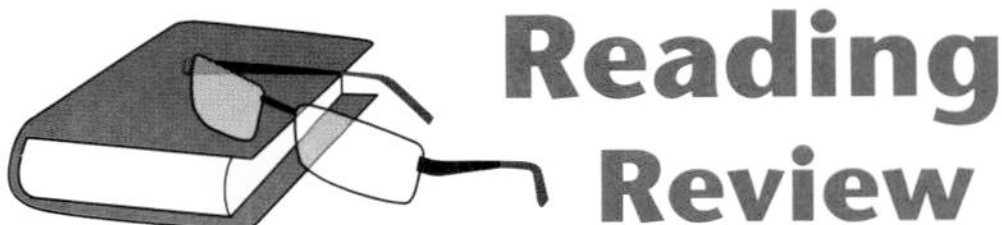

Reading Review

1. Why should all family members share in the care of the home?
2. What factors should be considered when making a cleaning schedule?

Section Summary

- Having a clean home is important. It can make you feel better and help you enjoy your home more.
- Perform cleaning tasks on a regular basis.
- A cleaning schedule helps divide these tasks fairly among all family members.

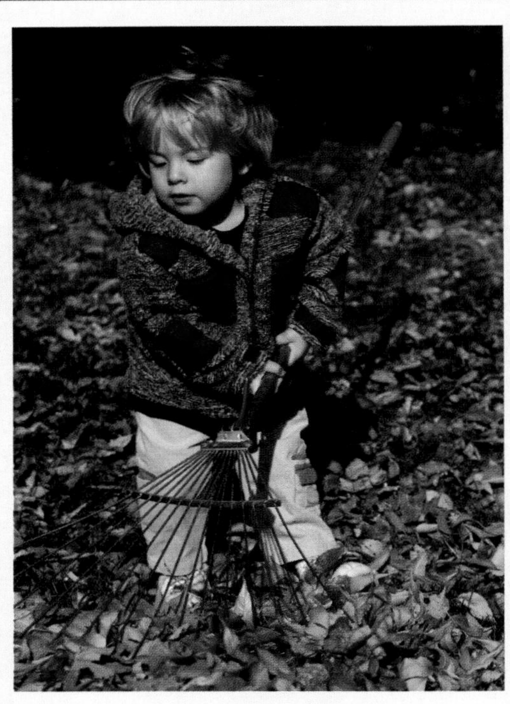

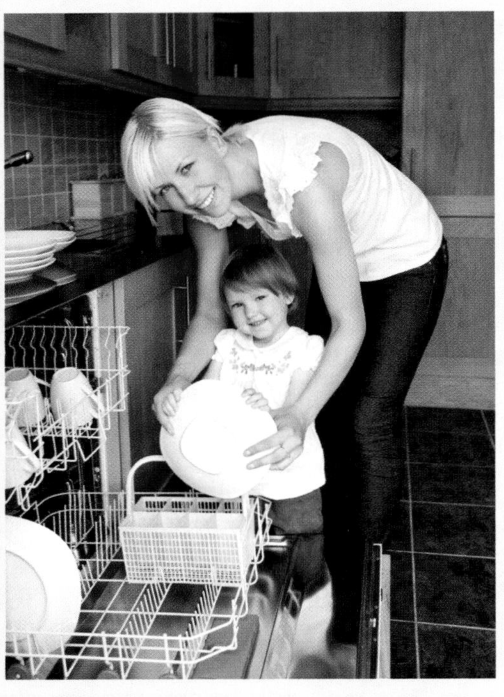

5-16 Young children often enjoy helping other family members complete indoor and outdoor tasks.

Chapter Summary

Your home helps meet some of your physical, emotional, and social needs. Managing your home, or living space, can help you enjoy it more. Some living space is shared. Keeping this space clean and comfortable lets you and your family enjoy it more. Each family member should help keep it clean and comfortable.

Private space is an area that is only yours. By planning carefully, you can use and decorate your private space wisely. Use a scale floor plan to arrange the furniture in your room. Use hidden and displayed storage to store your belongings. You should discuss your decorating plans with your parents. If you share a bedroom with a brother or sister, also discuss this with him or her. Moving can be a stressful experience for the entire family. There are tasks you can perform to make it easier.

To feel safe and secure in your home, help prevent accidents and break-ins. Most household accidents result from falls, fires, poisonings, and electricity. Follow safety rules to prevent these accidents. Certain steps can also be taken to protect your home from break-ins.

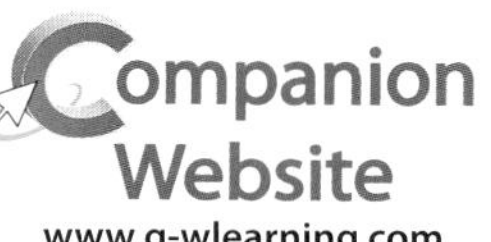

Review Key Terms and Main Ideas for Chapter 5 at the website.

Chapter Review

Write your answers on a separate sheet of paper.

1. What is the difference between a house and a home?
2. List three types of needs that a home can meet.
3. What is universal design?
4. True or false. Shared space is the area that belongs to one person in a home.
5. List three hints for sharing space in a home.
6. Draw the housing symbols for a door, window, and wall.
7. True or false. Allow at least five feet of space between pieces of furniture.
8. List the four causes of common household accidents. Then describe ways they can be prevented.
9. What is the most common household accident?
10. True or false. Labels tell you how to safely use products.
11. Name two types of accidents that can be caused by electricity.
12. List four ways to keep your home secure.
13. List three benefits of a clean home.
14. Give two examples each of daily, weekly, and occasional cleaning tasks.
15. Explain how to make a cleaning schedule.

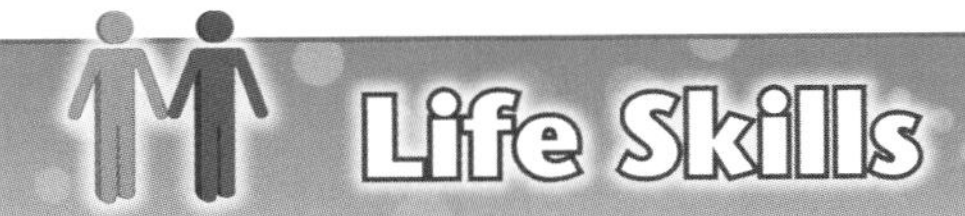

16. Your local newspaper is sponsoring a contest for teens who want to improve their homes. You must submit a plan for making your home more attractive and usable, safer, and easier to maintain. The first place prize is $500. Write a plan for improving your home. Describe how you would spend the $500 to make improvements. In your plan, also list ways you could improve your home without spending money.
17. Find out if your family has a fire escape plan. If not, make one for each member of your family for both day and night. Hold family fire drills to practice both plans.

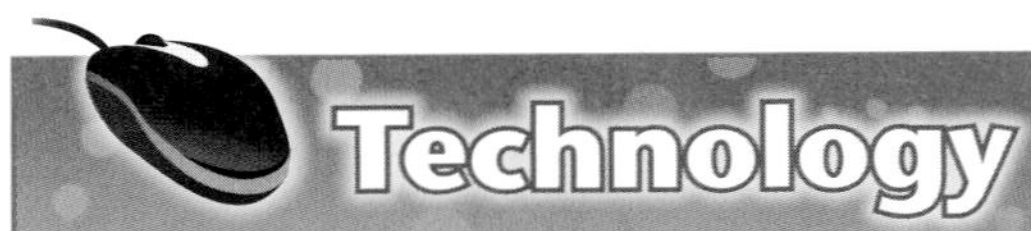

18. Research cleaning supplies and products that are considered *not harmful* to the environment. Use the terms *nontoxic cleaning supplies* and *eco-friendly household products* in a search engine for your online research. In addition, make a list of cleaning supplies and air fresheners that are *most toxic* to the environment. What are some of the easy ways toxic cleaning products can be eliminated from homes? Use word processing software to prepare a report of your findings.

19. Write in your journal about a stressful time and how you resolved it. Maybe you had to change schools or move to a new town. You may share a room with a sibling and have had differences about how to use the space or privacy issues. It could even involve a difference of opinion with someone close to you. There are many ways to handle stressful situations. Were you satisfied with how you handled this one? Looking back, were there other ways that might have worked better for you? What did you learn about yourself?

Academics

20. **Math.** Measure your room or another room in your home that you use. Also, measure the furniture in the room. Draw a scale floor plan. Use the scale floor plan to show three new furniture arrangements, keeping traffic patterns in mind.
21. **Social Studies.** Use the principles and elements of design to redecorate your room. Find different design elements you like in magazines or print them from online sources. Make a presentation board with your ideas and show how each one relates to a design principle and element.
22. **Science.** Look through your home for toxic substances. Be sure they are in a safe place. Then make a chart of the products you found. List what each label tells you to do in case of accidental poisoning. Keep this list near the emergency phone numbers in your home.
23. **Writing.** List your responsibilities to assist with caring for your home. With other family members, make a schedule showing each person's responsibilities and when they are to be done.

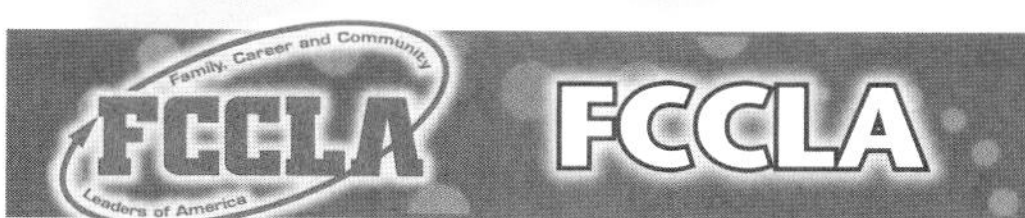

24. Identify an area of environmental concern in your school or local community. Brainstorm some ways to address the problem—either by yourself or in a group. Make sure you get the proper approval before starting the project. Write a short paper about the experience and what you learned. Complete an FCCLA *Create Your Own Service Project* for the *Community Service* program. Obtain further information about this program from your FCCLA advisor.

Chapter 6
Managing Your Environment

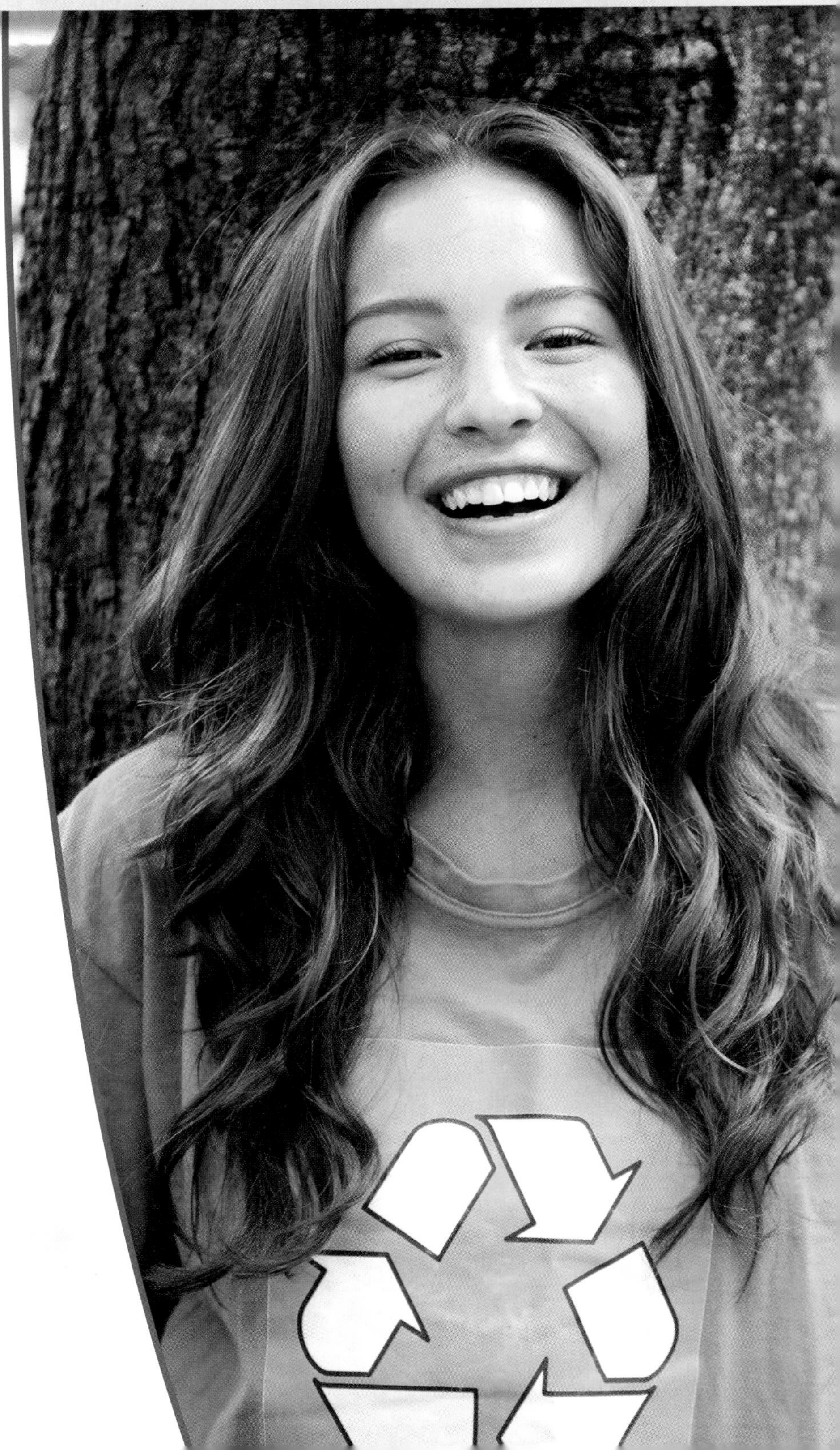

Sections

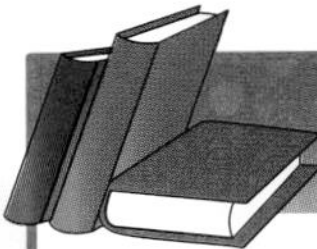

Sharpen Your Reading

Find a magazine article on www.magportal.com that relates to this chapter. Read the article and write four questions you have about the article. Next, read the textbook chapter. Based on what you read in the chapter, see if you can answer any of the questions you had about the magazine article.

Concept Organizer

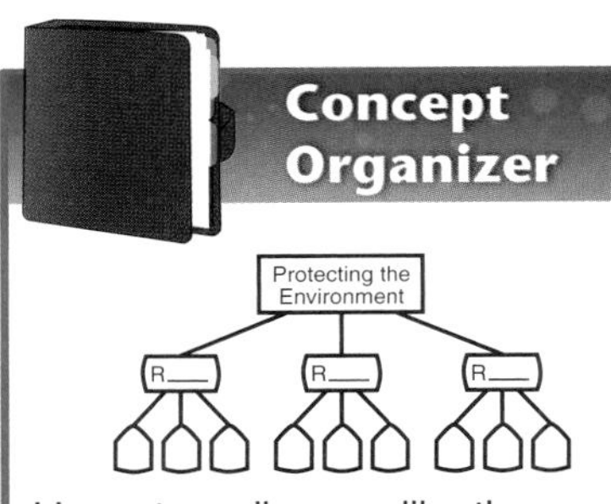

Use a tree diagram like the one shown to list the *three Rs* discussed in this chapter that can help protect the environment. List three activities you can do under each of the *three Rs*.

Companion Website
www.g-wlearning.com

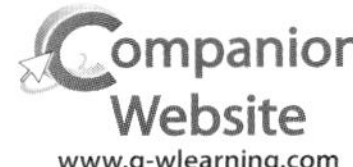

Print out the concept organizer at the website.

Technology is the use of new knowledge, tools, and systems to solve problems and make life easier. It affects your family and your home.

Impact of Technology on the Family

There are many ways that technology impacts your family, home, school, and future career. See **6-6**. Think of all the ways in which you use electronic technology in a given day. There are both advantages and disadvantages to relying on technology. How is your life better because of technology?

How would your family react to a day without technology? That would mean no television, computers, or other electronic devices. You would not listen to music, play video games or DVDs, or even use a phone for 24 hours. What would you do with the time? How would you relate differently to others? Much of this technology is recent. Many older adults still remember a time before TV.

Consider all the places in your home where computer controls are used. From microwave ovens to sewing machines, computers have improved the use of appliances. Lighting and heating can also be controlled by computers. This kind of technology makes housework easier for families. It makes tasks faster, as well. Families have more leisure time.

Technology affects the way people work. Many people now work at home from their computers. They do not have to waste time or energy commuting. They can spend more time with their families and help conserve natural resources. As this trend continues, more and more people may be working from home.

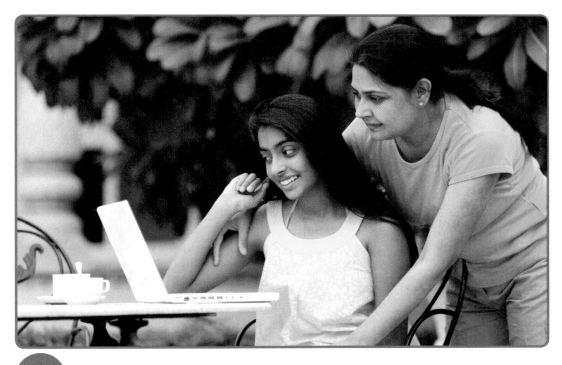

6-6 Families use technology to keep in touch with each other.

Succeed in Life

Protecting Your Computer

Computers are expensive. It is wise to learn how to protect them from harm. A *computer virus* is a computer program that can copy itself and damage computers. Some viruses can even track and give personal and credit card information to thieves.

Often, several family members use the same computer. It is important for all users to know how to prevent these viruses. Make sure your computer has antivirus software. Never open e-mail attachments from people you do not know.

Sometimes viruses can infect the computers of people you know. Viruses can even create and send harmful messages from those people. That is one way viruses spread quickly. Check with your parents first, or ask that person if they really sent you the e-mail before opening.

Never give personal information (or your e-mail address) online to people you do not know. Also, check with your parents before downloading anything from the Internet. That is another common way computer viruses spread.

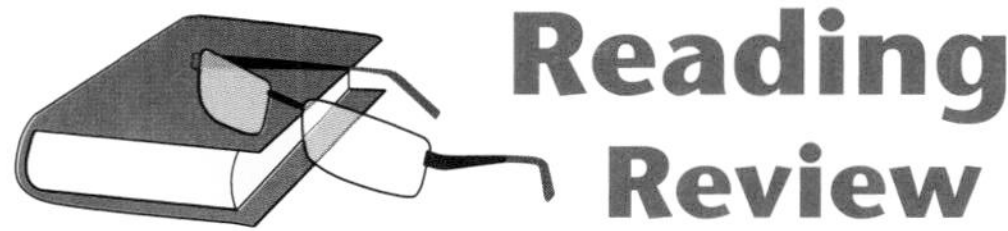

1. What types of technology do you use most?
2. How has technology affected your home and family?

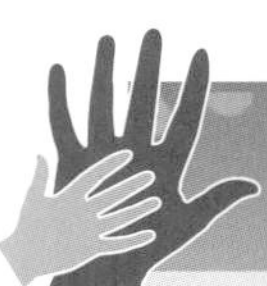

Safety Link

Social Networking Sites

It is important to get your parents' permission before joining a social networking site. Learn how to use the site carefully. Not everyone is honest on their profiles and not all people are your true friends. These sites use advertising to generate a profit. They also encourage other businesses to post websites for you to join. This is a growing form of marketing to teens. You may not want companies to have all the same information your friends have about you. Be very careful about giving out and posting your personal information.

Communicating with Technology

Technology has increased our opportunities to interact with each other. Computer technology makes it possible to communicate with almost anyone at any time by e-mail.

Some families who live in different places communicate online through video calling programs. To make and receive video calls, each person needs a webcam. **Webcams** are small video cameras showing live images through the Internet. They are connected to computers or other devices with Internet access.

Many people use social networking websites to keep in touch with friends and family. On these sites, you must join and create a profile online. You invite others to join that site and search for friends who are already registered. Some family members are using social networking sites to share photos and family stories.

Others are writing their thoughts and opinions about nearly everything online through a blog. A **blog** is a public online journal. Some people have travel blogs where they share their experiences. Blogs can be managed by an individual or by a group.

There are other programs, in addition to blogs, that allow users to post short instant messages online. Multiple people can read what you have to say and also comment on it. Remember to use care in what you write on blogs or other websites. Consider them public online conversations. Once posted, you generally cannot take your words back.

Many people now have cellular (cell) phones. Cell phones work through wireless technology. Some are called *smart phones* because they access the Internet and have many uses. Cell phones can be used as an alarm clock, camera, calendar, photo album, and music player. Texting is a quick way to communicate without talking to or seeing the person. See **6-7**. How has texting changed the way in which we communicate with others? Have you ever texted someone in your house instead of talking to him or her in person?

As you learned earlier, relationships depend on communication. Some research suggests that families now spend more time communicating as a result of technology. Other studies show, however, that less time is spent talking face-to-face. Some families text each other instead of talking in person. Remember that personal contact strengthens relationships. Be sure to balance other forms of communication with personal contact.

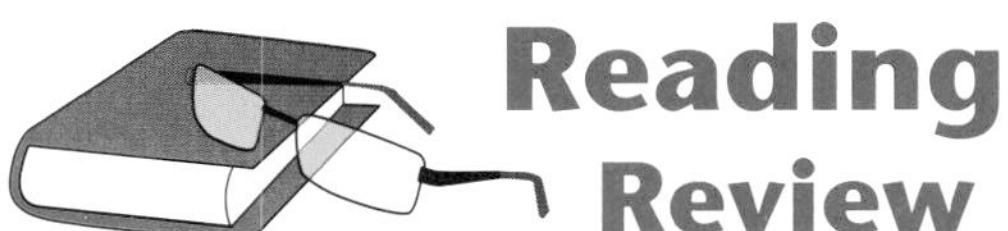

Reading Review

1. What are some ways to communicate through technology?
2. How do you protect your personal information when you are online?

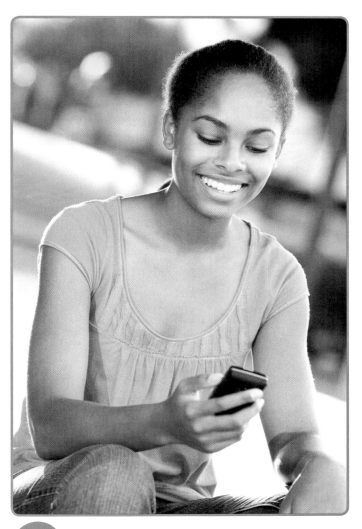

6-7 Using abbreviations can make texting quicker. What abbreviations do you know?

Using Technology for Entertainment and Learning

Cable and satellite TV give you more viewing choices than ever. DVDs and digital video recorder (DVR) technology let you decide when and what you want to watch. You can also use your computer or other devices to download and watch your favorite shows and movies. You can even read books through the Internet. There are a number of video-sharing websites on the Internet. These sites allow users to upload, share, and view personal videos.

A wide selection of video games has better graphics. Some game systems encourage physical interaction through motion-controlled gaming. With more choices, family members may not spend as much time together. It is easy to go to different rooms to watch different shows or play video games. Has technology increased or decreased the time your family spends together?

Computers work through software. **Software** is a set of instructions telling a computer what to do. There are two categories of software. *Systems software* includes everything that makes your computer run and keeps it working. *Applications software* includes the programs you use to do work or other activities. The most common types of applications software are listed in **6-8**. You can now buy some applications software, or *apps*, online for your computer, smart phone, or other electronic devices.

Types of Applications Software

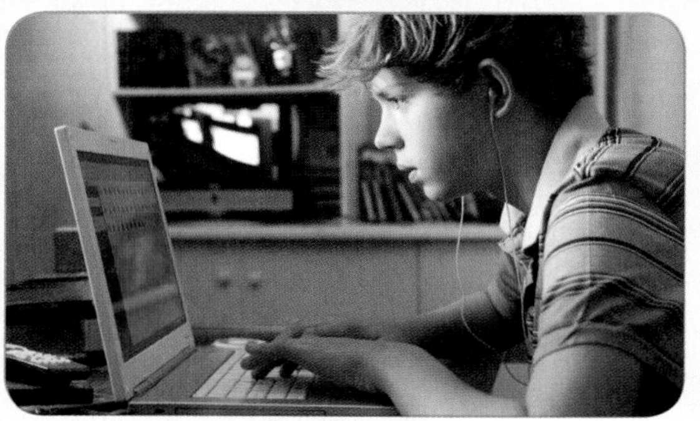

Word Processing allows you to type, edit, and print materials. You can use this program to do homework and write letters.

A *database* is a collection of data organized so you can quickly select desired information. It is often called an *electronic filing system.* You can use it to store lists such as your friends' birthdays and addresses.

Spreadsheets let you create tables of numbers. You can then use math functions to add, subtract, multiply, or divide the numbers. Families can use this software to monitor household budgets, prepare tax forms, and pay bills.

Graphics software allows you to draw, paint, or draft images. Most can be used with other programs to add graphics to text.

6-8 A variety of software is available for personal computers.

The World Wide Web is accessed through the Internet. People, companies, and organizations create their websites on the World Wide Web. Each website is a source of information and can be linked to others. You can find websites on almost any topic. You can read newspapers and e-books online. Weather forecasts from other parts of the world are listed. College catalogs are available online. You can even do research from library databases.

Many companies advertise and sell products on the Internet. Website addresses are listed in TV commercials. Consumers are directed to use their computers to learn more about products and can order them at the same time. Some companies only sell their products online. They may not have physical stores.

When you are doing research, it is important to check the accuracy of a website. Just because something is on the Internet does not mean it is true or correct. Anyone can create a website. This does not mean the person is an expert in the subject. Websites created by the government or educational agencies are likely to be more reliable.

The Internet allows you to do much more than homework research. You can also use your computer to bank, shop, and play games. In fact, grocery stores in some large cities have online services. You can place an order through your computer and arrange to have your groceries delivered to your home. These kinds of services often cost a small fee.

Reading Review

1. Describe different sources of entertainment with technology.
2. Explain the two types of software.
3. What are three ways application software can be used in the home?

Using Technology Responsibly

Remember to be polite when communicating through technology. **Netiquette** is a term for proper etiquette on the Internet. There are also guidelines for polite behavior when using cell phones. See **6-9**.

Proper Behavior When Using a Cell Phone

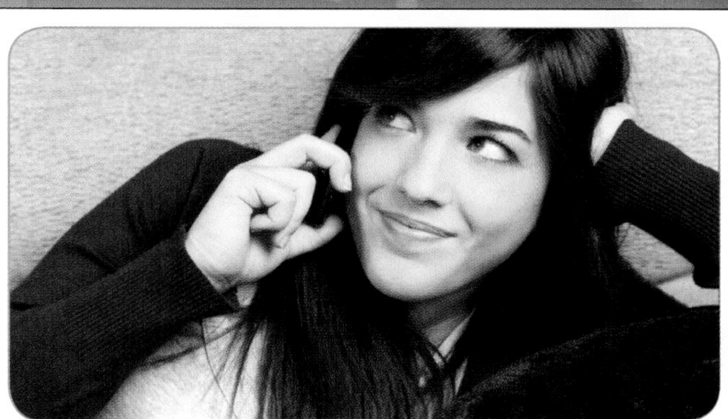

- Respect people around you when using a cell phone.
- Turn off the phone in public places such as classes, restaurants, and movies.
- In public, take calls in a private or separate area.
- Keep your voice down.
- Avoid taking a call when you are talking personally with someone. If you are with someone and must take the call, keep the conversation brief.
- Do not discuss private matters in public places.
- Do not talk about others.
- Use appropriate language.
- Never talk on the phone while driving.

6-9 When using a cell phone, be considerate of the people around you.

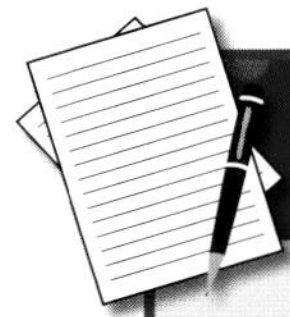

Writing Link

Sending E-mails

You may use e-mail for personal or business communication. In either case, use proper grammar, punctuation, and spelling. You want the person who receives your message to clearly understand your meaning.

Remember that the other person cannot see your facial expressions and may misunderstand what you are writing. In personal e-mail, you can use *emoticons*, or creative punctuation and letters to express emotions. Do not use emoticons, however, in business e-mail.

Avoid sending e-mails when you are angry. Sending a message quickly does not give you time to reflect on what you wrote. Others may read and even forward your e-mail. Do not send anything you would not want posted. Avoid sending chain letters through e-mail.

Netiquette helps you communicate better with others. When e-mailing, keep your message short. Use meaningful subject lines. Do not use all capital letters, unless you want to shout your message.

Many Internet providers have instant messaging. This service allows you to have a private chat with someone when you are both online. The system alerts you when a person from your list is online when you are.

Some Internet providers have *chat rooms*. You can chat with a group of people who are online at the same time. Treat people in a chat room as if you were meeting strangers. Treat them with respect and courtesy, but never give out personal information. Do not agree to meet anyone in person whom you have met online. It is easy for others to hide their true identities. If someone asks you to meet with him or her, talk about it with your parents.

It is important to use technology responsibly. On social networking sites, avoid making friends with people you do not know. Be honest when creating your profile. Treat people through these websites as you would like to be treated.

Unfortunately, some schools are having problems with cyberbullying. **Cyberbullying** is when a person is negatively targeted by another through technology. This can include cell phones, Internet use, or interactive digital technologies. There can be rude and embarrassing comments made that hurt the other person. Some teens have lost their Internet provider service as a result of cyberbullying. This behavior violates the service providers' contracts.

It is important that you report any cases of cyberbullying you witness. Tell a parent or a teacher. Refuse to join others who are bullying. If someone sends you a hateful or hurtful comment, just delete it. If cyberbullies cannot hurt or torment others, then they will often stop.

Learn how to control technology and not be controlled *by* it. Technology produces machines. Machines are designed to make people's lives easier. They are not designed to replace people. Machines can do only what you tell them to do. It is important for families to choose what types of technology to use.

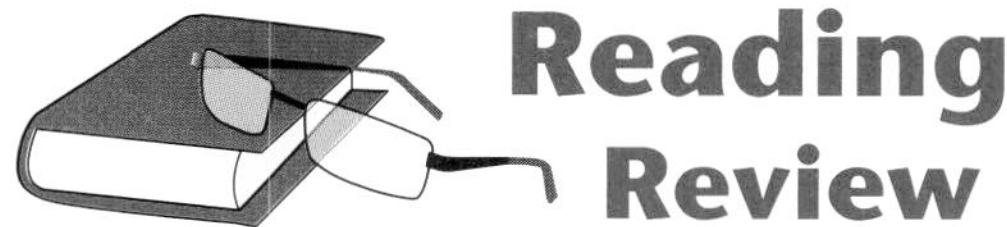

1. List three rules for netiquette.
2. Why should you check the accuracy of a website?
3. Why should you never agree to meet anyone in person whom you have met online?

Section Summary

- Your home and lifestyle have been affected by technology.
- Technology has changed the way we communicate, learn, and relate to each other.
- You should learn as much as possible about technology now to prepare for the future.

Chapter Summary

To be able to enjoy the future, take care of what you have today. It is very important to protect the environment. If the environment is not protected, the natural resources all living beings need will be used up or damaged. Energy crises are the result of people using too many natural resources. Air and water pollution are caused by people abusing natural resources.

There are many ways for you and your family to help protect the environment. Laws are made to prevent pollution. They also help protect natural resources. Glass, paper, aluminum, and other materials can be recycled and used again.

Another way to protect natural resources is to improve energy efficiency. When you conserve energy, you are not using as much as before. There are many ways to conserve heating fuels. You can learn to cool homes and use appliances more efficiently, too.

Technology makes your life easier. Computers can help you do homework and keep track of budgets. Many people use technology to communicate with friends and family. Be polite when talking with others online or through e-mail. Also, be careful to never meet in person with anyone you have met online. It is harmful to become involved in any cyberbullying activities.

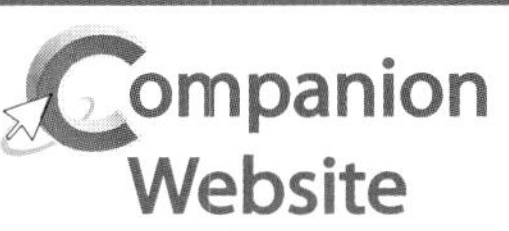

Review Key Terms and Main Ideas for Chapter 6 at the website.

Chapter Review

Write your answers on a separate sheet of paper.

1. What is the relationship between ecology and the environment?
2. True or false. The waste from producing nuclear power is nontoxic.
3. Give two examples of natural resources in your environment.
4. True or false. Cars use fuel made from petroleum.
5. Which of the following is a cause of an energy crisis?
   A. Limited natural resources.
   B. Greater demand for energy than supply.
   C. Misused natural resources.
   D. All the above.
6. What does the term sustainability mean?
7. What are the *three Rs*? Give two examples of each one.
8. What is the advantage of using solar energy?
9. List four ways to conserve energy when heating your home.
10. List four ways to conserve energy when cooling your home.
11. True or false. Not everyone is honest on their profiles and not all people are your true friends.
12. Give three ways in which people communicate using technology.
13. What is a blog?
14. What are three rules for netiquette?
15. What should teens do when they see cyberbullying?

Life Skills

16. There is a center for older adults two blocks from your school. The director of the center would like to start a recycling program that would involve the center's members and students from your school. Develop a plan for this recycling program. Then create a presentation you can show to the center's advisory board.
17. Work with your parents to make a list of ways to conserve energy in your home. Choose two strategies and try them. How will you evaluate their efficiency? After two months, determine how well they worked. If necessary, make any changes and try them again. If they worked well, try some of the other strategies. Report you findings to the class.

Technology

18. Conduct online research about new sources of energy. You might choose solar or wind power as your topic, or find even newer sources. How long has the source of energy you are researching been available? Why are alternative energy sources being researched and developed at this point in time? When will they be more common than the current energy sources? Write a short report based on your research.

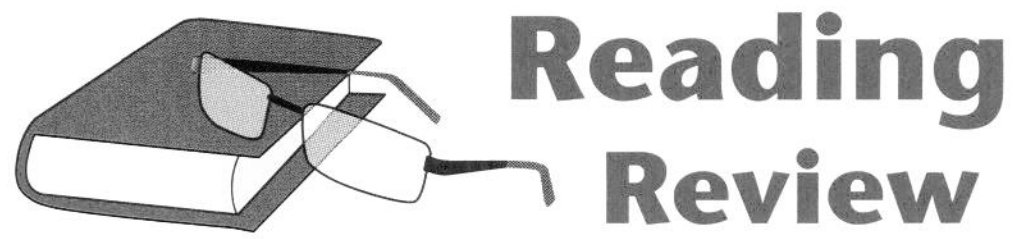

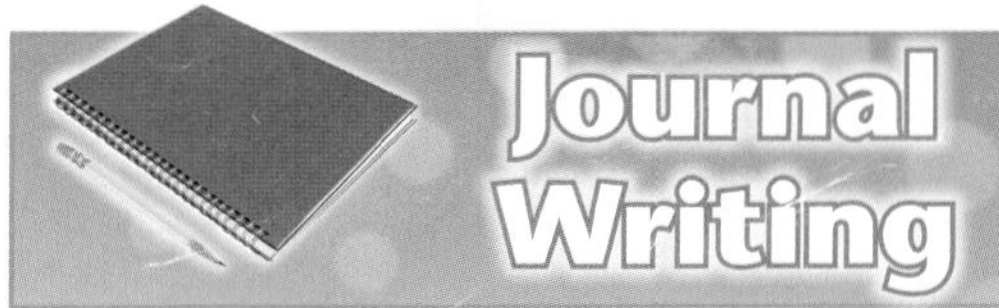

19. Write a journal for two days of your life in the year 2025. Describe your home, family, and work. Does the world look very different than it does now? How and why? Also, describe the kinds of technology you think will be available.

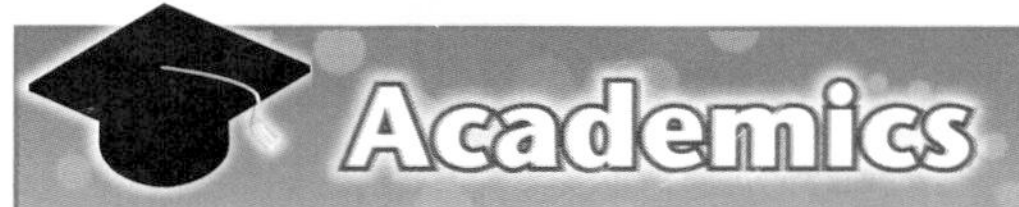

20. **History.** Interview your parents about the increased costs of electricity, heating fuel, and gasoline. Ask them how much these cost when they were your age. Ask them how much costs have risen in your lifetime. What do you expect energy costs to be when you are an adult? Why?
21. **Reading.** Use print or online sources to find a recent article about an environmental problem. Read your article to the class. Discuss the effects this problem might have on the earth both now and in the future.
22. **Writing.** Write an article about netiquette and cell phone etiquette for your school's newspaper. Discuss the common social networking sites and the issues to look for when using those sites. In addition to general cell phone etiquette, list your school's rules for cell phone use.

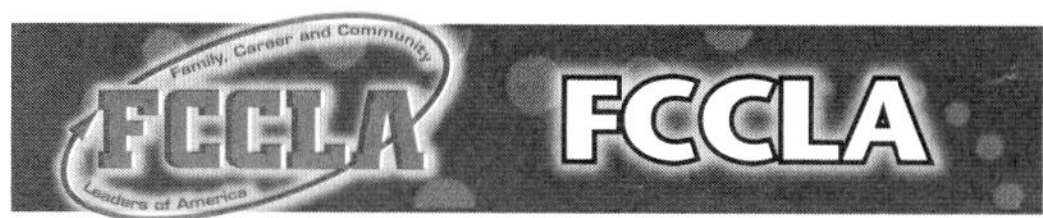

23. As a class, brainstorm about the reasons that bullying occurs and the consequences for both the bully and the victim. What are the signs of bullying? Make *Anti-Bullying* posters listing the different types of bullying and the various ways it can be stopped. Get permission to display informational posters in your school. Then develop an FCCLA project for the *STOP the Violence* program. Obtain further information about this program from your FCCLA advisor.

Unit 3
You and Food

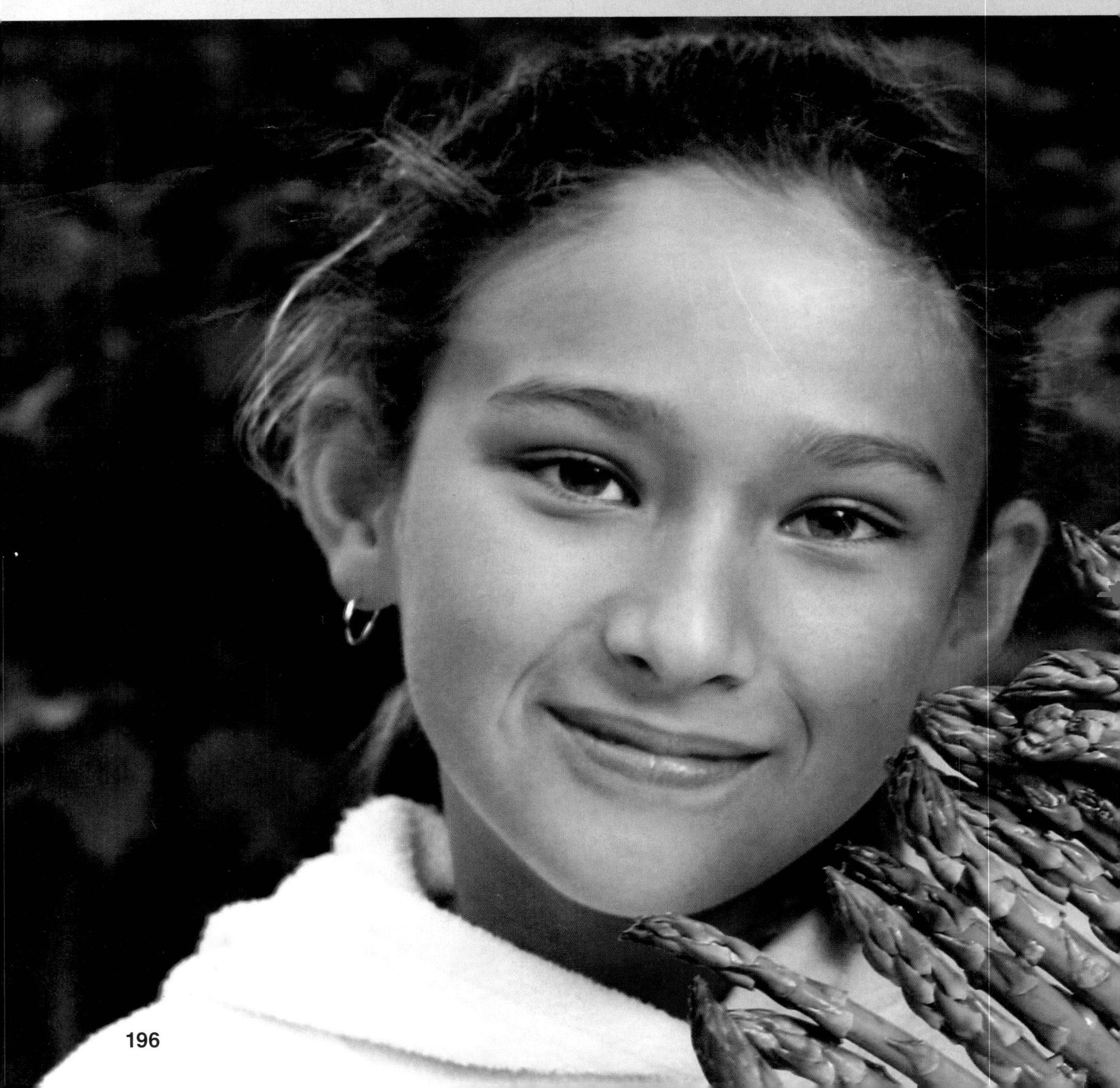

Chapter 7	The Foods You Eat
Chapter 8	Planning Meals
Chapter 9	You in the Kitchen

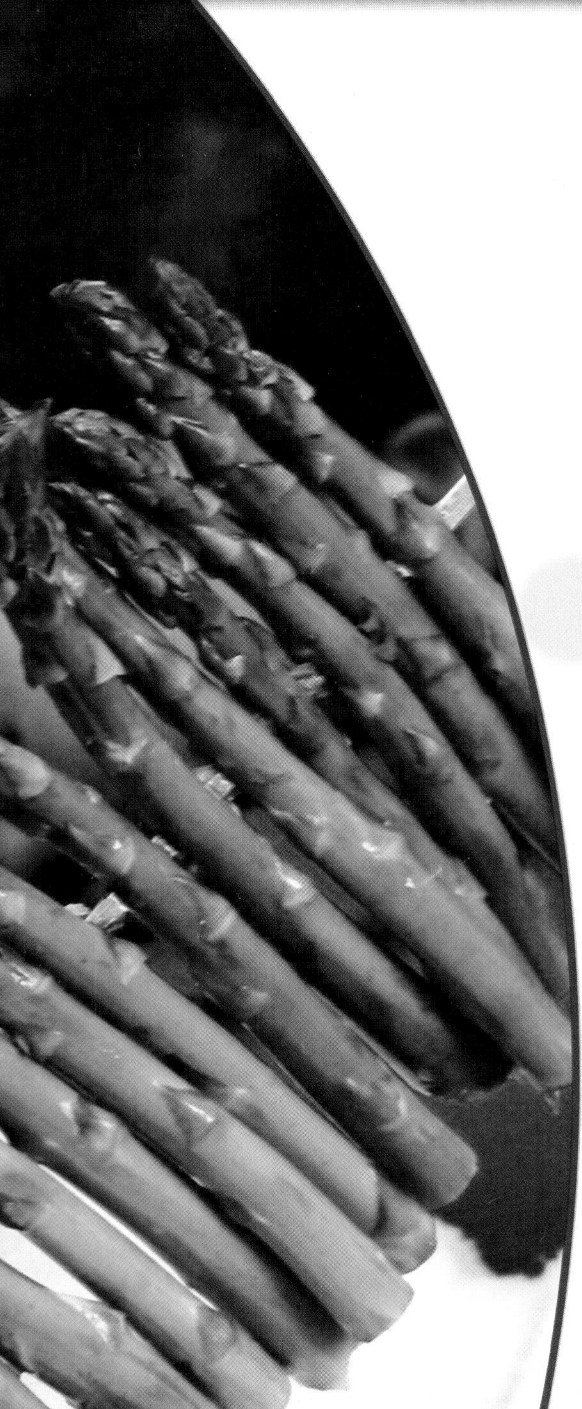

Exploring Careers

The following careers relate to the information you will study in Unit 3. Read the descriptions and then complete the activity to learn more about the careers that might interest you.

Career	Description
Server	Takes orders and serves food to restaurant diners
Dietitian	Plans nutrition programs and supervises the preparation and serving of meals
Caterer	Prepares, delivers, and serves food
Chef	Oversees food preparation, develops recipes, and manages a restaurant's kitchen
Food stylist	Prepares and arranges food for presentation and photography
Baker	Prepares breads, cakes, cookies, and pastries
Sanitation supervisor	Maintains a clean, hygienic environment
Food scientist	Creates and improves food products

Activity: Pick three of the eight careers listed and briefly research each one. Write a list of eight words describing the skills and traits a person needs to be successful in each career.

Chapter 7
The Foods You Eat

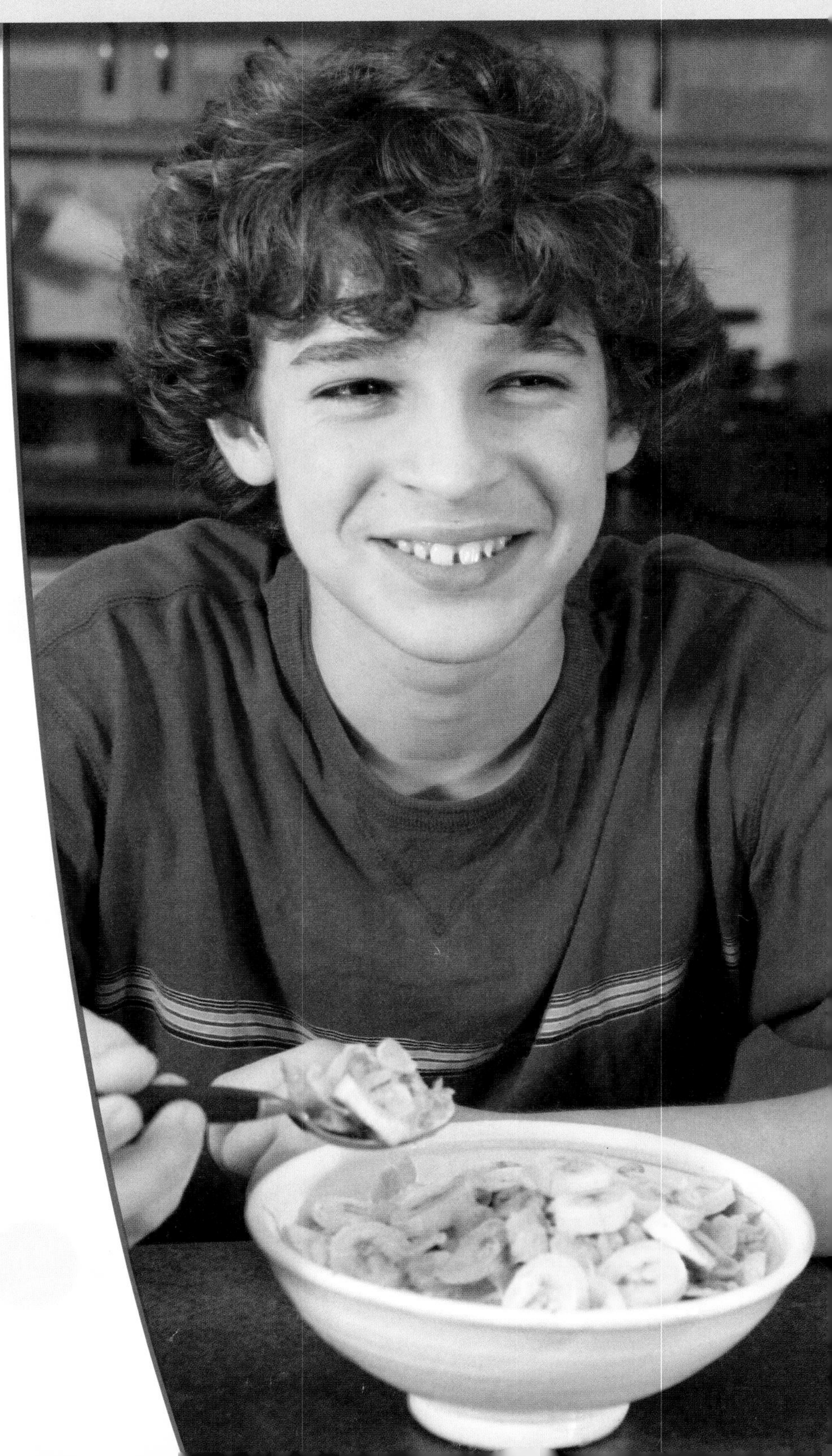

Sections

Sharpen Your Reading

After reading each section, answer this question: If you explained the information to a friend who is not taking this class, what would you tell him or her?

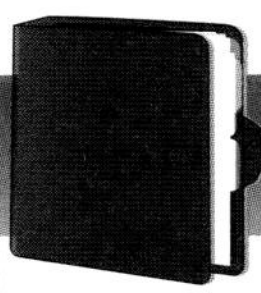

Concept Organizer

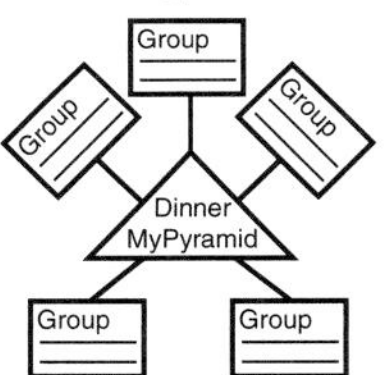

Use a star diagram like the one shown to plan a healthful dinner using a food from each of the food groups in MyPlate.

Companion Website
www.g-wlearning.com

Print out the concept organizer at the website.

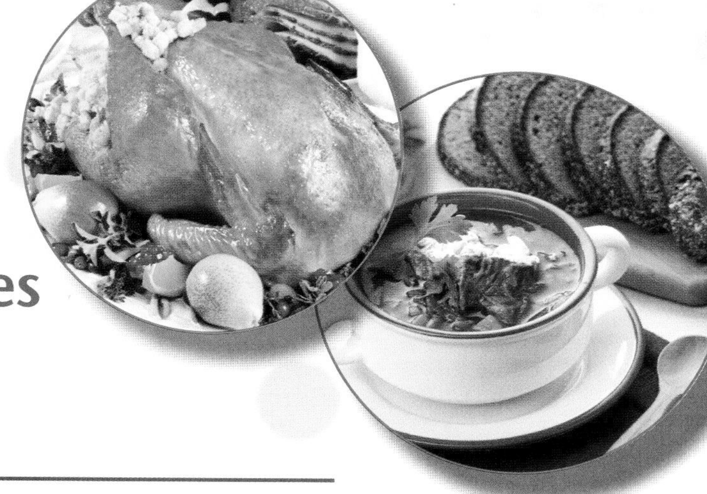

Section 7-1
Nutrition and Food Choices

Objectives

After studying this section, you will be able to
- **define** *nutrition*, *nutrients*, *diet*, *saturated fat*, *trans fat*, *cholesterol*, and *traditions*.
- **give examples** of the functions and sources of the six types of nutrients.
- **explain** how your diet affects your performance in school, sports, and social activities.
- **explain** how food choices are individual and influenced by many factors.
- **describe** how ethnic and cultural traditions influence foods that families enjoy.

Key Terms

nutrition: the study of how your body uses food and the effects food has on it.

nutrients: chemicals and other substances from foods needed for the body to function.

diet: the food and beverages consumed each day.

saturated fat: a fat that is solid at room temperature.

trans fat: a type of fat found in vegetable shortening, some margarine, baked goods, and many processed foods.

cholesterol: a fatty substance found in foods from animal sources.

traditions: customs passed from one generation to another.

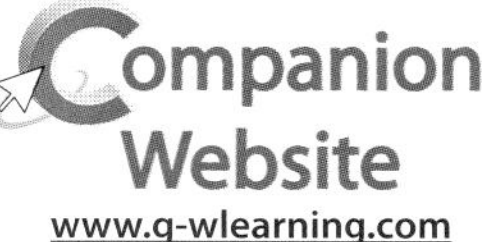

Study the Key Terms by completing crossword puzzles, matching activities, and e-flash cards at the website.

Main Ideas

- Nutrients in food help your body grow, develop, and be healthy.
- Your diet affects your performance in daily activities.
- Food choices are individual and influenced by many factors.
- Personal preferences and habits guide food choices.
- Ethnic and cultural traditions influence foods that families enjoy.

Nutrition is the study of how your body uses food and the effects food has on it. **Nutrients** are the chemicals and other substances from foods needed for the body to function. Your body needs nutrients to grow, develop, and be healthy. Nutrients are used by your body to provide for growth and repair. They also furnish energy and regulate body processes.

A **diet** is the food and beverages consumed each day. Your diet affects how you perform in school, in sports, and at social activities. Your diet provides the nutrients your body needs. Learning is hard work. A diet high in nutrients can give you the energy for learning, as well as physical activities.

The Nutrients

There are six types of nutrients. They are proteins, carbohydrates, fats, vitamins, minerals, and water. You can get the nutrients you need by eating many kinds of foods. See **7-1**.

Proteins can be found in both meat and meat substitutes. They give your body energy. They also help your body grow and repair body tissues, such as hair, skin, muscles, and nerves. Your heart, liver, lungs, and brain also need protein to function and stay in good shape. People of all ages need protein in their diets.

Carbohydrates provide energy. Starch, sugar, and fiber are the three kinds of carbohydrates. They can be found in breads and cereals, fruits and vegetables, and products containing sugar.

Fats add flavor to food and help satisfy your hunger. You need some foods containing fat in a healthful diet. **Saturated fat** is a fat that is solid at room temperature. **Trans fat** is a type of fat found in vegetable shortening, some margarine, baked goods, and many processed foods. **Cholesterol** is a fatty substance found in foods from animal sources, such as meat and eggs. Many people eat too much fat for their body frames. This can lead to health problems such as heart disease, high blood pressure, and obesity.

Vitamins are used by your body for the growth and repair of tissues. Fat-soluble vitamins, such as vitamins A and D, are stored in your body. You can eat foods rich in these every other day and still get the amount you need. Most water-soluble vitamins, such as vitamin C, are not stored in your body. You need to eat foods rich in these every day.

Minerals help regulate body processes. Two important minerals are calcium and iron. Calcium is needed to build strong bones and teeth. Iron helps blood cells function.

Water is a very important nutrient. Your body can survive only a few days without water. It carries the other nutrients to every cell in your body and then carries away the waste.

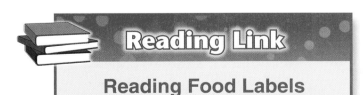

Reading Food Labels

Get into the habit of reading the nutrition facts on your food's packaging. Check the levels of those nutrients it is best to limit. It is also helpful to know the specific ingredients in your food before you eat.

The Nutrients	
Functions	**Sources**
Proteins	
• Needed for growth and repair of body tissues. • Help body organs function and stay in good condition. • Supply energy.	Meat, eggs, poultry, fish, legumes, peanuts, nuts, seeds, milk, cheese, and yogurt.
Carbohydrates	
• Supply energy. • Provide fiber to aid in digestion and remove body wastes.	Breads, cereals, rice, pasta, fruits, vegetables, legumes, and sugar and other sweets.
Fats	
• Provide energy. • Insulate the body. • Cushion body organs. • Help promote growth and healthy skin.	Oil, butter, margarine, salad dressing, meat, poultry, eggs, cheese, nuts, and peanut butter.
Vitamins	
Vitamin A • Helps with normal vision. • Helps keep body tissues healthy. • Helps with growth.	Dark green vegetables, deep yellow or orange vegetables and fruits, and eggs.
B Vitamins (thiamin, riboflavin, niacin) • Help your body use other nutrients in food for energy. • Help keep skin, hair, muscles, and nerves healthy. • Help keep appetite and digestion normal. • Help your body use oxygen more efficiently.	Meat, poultry, fish, eggs, whole-grain and enriched breads and cereals, milk, cheese, yogurt, and ice cream.
Vitamin C • Helps keep gums healthy. • Helps cuts and bruises heal. • Helps your body fight infections. • Helps with growth.	Oranges, grapefruit, lemons, limes, tangerines, berries, papaya, melons, broccoli, spinach, peppers, kale, collards, mustard greens, turnip greens, potatoes, tomatoes, and cabbage.
Minerals	
Calcium • Helps build strong, healthy bones and teeth. • Helps the heart beat properly. • Helps muscles move.	Milk, cheese, yogurt, ice cream, leafy green vegetables, and fish with tiny bones.
Iron • Helps blood carry oxygen. • Helps cells use oxygen.	Meat, eggs, liver, legumes, and whole-grain and enriched breads and cereals.
Water	
• Carries nutrients to the cells and wastes away from cells. • Helps regulate body processes such as digestion. • Helps maintain normal body temperature. • Helps cells operate.	Milk, juices, soups, drinking water, juicy fruits and vegetables, and some solid foods.

7-1 Knowing the functions and sources of nutrients can help you eat nutritiously.

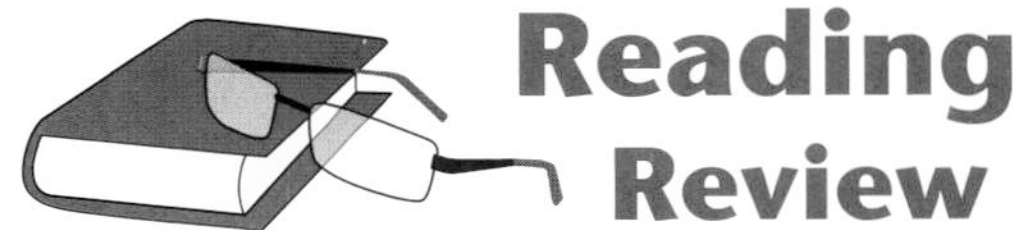

1. What is the difference between nutrition and nutrients?
2. What are the three kinds of carbohydrates? In what foods are carbohydrates found?
3. Why is water such an important nutrient? What does it do in your body?

Personal Preference and Habit

Eating is one of life's greatest pleasures. It is often part of holidays and special events. See **7-2**. The food choices you make several times a day are unique and influenced by many factors. You may not think much about why you like or select certain foods. Your choices are important, however, because they can benefit or harm your health. The secret is to balance foods that give you pleasure with those that offer health benefits. Knowing why you choose certain foods can help you make wise decisions.

The most common reason people choose certain foods is because they like the flavors. Some people like the hot, peppery taste of chili. Others prefer the bland flavor of plain rice. You may select some foods because of habit. Perhaps you often enjoy eating cereal for breakfast and a piece of fruit after school. Food habits are comforting. You do not have to think about choices.

It is also fun to try different foods for meals or snacks. For instance, you may enjoy trying new foods when you eat out with family or friends. You might decide you like these new foods. Making a habit of eating a wider variety of foods can make a diet more interesting.

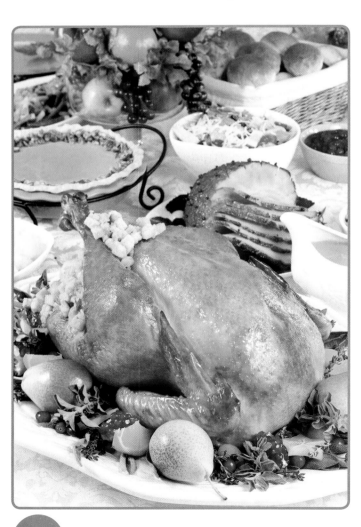

7-2 These are traditional foods for Thanksgiving dinner.

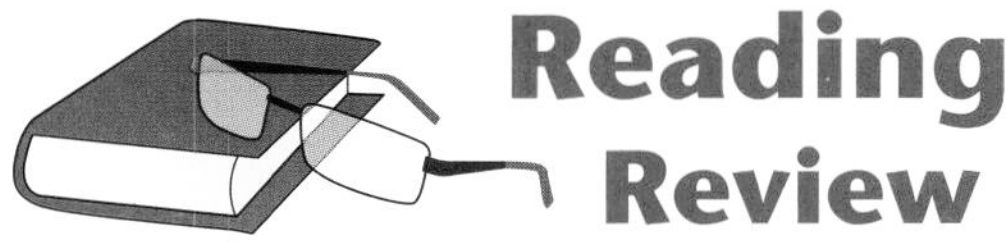

1. Name six of your favorite foods. Describe the flavors and tastes.
2. How do likes and dislikes affect family food choices?

Cultural and Social Influences

Another strong influence on your choice of food is your ethnic or cultural heritage. When people talk about their culture, they often describe special foods that are part of their background. Throughout the world, people enjoy foods that reflect their local cultures. In England, people might dine on fish and chips. In Italy, pasta dishes are part of the culture. In the Middle East, people often eat hummus, which is a food made from chickpeas. See **7-3**.

A wide variety of foods is part of the culture in the United States. People from many different cultures contributed these foods. Native Americans were one of these cultural groups. Hundreds of years ago, Native Americans raised corn, beans, pumpkins, and squash. These foods are still part of the culture in the United States.

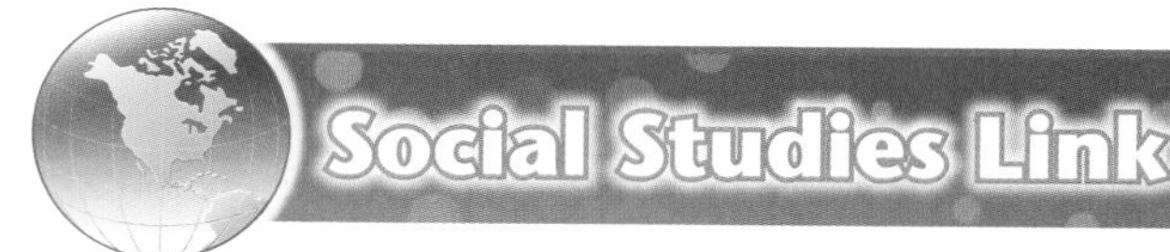

Cultural Influences and Food Choices

Some of the foods your family eats may relate to your culture. They may be foods your relatives brought from another country. The region where you live is also part of your culture. Some of the foods you enjoy may be special to your region. Southern fried chicken and New England clam chowder are examples.

Bring a special family food to class and have a *tasting party*. Along with the food, include a brief summary of the origin of the food and the recipe. Bring enough copies of the recipe to share with the class.

Each cultural group that settled in the United States brought its own eating habits and food customs. For instance, people from China brought the cooking technique of stir-frying. People from Mexico brought foods such as tacos and burritos.

Sometimes people could not find foods from their culture. Therefore, they adapted available foods to their ways of cooking. They also created new ways to prepare these foods. For instance, French people in Louisiana developed Cajun cooking.

As the United States grew, many people moved from one region to another. They again brought their food customs with them. As a result, you can now find many cultural foods throughout the United States.

Traditions are customs passed from one generation to another. Family traditions affect foods children learn to like and enjoy. Typical breads on your family table may be bagels, biscuits, or tortillas. Special meats, fish, or baked goods may be prepared for family celebrations. Some families adapt traditional foods to meet the changing likes and dislikes of family members. Some families and individuals follow vegetarian meal patterns. See **7-4**.

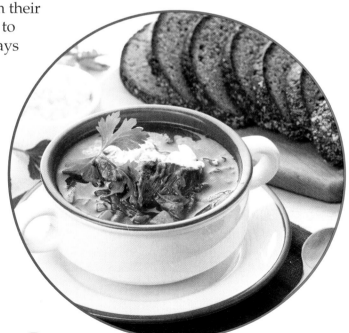

7-3 Borscht, a beet soup, is popular in Russian culture.

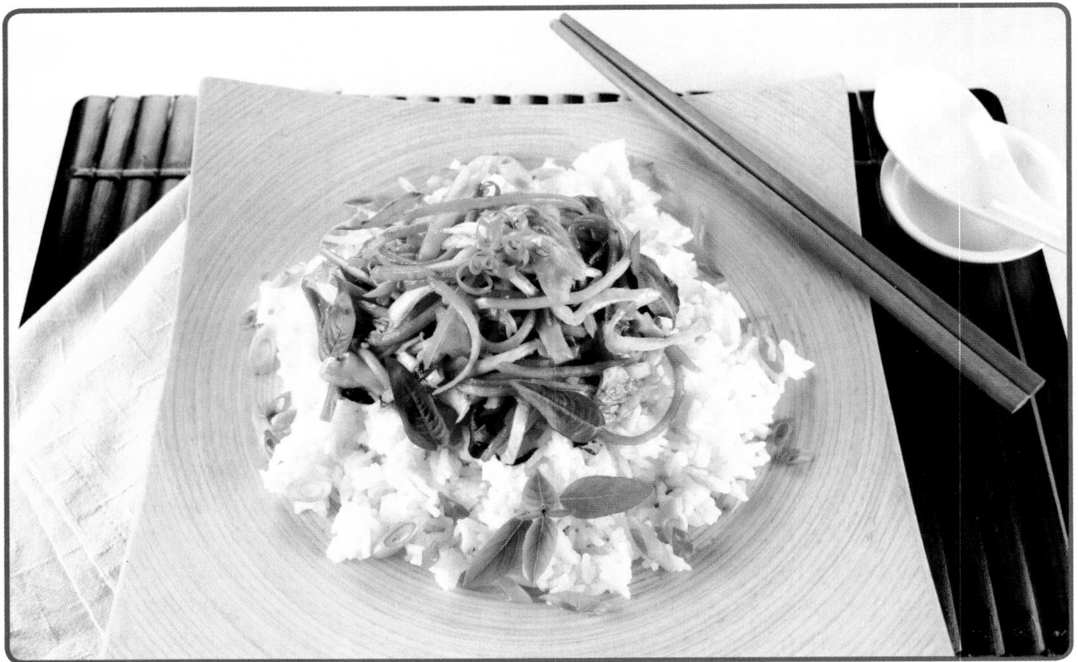

7-4 A vegetarian meal might include an Asian stir-fry on rice with Thai basil and Vietnamese mint.

Your food choices are also affected by social contacts. It is fun to share food with friends at a party. You can make wise food choices in social situations. Instead of chips, choose crisp, crunchy vegetables. Suppose you are trying to maintain your best weight, but find it difficult to say *no* when friends are going for ice cream. Maybe having a small ice cream cone instead of a large hot fudge sundae is a better choice.

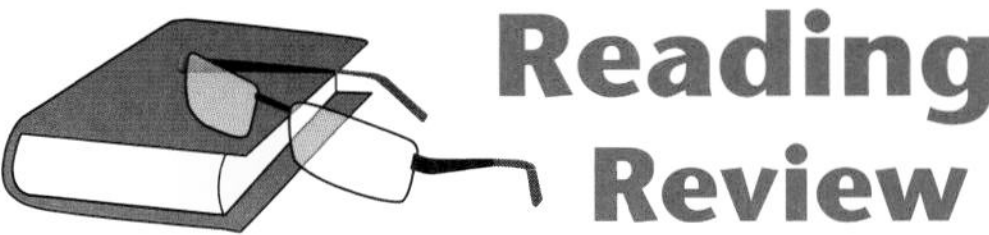

Reading Review

1. Describe the cultural heritage of your family. Are there special foods that are common to your family heritage?
2. Why are there so many food choices in the United States?
3. Name three social situations that might affect your food choices.

Section Summary

- The six types of nutrients are proteins, carbohydrates, fats, vitamins, minerals, and water.
- Many factors can influence your daily food choices.
- Your personal preferences and habits affect your food choices.
- Your ethnic and cultural heritage influences the foods your family eats.

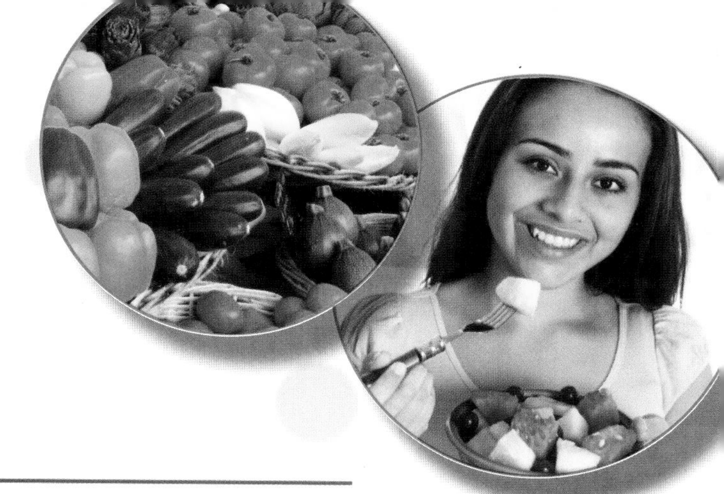

Section 7-2
Using MyPlate

Objectives

After studying this section, you will be able to

- **define** *Dietary Guidelines for Americans*, *nutrient dense*, *SoFAS*, *MyPlate*, *balanced diet*, and *enriched*.
- **list** the two main messages of the *Dietary Guidelines for Americans*.
- **name** the food groups in MyPlate.
- **describe** how foods from each group help meet your body's needs.

Key Terms

Dietary Guidelines for Americans: document developed by experts to promote a healthful lifestyle through improved nutrition and physical activity.

nutrient dense: foods that provide vitamins, minerals, and other substances that have positive health effects, with relatively few calories.

SoFAS: foods that are high in solid fats and/or added sugars.

MyPlate: the United States Department of Agriculture's (USDA) new food guidance system based on the *Dietary Guidelines for Americans*.

balanced diet: a diet that provides all the nutrients your body needs for good health.

enriched: to have nutrients added to a product to replace those removed during processing.

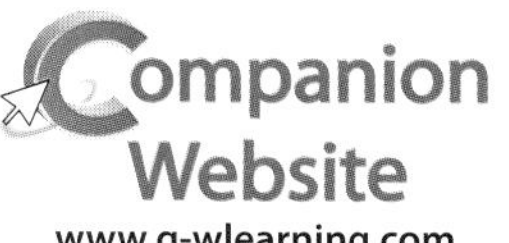

Study the Key Terms by completing crossword puzzles, matching activities, and e-flash cards at the website.

Main Ideas

- Following the *Dietary Guidelines for Americans* can help you achieve good health and avoid certain diseases.
- Selecting the recommended daily amounts from each food group in MyPlate will help you eat a balanced diet.

Most teens want to know how to eat better to stay active and healthy. You are a growing teen. What foods should you eat to look and feel your best? There are many tools available to help you make healthful choices. In this section, you will learn about a few of the resources that can help keep you healthy and fit for enjoying life and doing well in school.

Dietary Guidelines for Americans

The **Dietary Guidelines for Americans** is a document developed by experts to promote a healthful lifestyle through improved nutrition and physical activity. The *2010 Guidelines* provide dietary advice for Americans two years and older. This includes people at increased risk of chronic disease.

The two main messages of the *Guidelines* focus on maintaining a healthy weight and choosing nutrient-dense foods and beverages. Foods that are **nutrient dense** provide vitamins, minerals, and other substances that have positive health effects, with relatively few calories.

To achieve and maintain a healthy weight, follow these tips:

- Get plenty of physical activity.
- Enjoy your food, but eat less.
- Avoid large portions.

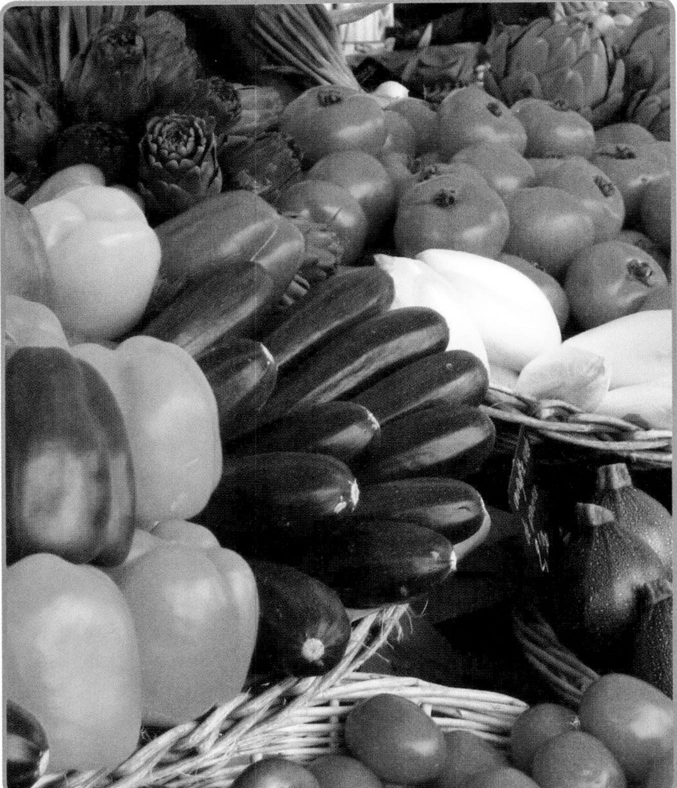

7-5 Dark-green vegetables, red and orange vegetables, and beans and peas are all good vegetable choices.

To consume a more nutrient-dense diet, follow these tips:

- Make half your plate fruits and vegetables. See **7-5**.
- Switch to fat-free or low-fat (1%) milk and milk products.
- Compare sodium in foods and choose the lower sodium foods.
- Drink water instead of sugary drinks.

To achieve dietary goals, Americans must become conscious eaters. Select the most nutritious foods packed with vitamins, minerals, fiber, and other nutrients. Choose more fresh fruits and vegetables, protein-rich meats, poultry, lean fish, beans, and nuts. Avoid foods that are high in solid fats and/or added sugars, called **SoFAS**. Cookies, cakes, and doughnuts are all examples of foods that are high in SoFAS.

Good health depends on daily physical activity as well as nutritious food. You can find the balance between food and activity that is right for you. The *2010 Dietary Guidelines* recommend you follow the advice given in the *2008 Physical Activity Guidelines for Americans*. These guidelines help

Americans six years old and older to gain health benefits by doing physical activity.

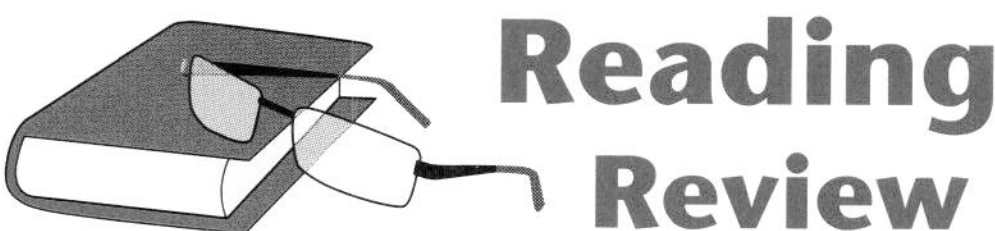

1. How can you achieve and maintain a healthy weight?
2. What is a nutrient-dense diet? Give examples.

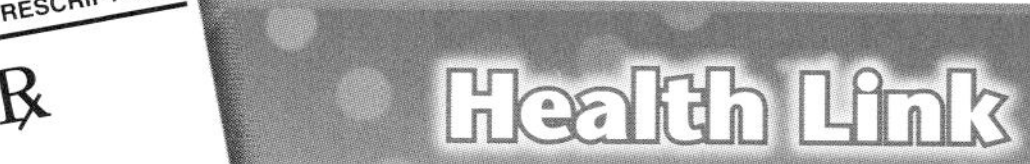

Choosing Nutrient-Dense Foods

What kinds of foods do you often choose when you get hungry and want a snack? Do you choose an orange or a chocolate chip cookie? Hopefully you will choose the orange. The orange has lots of vitamins and is nutrient dense. It will help you feel full, which can satisfy your hunger until your next meal. The cookie has much more sugar and fewer nutrients. It probably will not satisfy your hunger, but can often leave you wanting more. Next time you are choosing a snack, consider foods that are nutrient dense such as nuts, seeds, whole grains, fruits, and vegetables.

MyPlate

MyPlate is the United States Department of Agriculture's (USDA) new food guidance system based on the *Dietary Guidelines for Americans*. It divides commonly eaten foods into five main groups. These groups are grains, vegetables, fruits, dairy, and protein. Oils are also included.

MyPlate helps you select the right foods for a balanced diet. A **balanced diet** is one that provides all the nutrients your body needs to maintain good health.

You can create a personalized food plan by going to the website chooseMyPlate.gov. Enter your age, gender, and amount of physical activity. To get a more accurate food plan, you can also enter your height and weight. After entering this data, the program selects the food plan that is right for you. Your plan will recommend daily amounts from each of the five food groups, calories, oils, and physical activity. See **7-6**. Each family member can create a food plan. MyPlate can be used for people two years and older. Vegetarians can also follow MyPlate.

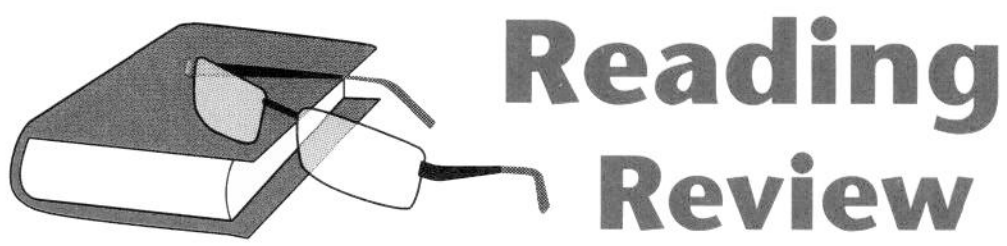

1. How can you get a more accurate food plan from MyPlate?
2. How can you make sure the nutritional needs of each family member are met?

Grains

Grains include bread, cereal, rice, and pasta. Foods in this group are made from grains such as wheat, oats, corn, rice, and barley. These foods are good sources of carbohydrates and the B vitamins. Protein and iron can also be found in many grain products.

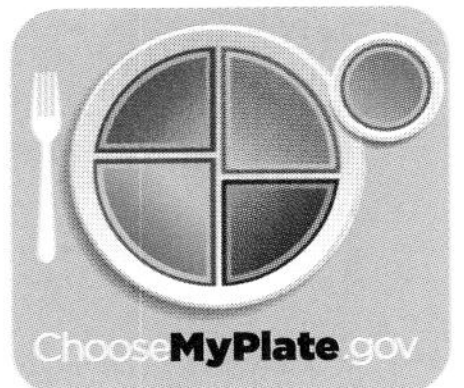

My Daily Food Plan

Based on the information you provided, this is your daily recommended amount from each food group.

GRAINS 6 ounces	VEGETABLES 2½ cups	FRUITS 2 cups	DAIRY 3 cups	PROTEIN 5½ ounces
Make half your grains whole Aim for at least 3 ounces of whole grains a day	**Vary your veggies** Aim for these amounts each week: Dark green veggies = 1½ cups Red and Orange veggies = 5½ cups Beans & peas = 1½ cups Starchy = 5 cups Other = 4 cups	**Focus on fruits** Eat a variety of fruits Choose whole or cut-up fruits more often than fruit juice	**Get your calcium-rich foods** Drink fat-free or low-fat (1%) milk, for the same aount of calcium and other nutrients, but less fat Select fat-free or low-fat yogurt and cheese, or try calcium-fortified soy products	**Go lean with protein** Twice a week, make seafood the protein on your plate Vary your protein routine—choose beans, peas, nuts, and seeds more often Keep meat and poultry portions small and lean

Find your balance between food and physical activity	Know your limits on fats, sugars, and sodium
Be physically active for at least 60 minutes each day.	Your allowance for oils is 6 teaspoons a day. Limit calories from SoFAS to 260 calories a day. Reduce sodium intake to less than 2,3000 mg a day.

Your results are based on a 2000 calorie pattern Name: ____________

This calorie level is only an estimate of your needs. Monitor your body weight to see if you need to adjust your calorie intake.

7-6 This personalized MyPlate plan is for a fourteen-year-old girl who is physically active 30–60 minutes daily.

Read bread and cereal labels to see if the product is whole grain or enriched. **Enriched** products have nutrients added to them to replace those removed during processing. Refined grains are often enriched.

Whole-grain products are healthier choices. They provide natural grain fiber that aids in digestion and ridding the body of waste. Your goal is that at least half the grains you eat are whole grains.

You need to follow the recommended amounts in your food plan. Use ounces to count the amount of grains you eat. An *ounce-equivalent* of grains is one slice of bread, one-half cup cooked cereal, one small tortilla, or one-half cup cooked pasta or rice.

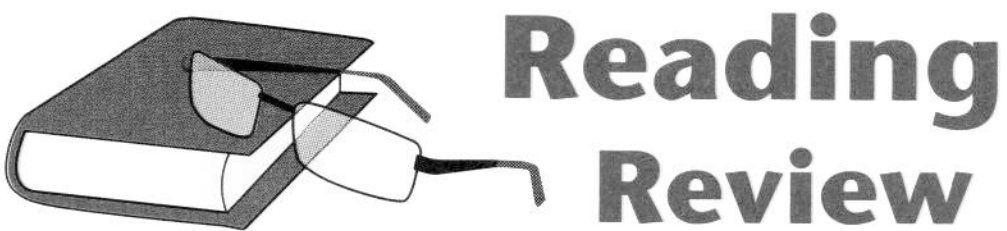

Reading Review

1. Which nutrients are found in foods from the grains group?
2. Why are whole-grain and enriched bread and cereal products good for you?

Vegetables

Vegetables provide important fiber and essential nutrients, such as vitamins A and C. It is easy to remember which vegetables are high in vitamin A by their color. Vitamin A is found in deep yellow or orange vegetables such as carrots and sweet potatoes. This group includes fresh, frozen, and canned vegetables, and vegetable juices.

Use cups to count the amount of vegetables you eat. Two cups of raw, leafy vegetables count as one cup from the vegetables group. One cup of cooked vegetables or juice is also equal to one cup from this group.

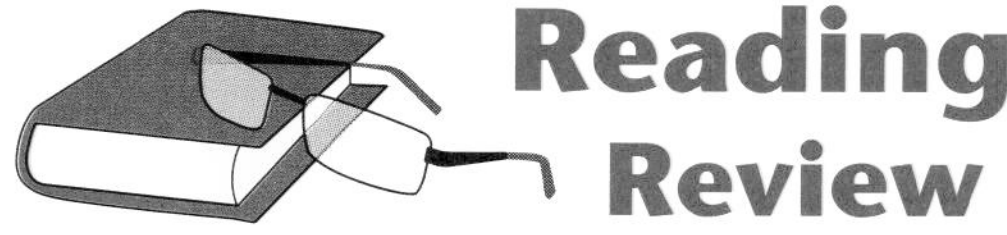

Reading Review

1. What color are vegetables that are rich in vitamin A?
2. How should you count the amount of vegetables you eat every day?

Succeed in Life

Buying Vegetables

It is good to remember that when buying vegetables, the more colorful ones have the most nutrients. The vegetable group is broken into the following five subgroups:

- green vegetables, such as broccoli, spinach, and kale
- orange vegetables, such as carrots, winter squash, and sweet potatoes
- dry beans and peas, such as kidney beans, tofu, and lentils
- starchy vegetables, green peas, corn, and potatoes
- other vegetables, such as celery, onions, and tomatoes

You do not need to eat vegetables from each of these subgroups daily. You should, however, try to eat vegetables from all the subgroups weekly. Your personalized MyPlate plan will tell you how many cups you need weekly from each vegetable subgroup.

Fruits

Fruits include fresh, canned, frozen, and dried fruits, and fruit juices. Make most of your choices whole or cut-up fruit, because fruit juice provides little fiber and often has added sugar. See **7-7**. Fruits are important sources of many nutrients including vitamin C and potassium. Those richest in vitamin C are the citrus fruits, such as oranges and grapefruit. Strawberries, apples, cantaloupe, and kiwi also contain vitamin C. Bananas are a good source of potassium. Your plan recommends a number of cups from the fruit group daily as a guide.

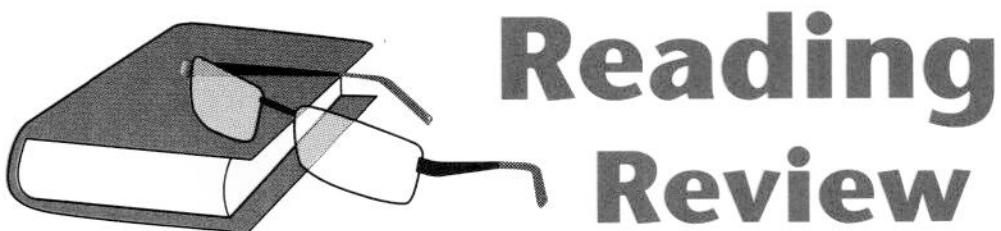

Reading Review

1. Why should you select whole or cut-up fruit more often than juice?
2. What are some fruits that are good sources of vitamin C?

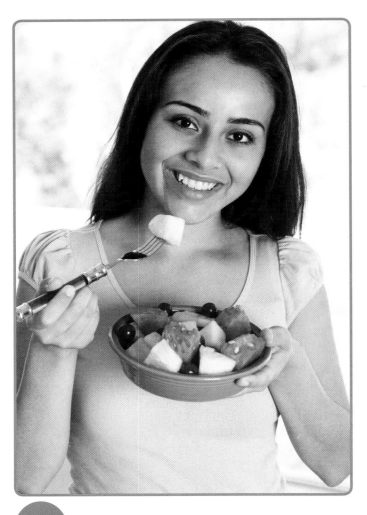

7-7 Fruits are an important source of many nutrients.

Dairy

The dairy group includes foods that are good sources of vitamins and protein. These foods are also rich in minerals, especially calcium.

Teens need three cups from the dairy group every day. Choose fat-free or low-fat milk products most often. One and one-half ounces of natural cheese, one cup of yogurt, or two ounces of processed cheese count as one cup of milk. Some foods made from milk are low in calcium and high in fat and sugars. Ice cream, cream cheese, and butter are examples. These foods are not in this food group.

Foods from the dairy group are important when your body is growing. When children do not get enough calcium in their diets, their bones may be weak or misshapen. Older adults who did not get enough calcium when they were young may also have problems. Their bones may break easily and mend slowly. When you prepare foods for your family, be sure to choose foods that are good sources of calcium.

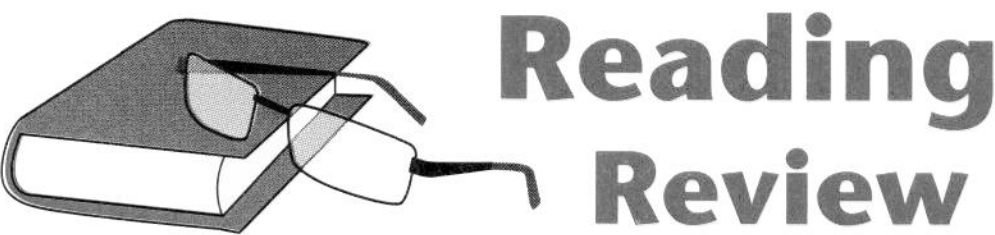

1. Why do you need milk or other dairy products every day? What nutrients do these foods provide?
2. What can happen to children who do not get enough calcium in their diet?

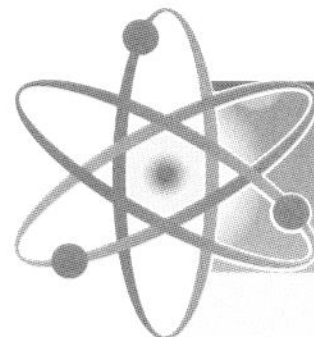

Science Link

Amino Acids

Your body digests the proteins from food and breaks them down into *amino acids*. Your body then reuses the amino acids to make the proteins it needs to function properly. There are many amino acids in proteins. Your body can make some of these amino acids. You must get other amino acids, however, from the foods you eat. Complete proteins contain all the amino acids your body needs to function. Incomplete proteins, however, lack one or more of these amino acids. To get all the amino acids you need, eat a variety of protein-rich foods throughout the day.

Protein

This group includes meat, poultry, fish, dry beans, eggs, seeds, and nuts. It provides a variety of protein-rich foods. Other important nutrients are the B vitamins and iron.

Protein foods are divided into two main groups. Animal sources of protein are called *complete proteins*. Most plant sources of protein, such as nuts and dry beans, are called *incomplete proteins*. They need to be combined with certain other foods to make complete proteins. A balance of complete and incomplete proteins will provide your body with the nutrients it needs.

Many foods in this group are also rich sources of iron. Iron is an important part of blood. It helps your blood carry oxygen to all the cells in your body. If you do not eat foods that supply iron, your body will not get enough oxygen.

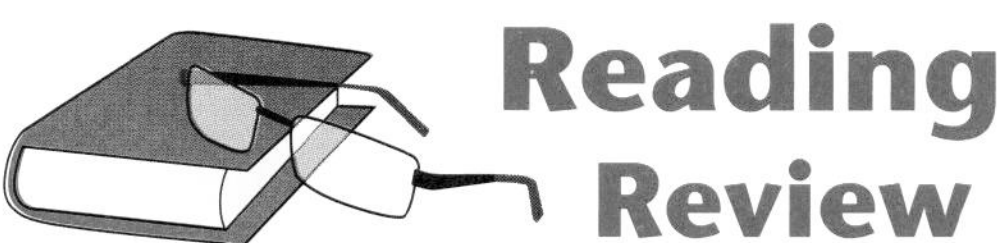

1. What nutrients are provided by foods from the protein group?
2. Why is getting enough iron from the foods you eat important?

Oils

Oils are fats that are liquid at room temperature. Oils come from many different plants and from fish. Some oils are needed in the diet to provide essential nutrients. Foods that contain oils and solid fats are often high in calories. Foods such as butter, margarine, and salad dressing are examples. Many of these foods are nutrient-poor, and provide little more than calories.

Too many foods containing oils and solid fats result in a diet that has more calories than are being used in activity. This imbalance causes weight gain. MyPlate recommends replacing solid fats with oils when possible and limiting oils in your diet to balance calories.

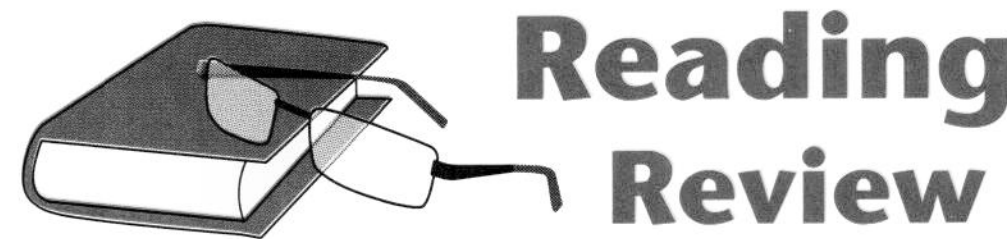

1. Why should you avoid eating too many oils and solid fats or foods containing oils and solid fats?
2. Which foods should you add to your diet to get the most nutrients out of your calories?

Meals to Meet Your Needs

When counting the amount of food you eat, use cups or ounce-equivalents. See **7-8**. Measure one cup of pasta or one ounce of cheese so you are familiar with what these amounts look like. Many dinner servings of spaghetti may be two cups of pasta. Suppose you eat two slices of bread with your spaghetti. This would equal the entire recommended daily amount from the grain group for a 2,000-calorie plan in just one meal.

Remember, snacks like fresh fruit and low-fat milk also help meet your recommended daily amounts. Save chips and cookies for a special treat and be mindful about how much you eat of these foods. Choose nutritious snack foods most of the time. Apples, oranges, carrot sticks, yogurt, and peanut butter sandwiches are all healthful snack choices.

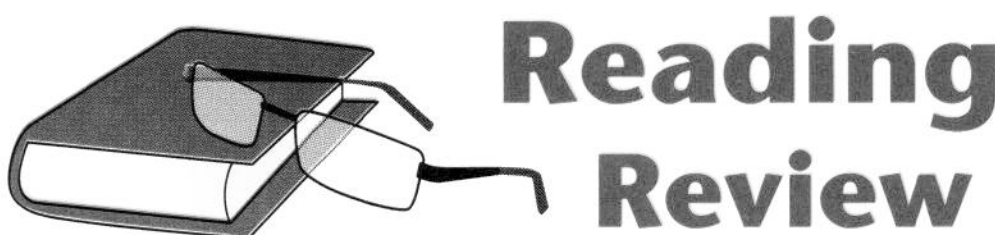

1. Why should you think about what an ounce or a cup of food looks like when counting the amount of food you eat?
2. What are three nutritious foods you could eat as snacks?

Section Summary

- Following the *Dietary Guidelines for Americans* will help you enjoy good health and be physically fit.
- MyPlate is a good tool to help you decide what to eat each day. It divides foods into five main groups. They are grains, vegetables, fruits, dairy, and protein.
- Your daily meals and snacks should include the recommended amounts from the MyPlate food groups.

Cup and Ounce-Equivalents

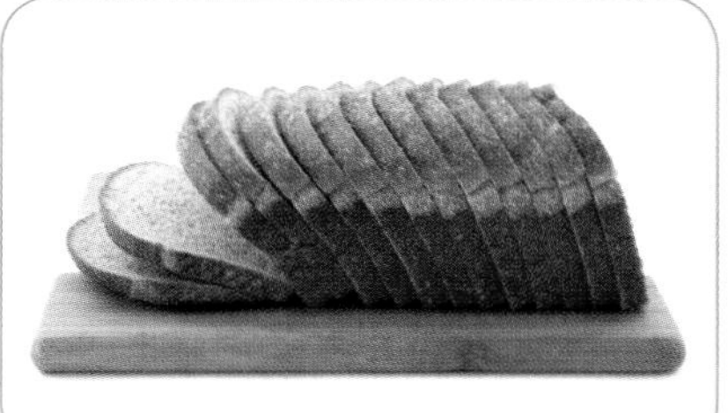	**Grains** *Count as one ounce-equivalent:* 1 slice of whole-wheat bread 1 cup of ready-to-eat cereal 5–7 small crackers ½ cooked pasta or rice
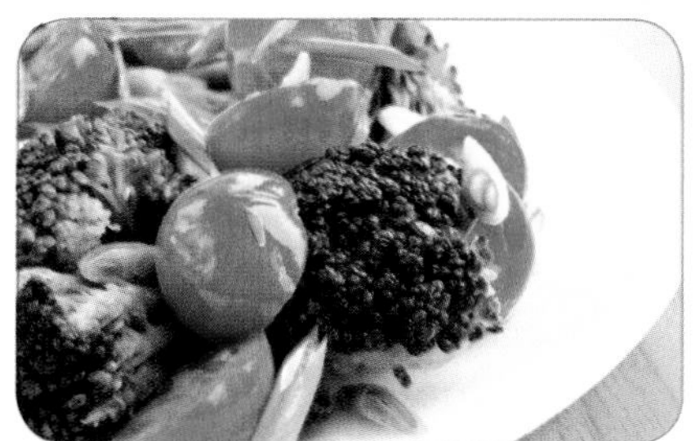	**Vegetables** *Count as one cup:* 1 cup broccoli, raw or cooked 1 large tomato 1 medium baked potato 2 cups romaine lettuce
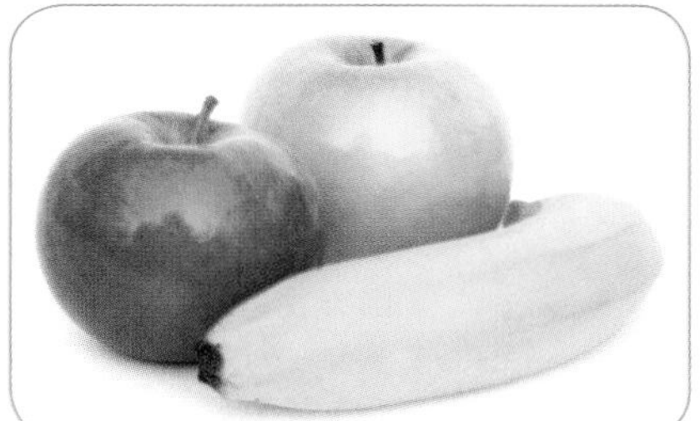	**Fruits** *Count as one cup:* 1 cup canned fruit or fruit juice 1 small apple or medium banana ½ cup dried apricots ¼ of a medium cantaloupe
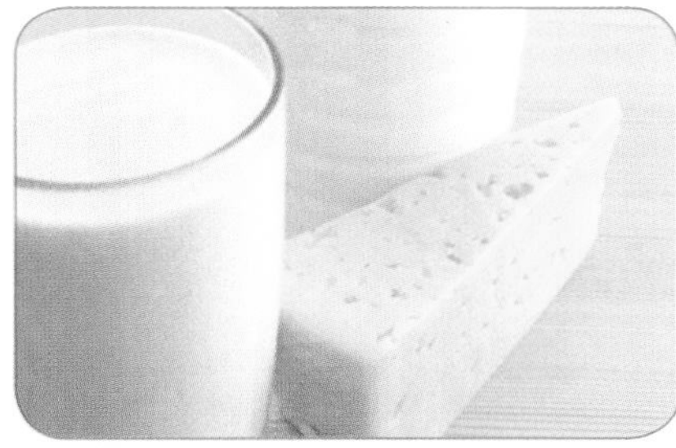	**Dairy** *Count as one cup:* 1 cup fat-free or low-fat milk or yogurt 1½ ounces natural cheese 2 ounces processed (American) cheese ⅓ cup shredded cheese
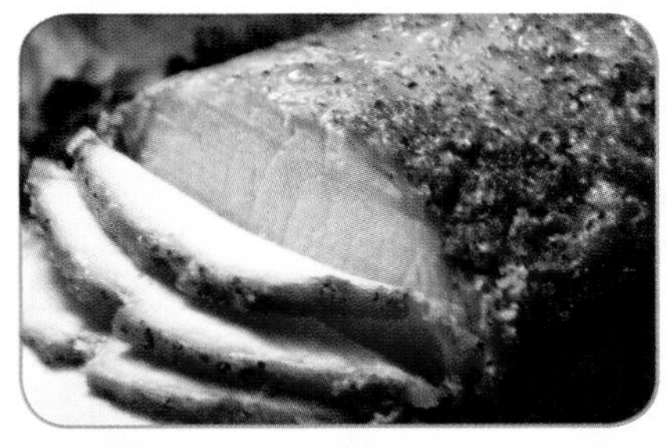	**Protein** *Count as one ounce-equivalent:* 1 ounce cooked lean meat, poultry, or fish 1 egg ½ ounce of nuts 1 tablespoon peanut butter ¼ cup dried beans or peas ½ ounce sunflower seeds, hulled

7-8 You need to know how to count the foods you eat from each of the food groups in MyPlate.

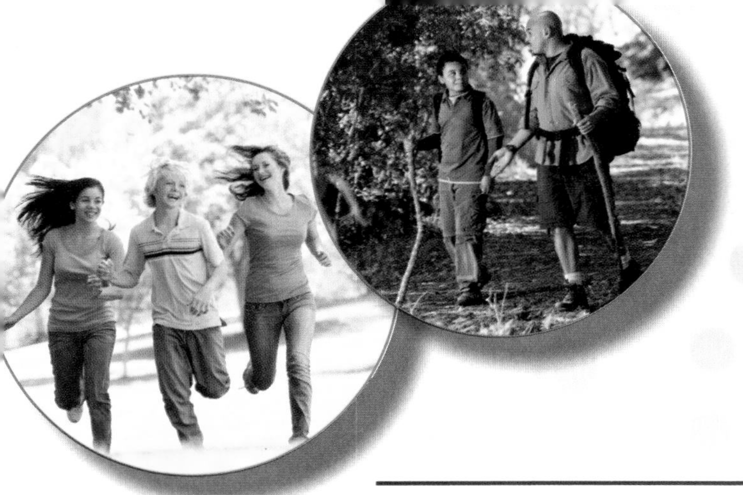

Section 7-3
Managing Your Weight

Objectives

After studying this section, you will be able to
- **define** *energy*, *calories*, *appetite*, *anorexia nervosa*, *bulimia*, and *binge eating*.
- **explain** why your body needs calories.
- **describe** how calories, body weight, and physical activity are related.
- **give examples** of healthful ways to manage your weight.

Key Terms

energy: the capacity for doing work.

calories: units of energy provided by proteins, carbohydrates, and fats.

appetite: the desire to eat.

anorexia nervosa: an eating disorder in which the fear of weight gain leads to poor eating patterns, malnutrition, and excessive weight loss.

bulimia: an eating disorder in which people eat large amounts of food and then purge themselves of the food.

binge eating: an eating disorder in which people eat large amounts of food in a short time without taking measures to rid the body of unwanted food.

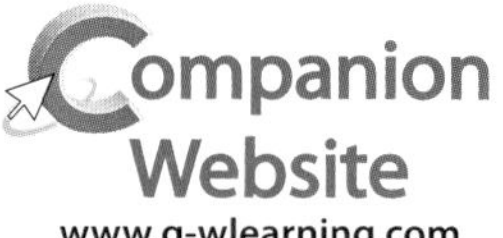

Study the Key Terms by completing crossword puzzles, matching activities, and e-flash cards at the website.

Main Ideas

- Your body needs calories to work, play, grow, and be healthy.
- The amount of calories you take in and your body weight are related.
- A healthful way to manage your weight is to be physically active and eat the proper amounts of nutritious foods.

Most teens want to look and feel their best. Every person's natural size is different. There is no one size that is *better* than another. You may, however, want to gain or lose a few pounds. You may want to maintain your current weight. To manage your weight, you need to learn how to balance the healthful foods you eat with physical activity.

PRESCRIPTION

℞

Health Link

Planning a Healthful Diet

When planning a diet, remember to choose foods from the five main groups in MyPlate. You should also eat regular meals that include a variety of foods. Be sure to choose lower calorie foods and eat smaller amounts to lose weight. If you want to gain weight, choose nutritious higher calorie foods and eat larger amounts. Be sure to check with a doctor, nutritionist, or school nurse before beginning any diet program.

Calories

Energy is the capacity for doing work. The energy you get from food helps you stay alive, work, play, grow, and be healthy. **Calories** are units of energy provided by proteins, carbohydrates, and fats. For instance, an orange has around 60 calories. This means it will supply your body with that much energy for activity. You need to eat a certain number of calories each day. They provide your body with the energy it needs to function.

You need to learn about calories. Your MyPlate plan tells you how many calories you need. This amount depends on your age, sex, and level of physical activity. See **7-9**. Physical activity helps you use calories.

You should also find out how many calories are in the foods you eat. Some cookbooks and nutrition books have calorie charts. You can record your physical activity and the food you eat on choose**MyPlate**.gov. It will keep track of your calories .

Reading Review

1. Why might you and your friends have different calorie needs?
2. How can you find out how many calories are in your favorite foods?

Calories and Weight

The food you eat provides your body with the calories it needs. If you eat a balanced diet and are at a healthy weight for your body build, you are probably eating the right number of calories. This means your body uses all the calories you take in from the foods you eat.

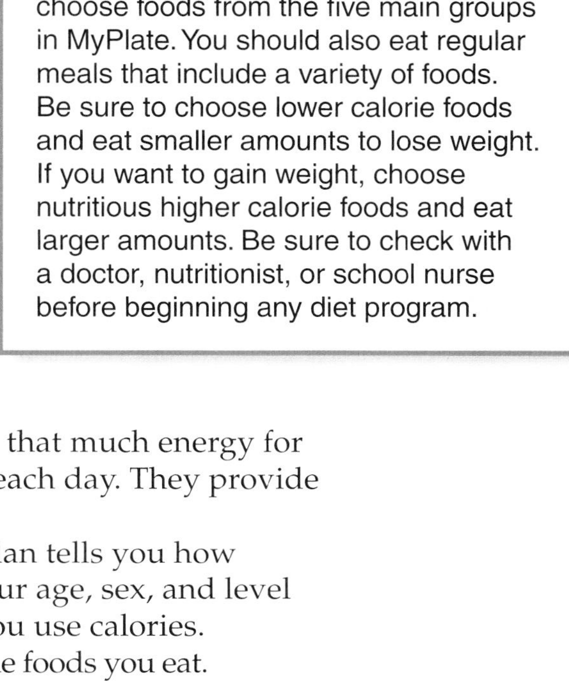

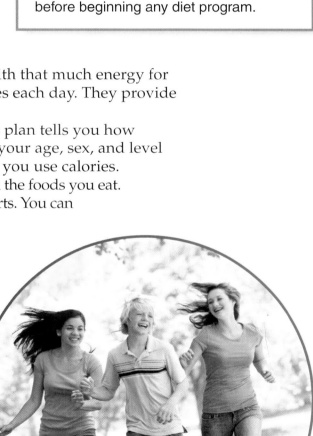

7-9 Your body needs more calories to run than it does to watch TV.

When your body uses fewer calories than you take in, you gain weight. The extra calories are turned into fat and stored by your body. When you take in fewer calories than your body needs, you lose weight. Your body uses the stored fat for energy.

One way to lose weight is to reduce calories. A good rule to follow is *cut down, not out*. You can still eat many of the foods you like, but in smaller amounts. It is the total number of calories you eat each day that affects your weight.

Fat and sugar contain very few nutrients, mostly calories. Avoid choosing foods with added fat and sugar. Choose more nutrient-dense foods from the fruit, vegetable, and grain groups, especially whole grains. Be mindful about the foods you eat.

Do not try *fad diets*, which claim you will lose a lot of weight fast. They usually do not include enough of the right kinds of food. They can be harmful to your health.

Your **appetite**, or desire to eat, may be a good guide to how much food you need. Your appetite may not guide you to the kinds of food you need, such as low-fat, nutrient-dense foods. If you have been eating second servings, eat one instead. Eat smaller portions. Fruit and low-fat or fat-free milk are good choices. Drink water instead of drinks filled with added sugars. Be physically active. See **7-10**.

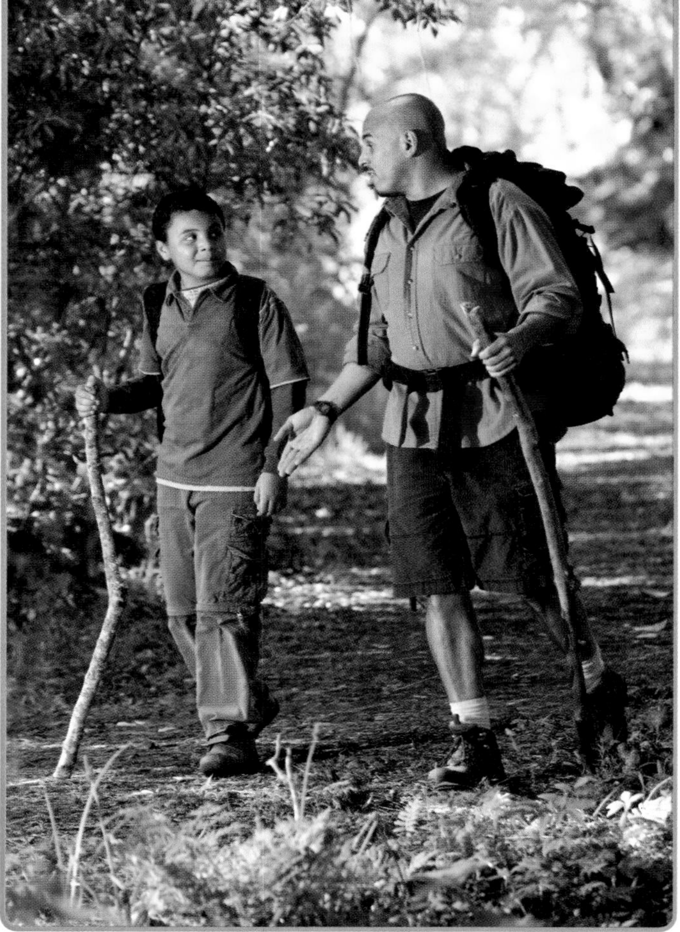

7-10 Physical activities such as hiking can help families have fun and manage their weight.

To gain weight, you need to take in more calories than your body uses. Once again, use the food groups as a guide. Try eating more foods from each of these groups. Sometimes, it may be hard to eat a lot at one meal. Instead, try eating several small meals throughout the day. Also, be sure to get plenty of rest.

If you want to change your weight, talk to a dietitian, doctor, or school nurse. Follow the advice you are given. They may suggest you change your diet and eating habits. Learning to count calories is important.

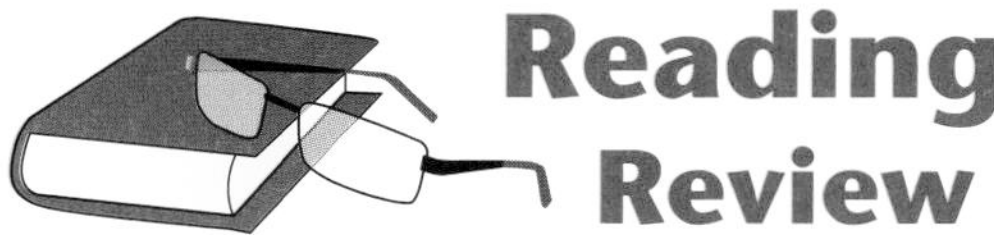

Reading Review

1. How does the statement *cut down, not out* apply to losing weight?
2. Why should you not go on a fad diet to try to lose weight?

Calories and Physical Activity

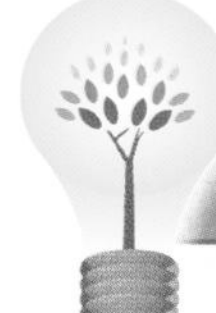

Think Green

Physical Activity Choices

When you develop a physical activity program, think of different ways you can *go green*. For instance, before you decide to join the local gym, consider the type of equipment available and how much electricity it uses. Also, consider the gas you will use to drive to the gym. Going for a walk or a bike ride saves electricity and gas, but still helps you burn calories. What other *green* ideas can you add into your physical activity program?

Daily physical activity is important to manage your weight. Physical activity can affect your weight because the calories you use are increased. Walking, bicycling, basketball, and swimming are all good forms of physical activity. Nutritionists, doctors, or school nurses can help you plan a diet and physical activity program.

Regular physical activity burns extra calories. Being active keeps your muscles in good shape. This helps your appearance and makes you feel energetic.

Physical activity can also help you build well-toned muscles. Adding muscle can also add weight. Physical activity may help increase your appetite and improve how you feel.

When you start a new physical activity, begin slowly. Otherwise, you may damage your muscles. Give your muscles time to get used to the new activity. If you have health problems, check with your doctor before you start physical activity.

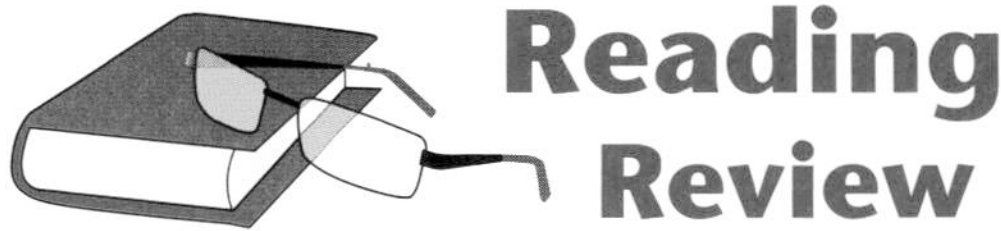

Reading Review

1. How can regular physical activity help you manage your weight?
2. Why should you start slowly when you begin a new physical activity?

Eating Disorders

Some teens, mostly girls, can develop abnormal, unhealthy eating patterns known as *eating disorders*. Eating disorders are often linked to the mistaken belief that people must look a certain way to be happy. Not everyone can, or should, look like very tall and too-thin models. All body build types can be attractive.

The most common eating disorders are anorexia nervosa, bulimia, and binge eating. **Anorexia nervosa** is an eating disorder in which the fear of weight gain leads to poor eating patterns, malnutrition, and excessive weight loss. Sometimes exercising too much for the amount of food eaten is part of the disorder. A person with anorexia nervosa often feels overweight even though they really may be underweight for their body build. If anorexia nervosa remains untreated, it can cause severe health problems or even lead to death.

Recognizing Eating Disorders

In the United States, millions of people struggle with eating disorders. Would you notice if your best friend developed an eating disorder? What would you say to your friend? How could you try to help him or her? Could you talk with one of your friend's parents? Research one of three eating disorders for ideas about how to help people you care about with an eating disorder. Write a one-page narrative describing what your options might be to help your friend.

Bulimia is an eating disorder in which people eat large amounts of food and then purge themselves of the food. People with bulimia binge and purge to prevent weight gain. *Bingeing* means eating large amounts of food in a short time. *Purging* means ridding the body of unwanted food by self-induced vomiting or taking too many laxatives. People with bulimia may often have frequent changes in their weight. Like anorexia nervosa, bulimia can lead to severe health problems and death.

Binge eating is an eating disorder in which people eat large amounts of food in a short time without taking measures to rid the body of unwanted food. People who are binge eaters may often gain or lose weight frequently. Binge eating can cause heart problems, high blood pressure, or even diabetes.

Eating disorders often develop from emotional stresses and social or physical issues. They are considered diseases, which need unique treatment plans. Early treatment helps improve chances of getting better. A physician, a psychiatrist, and a dietitian often work together to provide care. The emotional and physical aspects of eating disorders must be treated together.

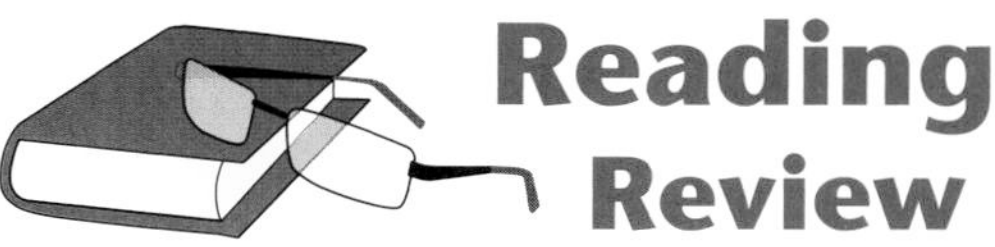

1. What health problems can develop if eating disorders remain untreated?
2. What helps improve chances of recovering from an eating disorder?

Section Summary

- Calories are units of energy in food.
- You should learn about calories because they can make a difference in your weight and health.
- If you take in more calories than your body needs, you gain weight. If you take in fewer calories than your body needs, you lose weight.
- Eating disorders are life-threatening conditions related to unhealthy eating.
- Nutritionists, doctors, or school nurses can help you plan diet and physical activity programs to manage your weight.

Chapter Summary

Your diet affects how you perform in school, in sports, and at social activities. The food choices you make several times a day are unique and influenced by many factors. Your personal preferences and habits affect your food choices. Your ethnic and cultural heritage influences the foods that are eaten in your home. Your food choices affect your health, fitness, and appearance.

Following the *Dietary Guidelines for Americans* can help you make healthful food choices and decrease your chances of getting certain diseases. The foods and beverages you consume each day provide your body with the nutrients it needs to function. Choose nutrient-dense foods that contain many nutrients and are low in calories. Avoid nutrient-poor foods that provide large amounts of calories, but few nutrients.

MyPlate is based on the *Dietary Guidelines* and can help anyone over the age of two develop a healthful eating plan. MyPlate includes the five basic food groups plus oils, which you should use sparingly. Limit other fats and sweets as well.

Knowing how many calories are in foods can help you manage your weight. To lose weight, you need to take in fewer calories than your body needs. To gain weight, you need to take in more calories than your body needs.

Physical activity can help you manage your weight. Choose a type of physical activity you enjoy and will do often. Also, be aware of eating disorders, which can seriously harm your health. Nutritionists, doctors, or school nurses can help you plan healthful diet and physical activity programs.

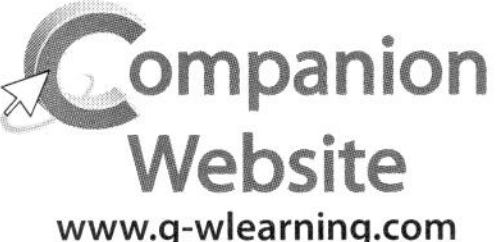

Review Key Terms and Main Ideas for Chapter 7 at the website.

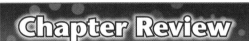

Chapter Review

Write your answers on a separate sheet of paper.

1. A(n) _____ is the food and beverages consumed each day.
2. Name the six types of nutrients and list five food sources for each.
3. Give the name of a food you associate with the following events:
   A. Birthday party.
   B. Wedding reception.
   C. Graduation party.
   D. Thanksgiving.
4. Give three examples of cultural foods found in the United States.
5. Give an example of how food can be a part of family traditions.
6. List the two main messages from the *2010 Dietary Guidelines for Americans*.
7. List two ways to consume a more nutrient-dense diet.
8. A diet that provides all the nutrients your body needs for good health is a(n) _____ diet.
9. List the five main food groups in MyPlate.
10. _____ breads have nutrients added to replace those removed during processing.
11. True or false. Butter and ice cream are in the dairy group.
12. True or false. All teens need the same number of calories each day.
13. One way to _____ weight is to reduce the calories you take in.
14. True or false. Physical activity can affect your weight because the calories you use are increased.
15. What are the three most common eating disorders?

Life Skills

16. Prepare a three-part article entitled *Wellness Tips for Your Good Health.* Create a list of 10 tips for each of the following topics: *Make Wise Food Choices for a Healthful Lifestyle, Follow MyPlate for Good Nutrition*, and *Staying Active to Manage Your Weight*. Also, include information you think other students may need to know about wellness. Find photo suggestions to accompany the articles. Ask your teacher to review the articles and discuss them with you before presenting them to the class.

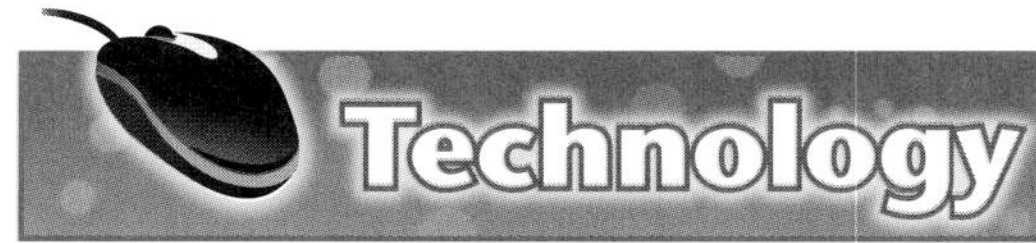

Technology

17. Work with a partner to research vegetarian diets on the Internet. Use the website, www.vrg.org. Click on the *Teens, Family & Kids* link; then click on *Vegetarian Nutrition for Teens*. Prepare a report to share with class about how teen vegetarians might meet their nutritional needs for protein, calcium, vitamin B_{12}, and iron.
18. Using online or print sources, find information showing the calories used in various physical activities.

How many calories would you use in 30 minutes of walking? dancing? playing basketball? Use the software of your choice to create a table of your findings.

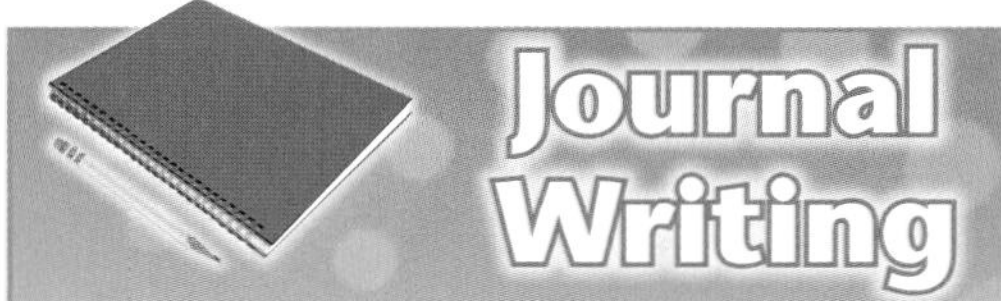

19. Keeping a food diary is a good way to learn more about your eating habits. In your journal, write every item you eat and drink for 10 days, including the amounts and time of day. You will start to see a pattern to your eating habits. Some patterns may be healthy, but others may not. Your food diary will help you determine any eating habits you would like to change.

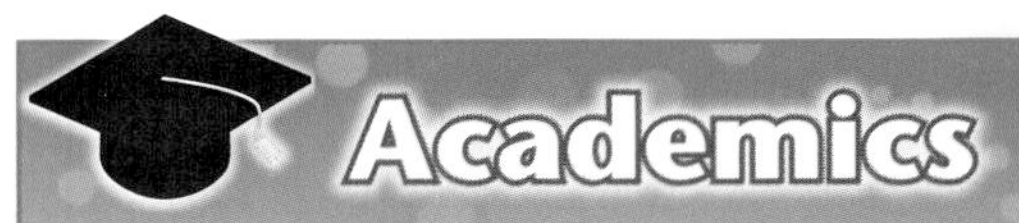

20. **Science.** The B vitamins and vitamin C are water-soluble vitamins the body needs regularly. Research the foods that give your body essential B vitamins and vitamin C. Is it better to get these vitamins from foods or from taking vitamin pills? Why? Discuss your findings with the class.
21. **Writing.** Write a short essay about a family food tradition that has been passed down from one generation to another. Share your story with the class and your family.
22. **Science.** What are the functions of protein in your body? Why are foods containing protein important for teens to have daily?
23. **Math.** Check a calorie guide for the number of calories in an apple, banana, orange, and a glass of fat-free milk. What nutrients do these foods provide? Then look up the calories in two chocolate chip cookies, one cola drink, one cup of buttered popcorn, one bagel, and one small bag of potato chips. What nutrients do they provide? Why are fresh fruits and fat-free milk healthful choices for snacks?

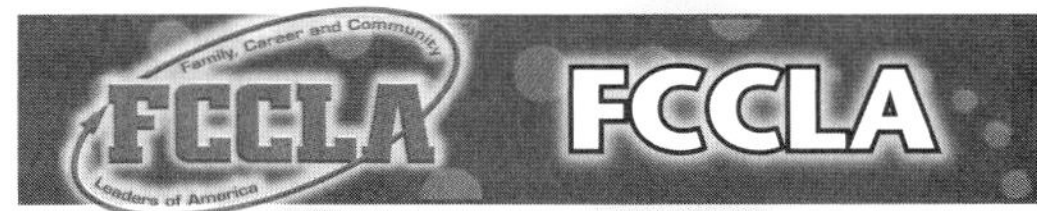

24. Regular physical activity is a large part of living a healthful lifestyle. To stick with a physical activity routine, it is best to find those activities you really enjoy. Do you like to play a team sport, or are you happier in fitness or yoga classes? Would you rather be running or lifting weights? How much time can you spend each week on a physical activity? These are just a few of the many questions you can answer to help you find the best fitness program for you. After making your own physical activity program, develop an FCCLA *A Better You* project for the *Power of One* program. Obtain further information about this program from your FCCLA advisor.

Chapter 8
Planning Meals

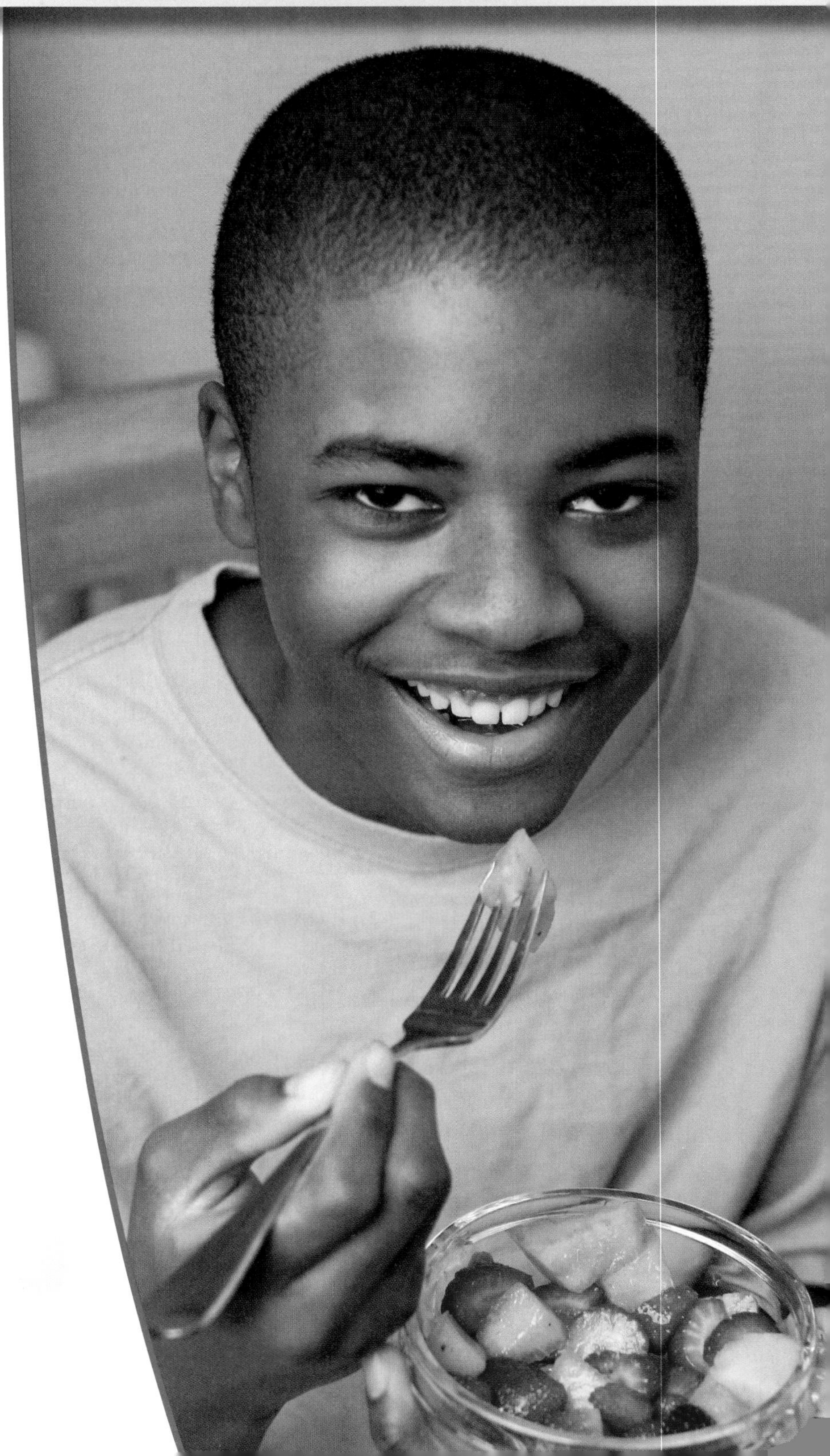

Sections

8-1 Planning Menus
8-2 You—A Food Shopper
8-3 Buying and Storing Food
8-4 Serving Meals
8-5 Caring About Behavior

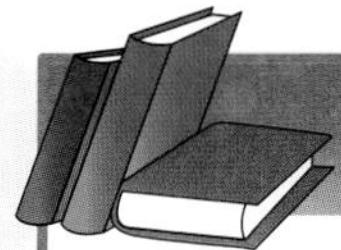

Sharpen Your Reading

On a separate sheet of paper, write the main headings in each section of this chapter. Be sure to leave space under each heading. As you read, write three main points you learn about each section.

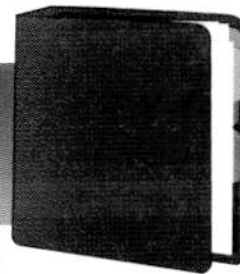

Concept Organizer

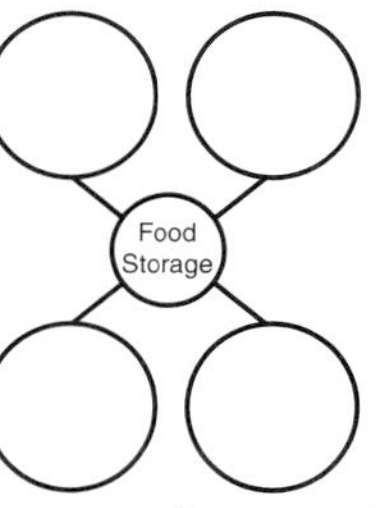

Use a star diagram like the one shown to identify the best ways to store food in the four food groups discussed in this chapter. Briefly explain why foods should be stored in this way.

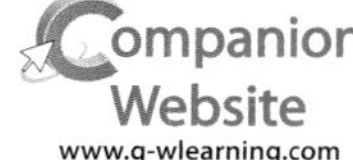

Print out the concept organizer at the website.

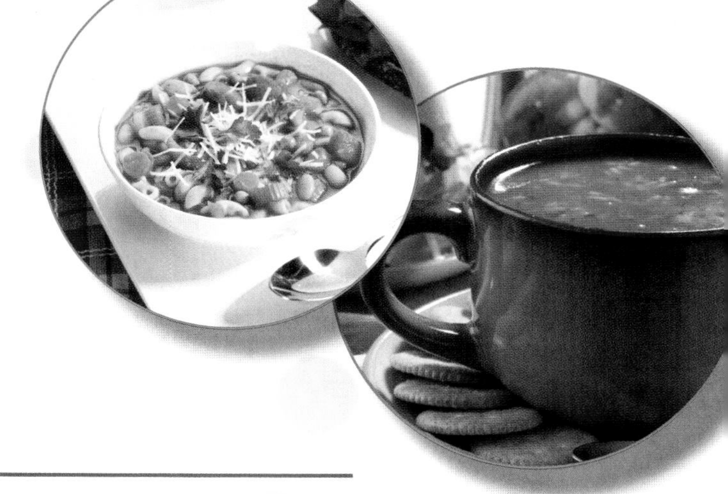

Section 8-1
Planning Menus

Objectives

After studying this section, you will be able to
- **define** *menu*, *meal patterns*, *course*, and *appetizer*.
- **give examples** of meal patterns.
- **plan** menus that include foods your family will like.
- **plan** menus that are nutritious and attractive.

Key Terms

menu: a list of foods to be prepared and served.

meal patterns: the number of times and types of foods you eat daily.

course: all the foods served as one part of a meal.

appetizer: a light food or drink served before the meal.

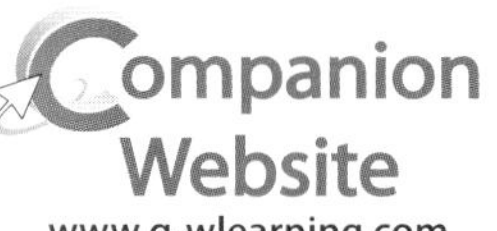

Study the Key Terms by completing crossword puzzles, matching activities, and e-flash cards at the website.

Main Ideas

- Meal patterns can help you achieve nutrition goals.
- Think about your family's likes and dislikes when planning menus.
- Consider nutrition and the appearance and taste of food when planning menus.

A **menu** is a list of foods to be prepared and served. When planning menus for your family, you should keep your culture and family customs in mind. You should also consider the likes and dislikes of the people you are serving. People like different foods for many reasons, which often include taste, variety, convenience, cost, and nutrition. When you plan menus, be sure to consider these factors.

Daily Meal Patterns

Meal patterns are the number of times and types of foods you eat daily. Meal patterns serve as guides for planning menus. Three common meal patterns include breakfast, lunch, and dinner. See **8-1**. Snacks are foods you eat between meals.

Breakfast provides nutrients and energy to start the day. At breakfast, take in about one-fourth to one-third of the nutrients and calories you need for the day.

Lunch is eaten at midday. This meal provides about one-fourth to one-third of the food you need each day.

Dinner is a heavy meal eaten at noon or in the evening. It is the meal people most often share with their family and friends. Dinner may be plain or fancy. Special events often call for special dinners. Dinner should provide about one-third of the calories for the day.

In all meal patterns, especially dinner, food may be served in courses. A **course** is all the foods served as one part of a meal. For instance, the main course includes the meat or meat alternate dish. A vegetable and rice or pasta might also be part of the main course. An **appetizer** is a light food or drink, such as soup or juice, served before the meal. An appetizer is supposed to stimulate the appetite.

Be mindful of the beverages you consume and serve throughout the day. Sweetened colas add calories from sugar. Corn syrup or other sugars are often added to pure fruit juice, which increases calories. Plain water (tap water) is the best choice. Tap water has no calories, is important for the body's good health and fitness, and costs much less than bottled water. You can add your own flavorings to tap water for variety.

In addition to the three common meal patterns, snacks can also help meet your

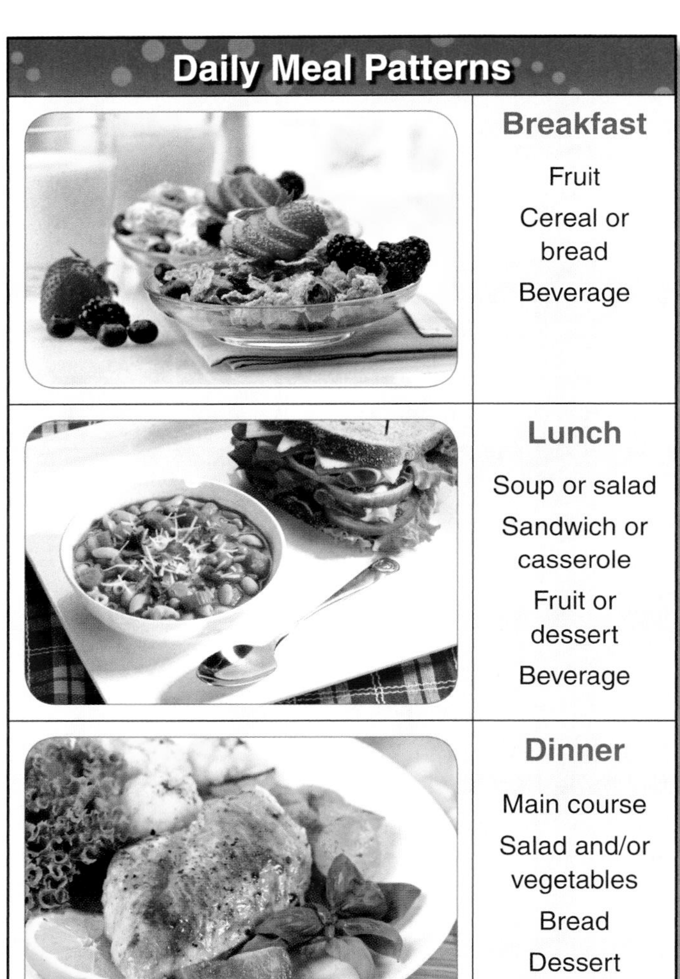

8-1 Using meal patterns can make menu planning easier.

daily nutritious needs. Avoid snacks that are high in fat, sugar, and sodium. Instead, choose healthful snacks such as fruits, vegetables, or nuts. Do not get too many of your daily calories from snacks.

Family members need food energy throughout the day. This means they should eat balanced meals at set times during the day. Follow the MyPlate guidelines when you plan menus. It tells you what foods need to be included each day. Do not skip an important meal, such as breakfast. This can make it harder for family members to function their best at school or work.

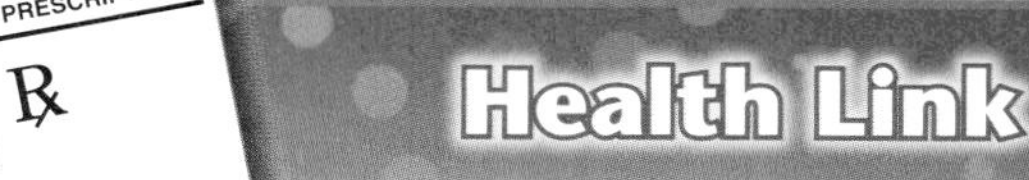

Balancing Nutritional Needs

Create menu plans that meet your family's nutritional needs. Be mindful about the calories in meals you plan. It is important to balance your nutritious needs throughout the day. Do not try to get all your calories in one meal. For instance, the calories for a sandwich loaded with meats, cheeses, and mayonnaise could equal one-half of your daily needs. It could also provide your total daily fat and sodium intake. Healthful meals include foods from MyPlate.

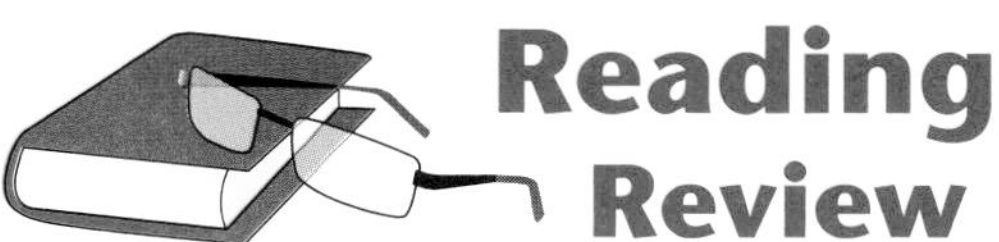

Reading Review

1. What dishes may be included in the main course of a dinner?
2. Why is it important to eat balanced meals throughout the day?

Planning Tips

Keeping certain tips in mind can help you plan any meal. These tips include your family's food likes and dislikes, variety, and nutrition.

Your family's likes and dislikes may be affected by your cultural heritage and family customs. Taste, convenience, and cost may also affect which foods your family enjoys.

Serving new foods adds variety to meals. Help your family try different foods along with old family favorites. You might want them to try foods you have had at a friend's home or when eating out. These foods that offer different tastes may soon join the list of favorites.

Keep nutrition in mind when planning meals. The kinds and amounts of food people need depend on their age, health, work, and activities. Babies need foods to help them grow. Sick people need food to get well. Active people need more food than those who are less active. Count calories every day so the intake is right for you and your family. If you plan carefully, menus can meet the whole family's nutritional needs.

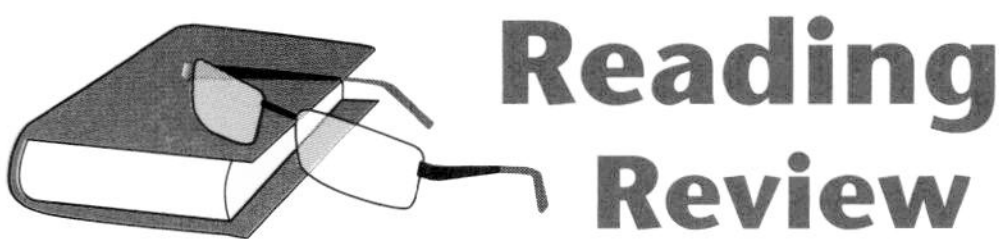

Reading Review

1. What factors can affect the foods your family chooses?
2. Why do you need to keep nutrition in mind when planning meals?

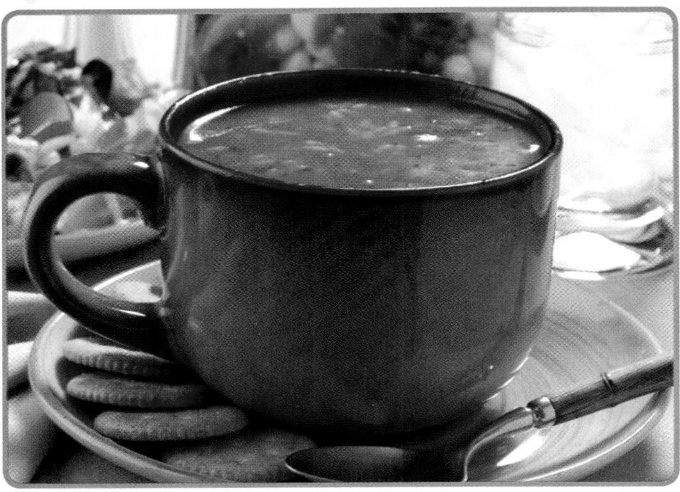

8-2 Homemade hot chicken gumbo soup and salad offer variety of texture and temperature.

Appearance and Taste

The appearance and taste of food often affects whether it is eaten. When you plan menus that look and taste good, your family will usually eat them.

When planning a menu, ask yourself if the foods look appealing. Foods that are all the same color are not appealing. There should be a variety of colors on the plate for the meal to be interesting visually.

Think about the textures and temperatures of foods. Avoid serving too many soft or crisp foods in the same meal. A grilled cheese sandwich mixes both soft and crisp textures. Serve hot and cold foods at the same meal for variety and interest. See **8-2**. Soup with a green salad is a good example.

The shape of food also makes a difference. Think about how it looks on a plate. A variety of shapes can make a meal more appealing.

Also, think about the flavors of foods when planning menus. There are many foods that taste better when eaten with other foods. Often, highly seasoned, strong-tasting foods should be eaten with mild-tasting foods. This makes each food taste more enjoyable. For instance, spicy chili may be served with mild cornbread.

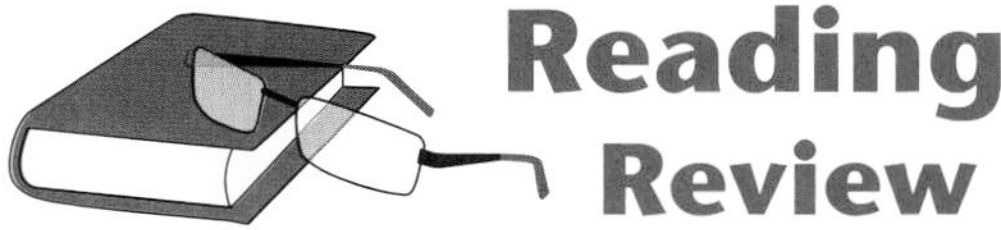

Reading Review

1. How can you make a meal more attractive? Why is the appearance of food important?
2. Why should you avoid serving too many soft or crisp foods in the same meal?

Section Summary

- Meal patterns serve as guides when planning menus.
- The three common meal patterns include breakfast, lunch, and dinner.
- Plan menus according to your family's food choices and nutritional needs. Follow the MyPlate guidelines to help meet your family's nutritional needs.
- Consider appearance and taste when planning menus.

Section 8-2
You—A Food Shopper

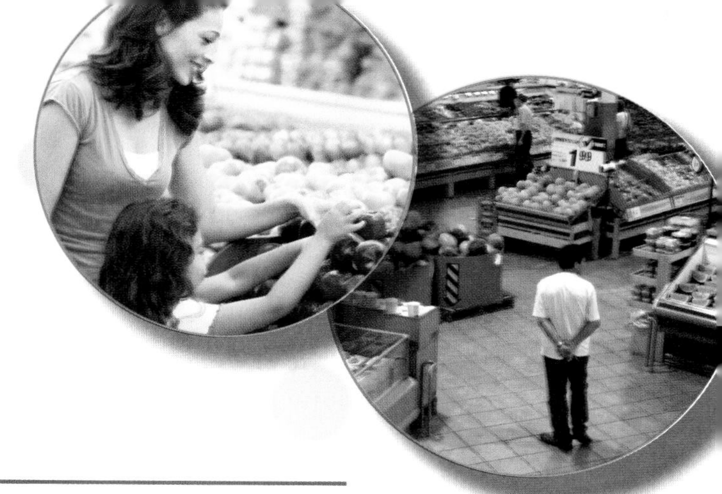

Objectives

After studying this section, you will be able to
- **define** *food shortage*, *allergens*, *nutrition label*, and *Daily Values (DV)*.
- **explain** what affects the cost of food.
- **give examples** of how to be a skillful shopper.
- **discuss** how information on food labels can be used by shoppers.

Key Terms

food shortage: a condition in which there is not enough to meet the demand.

allergens: substances that cause an allergic response in people that can be fatal.

nutrition label: a panel on a food product package with information about the nutrients the food contains.

Daily Values (DV): reference figures on nutrition labels that help consumers see how food products fit into a total diet.

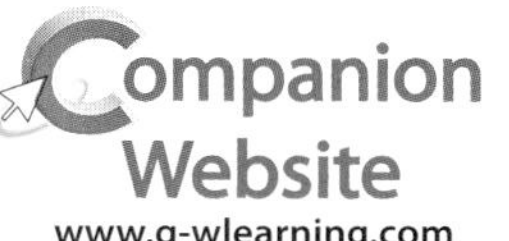

Study the Key Terms by completing crossword puzzles, matching activities, and e-flash cards at the website.

Main Ideas

- You can learn skills to become a better food shopper.
- There are many factors that affect food costs.
- Food labels include information that can help consumers make wise food purchases.

As a food shopper, you have power. When you shop, you can decide how much you want to spend for food. You can also choose where and when you will shop. You can use package labels to help you make wise food choices.

Be aware of outside pressures that affect your food-buying decisions in a negative way. Your peers may introduce you to unhealthful food products they enjoy. Advertisements and commercials might persuade you to try new products. Developing good shopping skills will help you avoid these pressures. Learn to use peers and advertisements as sources of information. Resist the urge to buy foods that are unhealthful for you and your family, such as those loaded with sugar, fat, and sodium.

Making Shopping Decisions

To be a skillful shopper, you must be able to make important decisions. First, you must decide how much to spend and what to buy. It is important to consider your income and expenses when developing a food budget. Base your shopping list on your menu plans. Also, be sure your menu plans include only foods you can afford to buy.

The next decision you must make is where to shop. Location, quality, price, and variety are several factors that may influence your choice of stores. Supermarkets, specialty food stores, and convenience stores are three types of food stores.

Supermarkets are often part of a chain that lets them buy food in large amounts. This means they pay lower prices for food. The price they pay affects what you pay. See **8-3**.

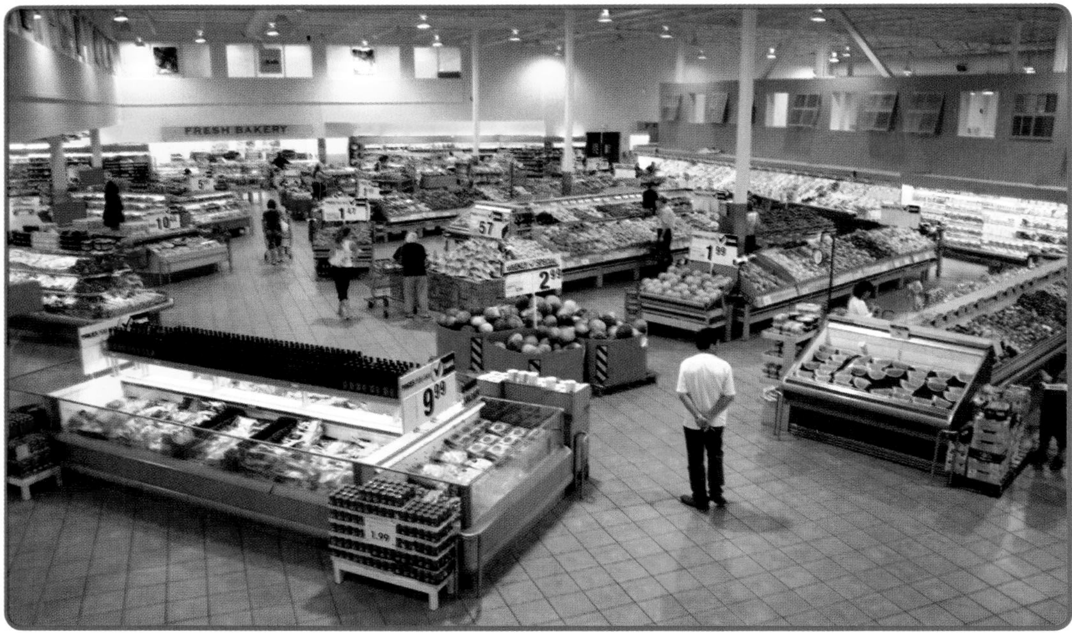

8-3 Supermarkets are large stores that offer a wide variety of foods.

Specialty food stores offer one type of food such as baked goods, meats, or imported products. The prices are often high. Many shoppers, however, think the freshness and high quality of the food is worth the cost.

Convenience stores are often small and stay open longer hours than other stores. They offer less variety, and their prices are often high. When stores buy in small amounts, they pay higher prices. If they are part of a chain, their prices may be lower.

You may also choose to shop at outdoor markets and food co-ops. Compare the prices, quality, and variety of foods in each type of store.

The third decision you must make is when to shop. You might pick a time when the stores are not crowded. To avoid browsing and picking up extra items, shop when you do not have much extra time. Also, it is best to shop at a time when you are not hungry.

The more you shop, the more skilled you can become. Shopping for food often helps you learn to make better choices. You can learn many skills to become a better food shopper.

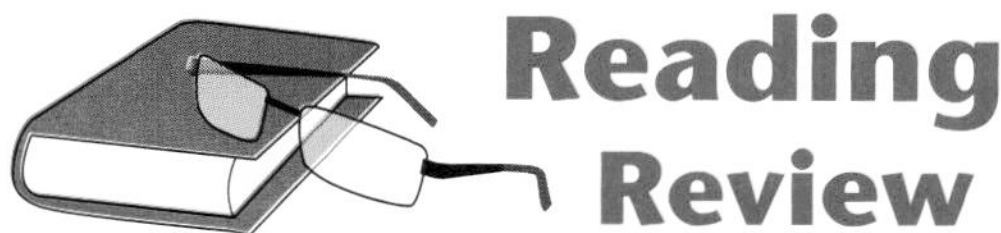

Reading Review

1. What are three decisions you should make before shopping for food? How can they help you be a better shopper?
2. Why should you shop at a time when you are not hungry?

Controlling Food Costs

The cost of food affects how much you buy with the money you decide to spend. A number of factors affect food costs. Being aware of these factors can help you get the most from your food dollar.

Succeed in Life

Choosing a Quality Food Store

You may have certain reasons for choosing one store over another. Your decision about where to shop should depend on prices, services offered, and the location of the store. Wherever you shop, get to know the store. The following list tells you what to look for in a good store.

- fresh, clean fruits, vegetables, and meats
- well-packaged foods with prices clearly marked
- clean, airy surroundings with good lighting
- well-groomed, polite staff who handle food carefully
- well-organized display counters
- state- or city-inspected and approved store conditions

The amount of food available affects food costs. When food is plentiful, there is enough or more than enough to meet demand. A **food shortage** occurs when there is not enough to meet the demand. When food shortages occur, prices often increase. For instance, colder weather than usual may affect a crop of lettuce or oranges, which can cause a shortage of those items. If the prices of these foods increase, you can substitute other less expensive items.

Where you shop affects the price of food. If you shop in different stores, you may notice foods are not always priced the same. Prices vary because stores pay different prices for the food they buy. The services they offer also affect prices.

Each type of store has different services to offer. For instance, some may offer carry-out service to your car. Others deliver groceries to your home. Some have bakeries or delis. Others offer lower prices for buying large amounts. Some stay open later than others. A store may even offer all these services. Stores pass along the costs of these services to you through food prices.

The season of the year can also affect food costs. In some parts of the country, fresh fruits and vegetables can be grown only part of the year. Some fruits and vegetables cannot be grown at all. This means they must be shipped in from other parts of the country and from other countries. Shipping costs add to the price of food. See **8-4**.

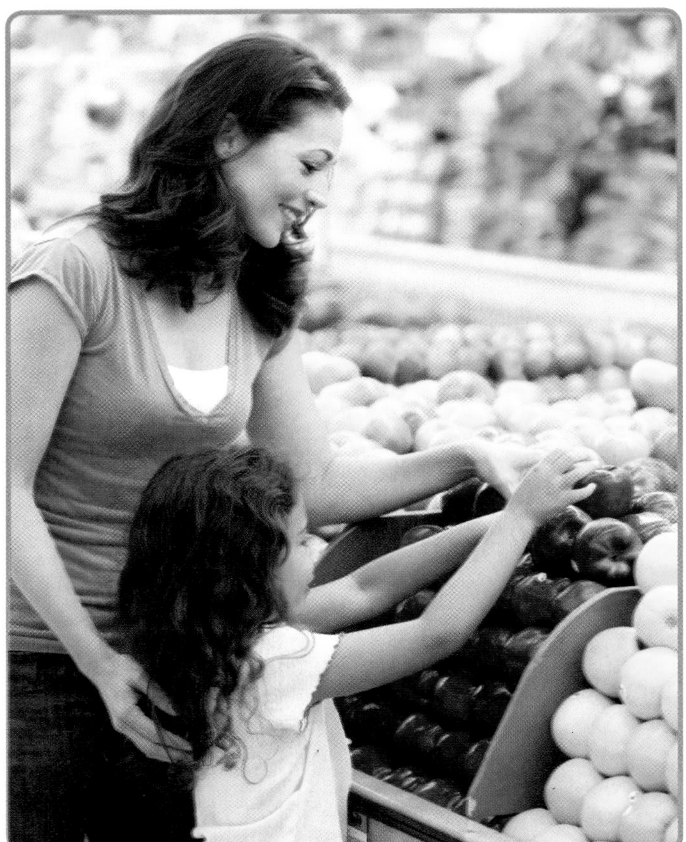

8-4 The price of fresh fruits and vegetables depends on the season.

How foods are sold and who makes them are factors in the cost. Fresh, frozen, and canned foods have different prices. Larger packages may be better values than small packages. Buying in bulk quantities can often save dollars and packaging waste. Store brands may be better buys than name brands. Comparing prices of food items will help you get the best buys. Learn to get the most nutritious food for your money.

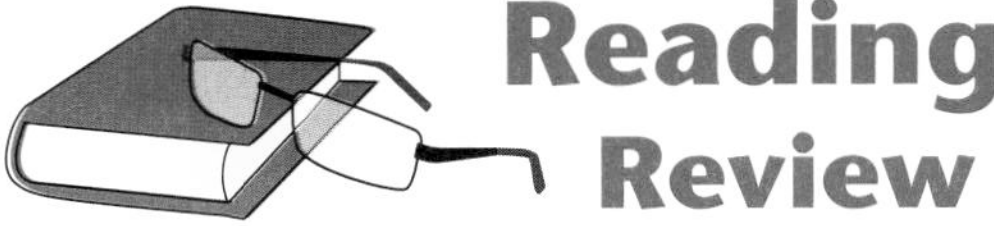

Reading Review

1. What are three factors that affect food prices? How do shortages affect food prices?
2. How can the type of store you shop at affect the price of the food?
3. Why do fruits and vegetables need to be shipped to certain parts of the country?

Creating a Shopping List

Having a shopping list can help you control food costs. When making a list, include all the items you need. Then buy only what is on the list. If you follow the list, you will not have to make extra shopping trips. When you make fewer trips to the store, you often spend less money. Shopping lists also help prevent impulse buying.

Making a shopping list can save you time. If you only shop in one store, you can list the foods in the order they are found in the store. This helps you avoid retracing your steps.

It is easy to make a shopping list at the same time you plan menus. When you plan menus several days in advance, include in your shopping list the foods you need for those menus. You can develop a routine such as the following for planning and making a shopping list:

1. Write menus for several days at a time.
2. Check the foods you already have available.
3. List what you need to buy.
4. Take your shopping list with you to the store.
5. Avoid impulse buys, or foods not on your list.

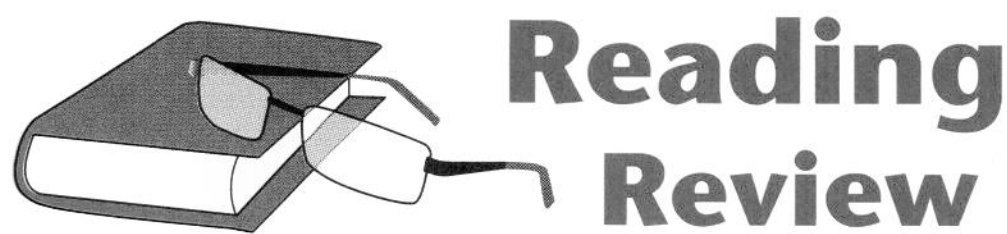

Reading Review

1. How can making a shopping list help you spend less money?
2. What are the steps in the routine for planning and making a shopping list?

Reading Labels

Be sure to read the labels on packages to obtain important information about products. Labels must include the name and weight of the product. The manufacturer's name and address must also be included, as well as a list of ingredients. The *ingredients labeling* must identify the presence of any major food allergens in the product. **Allergens** are substances that cause an allergic response in people that can be fatal. There are eight major food allergens. They are milk, eggs, fish, crustacean shellfish, tree nuts, peanuts, wheat, and soybeans.

A **nutrition label** is a panel on a food product package with information about the nutrients the food contains. See **8-5**.

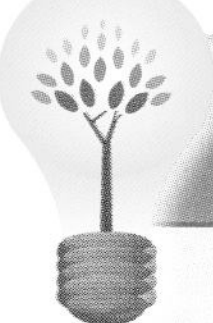

Think Green

Organic Foods

Some people choose to purchase organic foods because they do not have a negative effect on the environment. Organic foods are grown without the use of synthetic pesticides or fertilizers. This also means animals are not given antibiotics, hormones, or other artificial drugs. Organic foods have an organic seal. The *organic seal* means the product follows the USDA requirements for use of chemicals. The organic seal does not tell you the product has more nutrients than those conventionally grown. You can learn more about organic food production by visiting the USDA website at www.usda.gov.

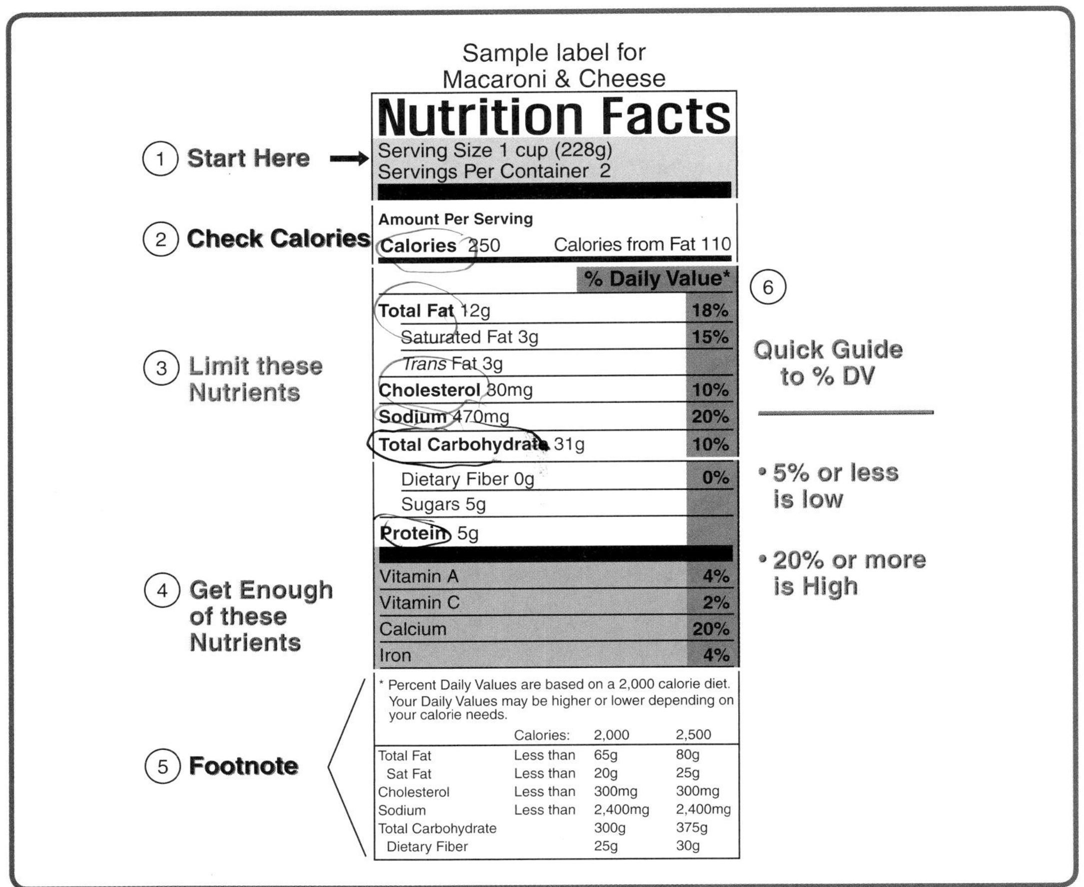

Sample label for
Macaroni & Cheese
Nutrition Facts
1 Start Here
Serving Size 1 cup (228g)
Servings Per Container 2
2 Check Calories
Amount Per Serving
Calories 250 Calories from Fat 110
% Daily Value*
6
Total Fat 12g 18%
Saturated Fat 3g 15%
3 Limit these Nutrients
Trans Fat 3g
Cholesterol 30mg 10%
Sodium 470mg 20%
Total Carbohydrate 31g 10%
Quick Guide to % DV
Dietary Fiber 0g 0%
Sugars 5g
Protein 5g
• 5% or less is low
• 20% or more is High
4 Get Enough of these Nutrients
Vitamin A 4%
Vitamin C 2%
Calcium 20%
Iron 4%
5 Footnote
* Percent Daily Values are based on a 2,000 calorie diet. Your Daily Values may be higher or lower depending on your calorie needs.
Calories: 2,000 2,500
Total Fat Less than 65g 80g
Sat Fat Less than 20g 25g
Cholesterol Less than 300mg 300mg
Sodium Less than 2,400mg 2,400mg
Total Carbohydrate 300g 375g
Dietary Fiber 25g 30g

Food and Drug Administration

8-5 Reading nutrition labels can help you choose healthy foods for a balanced diet.

It can help you see how a certain food fits into your total daily diet. All manufacturers must follow labeling guidelines set by the Food and Drug Administration. Make it a habit to read labels as you shop.

Nutrition labels are required to include certain kinds of information. This information is listed under the heading *Nutrition Facts*. The first item found under the heading is the *serving size*. This is the amount a person would normally eat. Similar products have the same serving size. This allows you to easily compare products. Serving sizes are given in both household and metric measurements.

Following the serving size is *servings per container*. This is the number of portions that are in the food package.

Calorie information appears next. The number of calories in one serving of the food is stated. The number of those calories that come from fat is also given. This can help you limit fat to no more than 30 percent of your total calories.

The next type of information is a list of *dietary components*. This is a list of nutrients found in each serving of the food product. The list includes total fat, saturated fat, trans fat, cholesterol, sodium, total carbohydrate, dietary fiber, sugars, and protein. Vitamin A, vitamin C, calcium, and iron are also listed. Some food products may list other nutrients as well.

Beside the dietary components, *percent Daily Values* are given. **Daily Values (DV)** are reference figures on nutrition labels that help consumers see how food products fit into a total diet. The footnote at the bottom of the nutrition label is a *reference of Daily Values.* This information shows the greatest amount of fat, saturated fat, cholesterol, and sodium most people should consume each day. It also shows the smallest amount of total carbohydrate and dietary fiber people should consume. Daily Values are given for two calorie levels: 2,000 and 2,500.

Many food packages have a group of bars and numbers on them. This is the *universal product code (UPC).* It provides pricing and other product information to a computer scanner. Each product has its very own code. Most stores have computerized checkout equipment that reads the code and rings up the sale. This also tells the store manager how much of that item is on hand. The manager knows how fast items are being sold and when and how much to order.

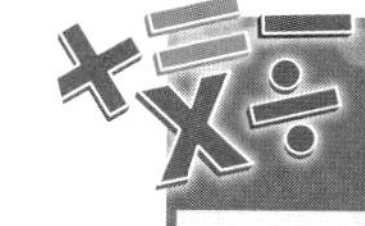

Math Link

Percent Daily Values

The percent Daily Values on nutrition labels are based on a 2,000-calorie diet. Most active teens need more than 2,000 calories per day. Therefore, their Daily Values are higher. The percent of their Daily Values met by a food product is lower than figures shown on the label. For instance, the Daily Value for total fat for a 2,000-calorie diet is 65 grams. If you need 2,800 calories per day, you can consume up to 93 grams of total fat. Determine how many grams of total fat you should consume based on your daily calorie needs.

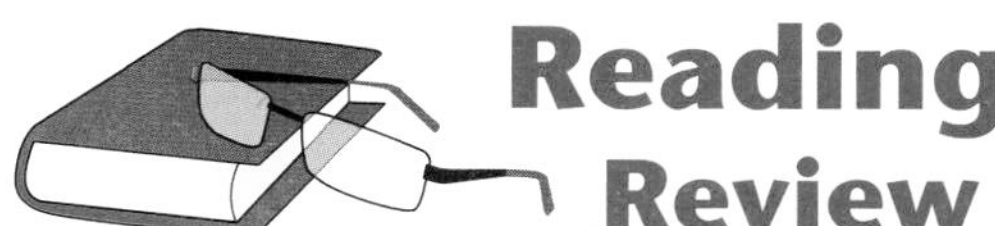

Reading Review

1. What is the first item found under the heading *Nutrition Facts* on a nutrition label?
2. On what calorie level are the percent Daily Values on nutrition labels based?

Section Summary

- To be a skillful shopper, you must be able to decide how much to spend and what to buy. You must also decide where and when to shop.
- Several factors determine the cost of food. They include how plentiful food is, how it is packaged, and where it is purchased.
- You should make shopping lists at the same time you plan menus. This can save you time and money.
- Labels provide important information about the foods you are buying.
- Using the information on nutrition labels will help you make nutritious food choices.

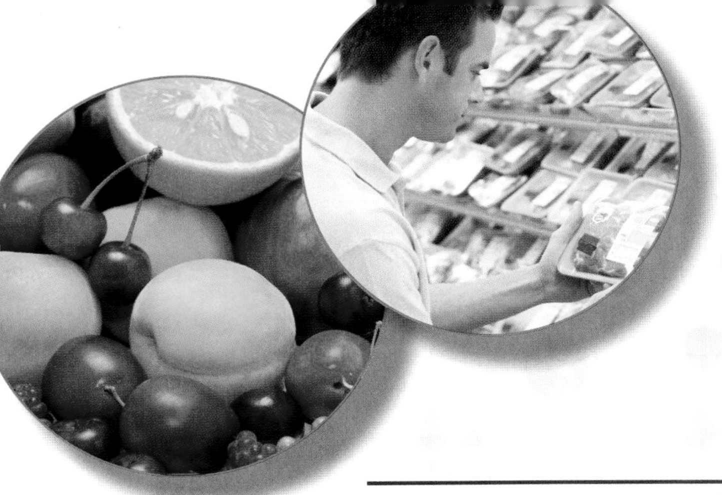

Section 8-3
Buying and Storing Food

Objectives

After studying this section, you will be able to
- **define** *produce*, *ripe*, *pasteurization*, *homogenization*, and *grade labeling*.
- **state** what to look for when buying various types of foods.
- **describe** how to properly store foods to preserve their nutrients, quality, flavor, and freshness.

Key Terms

produce: fresh fruits and vegetables.

ripe: fully grown and developed.

pasteurization: a process in which a liquid such as milk is heated to destroy harmful bacteria.

homogenization: a process in which milk fat is broken into tiny pieces and spread throughout the milk.

grade labeling: a rating of quality determined by the USDA for meats, poultry, and eggs.

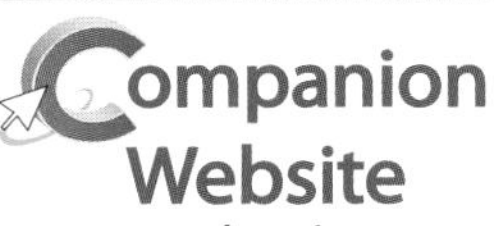

Study the Key Terms by completing crossword puzzles, matching activities, and e-flash cards at the website.

Main Ideas

- You can learn how to buy good quality foods.
- Storing foods carefully protects quality, nutrients, flavor, and freshness.

Shop carefully for good quality foods. Once you buy food, store it as well as possible. This helps protect its nutrients, quality, flavor, and freshness. When shopping for signs of quality in different foods, look at various factors. The type of food also makes a difference in how it is stored.

Buying and Storing Fruits and Vegetables

Fresh fruits and vegetables are called **produce**. Buy produce from a store or market where many fresh fruits and vegetables are sold. They are more likely to be fresh. Try to buy produce when it is *in season*. That is the time of year when a new crop is being harvested. See **8-6**. Handle produce carefully when choosing it. If you squeeze or pinch produce, it can bruise easily.

Choose produce that looks tasty. How ripe produce is makes a difference in its taste. **Ripe** means fully grown or developed. Fully ripened fruits and vegetables taste better than unripe produce. Two signs of ripe produce are good color and a firm texture that yields slightly to gentle pressure. If you buy unripe produce, keep it at room temperature until it ripens. Then store it in the refrigerator.

Wash produce carefully before storing it. Use cold water and a vegetable brush to get rid of dirt. To keep produce fresh and crisp, drain and store it in plastic bags or covered containers in the refrigerator. If you store produce in water, it will lose nutrients. Do not wash berries until you are ready to eat them. Store them loosely covered in the refrigerator. Some vegetables, such as potatoes and onions, keep best in a cool, dry place.

When fresh items are not in season, choose canned or frozen fruits and vegetables instead. Look for cans that are not bulging, dented, or leaking. Store cans on shelves in clean, dry cupboards. Look for frozen packages that are frozen solid. Store them in the freezer until you are ready to use them.

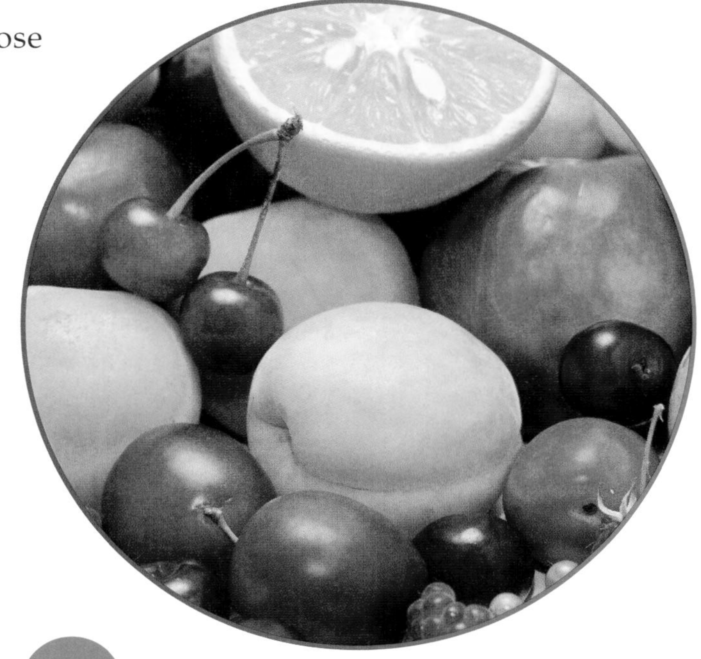

8-6 Produce is freshest when it is in season.

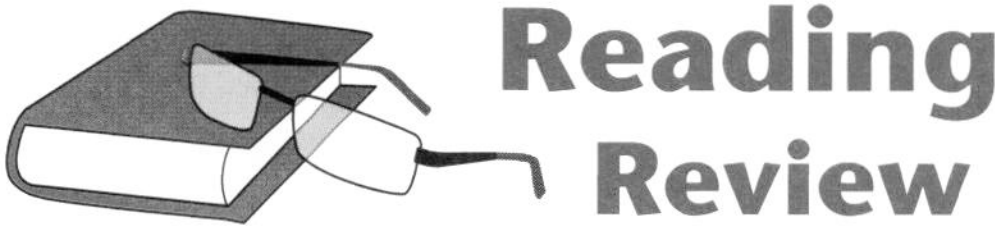

Reading Review

1. How can you tell if produce is ripe? What should you do if you buy produce that is not ripe?
2. How can you store most produce to keep it fresh and crisp?

Buying and Storing Grain Products

When buying bread, cereal, rice, or pasta, choose enriched or whole-grain products. These items are more nutritious. Packages for these foods should be clean and tightly sealed. Bread should be fresh and free from mold.

Rice, pasta, and most flours should be stored in sealed containers in cool, dry places. Store whole wheat flour in a tightly sealed container in the refrigerator or freezer to maintain freshness. Bread should be wrapped tightly to keep it fresh. Open cereal packages should be kept closed when not in use. This helps the cereal stay crisp and fresh.

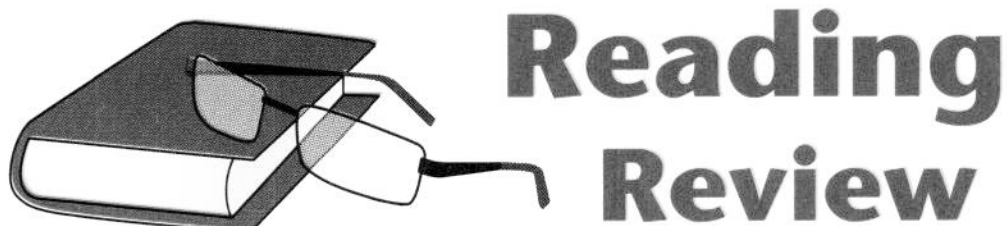

1. Why should you buy enriched or whole-grain bread or cereal products?
2. Where should whole wheat flour be stored to maintain freshness?

Buying and Storing Dairy Products

Milk and other dairy products sold in stores are pasteurized. **Pasteurization** is a process in which liquid such as milk is heated to destroy harmful bacteria. Whole milk is usually homogenized. **Homogenization** is a process in which milk fat is broken into tiny pieces and spread throughout the milk. There are many different types of milk available. See **8-7**.

The two main types of cheese are natural and process. The difference between natural and process cheese is how they are made. *Natural cheese* is made from milk. Natural cheese may be either hard or soft. *Process cheese* is made by melting and blending natural cheeses. Process cheese melts well and has a mild flavor. American cheese is probably the most common process cheese.

Cheese comes in many forms. You can buy it in chunks or sliced, cubed, shredded, or grated. In addition to packages, cheese also comes in jars and pressurized cans. These are convenient, but often cost more.

Types of Milk

- **Whole milk:** milk containing 3 to 4 percent butterfat.
- **Low-fat milk:** milk containing 1% butterfat.
- **Fat-free milk:** milk with all the butterfat removed.
- **Nonfat dry milk:** fat free milk with all the water removed.
- **Evaporated milk:** whole or fat-free milk with about half the water removed. It is sealed in cans.
- **Buttermilk:** made by special processes from whole or fat-free milk.

8-7 There are many types of milk from which to choose.

Store fresh milk in the refrigerator or it will spoil. Store nonfat dry milk in an airtight container in a cool place. After it is mixed with water, store it in the refrigerator. Unopened cans of evaporated milk can be stored on a shelf. After cans are opened, unused portions of evaporated milk should be refrigerated.

Cheese should be stored in the refrigerator to preserve nutrients and to prevent spoilage. Soft cheeses do not stay fresh as long as hard cheeses. Store soft cheeses, such as cottage cheese, in tightly covered containers. Wrap hard cheeses, such as Swiss and Cheddar, tightly to prevent drying.

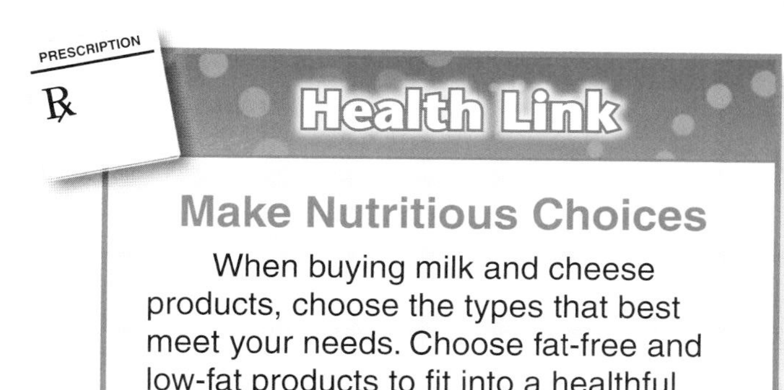

Make Nutritious Choices

When buying milk and cheese products, choose the types that best meet your needs. Choose fat-free and low-fat products to fit into a healthful diet. Check the freshness date stamped on cartons and packages. Be sure you will be able to use these products within a few days after this date.

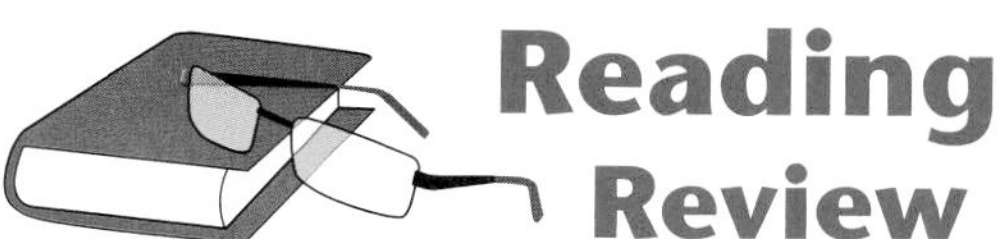

Reading Review

1. What does pasteurization do to milk? What does homogenization do?
2. What are the differences between the two types of cheese?

Buying and Storing Protein Foods

A large part of the money spent on food often goes toward protein-rich foods. Smart shopping can help you get your money's worth.

Choose meat, poultry, and fish carefully. Look for lean meat cuts that have fresh coloring. Choose poultry that is free of defects, such as cuts, bruises, and feathers. Select fish that has firm flesh and no strong odor. See **8-8**.

Meat, poultry, and fish can also be purchased canned or frozen. Choose these products with the same care you use when buying other canned and frozen foods. Select cans that are not dented or do not have a bulging shape. Frozen packages should be frozen solid and free from ice crystals.

Eggs come in many sizes. Check to be sure they have smooth shells and regular shapes. Do not buy eggs if the shells are cracked.

Look for grade labeling on meats, poultry, and eggs. **Grade labeling** is a rating of quality determined by the USDA. For instance, eggs may be graded AA, A, or B. Eggs of the highest quality are grade AA. Each type of meat has its own grade labeling system.

Beans are also a high-protein food. They can be bought in both dry and ready-to-use canned forms. There are many kinds of dry beans and peas you can use to prepare tasty meals.

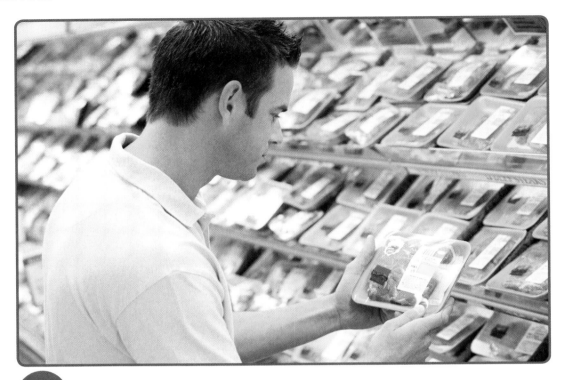

8-8 Look on fresh meat packages for information about how to handle products safely at home.

Fresh meat, poultry, and fish spoil quickly if not stored promptly. For short-term storage, loosely wrap meat and poultry in waxed paper and tightly wrap fish. Store these foods in the coldest part of the refrigerator or in the meat drawer. For long-term storage, store fresh and frozen foods in the freezer. Eggs should be stored in their original carton in the coldest part of the refrigerator. Dry beans should be stored in tightly covered containers. Colored glass or plastic containers help preserve the nutrients. See **8-9**.

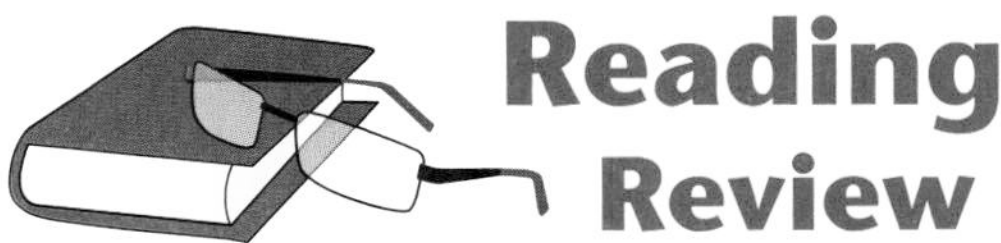

Reading Review

1. What should you look for when buying fresh meat, poultry, and fish?
2. In what part of the refrigerator should fresh meat, poultry, and fish be stored?

Section Summary

- There are useful guidelines for buying and storing different types of food.
- Learning these guidelines will help you buy foods that give you the best quality for your money.
- Following guidelines will help you store foods safely to protect nutrients, flavor, and freshness.

Cold Storage Chart

Product	Refrigerator (40°F, 4°C)	Freezer (0°F, -18°C)
Eggs		
Fresh in shell	3 weeks	Do not freeze
Hard cooked	1 week	Do not freeze well
Salads		
Egg, chicken, ham, tuna, and macaroni salads	3 to 5 days	Do not freeze well
Hot Dogs		
Opened package	1 week	1 to 2 months
Unopened package	2 weeks	1 to 2 months
Luncheon Meat		
Opened package or deli meat	3 to 5 days	1 to 2 months
Unopened package	2 weeks	1 to 2 months
Bacon and Sausage		
Bacon	7 days	1 month
Sausage, raw (chicken, turkey, pork, beef)	1 to 2 days	1 to 2 months
Hamburger and Other Ground Meats		
Hamburger, ground beef, turkey, veal, pork, lamb, and mixtures	1 to 2 days	3 to 4 months
Fresh Beef, Veal, Lamb, and Pork		
Steaks	3 to 5 days	6 to 12 months
Chops	3 to 5 days	4 to 6 months
Roasts	3 to 5 days	4 to 12 months
Fresh Poultry		
Chicken or turkey, whole	1 to 2 days	1 year
Chicken or turkey, pieces	1 to 2 days	9 months
Soups and Stews		
Vegetable or meat added	3 to 4 days	2 to 3 months
Leftovers		
Cooked meat or poultry	3 to 4 days	2 to 6 months
Chicken nuggets or patties	3 to 4 days	1 to 3 months
Pizza	3 to 4 days	1 to 2 months

USDA Kitchen Companion: Your Safe Food Handbook

8-9 Use this information as a guide to help you store food safely in your refrigerator and freezer.

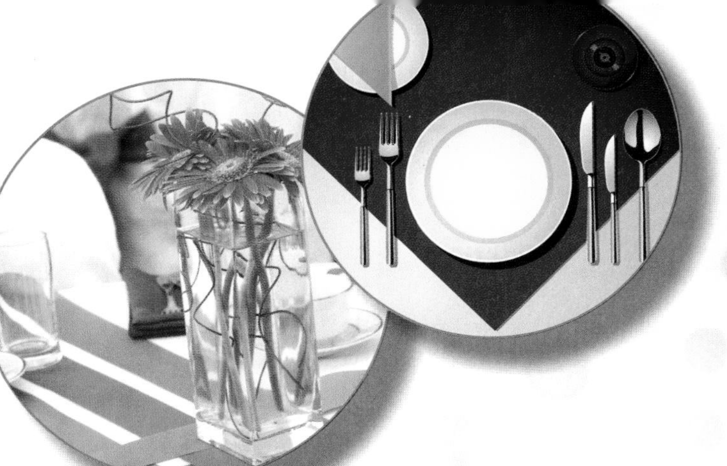

Section 8-4
Serving Meals

Objectives

After studying this section, you will be able to

- **define** *tableware*, *flatware*, *centerpiece*, *cover*, *family service*, *buffet service*, and *plate service*.
- **describe** items found in a table setting.
- **demonstrate** how to correctly set a table.
- **describe** different ways to serve meals.

Key Terms

tableware: dishes, flatware, and glassware.

flatware: forks, knives, and spoons used for serving and eating.

centerpiece: a decorative object placed in the middle of the table.

cover: the table space in front of a person's seat.

family service: a style of meal service in which people serve themselves as dishes are passed around the table.

buffet service: a style of meal service in which people help themselves to food set on a serving table.

plate service: a style of meal service in which plates are filled in the kitchen. They are then carried to the table and served to each person.

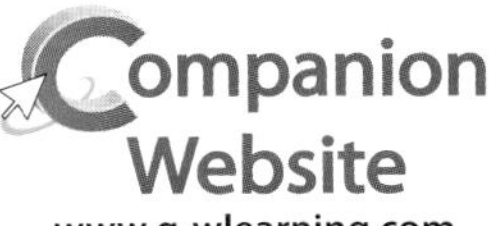

Study the Key Terms by completing crossword puzzles, matching activities, and e-flash cards at the website.

Main Ideas

- You can use creative table settings to add color and pleasure to the types of meals you serve.
- Different styles of meal service increase the pleasure of serving food.

There are as many ways to set a table as there are different kinds of meals to serve. For instance, you may use a simple table setting when serving a sandwich and a bowl of soup. You may want to be more creative for a special dinner.

Meals can be casual or formal depending on the event. For instance, meals are often more formal for special events and may require more complex table settings. Family customs often affect how the table is set and the meal is served.

Setting the Table

The items needed to set a table include tableware, table covers, and centerpieces. **Tableware** is dishes, flatware, and glassware. Dishes include plates, bowls, mugs, cups, and saucers. They can be made from glass, pottery, wood, plastic, china, metal, or paper. Dishes come in many colors, shapes, and patterns. Forks, knives, and spoons are called **flatware**. They are often made from metal or plastic. Glassware includes all types of drinking glasses. They are available in glass, metal, plastic, or paper in many different sizes, styles, and colors.

Tablecloths or place mats are used to protect the table from food spills. They also reduce the noise of dishes and other items being placed on the table. Special pads or old sheets can be placed under tablecloths to protect the table from hot dishes.

A **centerpiece** is a decorative object placed on the table. See **8-10**. Centerpieces are often made from flowers. They can also be made using many other types of materials. The centerpiece should add color and pleasure to the type of meal you serve. For instance, a basket of noisemakers and black and white balloons would be a fun centerpiece for a New Year's Eve dinner. Choose centerpieces that are low enough for people to see one another when seated.

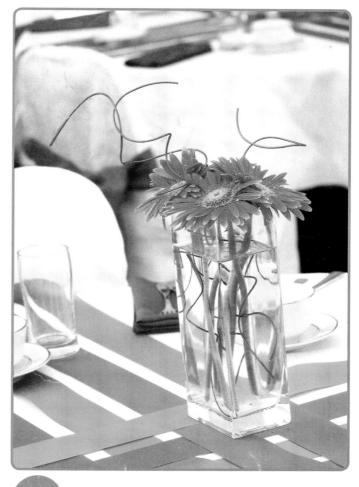

8-10 Centerpieces add color and make tables look attractive.

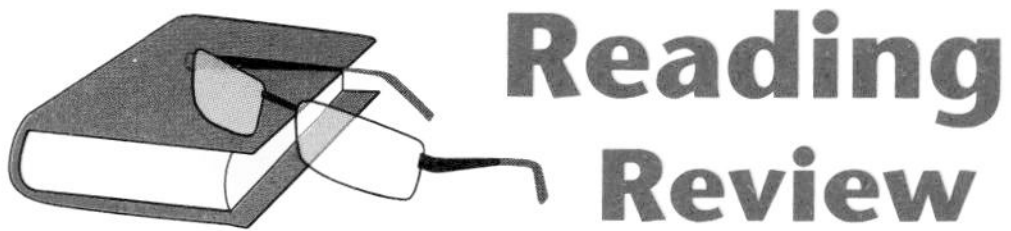

Reading Review

1. What are table covers? Why should you use them?
2. How can centerpieces make your table more attractive?

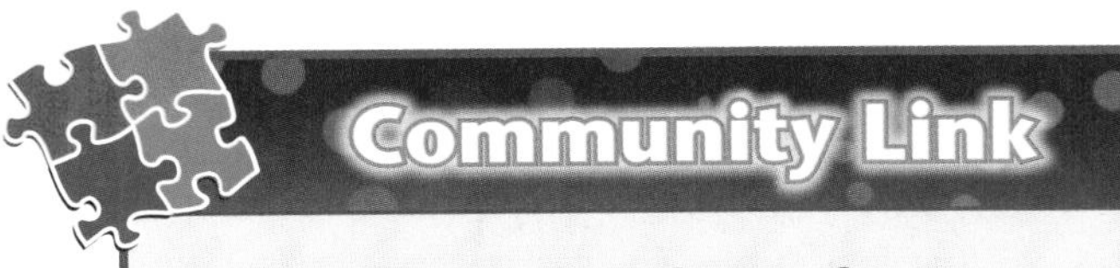

Table Settings for Special Events

Birthday parties or family holidays are good times to use special table settings. You can use creative centerpieces and table covers. When you eat out, you may notice that tables are set differently from the way they are at home. Pay attention to the type of meal service used in restaurants. This can make you feel more at ease when you eat at different restaurants. You may also be able to get ideas for table settings you might like to use when entertaining at home.

Making a Table Attractive

To set an attractive table, you must first learn to prepare a cover. The **cover** is the table space in front of a person's seat. It is large enough to hold a person's dishes, flatware, and glassware. Meals can be more enjoyable when the cover is arranged in a visually pleasing way.

Whether your table is large or small, round or square, it can be attractively set. Clean the table before and after each meal. Make sure the tableware is clean. Choose the correct dishes, glassware, and flatware for the food you are serving. Also, choose colors that go well together.

No matter how fancy or simple your meal is, the basics for setting a cover are the same. More tableware is often added as meals become fancier. Begin setting the table by selecting a tablecloth or place mats. Center tablecloths evenly over pads or sheets. If you are using place mats, be sure to line them up evenly with the edges of the table.

The dishes for the main course should be put on the table first. Set plates in the center of each person's cover. Place the knife on the right side of the plate with the blade facing the plate. Place the spoon to the right of the knife. Set the fork on the left side of the plate. (If extra flatware is used, place the flatware to be used first farthest from the plate.) Line flatware up with the bottom of the plate. Glassware should be placed at the point of the knife. Salad plates should be placed above the fork. See **8-11**.

Use only the dishes, flatware, and glassware you need. This saves you the extra work of setting and cleaning unnecessary tableware. People may often feel more comfortable when there is not excess tableware on the table.

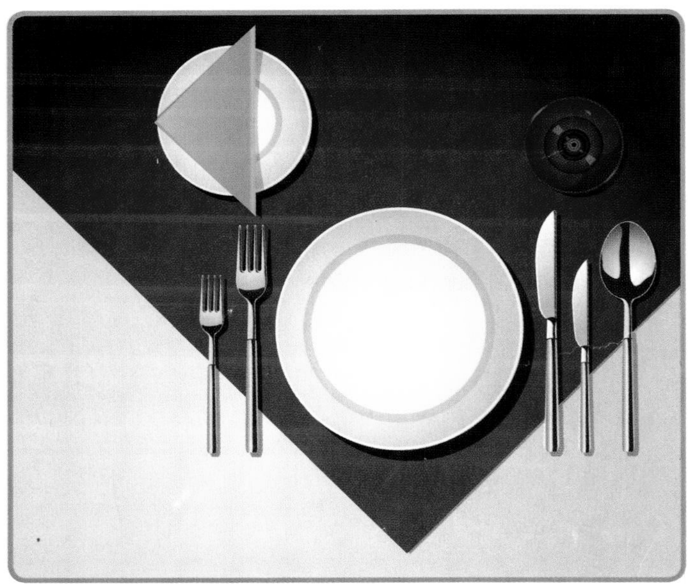

8-11 Other cover settings are based on this basic cover.

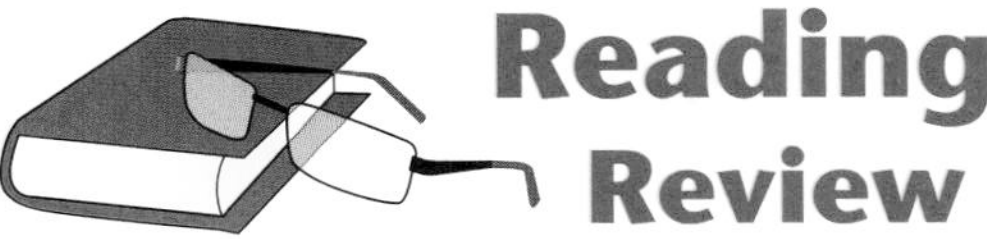

1. Why are plates the first dishes to be placed on the table?
2. Where should glassware be placed when setting a table?
3. Why should you use only the dishes, flatware, and glassware you need?

Serving the Meal

There are many ways to serve a meal. The type of service you choose depends on the event and the food served. Family customs and the number of people to be served also affect meal service. When you eat out, you may find restaurants have their own style of meal service.

Family service is a style of meal service in which people serve themselves as dishes are passed around the table. This is how meals are often served at home.

Buffet service is a style of meal service in which people help themselves to food set on a serving table. They may eat while standing or holding plates in their laps. Desserts and beverages may be served at a different time. Buffet service is a good way to serve large groups of people and offer variety.

Plate service is a style of meal service in which plates are filled in the kitchen. They are then carried to the table and served to each person at the table. This kind of service is often used in hotel dining rooms, restaurants, and banquet halls. The guests are seated first and then the food is placed on the table. This type of service needs more planning and effort. It makes certain events, however, seem more special.

Some people like to eat smaller servings at social events and family celebrations. If you are entertaining, you may want to choose a type of meal service that will allow others to eat less food. Family service and buffet service allow you to take a smaller serving.

Plate service means you will need to ask for smaller servings. For instance, you may have to ask to omit the gravy. You might ask for other changes in the food service. You might ask to have salad dressing served on the side so you can add as much as you want. If you are served more food than you want, you do not have to eat it. Leave items on your plate if you do not want them.

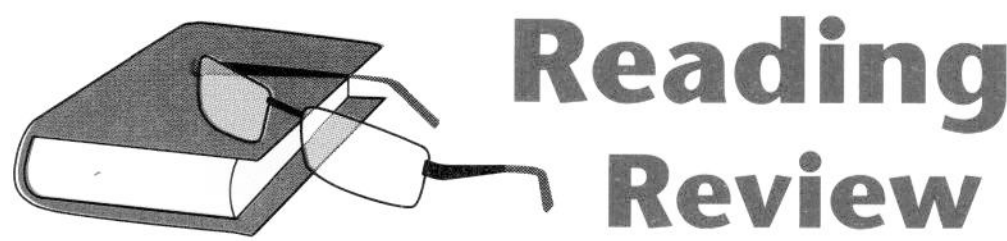

Reading Review

1. What are three factors that affect how you serve a meal?
2. What are the differences among the three types of meal service?
3. Which meal service would be best to allow guests to control serving sizes?

Section Summary

- Tableware should be clean and neatly arranged on the table.
- Choose a cover and style of meal service that best fits the needs of the people eating. Also, think about family customs, the menu, the kind of event, and number of people eating.

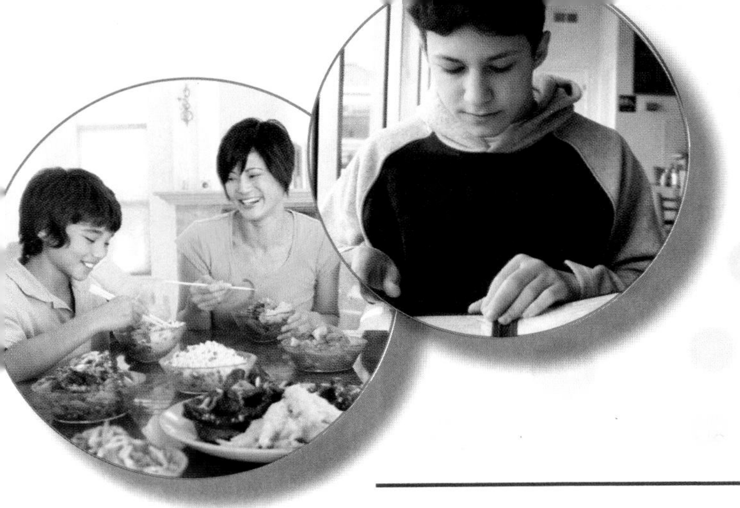

Section 8-5
Caring About Behavior

Objectives

After studying this section, you will be able to

- **define** *etiquette*, *manners*, and *à la carte*.
- **list** reasons it is important to use good manners every day.
- **state** why having good table manners can help you feel confident.
- **explain** how you can help guests feel welcome when entertaining.

Key Terms

etiquette: proper behavior in social settings.

manners: guidelines for behavior.

à la carte: a menu term meaning each food or course is listed and priced separately.

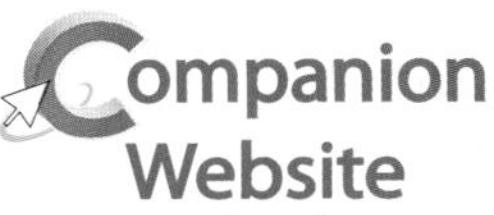

Study the Key Terms by completing crossword puzzles, matching activities, and e-flash cards at the website.

Main Ideas

- Good manners should be used every day.
- Knowing how to behave when eating out helps you feel confident.
- You can help guests feel welcome and comfortable when entertaining.

When you care about your behavior, you make meals more enjoyable for yourself and others. **Etiquette** is proper behavior in social settings. Etiquette is guided by **manners**, which are guidelines for behavior. Try to use good manners every day. Proper behavior will soon become a habit that is easy to use when you entertain or eat away from home.

Using Table Manners

Use good table manners at home as well as when you eat out. If you practice good manners at home, they will become a habit. They will help you feel at ease in any situation. You will not have to think about how to behave when you are with others.

Table manners can vary. Family and religious customs can affect table manners. What people do in one city or country may be different from what you do. It is easy to adjust to most situations when you use basic good manners.

Part of having good table manners is learning how to use tableware properly. You should practice using different types of tableware until you feel comfortable. See **8-12**.

Accidents will happen at the table. They may include dropping a piece of food or spilling a drink. If you are involved in an accident, apologize. You should also offer your help. Then you should forget about the matter. Do not keep talking about the accident. This only makes others feel uncomfortable.

Using Tableware Properly

- Place your napkin in your lap during a meal.
- Take the napkin from your lap to wipe your mouth. Wipe your fingers without taking the napkin away from your lap. At the end of the meal, place the napkin to the left of your plate.
- Use a fork to carry food to your mouth. Use a spoon if food is soft or liquid. Do not point or gesture with your flatware.
- Cut tender meats and salads with the side of a fork. Use a knife to cut food that cannot be cut easily with a fork.
- Spread butter or jam on bread with a knife.
- When you finish using a knife, place it across the rim of the plate. Do not put it on the table or tablecloth. It may be greasy or sticky.
- Dip a soup spoon away from you. Then move it from the back of the bowl to your mouth. Eat from the side of the spoon. Do not bend over the bowl, lift the bowl to your chin, or make any noise while eating soup.
- You can eat some foods with your fingers. They are often crisp or dry. Some finger foods are vegetable sticks, most fresh fruits, and snack chips. Fried chicken or barbecued ribs may be eaten with the fingers at informal events. Sandwiches are eaten with the fingers.
- After use, spoons should be placed on the saucers under cups and bowls.
- Place flatware across the center of the plate when you finish eating. This makes it easier to clear the table, and flatware will not fall off the plate.

8-12 Following these guidelines will help you feel comfortable using tableware.

Succeed in Life

Using Good Table Manners

Table manners are based on care and respect for others. When you eat, use the following guidelines. They can help make meals more pleasant for everyone.

- Wait in line quietly in a cafeteria or restaurant.
- Pass food to others carefully. Ask politely for food to be passed to you.
- Use good posture. Sit as quietly as possible. Relax and enjoy the meal.
- Eat slowly and quietly, taking small bites. Chew with your mouth closed. Do not talk when your mouth is full.
- Keep you plate neat. Be careful not to spill food.
- If you do not like a certain food, leave it on your plate. Do not make rude comments about it.
- Remain seated at the table until everyone is finished eating. If you must leave early, ask to be excused.
- When eating in a cafeteria or fast food restaurant, carry your tray and tableware to the proper place when you leave.
- Help keep the conversation pleasant and interesting when eating with others. In public places, keep your voice low so you do not bother other guests.

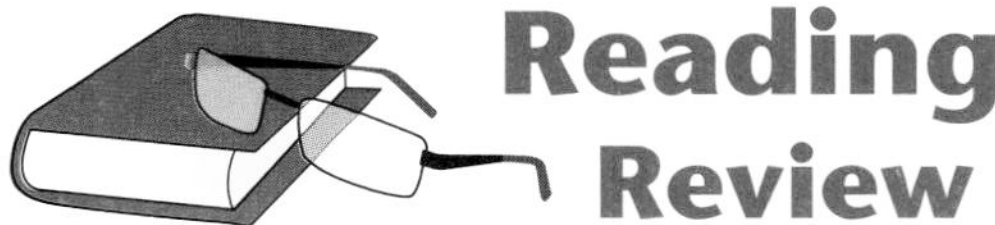

Reading Review

1. Why should you practice good table manners at home?
2. If someone sitting next to you spills milk on you, how should you behave?

Eating Away from Home

When eating out, good table manners include being able to properly order your food. Understanding how to read a menu can help you do this with ease. Menu forms vary from place to place. Menus often list foods and prices in standard ways, however.

Some family-type restaurant menus list food as complete meals. One price includes all the courses for a meal. For instance, the price for a full dinner might include the appetizer, main course, bread or rolls, and dessert. A beverage may not be included in the price. Drinks, however, are usually available at an extra cost.

Some menus may include à la carte items. **À la carte** means each food or course is listed and priced separately. Appetizers, soups, salads, main dishes, desserts, and beverages are all individually priced. It often costs less to buy a complete meal than it does to buy the same foods à la carte.

Menus may be different in specialty restaurants that feature cultural or ethnic foods. For instance, Chinese, Indian, Turkish, or Mexican restaurants may have their own ways of listing foods and prices.

Some menus are posted on bulletin boards with prices. Besides understanding how foods are priced, you need to recognize how they are prepared. Restaurant menus sometimes include terms that may not be familiar to you. Some of these are listed in **8-13**.

Some menus carry nutritional information about the food offerings. Read the menu carefully to select the foods that best meet your nutritional needs. Avoid excess sugar, fat, and sodium. To reduce fat, saturated fat, trans fat, and cholesterol, choose tasty fresh vegetable or fruit salads. Check if low-fat dressing is available or ask to have dressing served on the side. Avoid foods served with gravies, cheeses, or cream sauces. Check the preparation method for meat, poultry, and fish. Avoid fried dishes. Instead, select main dishes that are baked, roasted, broiled, grilled, poached, or steamed.

If the restaurant has servers, give your order to the server. Speak clearly. Your server may ask questions about how you would like your food prepared. You can also ask the server questions about items on the menu.

If you are with a group, tell the server how to make out the bill. Each group member may plan to pay for his or her food. If so, one member of the group should collect the money and pay the bill. It is usually easier for the

Menu Terms

à la mode: served with ice cream.

au gratin: served with cheese.

au jus: served with natural juices.

basted: prepared by spooning juices over the food to keep it moist and add flavor.

braised: cooked in a small amount of liquid.

browned: cooked to give the surface of the food a brown color.

deep-fried: cooked in a large amount of hot fat.

du jour: of the day, such as soup du jour, which means soup of the day.

garnished: decorated with small pieces of food, such as parsley sprigs or lemon twists, to add color.

grilled: cooked over hot coals.

julienned: cut into thin strips.

marinated: soaked in a flavorful liquid.

poached: cooked in simmering liquid.

pureed: blended to turn a solid food, such as fruit, into a thick liquid, such as a fruit sauce.

roasted: cooked in an oven.

sautéed: cooked in a small amount of hot fat.

steamed: cooked in steam.

stir-fried: cooked quickly in a small amount of fat until the food has a crisp-tender texture.

8-13 Being familiar with these menu terms will help you know how restaurant foods are prepared.

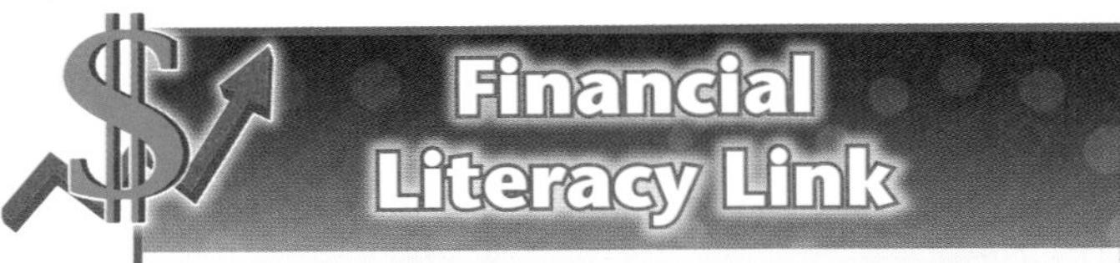

Figuring the Tip

When dining out, the percentage of tip you leave a server is based on several factors. These include the quality of your food, the service you receive, and the total bill amount. Servers earn less than minimum wage, so tips are their main source of income. Some expensive fine-dining restaurants add the server's tip to the final bill, but that is a rare practice. It is usually common to leave a 15 to 20 percent tip to a good server. For instance, when your total bill is $15 and you are tipping 15 percent, the tip would be $2.25. What would the tip be when the bill is $25 and you tip 20 percent?

server to write one bill. When everyone orders different food items, however, you might want to ask your server for individual bills or separate checks.

Paying for your meal differs at various types of restaurants. At fast food or some specialty restaurants, you often pay at the counter when you order.

Tipping is done to show a server you appreciate good service. Fast food restaurants do not have servers. Therefore, tipping is not necessary. Menu prices generally do not include the tip. You must decide how much to leave for a tip.

Using good table manners is especially important when you are eating in a restaurant. Talk quietly with the people at your table so you do not disturb other diners. If you have a problem with your food, quietly call it to your server's attention. If your server is unable to help you, ask to speak to the manager. Avoid making a loud scene.

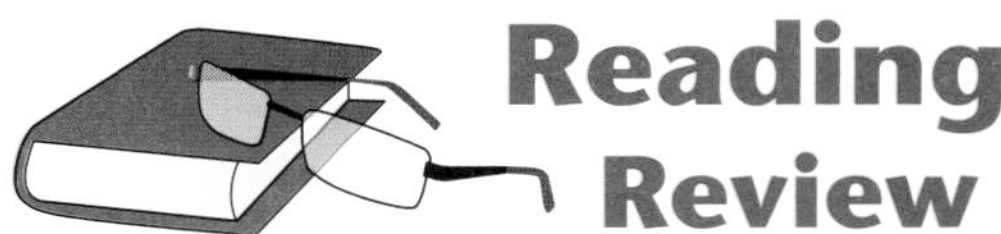

1. Why would ordering a complete meal cost less than ordering a meal à la carte?
2. How can you reduce fat, saturated fat, trans fat, and cholesterol when ordering from a restaurant menu? Give examples.
3. What should you do when you have a problem with your food in a restaurant?

Entertaining at Home

You may like to entertain at home. If so, plan and prepare for the event. Choose a menu of healthful foods. Having good manners is also necessary. Be ready when your guests arrive. You want your guests to have a good time and feel welcome.

When you have guests, introduce people to one another. You may feel uncomfortable when you first make introductions. Take your time and try to feel relaxed. To make an introduction, clearly state the names of your guests. If you forget a person's name, ask him or her to remind you. It is better to ask a person's name again than to hide the fact that you do not remember it.

Try to help start conversations. When you make introductions, say something interesting about each person. This may help your guests think of something to say to one another.

When you have guests in your home, you set the mood. This means planning activities and entertainment. Do not forget to show respect for your family and neighbors. Your guests will usually follow your example.

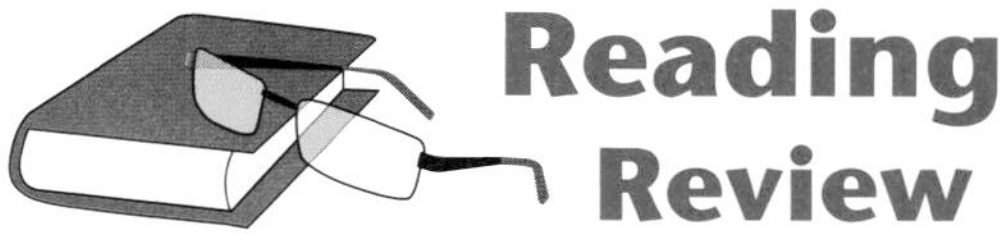

Reading Review

1. What tasks must you perform when you entertain at home?
2. How can you help start conversations among your guests?

Section Summary

- You can show care and respect for others by using good table manners.
- People will enjoy eating with you more when you use good table manners.
- You will often feel more comfortable eating out and entertaining when you practice manners daily.

Chapter Summary

When you are planning a meal, there are several factors to consider. They include planning the menu, shopping for the food, and buying and storing the food.

By planning carefully, you can make a meal that is nutritious, attractive, and tasty. You can make this process easier by following meal patterns.

When you buy food, shop skillfully. This will help you get the best quality food for your money. When you bring food home, store it properly. Otherwise, it may spoil. Then it will have to be thrown away.

After the meal has been planned, decide how you are going to serve it. You can choose from many different types of meal service. Set the table properly and use good table manners. This will give you more confidence when you eat out.

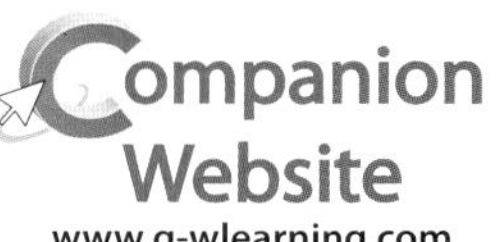

Review Key Terms and Main Ideas for Chapter 8 at the website.

Chapter Review

Write your answers on a separate sheet of paper.

1. What are the three common meal patterns?
2. List three tips to keep in mind when planning meals for your family.
3. What are five points you should consider when planning attractive and pleasing menus?
4. List three different types of food stores.
5. What happens to the price of food when there is a shortage?
6. True or false. Shop when you have extra time.
7. List three advantages of writing a shopping list.
8. How can a nutrition label help you?
9. What information must be on a nutrition label?
10. List three hints for buying and storing foods.
11. List two ways to tell when fruits and vegetables are ripe.
12. What is the difference between natural and process cheese?
13. Give an example of a centerpiece for a birthday party or special holiday dinner.
14. True or false. Forks are placed to the right of the plate.
15. What are three advantages of practicing good table manners at home?

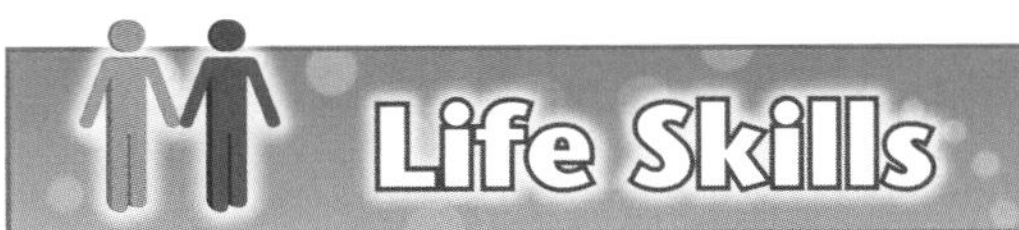

16. Plan a nutritious menu for your family for two days. List the ingredients you will need and the quantity of each one. Then check the refrigerator and cupboards to see which of the ingredients you have available. Create a shopping list for the ingredients you want to purchase. Present your plan to a parent for review and help in shopping.

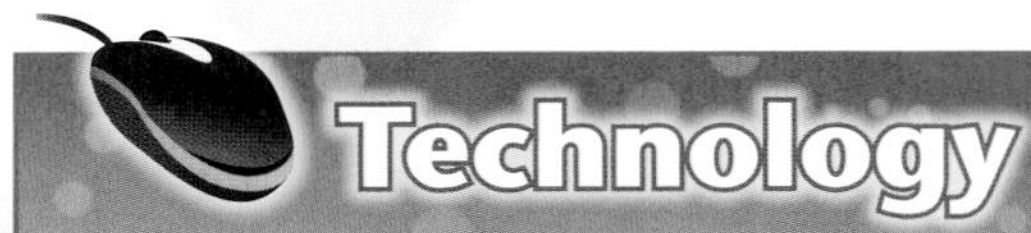

17. Many large fast-food restaurant chains have nutrition information available online. Use the Internet to research the nutritional value of your favorite fast-food items. Find out the calories, total fat, saturated fat, trans fat, cholesterol, and sodium content of various menu items. Decide which foods you could choose for a meal that would limit calories, total fat, saturated fat, trans fat, cholesterol, and sodium.

18. Keep track of the foods you eat each day by writing them in a food journal. You can also write entries showing the amount of physical activity you perform each day. Review your journal entries each week to learn how you can make more healthful food choices.

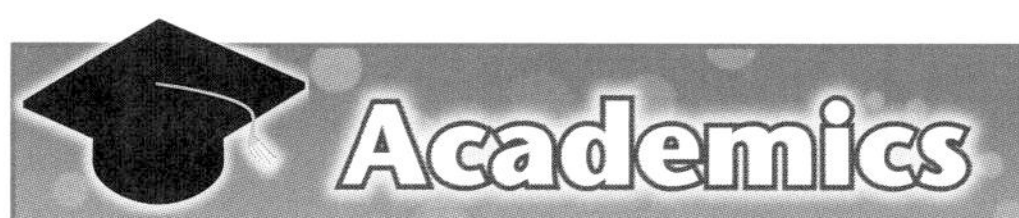

19. **Social Studies.** Obtain a copy of a lunch menu from your school cafeteria and one from a fast-food restaurant. Compare the foods they include. Use a calorie guide to estimate the calories in some of the menu items. Then decide which menu is the most nutritious. Share this information with the class.
20. **Reading.** Read food ads in magazines, in newspapers, and on the Internet. Identify those ads that attract your attention quickly and those that do not. Did the ads cause you to want to buy the product? In small groups, discuss why these ads attracted your attention.
21. **Writing.** Compare the nutrition labels for two similar food products. Write a brief summary stating which product you would choose based on the label information. Be sure to give reasons for your choice.

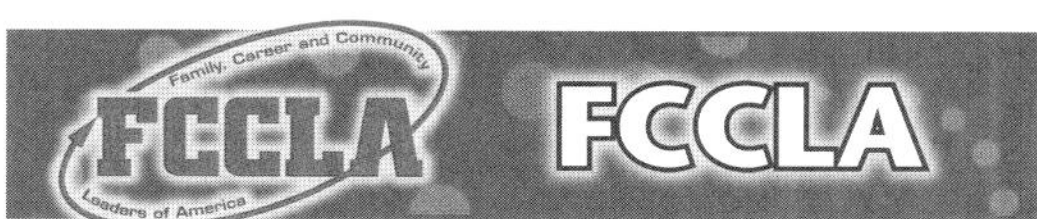

22. Develop a healthful menu plan for one week that includes nutritious items for breakfast, lunch, dinner, and a snack. Use the MyPlate guidelines to include the recommended daily amounts you need from each food group. Then get involved with the FCCLA *Student Body* program. Complete a project that relates to the *Eat Right* unit. Obtain further information about this program from your FCCLA advisor.

Chapter 9
You in the Kitchen

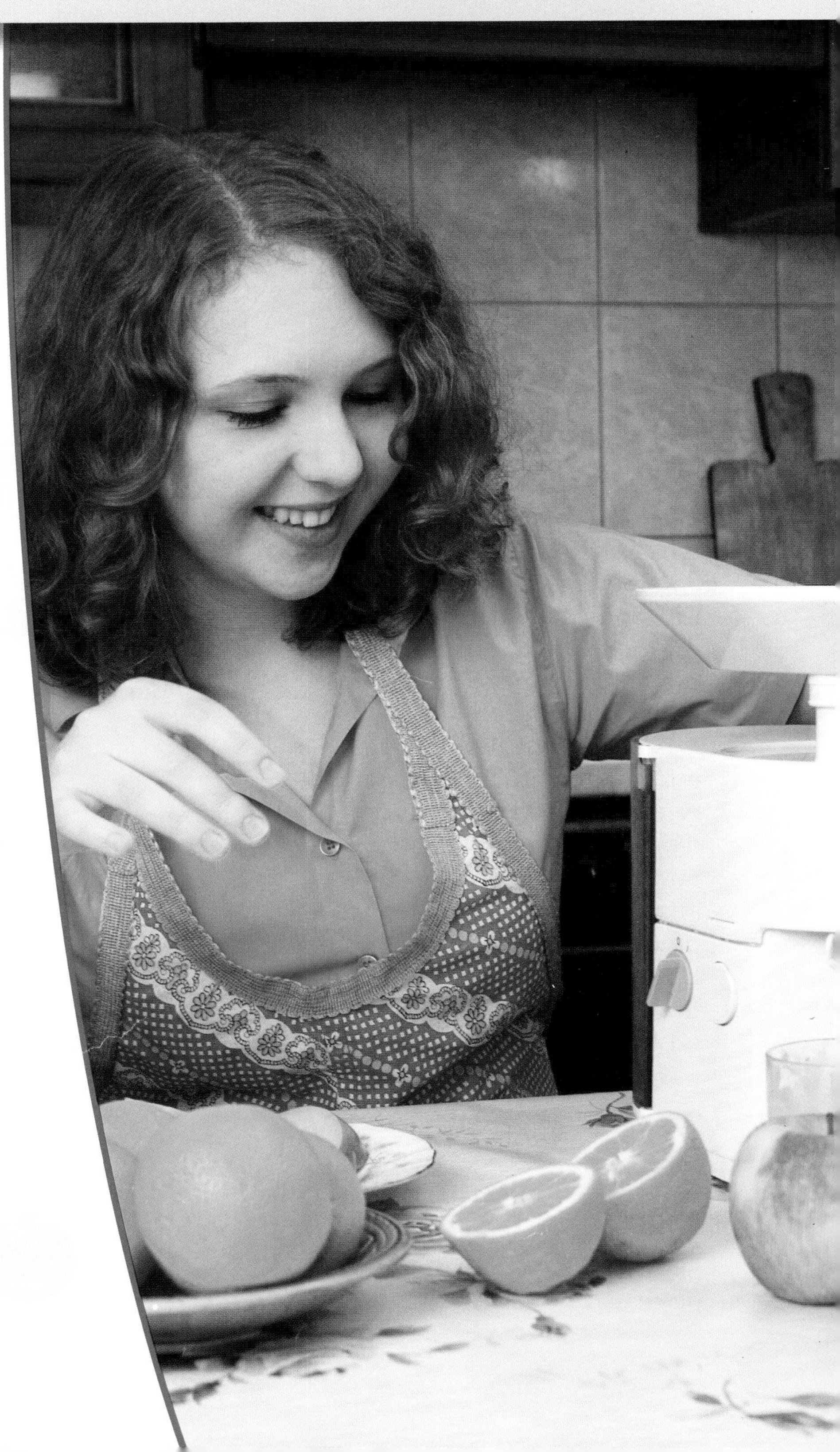

Sections

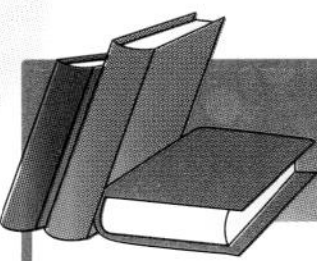

Sharpen Your Reading

Read the review questions at the end of the chapter *before* you read the chapter. Keep the questions in mind as you read to help you determine which information is most important.

Concept Organizer

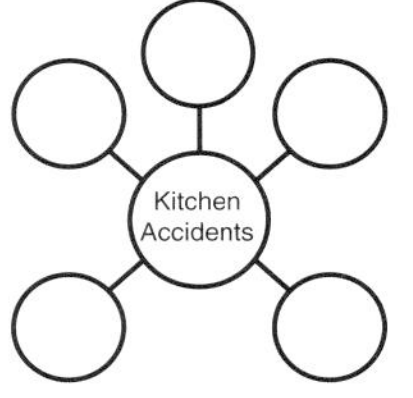

Use a star diagram like the one shown to identify the most common types of kitchen accidents. Why is safety awareness so important in the kitchen?

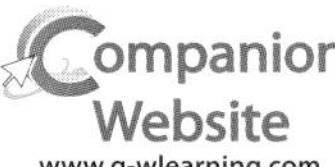

Print out the concept organizer at the website.

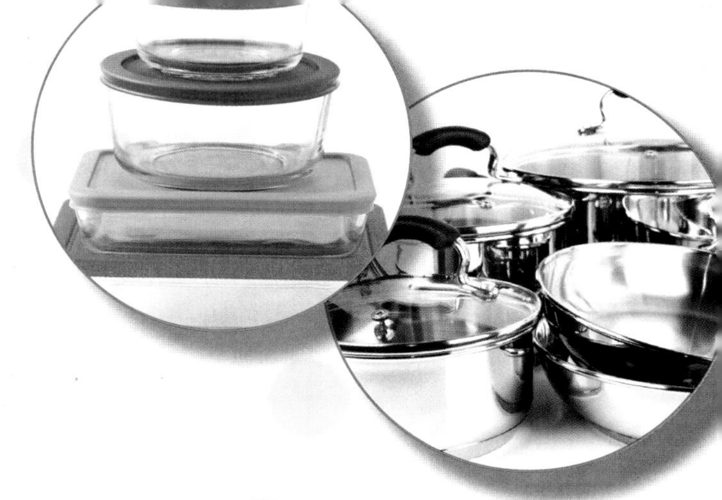

Section 9-1
Working with Kitchen Tools

Objectives

After studying this section, you will be able to
- **define** *utensil*, *use and care manual*, *cook, microwaves*, *cookware*, and *bakeware*.
- **identify** appliances and utensils used in the kitchen.
- **explain** why you should use and care for kitchen tools properly.

Key Terms

utensil: nonelectric, handheld kitchen tool used when preparing food.

use and care manual: a booklet of instructions for a tool.

cook: to prepare food for eating using heat.

microwaves: high-frequency energy waves often used to cook food.

cookware: pots and pans used on the stovetop.

bakeware: pots and pans used in conventional ovens.

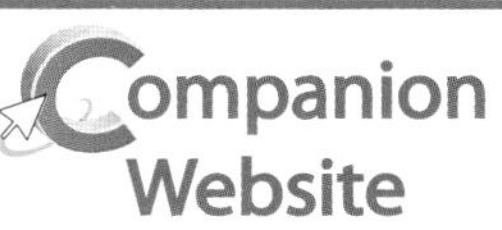

Study the Key Terms by completing crossword puzzles, matching activities, and e-flash cards at the website.

Main Ideas

- Appliances and utensils make preparing food easier.
- You should properly use and care for kitchen tools.

Appliances and utensils are important kitchen tools. A **utensil** is a nonelectric, handheld kitchen tool used when preparing food. Appliances and utensils are the backbone of your kitchen. They help you prepare food as well as save time and energy. As you become skilled at using kitchen tools, preparing food will become easier.

Kitchen Tools

To prepare food, use different kinds of kitchen tools. Kitchen tools include large and small appliances, pots and pans, and utensils. Large appliances are often costly and use a lot of energy. Small appliances are less costly and use less energy. Tools such as pots, pans, and utensils are also needed. Their costs vary and they do not use electricity.

The tools you choose will depend on many factors. They include the types of cooking you do and how much storage space you have.

Manufacturers provide a booklet of instructions for a tool called a **use and care manual**. It tells you how to safely operate the tool and the best ways to use it. Keep all use and care manuals handy.

Tools will last longer and work better when you use and care for them properly. You will avoid wasting energy. You may also reduce the cost of operating appliances.

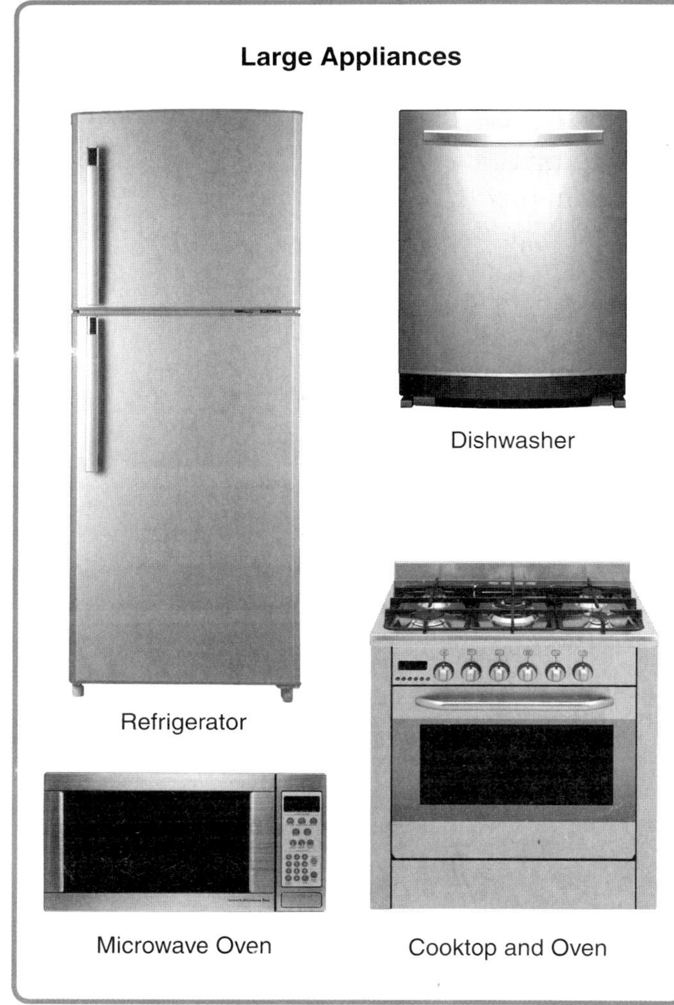

9-1 Large appliances come in many different styles. These are a few basic ones.

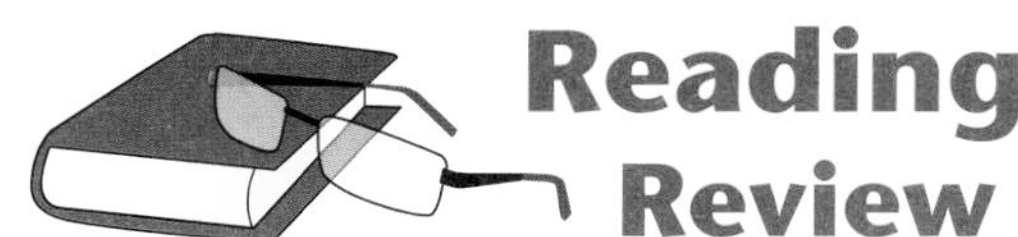

1. What information is included in a use and care manual?
2. Why is it important you take good care of your kitchen tools?

Large Appliances

Large appliances include refrigerators, freezers, cooktops, conventional ovens, microwave ovens, and automatic dishwashers. See **9-1**.

Certain foods should be stored in the refrigerator to keep from spoiling and becoming unsafe to eat. Refrigerator temperatures should be between 35°F and 40°F (2°C to 4°C). Higher temperatures

Succeed in Life

Use Microwave Ovens Correctly

In a microwave oven, you can speed cooking and promote even heating. You can cook, reheat, and defrost foods and prepare convenience foods that are already cooked. A microwave oven cooking guide or recipe book is useful. Always follow directions on a package or in a recipe. Only use microwave-safe utensils (glass or plastic), paper plates or towels, waxed paper, plastic wrap, cooking or storage bags. Do not use metal containers or aluminum foil for cooking. Metal can damage the microwave electronics. You can prepare foods such as meats, poultry, breads, seafood, vegetables, and hot cereals in a microwave oven. If foods need browning, use a conventional oven. Foods do not brown well in microwave ovens.

will cause foods to spoil. Lower temperatures will cause foods to freeze. Some refrigerators have special sections for storing milk products, meats, and vegetables. The temperature of each section is best for the type of food being stored there.

A freezer can be a part of the refrigerator or it can be a separate appliance. Freezers are used to keep foods frozen for later use. Freezer temperatures should be 0°F (-18°C) or below to maintain food quality.

Cook means to prepare food for eating using heat. The source of heat may be a cooktop, conventional oven, grill, or microwave oven. Microwave ovens use **microwaves**, which are high-frequency energy waves, to cook foods.

Cooktops may have from two to six surface cooking units on top of the oven. These units are called *burners* if they use gas and *elements* if they use electricity. Cooktops may be separate from the oven and built into a countertop. The oven may be built into a nearby wall or cabinet area.

Microwave ovens are often used in addition to stovetops and conventional ovens. They heat food quickly and evenly, saving you both time and energy. Microwave ovens may be placed on countertops or special carts, or be built into cabinets.

Automatic dishwashers save you the time and energy it takes to wash dishes by hand. This time can be spent on other tasks. Dishwashers are generally installed under a countertop near the sink. Some models are portable.

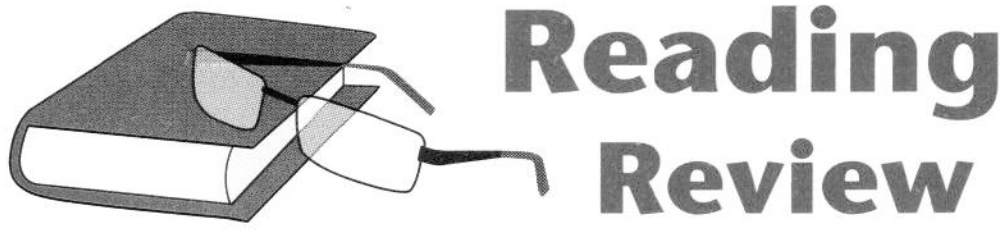

Reading Review

1. What are the correct temperatures for storing food in refrigerators and freezers?
2. How can microwave ovens save you time and energy?

Small Appliances

Small appliances help you perform tasks that would be much harder to do manually. Some common small appliances are electric skillets, toasters, electric mixers, blenders, slow cookers, and popcorn poppers.

Small appliances can help conserve energy when preparing food. For instance, when you cook food in an electric skillet instead of on a stovetop, you save energy.

Be careful when using small appliances. The outside finishes can be easily damaged. Glass or plastic parts can be broken with careless use. Follow the directions in the appliances' use and care manuals. The manuals explain how to use appliances without damaging them.

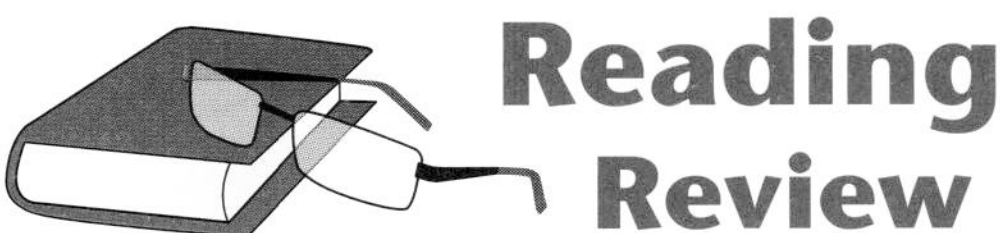

1. How can small appliances help you conserve energy?
2. Why should you be careful when using small appliances?

Pots and Pans

The pots and pans you use on a cooktop are called **cookware**. Examples of cookware are saucepans, pots, and skillets. Pots and pans are made with different materials. They include aluminum, cast iron, copper, stainless steel, enamel, glass, and pottery. Each material is used for a certain reason. For instance, aluminum conducts heat evenly.

Pots and pans used in conventional ovens are called **bakeware**. They include cake, pie, muffin, and pizza pans; cookie sheets; and roasting pans and racks. Items safe to use in microwave ovens are called *microwave cookware*. Glass is safe to use in microwave ovens, while metal is not. See **9-2**.

Types of Pots and Pans

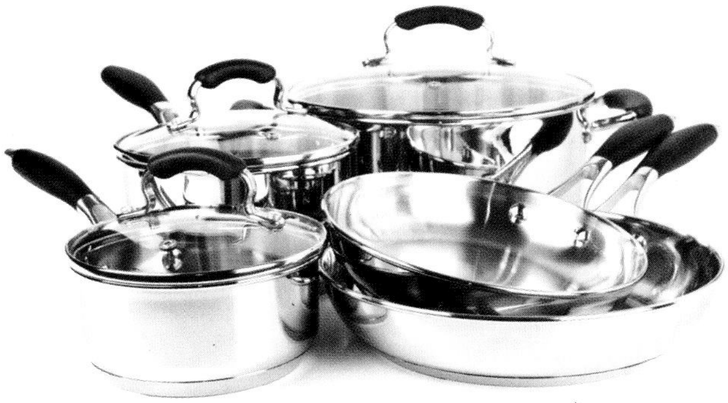

Cookware

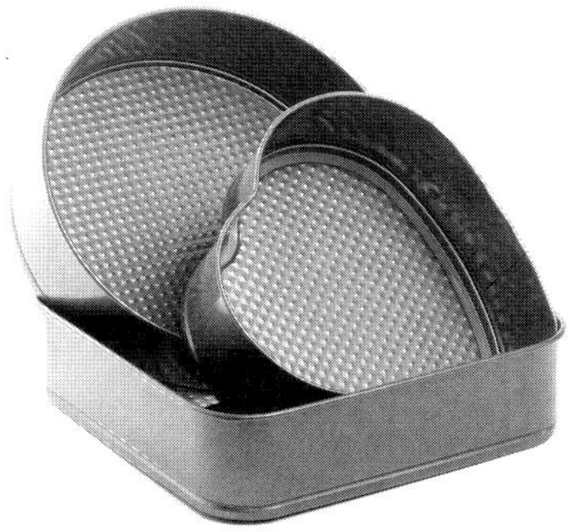

Bakeware

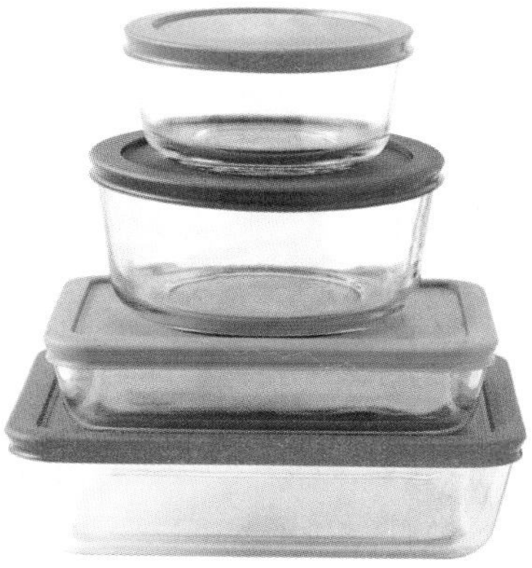

Microwave cookware

9-2 You will use different kinds of pots and pans when cooking on a cooktop, in a conventional oven, or in a microwave oven.

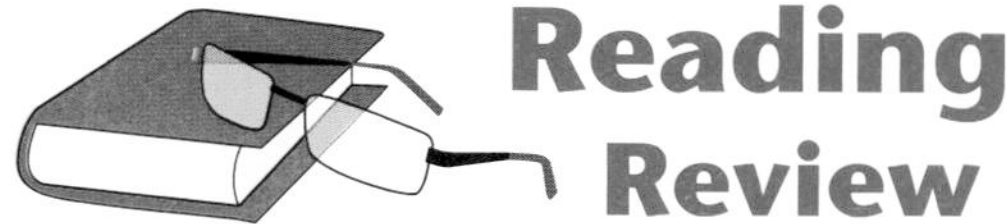

Reading Review

1. What are the differences among cookware, bakeware, and microwave cookware?
2. What are some materials that are used to make pots and pans?

Utensils

Utensils make preparing food easier. You can use them to measure, cut, mix, and prepare food for cooking. They can also be used to perform a variety of other tasks around the kitchen. Basic kitchen utensils include knives, cutting boards, mixing bowls, wooden spoons, rubber scrapers, spatulas, and colanders. Measuring spoons and cups are also basic utensils.

When you begin cooking, start with a basic set of utensils. As you cook more often, you may find you need other utensils, such as ladles and kitchen shears. Before buying any utensils, think about how you will use them. See **9-3**.

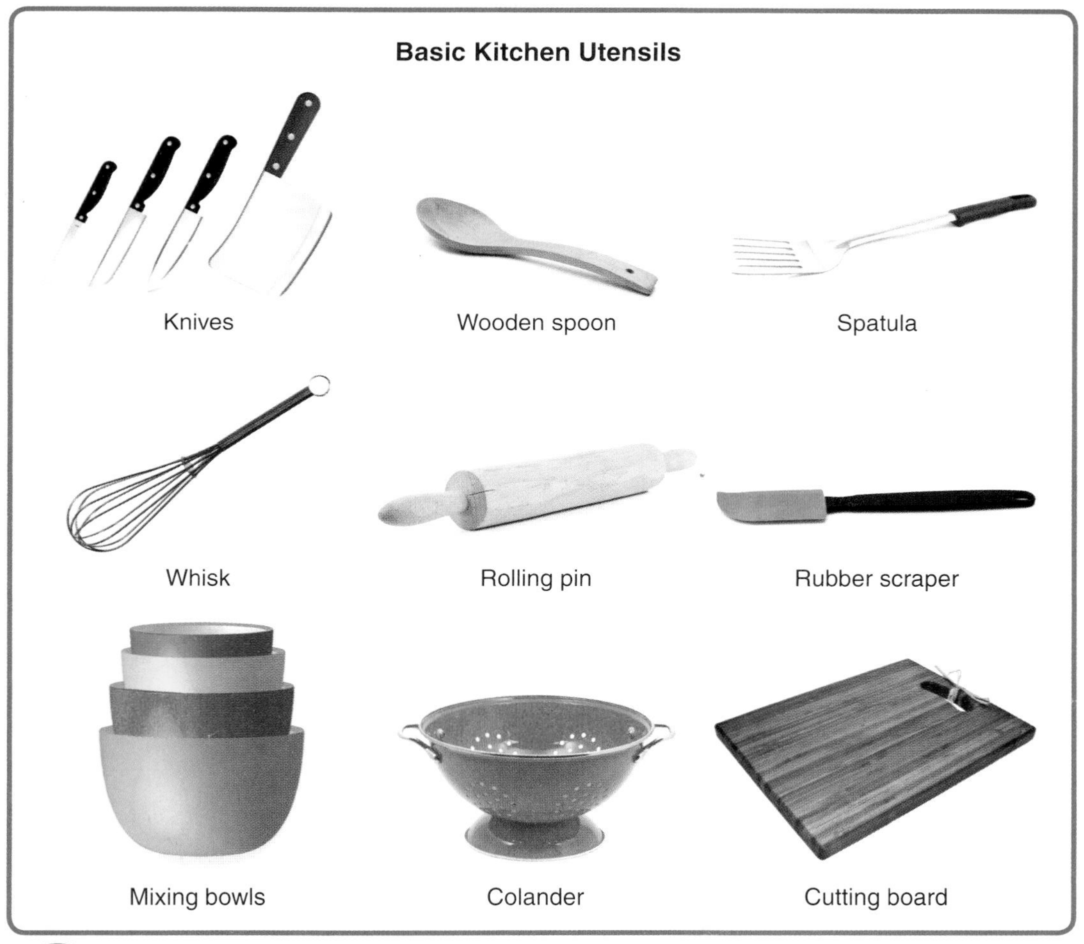

9-3 These are some basic utensils you may use for food preparation.

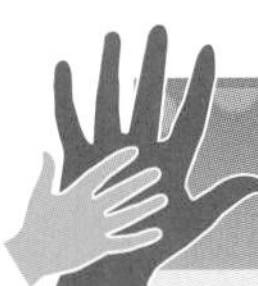

Safety Link

Safely Handling Knives

A good selection of stainless steel knives is very important when cooking. This may sound odd, but sharp knives are much safer than dull ones. It takes less force to cut through food with a sharp knife. This gives you greater control of the blade. Dull knives can easily slip off the food you are cutting and cut your fingers instead. Most cooking accidents are due to either the use of dull knives or using sharp knives incorrectly. Some tips for knife safety include the following:

1. Always cut with the knife blade angled away from you. Never try to open a can or bottle with a knife—or use a knife as a screwdriver. Use scissors instead of a knife to cut string, metal, or paper.
2. Always use a cutting board and keep it firmly in place. A damp towel or paper towel placed underneath will keep it from moving. Never cut anything in your hand. Use the cutting board, and make sure it has enough space for your task.
3. Make sure your hands are dry and stay focused on the job when using knives.
4. Do not use knives with broken or loose handles.
5. Wash your knives by hand and dry thoroughly. Never put knives into the dishwasher or drop them into a sink filled with sudsy water. Always hold a knife by its handle, never the blade.
6. Store knives properly. A knife block or magnetic knife rack is best. If you are storing knives in a drawer, make sure to keep them separate from other utensils.
7. Do not try to catch a knife you have dropped. Step away and wait until the knife comes to a complete rest before picking it up by the handle.

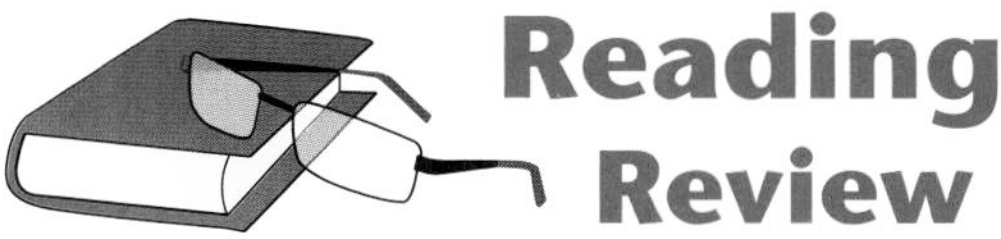

Reading Review

1. How can utensils be used to make preparing food easier?
2. Why should you start with a basic set of utensils?

Section Summary

- Kitchen tools consist of large and small appliances, pots and pans, and utensils.
- Each tool has its own purpose and use.
- Tools should be used according to their use and care manuals.
- Using kitchen tools correctly saves energy and prevents damage.

Section 9-2
Safety and Sanitation

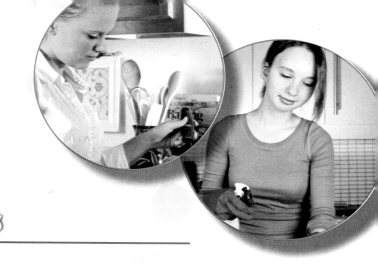

Objectives

After studying this section, you will be able to
- **define** *sanitation*, *foodborne illnesses*, and *toxins*.
- **explain** how to work safely in the kitchen.
- **state** how using proper sanitation can prevent foodborne illnesses.
- **describe** how to clean a kitchen to prevent the spread of bacteria.
- **explain** how to keep food safe when taking it to places away from home.

Key Terms

sanitation: the process of making conditions clean and healthy.

foodborne illnesses: illnesses caused from toxins produced by harmful bacteria in food.

toxins: poisonous substances.

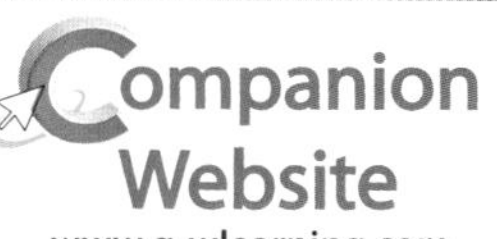

Study the Key Terms by completing crossword puzzles, matching activities, and e-flash cards at the website.

Main Ideas

- Kitchen accidents can be prevented.
- You can prevent foodborne illness from occurring.
- It is important to keep the kitchen clean.

When you work in the kitchen, you may be busy preparing food. You must, however, pay attention to safety and sanitation no matter how busy you are. Otherwise, the health and safety of everyone who uses the kitchen, or consumes food prepared in the kitchen, may be in danger. **Sanitation** is the process of making conditions clean and healthy.

Safety

Burns, fires, falls, cuts, and poisonings are the most common types of kitchen accidents. They can be prevented by following these guidelines.

Burns and Fires

It is important to be very careful when cooking food. Following are tips for preventing burns and fires in the kitchen:

- Turn pan, pot, and skillet handles toward the center of the cooktop.
- Use dry, clean potholders to handle hot kitchen tools. See **9-4**.
- Lift pot and pan lids away from you.
- Do not reach over open flames, hot burners, or steaming pans.
- Never leave food cooking on the cooktop unattended.
- Use appliances according to the use and care manual.
- Use low to medium heat when cooking. This prevents boilovers, burnt food, and fires.
- If a grease fire starts, turn off the burner and use an oven mitt to place a pan lid over the fire. You may also smother the fire with baking soda.
- Never put water on a grease fire. Water will cause both the grease and fire to spread.

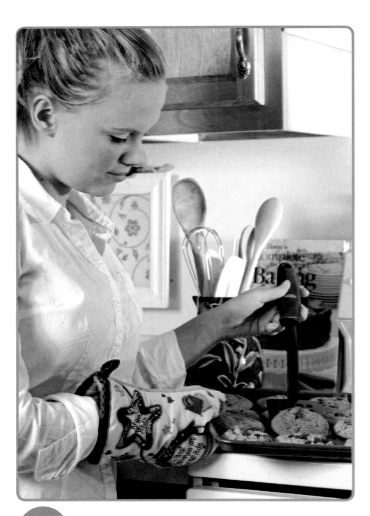

9-4 Oven mitts can protect you when you are removing hot pans from the oven.

Falls

Falls are the most common accident in the home. To help prevent them from happening in the kitchen, use the following hints:

- Wipe up spills right away.
- Use a sturdy step stool when reaching for objects from high shelves or cabinets.
- Make sure rugs have nonskid backings.
- Keep kitchen traffic areas free from objects that may block them.

Cuts

To prevent yourself from getting cut while in the kitchen, keep the following guidelines in mind:

- Carefully wash sharp knives one at a time.
- Keep knives sharp. Dull knives are not as safe as sharp knives.
- Always cut away from yourself.
- Use a cutting board for cutting and slicing.
- Store knives away from other utensils.
- Keep fingers away from blender and food processor blades.
- Do not put hands in the garbage disposal to try to dislodge food.
- Sweep broken glass on a piece of paper or cardboard to throw away. Use a damp paper towel to wipe up tiny slivers.

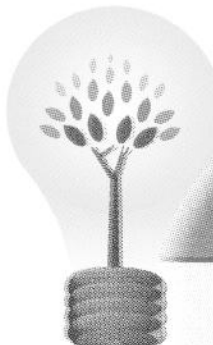

Think Green

Green Kitchen Cleaners

You can use common household products, such as table salt and baking soda, as inexpensive and nontoxic kitchen cleaners. For instance, combine about three tablespoons salt with one cup of boiling water to remove tough baked-on food stains in casserole dishes. Leave the mixture in the dish until the water is cool. Then wash as usual. You can use baking soda to clean counters as well as eliminate odors in the refrigerator or microwave.

Poisonings

Some poisonings can be fatal. The following are a few tips for preventing poisonings in the kitchen:

- Keep all medicines, cleaning supplies, and other household chemicals away from food storage areas.
- Keep food out of the way when spraying with chemical cleaners. Wash all work surfaces with hot, soapy water when you are finished spraying.

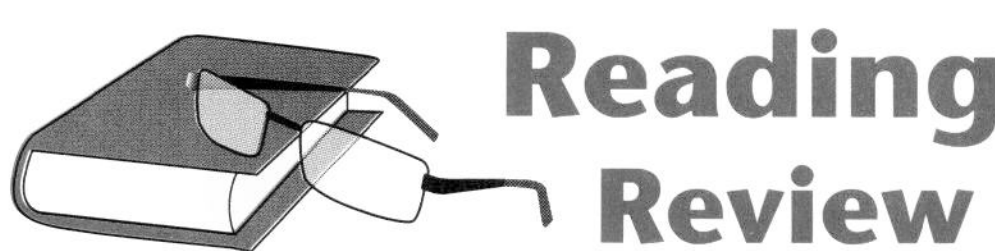

1. Why should you never put out grease fires with water? How should you extinguish them?
2. Why should you wash sharp knives one at a time?

Sanitation

Having a sanitary kitchen is important. Your food stays wholesome, and foodborne illnesses are prevented. **Foodborne illnesses** are illnesses caused from toxins produced by harmful bacteria in food. **Toxins** are poisonous substances. These illnesses are rarely fatal, but can be quite uncomfortable. This is sometimes called *food poisoning*.

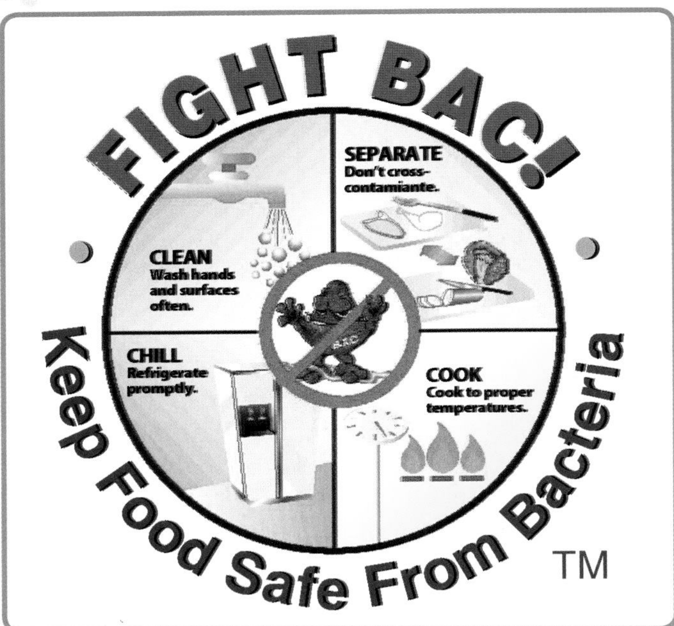

USDA/FSIS

9-5 These are the important steps to food safety.

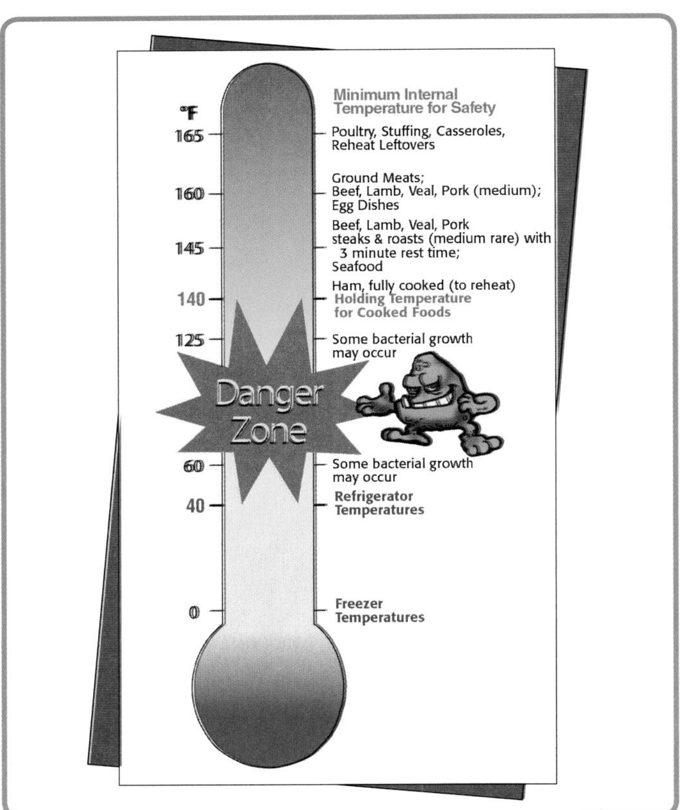

USDA/FSIS

9-6 Use these guidelines to cook foods to the proper temperature. Keep foods out of the temperature danger zone to prevent growth of harmful bacteria.

The *Fight BAC* program is sponsored by the USDA and the Food and Drug Administration (FDA). The purpose of Fight BAC is to educate consumers about the dangers of foodborne illnesses. They recommend four steps to prevent the spread of harmful bacteria in the kitchen. These steps are to *clean*, *separate*, *cook*, and *chill* foods properly. See **9-5**. To help keep your kitchen sanitary, follow these procedures:

- Wash your hands before handling food.
- If you handle unsanitary items, wash your hands again before touching food.
- Wash your hands after coughing, sneezing, blowing your nose, or going to the bathroom.
- Wear rubber gloves to protect any cuts on your hands.
- Keep your hands away from your face and hair.
- If your hair is long, keep it pulled back.
- Use only clean kitchen tools, containers, and work surfaces.
- Use one spoon for tasting and another for stirring.
- Separate raw meat, poultry, and seafood from other foods during grocery shopping and in the refrigerator. Raw meat contains the most harmful bacteria.
- Wash cutting boards with hot, soapy water after each use to prevent the spread of bacteria from raw foods to cooked foods.
- Thoroughly wash fresh fruits and vegetables with cool water.
- Thaw meat and poultry in the refrigerator.
- Keep hot foods hot and cold foods cold.
- Cook foods thoroughly. See **9-6**.
- Use separate towels for drying dishes and drying hands.

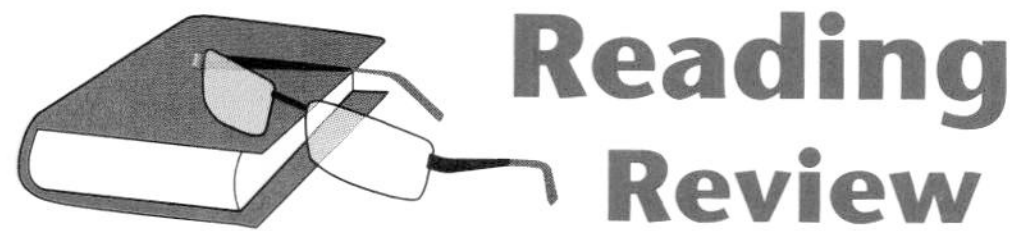

Reading Review

1. What are the four steps of the Fight BAC program? Give examples of each.
2. Why should you make sure your hands are kept clean?
3. Why should hot foods be kept hot and cold foods kept cold?

Cleaning Up

After a meal is over, clean the kitchen right away. A clean kitchen helps prevent the spread of bacteria. You can keep your tools, dishes, and appliances clean by following these guidelines:

- Repackage any unused food that does not need refrigeration.
- Store leftovers in tightly covered containers in the refrigerator immediately. Otherwise, the food may spoil.
- If you do not have an automatic dishwasher, wash dishes with dish detergent and hot water.
- Wash dishes in the following order: glasses, flatware, cups, plates, bowls, serving dishes, pots, and pans.
- Rinse dishes thoroughly with hot water to remove all bacteria and traces of detergent.
- Air dry dishes instead of towel drying them. Towel drying can spread bacteria.
- Place food waste in the garbage disposal, compost bin, or covered garbage container.
- Clean the sink and areas around the faucets, drains, and under the sink to get rid of grease and pieces of food. These can cause odors and produce bacteria.
- After washing the dishes, clean the table, countertops, and cooktop. See **9-7**.
- Sweep the floor daily and mop it on a regular basis.

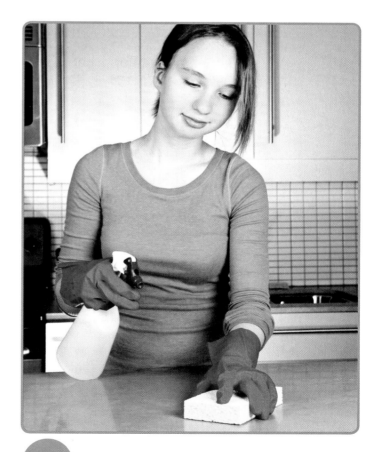

9-7 Clean the sink and countertops daily with a good cleanser. Avoid harsh cleansers that may scratch the surfaces.

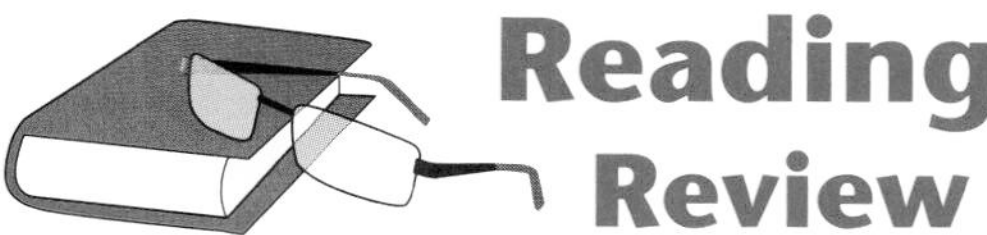

Reading Review

1. How can you prevent the spread of foodborne illnesses? Give examples.
2. In what order should you wash your dishes? Why?

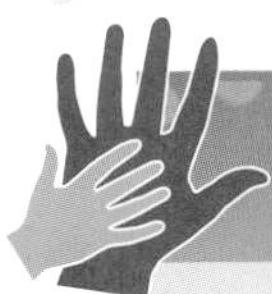

Safety Link

Proper Handling of Take-Out Foods

If you plan to purchase take-out foods for a picnic, eat them within two hours of pickup. This applies to foods such as fried chicken or barbecued meat. Otherwise, buy cooked foods ahead of time to chill before packing them in a cooler. You *must* keep foods with mayonnaise, such as potato salad, cold at all times. Bacteria grow readily in foods like potato salad or pies that contain eggs or dairy products.

Safe Food to Go

For bag lunches, picnics, or celebrations away from home, food must be kept safe for eating. This is necessary to prevent foodborne illnesses. First, you must handle and cook the food safely at home. Keep *perishable foods*, meaning those that will spoil, refrigerated until it is time to leave home. Then you must keep perishable food cold during transport and until eaten. Use the kind of containers that are designed to keep foods cold.

Some people like to take frozen, uncooked hamburger patties to a picnic. This helps keep them cold until cooking time. At the picnic, be sure to grill each burger according to the USDA recommendations. Make sure you bring the right-sized cooler and enough ice for those foods that need refrigeration.

Picnics are fun, but it is important to prevent foodborne illnesses that might result from picnic food. When taking food on a picnic, try to plan just the right amount of perishable foods to take. When it is all eaten, you will not have to worry about the storage or safety of leftovers.

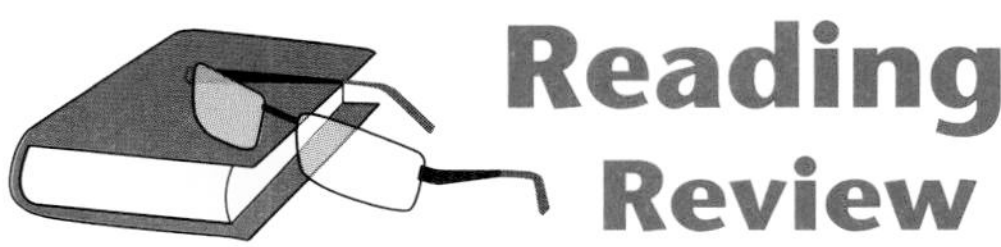

1. What is important to remember when preparing food at home to take for a school lunch, picnic, or family celebration?
2. Name five picnic food items that would need refrigeration.

Section Summary

- A safe and sanitary kitchen protects everyone who uses it from accidents and illness.
- When you follow safety guidelines, you can prevent burns, fires, falls, cuts, and poisonings.
- When you prepare food correctly and clean the kitchen well, you can prevent bacteria and food toxins that can cause foodborne illnesses from spreading.
- For bag lunches, picnics, or celebrations away from home, plan ahead to keep food safe.

Section 9-3
Reading Recipes

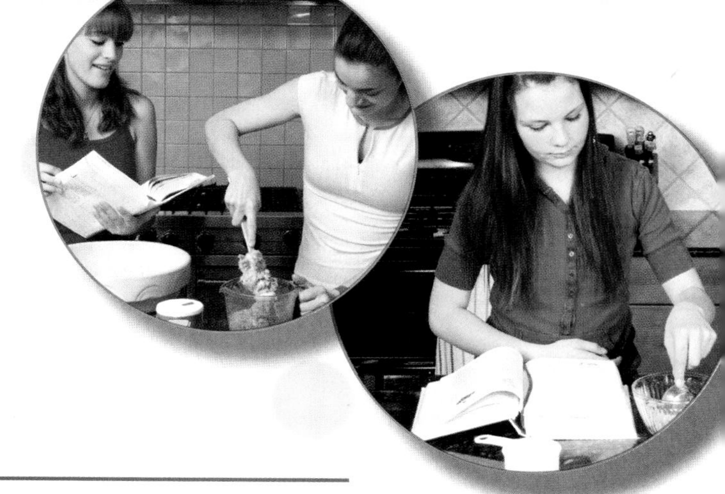

Objectives

After studying this section, you will be able to
- **define** *recipe*, *ingredients*, *abbreviation*, and *measure*.
- **list** the information that should be included in recipes.
- **identify** abbreviations used in recipes.
- **explain** why you should follow recipes carefully.

Key Terms

recipe: a set of directions used to prepare a food product.

ingredients: food items needed to prepare a food product.

abbreviation: shortened form of a word.

measure: to determine the amount of an item.

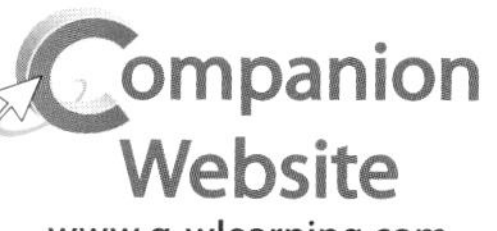

Study the Key Terms by completing crossword puzzles, matching activities, and e-flash cards at the website.

Main Ideas

- Recipes should include the information needed to create a food product.
- When choosing recipes, it is important to consider the food budget.
- Abbreviations are often used in recipes.
- To get good results, follow recipes carefully.

Knowing how to prepare food is a good skill to have. You can use this skill throughout your life. Recipes are an important part of preparing food. A **recipe** is a set of directions used to prepare a food product. Before you begin cooking, you must know how to read recipes. You should understand the terms used in a recipe to follow its directions properly.

Finding Recipes

You can find recipes in cookbooks and magazines, on the Internet, from TV cooking programs, in food stores, and from advertisers. If you eat something you like at a friend's home, ask for the recipe. See **9-8**.

When looking for recipes, be sure the recipe includes both the directions to prepare the food product and the ingredients. **Ingredients** are food items needed to prepare a food product. Sometimes, recipes call for costly or special ingredients you may not have at home. Buying these ingredients can place demands on your food budget. Think about the cost of all the ingredients when you choose recipes. You may decide to use recipes that do not call for these special ingredients.

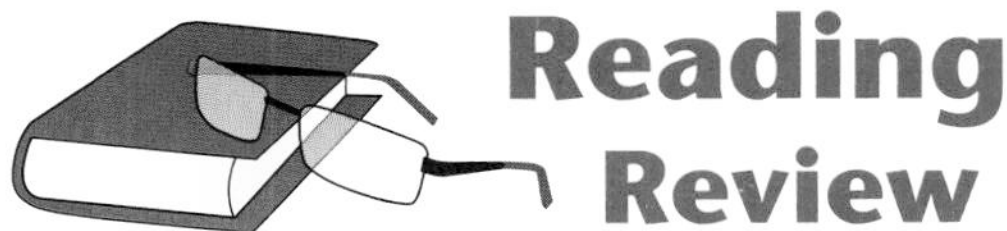

Reading Review

1. Name five places you can find recipes.
2. Why is it important to consider your food budget when looking for recipes?

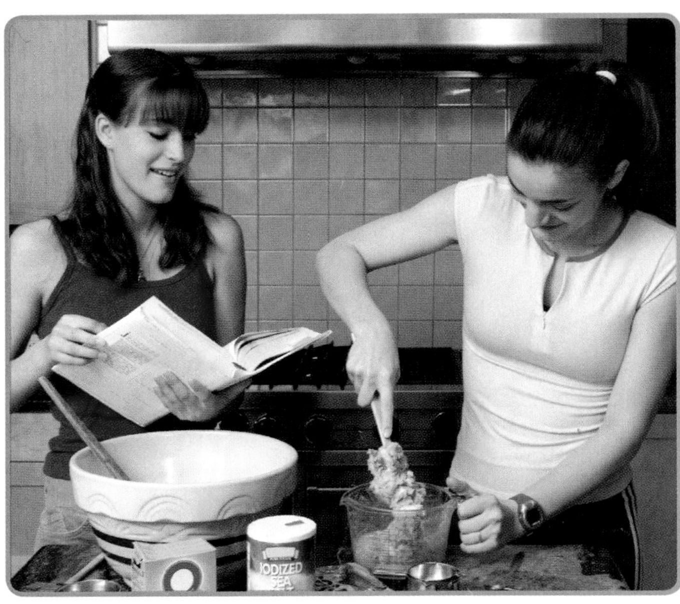

9-8 New recipes can be fun to try at home and they may even become new family favorites.

Understanding Recipes

When you first learn to prepare food, use recipes that are easy to read and understand. As you become more experienced with preparing food, you may want to try recipes that are more complex.

As you read recipes, you will note they include the following information:

- kind of food being prepared
- ingredients needed
- amount of each ingredient
- mixing directions
- cooking directions
- cooking time
- number of servings

Some recipes also include nutritional information for each serving. This helps you make healthful choices when deciding which recipes to prepare.

Recipes are broken into two parts. First, you will find a detailed list of the ingredients and the amounts needed for each one. Ingredients are often listed in the order they are used. To get the best results, use the exact amounts of ingredients stated in the recipe.

The next part is the directions for mixing and cooking. They are written in the order the ingredients are to be mixed. Follow this order to get good results.

Abbreviations

To understand recipes, you must also know how to read abbreviations. An **abbreviation** is a shortened form of a word. See **9-9**. Abbreviations are used instead of words. For instance, the letters *c*, *t*, and *T* are used in place of the words *cup*, *teaspoon*, and *tablespoon*. In food preparation, abbreviations stand for units of measure. **Measure** means to determine the amount of an item.

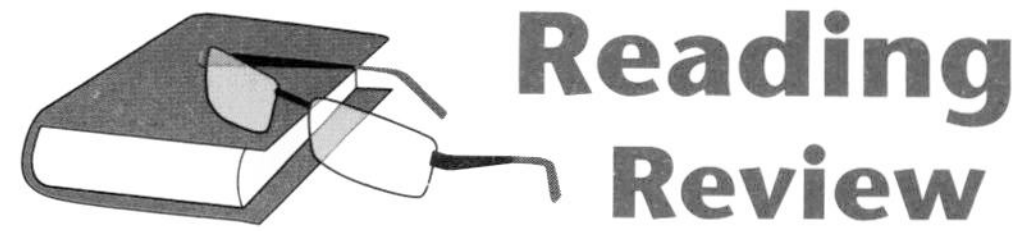

Reading Review

1. What information should recipes include? Give examples.
2. What do abbreviations stand for in food preparation?

Abbreviations Used in Recipes

f.g.	=	few grains
t. or tsp.	=	teaspoon
T. or Tbsp.	=	tablespoon
c.	=	cup
pt.	=	pint
oz.	=	ounce
qt.	=	quart
gal.	=	gallon
lb.	=	pound
°F	=	degrees Fahrenheit
°C	=	degrees Celsius

9-9 Understanding these abbreviations can help you follow recipes.

Writing Link

Copying Recipes Correctly

If you copy a recipe from a cookbook or magazine, check carefully to make sure you have copied it correctly. If you forget an ingredient, your product might not turn out right. Also, be careful not to change the letters in abbreviations or the numbers. For instance, two teaspoons (t.) of salt in whole wheat bread makes it taste good. Two tablespoons (T.) of salt, however, would make it taste so salty you could not eat it.

Following Recipes

Before you begin making a recipe, make sure you have all the ingredients and tools you need. Be sure to use the type and size of cookware and bakeware called for in the recipe. Make sure you understand the recipe. The following steps will help ensure your food product turns out the way you want:

1. Read the recipe all the way through. (If you are using a packaged mix, read the directions on the package.)
2. Collect the ingredients.
3. Collect the tools.
4. Complete preparation tasks.
5. Measure the dry ingredients.
6. Measure the liquid ingredients.
7. Add the ingredients and follow remaining directions.

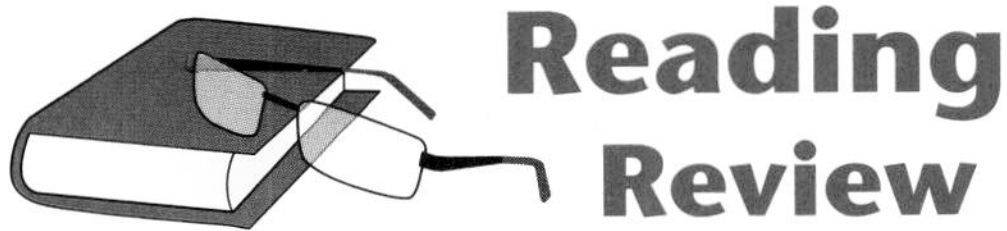

Reading Review

1. What should you do *before* you begin to make a recipe?
2. What could happen if you do not follow recipes correctly? Give an example.

Section Summary

- Recipes guide you in making food products.
- There are many places you can find recipes.
- It is important to consider your food budget when selecting recipes.
- Recipes include a list of ingredients needed and directions for mixing and cooking.
- To get good results when using recipes, be sure to understand the directions and follow them carefully.

Section 9-4
Basic Cooking Skills

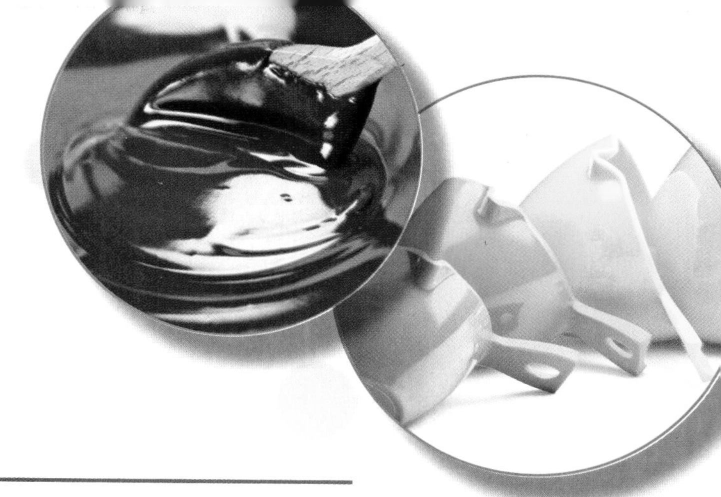

Objectives

After studying this section, you will be able to
- **define** *standard measuring tools*, *cut*, and *food processors*.
- **measure** liquid, dry, and solid ingredients correctly.
- **demonstrate** how to cut and mix ingredients according to recipes.
- **identify** basic cooking terms.

Key Terms

standard measuring tools: specially marked cups and spoons used to measure ingredients.

cut: to divide foods into small pieces.

food processors: electric kitchen appliances that cut ingredients in different forms and mix them.

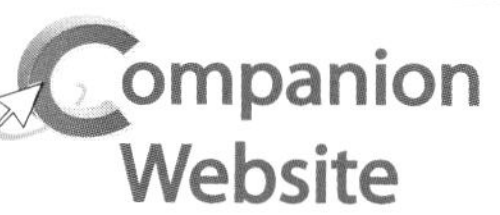

Study the Key Terms by completing crossword puzzles, matching activities, and e-flash cards at the website.

Main Ideas

- You must measure ingredients accurately when following recipes.
- Knowing which tools to use for cutting food correctly is important.
- Mixing ingredients correctly and in the right order is important.
- To get good results, follow the recipe's cooking directions carefully.

Certain skills are needed to get the results you want from your recipes. To follow the directions in a recipe, you must learn the measuring, cutting, mixing, and cooking terms used and know which tools to use.

Measuring Ingredients

Specially marked cups and spoons used to measure ingredients are called **standard measuring tools**. See **9-10**. They are marked to show exact amounts. Use standard measuring tools every time you prepare food. They will help make your recipes turn out just right.

There are three different types of standard measuring tools. The first type is *liquid measuring cups*. Use these to measure liquid ingredients, such as milk, water, and oil. They are made of clear glass or plastic with pouring spouts. They come in 1-, 2-, and 4-cup sizes. Lines on the sides of these cups measure fractions of a cup.

The second type of standard measuring tool is *dry measuring cups*. Use these to measure dry ingredients, such as flour and sugar. They often come in 1-, ½-, ⅓-, and ¼-cup sizes. They may come in other sizes, too.

The last type of standard measuring tool is *measuring spoons*. Use measuring spoons to measure both liquid and dry ingredients. You will want to use measuring spoons when the recipe calls for less than ¼ cup of any ingredient. They come in 1-tablespoon and 1-, ½-, and ¼-teaspoon sizes. They may also come in other sizes.

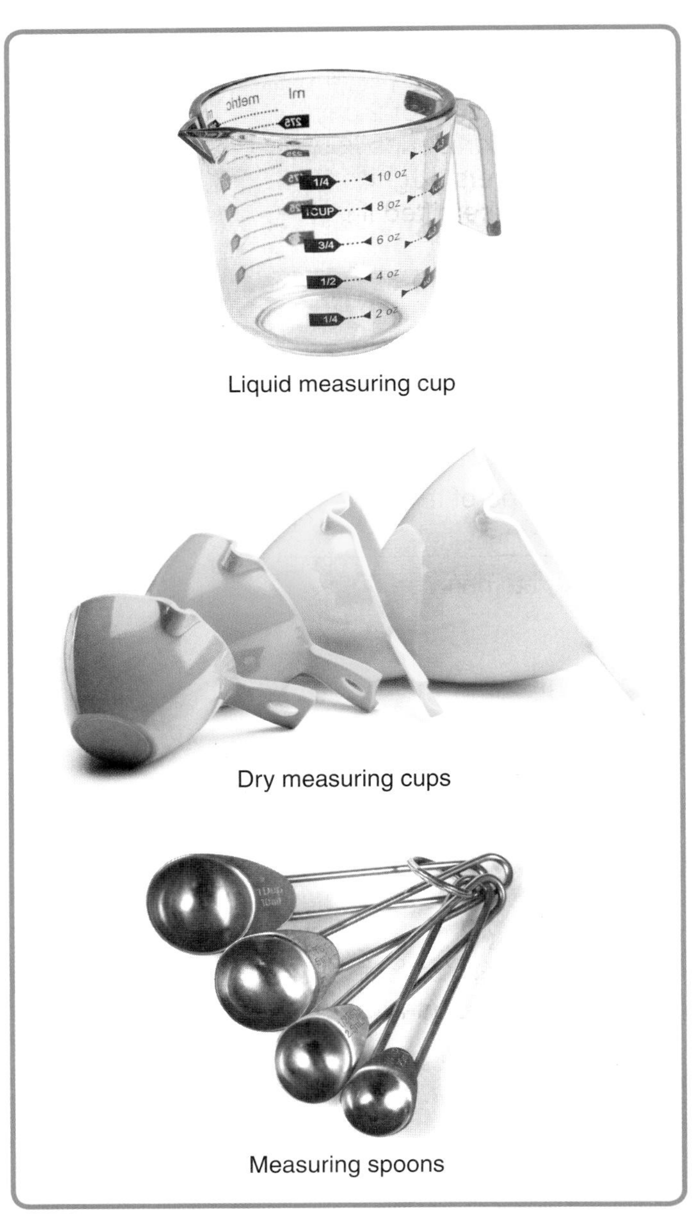

9-10 Standard measuring tools come in different sizes to help you measure ingredients accurately.

Measuring Methods

There are many ways to measure ingredients used in recipes. You will need to use different methods to measure different ingredients. For instance, ingredients such as brown sugar and peanut butter require special measuring methods. See **9-11**.

Equivalent Measures

Sometimes, you may need to make more or less of what your recipe tells you it makes. In that case, you may decide to double the recipe or cut it in half. You

Measuring Methods

To measure liquid ingredients, such as milk, water, juice, oil, and melted fat, follow these steps: 1. Place a liquid measuring cup on a level surface. 2. Pour the liquid into the cup to the correct line. 3. Check the measure at eye level to be sure you have measured the right amount.
To measure dry ingredients, such as flour, granulated sugar, salt, baking powder, cocoa, spices, and confectioners' sugar, follow these steps: 1. Use a dry measuring cup or spoon. 2. Use a spoon to fill the measuring cup or spoon to overflowing. Do not pack or shake the ingredient into the cup or spoon unless the recipe tells you to do so. 3. Level the measuring cup or spoon with a straight-edged spatula. 4. If needed, sift the ingredients before measuring. If the recipe calls for 2 cups sifted flour, sift the flour before measuring. If the recipe calls for 2 cups flour and then tells you to sift it, do so after measuring. Confectioners' sugar should be sifted before measuring. Granulated sugar should be sifted if it has lumps in it.
To measure brown sugar, follow these steps: 1. Use a dry measuring cup or measuring spoon. 2. Lightly pack the brown sugar into the cup or spoon. 3. Level the cup or spoon by packing the brown sugar, so that it is even with the top of the cup or spoon. You can also level the cup or spoon with a straight-edged spatula. 4. If it is measured correctly, the brown sugar will stay the shape of the cup or spoon when it is emptied.
To measure shortening and foods such as peanut butter and mayonnaise, follow these steps: 1. Use a dry measuring cup or measuring spoon. 2. Pack the food into the cup or spoon so there are no air spaces. 3. Level with a rubber scraper. 4. Use the rubber scraper to scrape all the food from the cup or spoon.

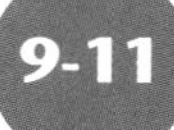

Using the proper methods is important when measuring ingredients.

will need to determine the new amounts of ingredients for more or less servings. An *equivalent measures chart* tells you how much of one measure equals a larger measuring amount. See **9-12**.

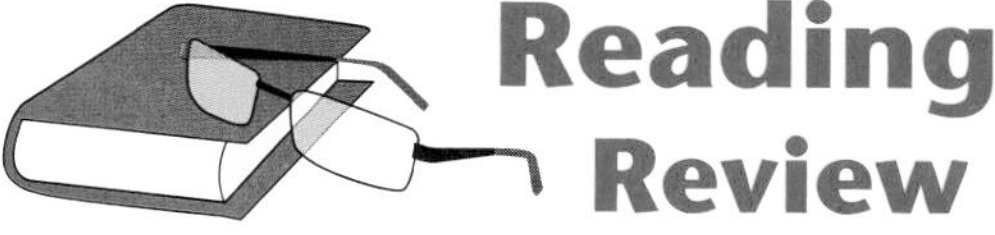

Reading Review

1. When should you use a measuring spoon instead of a measuring cup?
2. When would you refer to an equivalent measures chart?

Equivalent Measures	
Dry and Liquid Measures	3 teaspoons = 1 tablespoon 4 tablespoons = ¼ cup 8 tablespoons = ½ cup 12 tablespoons = ¾ cup 16 tablespoons = 1 cup few grains, dash, or pinch = less than ⅛ teaspoon
Liquid Measures	2 tablespoons = 1 fluid ounce 1 cup = 8 fluid ounces 2 cups = 16 fluid ounces = 1 pint 4 cups = 32 fluid ounces = 1 quart 2 pints = 1 quart 4 quarts = 1 gallon
Dry Measures	16 ounces = 1 pound 8 quarts = 1 peck 4 pecks = 1 bushel

9-12 Understanding how equivalent measures are used helps when doubling or halving recipes.

Cutting Ingredients

Some recipes call for ingredients to be cut. **Cut** is to divide food into small pieces with a sharp knife or kitchen shears. Other cutting tools may include vegetable peelers, graters, choppers, and food processors.

Food processors are electric kitchen appliances that cut ingredients in different forms and also mix them.

You must know which tool to use for the different types of cutting. For instance, cheese can be cubed, grated, or sliced. Recipes often refer to cutting in the following ways:

- **Chop:** cut into small pieces using a sharp knife, food processor, or blender.
- **Core:** remove the center, or core, of a food using a sharp knife.
- **Cube:** cut in small, even cubes using a sharp knife.
- **Grate:** rub a food back and forth against a grater to get very small pieces.
- **Mince:** cut into very small pieces with a sharp knife or kitchen shears.

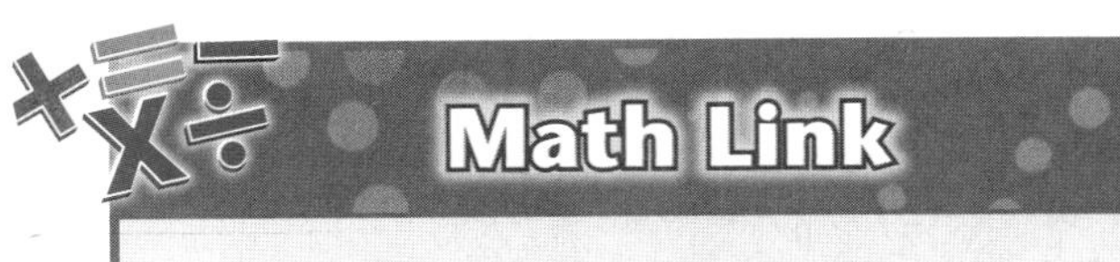

Doubling Recipes

There may be times when the recipe you want to use will not make enough for the number of people you need to serve. Sometimes, the recipe may make more than you need. You can double most recipes or cut them in half without problems. Select a recipe that has at least five ingredients. Refer to the *Equivalent Measures* in Figure 9-12 to help you double the recipe. Then practice cutting the same recipe in half.

- **Pare or peel:** remove the skin of a food using a paring knife or vegetable peeler. Peel fruits, such as oranges and bananas, by hand.
- **Slice:** cut food into even pieces using a knife or food processor. Slice vegetables before cooking. Slice bread and meat after cooking.

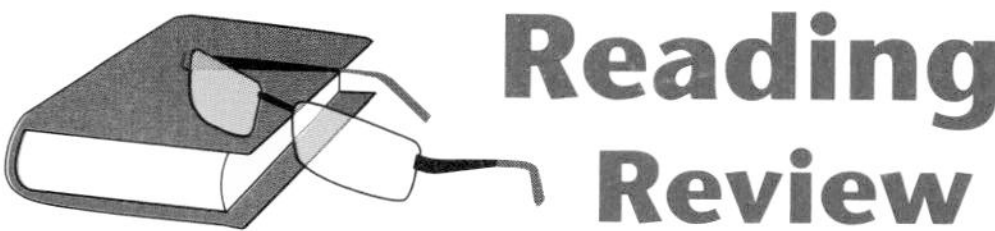

Reading Review

1. Why should you know how to cut foods correctly when following recipes?
2. What are some different tools that can be used for cutting?

Mixing Ingredients

Recipes use different mixing terms to tell you exactly how to combine ingredients. See **9-13**. They sometimes tell you which tools to use. When you mix ingredients properly, you will get good results. Mixing tools include spoons, whisks, hand or electric mixers, and food processors.

Mixing Methods

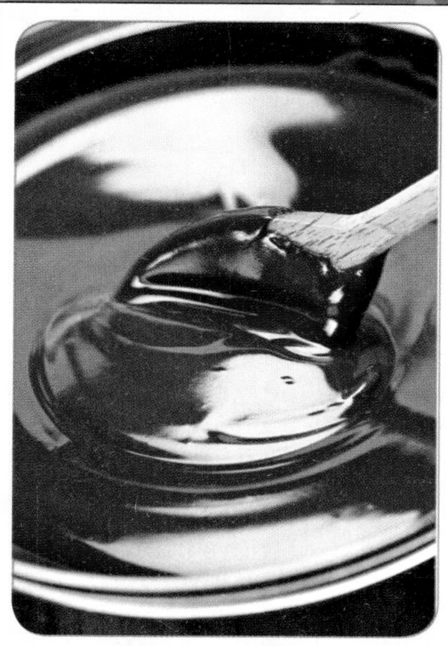

Blend: mix slowly using a spoon or an electric mixer on low speed.

Beat: mix fast bringing the contents to the top of the bowl and then back down again. Spoons, rotary beaters, or electric mixers are used for beating.

Combine: mix two or more ingredients together using a spoon.

Fold: mix a light, airy substance with a more solid substance by folding the two together with a rubber scraper. An example is mixing whipped cream with chocolate syrup. Use a very slow, careful over and over motion.

Cream: beat a mixture until it is light and fluffy using a spoon or electric mixer. This method is often used to mix sugar and shortening.

Stir: mix in a circular motion using a spoon.

Cut in: mix solid shortening into a flour mixture using two knives or a pastry blender to cut through the shortening.

Whip: beat quickly using a wire whisk or rotary beater to add air to one or more ingredients.

9-13 These are a few common ways to mix ingredients.

Sometimes, ingredients must be mixed quickly. Other times, they need to be mixed slowly. Ingredients can also be mixed for short or long periods of time. Recipes may tell you to mix all the ingredients together at once or to add a few ingredients at a time. Follow the recipes' directions. Otherwise, your food may not turn out right.

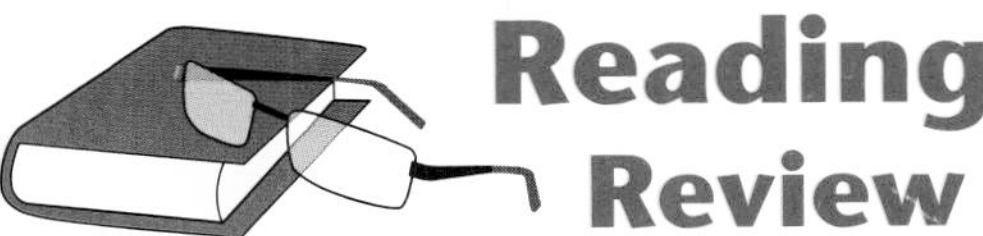

1. What are three common ways to mix ingredients?
2. What can happen if you do not follow a recipe's mixing directions?

Following Cooking Temperatures

Recipes give the proper temperature and length of time for cooking or baking. Read the directions carefully. Sometimes, you may need to use two different temperatures for one recipe. For instance, apple pie is baked at 425°F (218°C) for 10 minutes in a conventional oven. Then, the heat is lowered to 350°F (177°C) for 30 to 40 minutes. Cooking foods at the wrong temperature can burn the food or change the traits of the ingredients. The foods may not turn out as you expected.

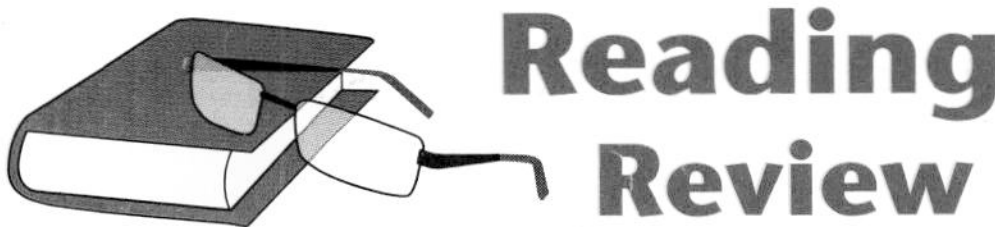

1. When might you need to use two temperatures for cooking? Give an example.
2. What can happen to food if you cook it at the wrong temperature?

Understanding Cooking Terms

Another way to help your food turn out right is to understand all the cooking terms used in recipes. These terms describe the different ways to cook food. See **9-14**. Be sure you carefully follow the directions for these terms. Otherwise, the food may be overcooked or undercooked.

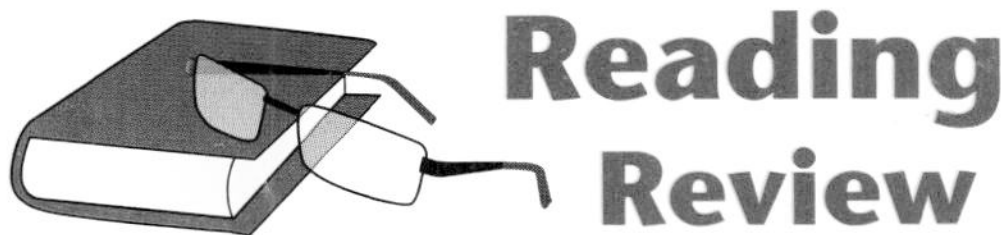

1. Name and briefly describe five different cooking terms.
2. Why is it important to understand all the cooking terms in a recipe?

Cooking Terms

Bake: cook in an oven in an uncovered container.

Boil: heat a liquid on a cooktop at a high temperature. Bubbles should constantly rise and break the surface.

Braise: cooking technique that combines browning and simmering. Brown food in a small amount of fat. Then, add a little liquid and simmer in a covered container.

Broil: cook by direct heat by placing the food under the heat source.

Brown: cook in fat until surface of food turns brown.

Cook: prepare food for eating using heat.

Deep fry: cook in enough hot fat to cover the food.

Dry-heat cooking: cook foods without liquids.

Fry: cook in fat or oil in a pan.

Grill: cook by direct heat by placing the food over the heat source. Heat sources can be gas, electric, charcoal, or wood.

Microwave: cook in a microwave oven.

Moist-heat cooking: cook foods by adding water or other liquids.

Panfry: cook in enough hot fat to cover the food halfway.

Poach: cook in liquid at a low temperature.

Roast: cook uncovered in an oven without liquid.

Sauté: cook small pieces of food in a small amount of fat, stirring often.

Simmer: cook in liquid at a temperature just below boiling. Bubbles form only along the edges of the pan and do not break the surface.

Steam: cook in a covered container on a rack above liquid that is boiling.

Stew: cook in enough liquid for ingredients to float freely.

Stir-fry: cook evenly cut pieces of food in a small amount of fat, stirring frequently.

9-14 These are just a few of the many cooking terms you will find in recipes.

Section Summary

- Ingredients must be measured carefully.
- Be sure to use the correct standard measuring tools for measuring liquid and dry ingredients.
- If the recipe calls for ingredients to be cut a certain way, this must also be done properly to get good results.
- When you mix ingredients, use the right tools.
- Cook foods at the proper temperature and for the amount of time in the recipe.
- You need to understand all the cooking terms in a recipe before you begin preparing food.

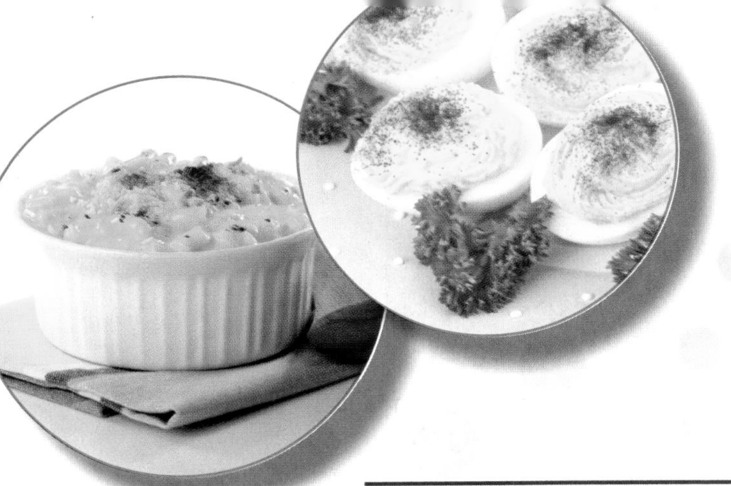

Section 9-5
Preparing Foods

Objectives

After studying this section, you will be able to

- **define** *leavening agent*, *curdling*, *scum*, *moist-heat cooking*, and *dry-heat cooking*.
- **discuss** how to prepare fruits and vegetables to be eaten raw or cooked.
- **explain** how to prepare grain products.
- **demonstrate** how to prepare milk and other dairy products.
- **describe** the cooking methods used to prepare protein foods.
- **state** tips for preparing desserts.

Key Terms

leavening agent: an ingredient that causes foods to rise during baking.

curdling: lumping of milk proteins caused by cooking with high heat.

scum: film that forms on the surface of heated milk.

moist-heat cooking: methods for cooking foods in which water or other liquids are added.

dry-heat cooking: methods for cooking foods without liquids.

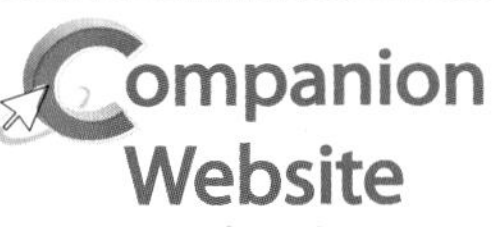

Study the Key Terms by completing crossword puzzles, matching activities, and e-flash cards at the website.

Main Ideas

- Using proper cooking methods makes foods taste better.
- Preparing foods correctly helps retain their nutritive value.

Now that you know how to measure, cut, mix, and identify cooking terms, the next step is to prepare the food. There are some simple rules for preparing food. If you follow these guidelines, your foods will not only look and taste good, but they will also be nutritious.

Science Link

Maintaining Textures and Flavors of Fruit

Fruit can be simmered, baked, or broiled. Cooking changes the flavor and texture of fruit. To get the best flavor, simmer peeled, cored fruits in small amounts of water. You may want to add a small amount of sugar to sweeten. To help fruit hold its shape, cook it for a short amount of time and add sugar. Dried fruit should soak in hot water for an hour before simmering. Canned fruits can be heated in their juices. Fruits may also be cooked in the microwave oven. Little or no water is needed for this method. If the skin is still on the fruit, be sure to pierce it with a fork before microwaving.

Fruits and Vegetables

You can serve fruits and vegetables raw or cooked. Always wash fresh fruits and vegetables before eating or using in recipes.

You can serve fruit as an appetizer, snack, or part of a dessert or side dish. See **9-15**. To prevent fresh fruits such as apples, peaches, and bananas from turning brown after you slice them, dip the slices in lemon or orange juice.

Be sure to thaw frozen fruit slightly before serving. If fruit is fully thawed, it will be too soft. You can serve canned fruit chilled or at room temperature. Dried fruit, such as raisins, can be eaten as is or used in baked products.

Fresh vegetables are crisp and flavorful. They add color to salads and appetizers. Some good vegetables to eat raw are carrots, celery, cucumbers, lettuce, mushrooms, and broccoli. To make fresh vegetables more attractive, you can cut them in different shapes and sizes before serving.

Cooked vegetables are often served as side dishes. They are also used in casseroles, stews, and soups. Vegetables can be simmered, steamed, microwaved, or stir-fried. Cook vegetables until they are tender, but crisp. Use only a small amount of liquid when cooking vegetables. This helps them retain their color, flavor, and nutrients.

Cook frozen vegetables while they are still frozen. Heat canned vegetables before serving. Dried beans should be soaked in cold water overnight or for an hour in boiling water before cooking. Cook dried vegetables for a longer amount of time than other vegetables.

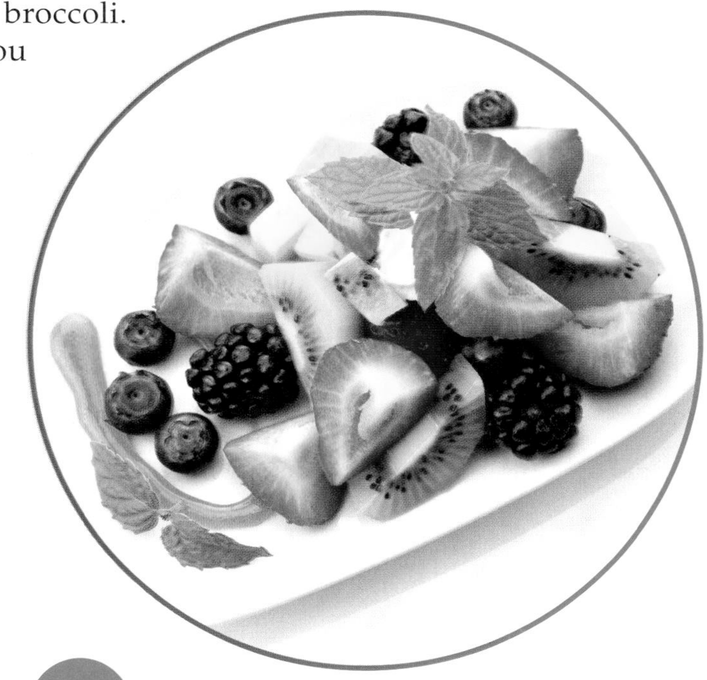

9-15 Fresh fruits can be served as a light dessert. Be sure to wash them first.

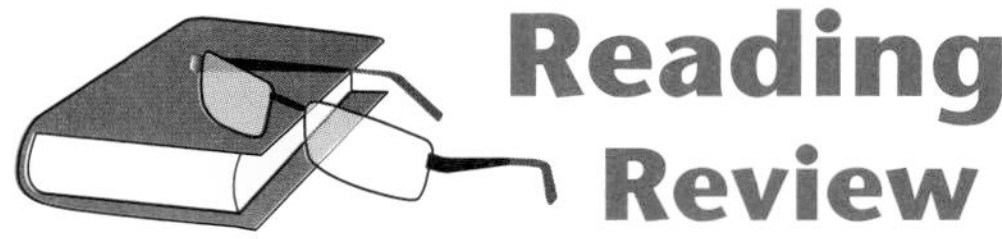

Reading Review

1. How can you help fruit keep its shape when cooking?
2. Why should you only cook fruits and vegetables in small amounts of liquid?

Grain Products

Grain products are often available at almost every meal. Bread is one of the most common grain products. You can purchase breads at the store or make them yourself. There are many kinds of bread, but just two basic types—quick breads and yeast breads. Muffins, biscuits, nut breads, and pancakes are examples of quick breads. Loaves of bread and dinner rolls are examples of yeast breads.

The ingredients for quick breads and yeast breads are similar, but their preparation methods are different. Both types of bread, however, must include a leavening agent. A **leavening agent** is an ingredient that causes the dough or batter to rise during the cooking process.

Baking soda and baking powder are the leavening agents in quick breads. They cause air bubbles to form during baking. This is what makes quick breads light and airy. Yeast is the leavening agent in yeast breads.

You can prepare quick breads in a short amount of time on the stovetop or in an oven. To make quick breads, mix the ingredients to form a thin *batter*. Then, pour the batter in a cooking pan.

Yeast breads take longer to make than quick breads. Preparation for yeast breads includes mixing ingredients to form thick *dough*. The dough must sit in a warm spot for about an hour to rise. Then, you must shape the dough into rolls or loaves and it must rise again. Finally, you bake the risen dough. See **9-16**.

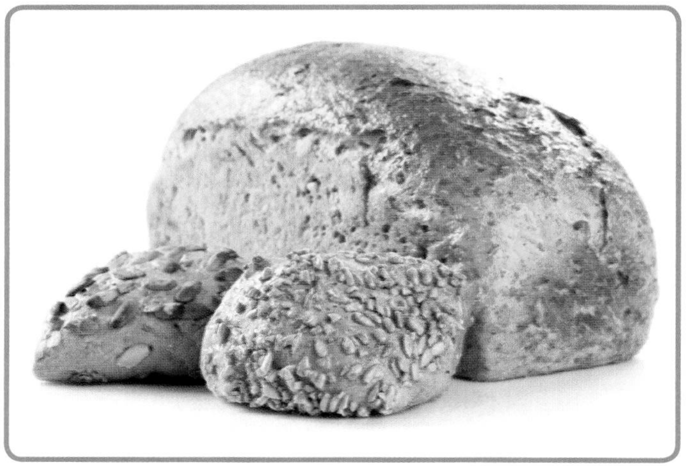

9-16 Whole grain yeast bread and rolls are shaped before baking.

Other grain products you may cook include cereals, pasta, and rice. The cooking time and temperature for each type differ. These products expand by absorbing liquid as they cook. Therefore, you may need a large amount of liquid for cooking.

You should cook breakfast cereals, such as oatmeal and farina, until they are soft enough to eat. If the temperature is too high, the cereal can become tough or lumpy. If the temperature is too low, the cereal will not swell enough to soften properly. Add liquid to cereals according to the recipe. Otherwise, they will not cook right.

When cooking pasta and rice, be sure to add water according to package directions. Pasta is done when it is a little chewy, but not crunchy. Rice should be tender and fluffy. Do not wash rice before or after cooking. Otherwise, you will wash away most of its nutrients.

You can also prepare cereals, pasta, and rice in the microwave. Follow the package directions. Always allow room for these products to expand while cooking.

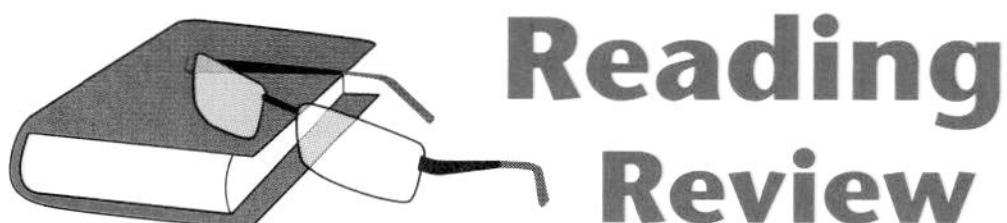

Reading Review

1. What is the difference between quick breads and yeast breads?
2. Why do you need to cook certain grain products in large amounts of water?

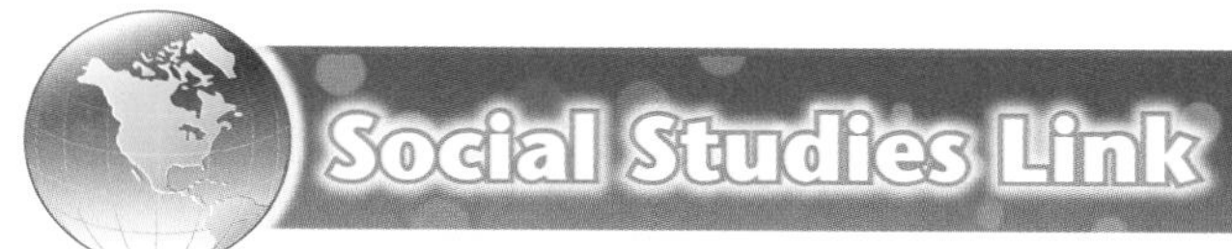

Breads and Cereals in Other Cultures

Every culture in the world has its own unique kinds of food products made from grains. Find two recipes for bread and pasta products from other cultures that you would like to share with the class. Perhaps your family has favorite cultural dishes that fall into this food category. Bring the recipes to class for sharing and if time allows, you can show the class how to make one.

Milk and Other Dairy Products

Recipes often call for milk and other dairy products. They add a rich flavor and creamy texture to many soups, casseroles, sauces, and desserts.

Be sure to use fresh milk in cooked foods. Also, use low cooking temperatures. The proteins in milk burn when they get too hot. This produces a bitter taste and a brown color. High temperatures can cause **curdling**, or the milk proteins to form small lumps. Curdling may also occur when milk is mixed with hot foods or acidic foods, such as oranges or tomatoes. Add these foods to milk slowly to help prevent curdling.

When heating milk, remove any **scum**, or film that forms on the surface. Scum will not dissolve. It can leave small particles in the milk that can affect the texture of the food product. Covering the pan or stirring milk gently during cooking can help keep scum from forming.

Be careful when cooking with cheese because it can overcook easily. Overcooking cheese makes it tough and rubbery. When using cheese in a recipe, cut in small pieces and add toward the end of cooking. See **9-17**. The cheese will be less likely to overcook, and it will melt faster.

Milk and other dairy products are often used to make desserts. When making desserts that need to be cooked,

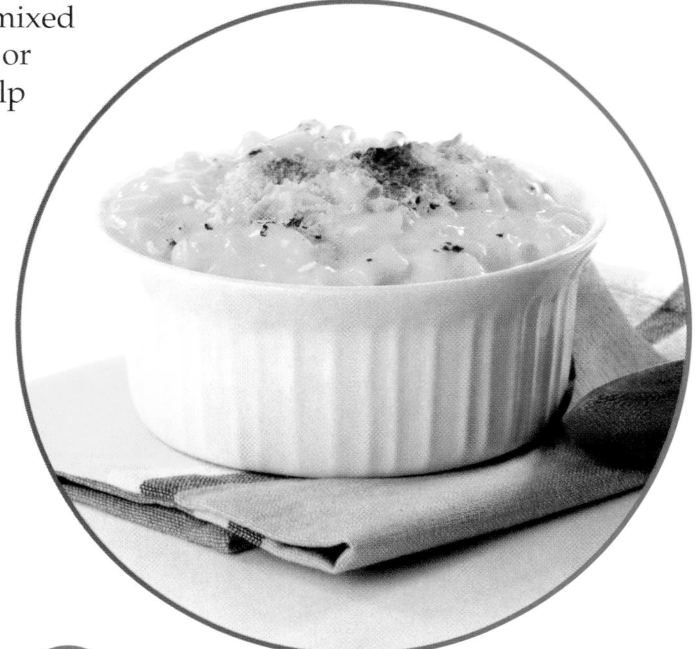

9-17 Prepare your own macaroni and cheese at home using a recipe rather than from a box or package. It has better flavor and saves money.

such as pudding or custard, use low cooking temperatures. Some people use ice cream freezers to make ice cream, frozen yogurt, and sherbet.

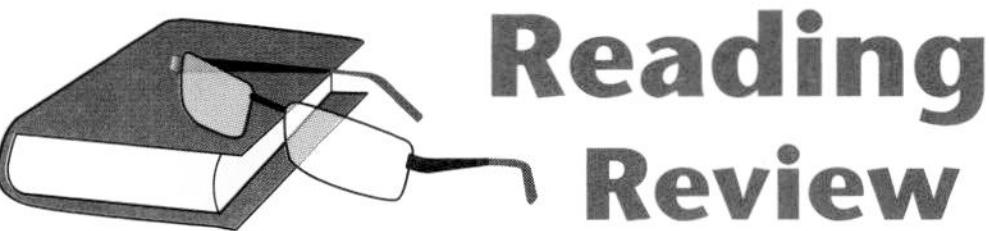

Reading Review

1. What are two reasons milk might curdle?
2. How can you prevent cheese from overcooking?

Protein Foods

When preparing meat, poultry, fish, and eggs, choose the best cooking method to increase the flavor and tenderness. The two main cooking methods are moist-heat cooking and dry-heat cooking.

Moist-heat cooking methods mean cooking foods in which water or other liquids are added. These methods include braising, poaching, and steaming. They are best for less tender cuts of meat. Moist-heat cooking helps make foods more tender and juicy.

Dry-heat cooking methods mean to cook foods without liquids. These methods include roasting, baking, broiling, grilling, and frying. They are best for tender meat, poultry, and fish.

The cut of meat affects which cooking method to use. Tender beef steaks, lamb chops, or pork chops can be broiled. Tender chicken and fish can be fried. Stewing chickens should be cooked in liquid to make the meat tender. Beef stew meat should be cooked in liquid to bring out flavor and tenderness. Some seafood, such as oysters and clams, must be cooked in liquid.

Be sure protein foods are thoroughly cooked. You do not want them to be overdone, however. Meat, poultry, and fish can become dry and tough if they are cooked too long. Meat cooked at too high a temperature can lose juices and shrink. Fish cooks quickly, so watch it carefully. Controlling cooking time and temperature keeps meat, poultry, and fish tender, moist, and flavorful.

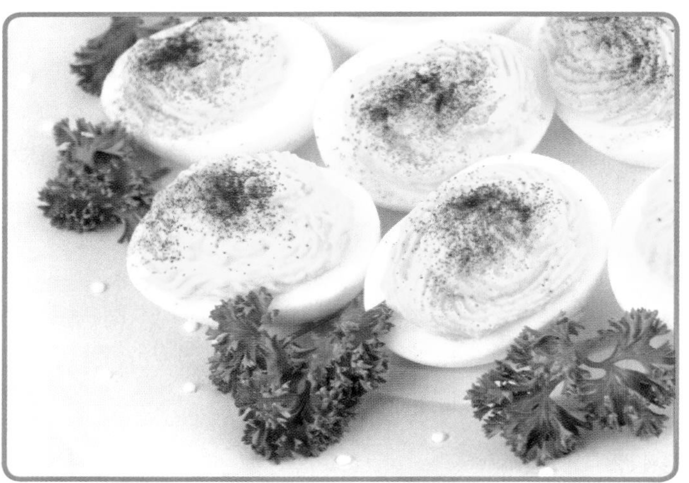

9-18 Deviled eggs are popular for some family gatherings. Cook eggs carefully to prevent overcooking.

Many people enjoy eating eggs for breakfast. Eggs are also an ingredient in many foods. These foods include mayonnaise, meat loaf, baked goods, ice cream, puddings, and custards.

Frying, scrambling, and cooking in the shell are common ways to prepare eggs. Eggs cook fast. If they are overcooked, they become tough and rubbery. See **9-18**. Always cook eggs before you eat them. This helps prevent food poisoning.

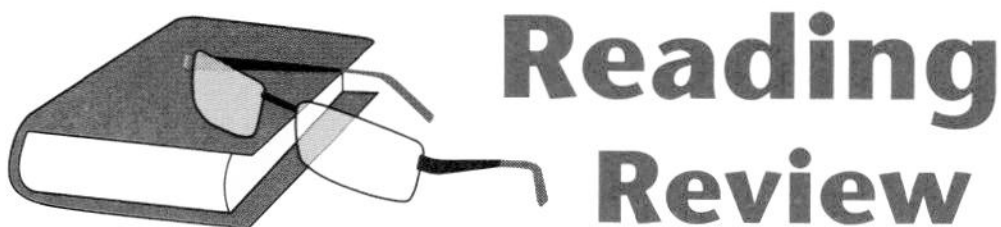

Reading Review

1. Which cooking methods are best for less tender cuts of meat? Which cooking methods are best for tender meats?
2. Why is it important to cook eggs before you eat them?

Desserts

Cakes, cookies, pastries, and doughnuts are just a few types of desserts. You probably like desserts. Their rich flavors often come from fat and sugar. Desserts, however, should not be the main part of your diet. Most are high in calories. Eat small servings.

Each type of dessert is prepared differently from the others. Therefore, follow the recipe carefully when making a dessert. Make sure you combine the ingredients properly. Use the right size pan. Cook at the correct temperature. Follow directions for storing and serving desserts. See **9-19**. By doing so, you can prepare a tasty dessert.

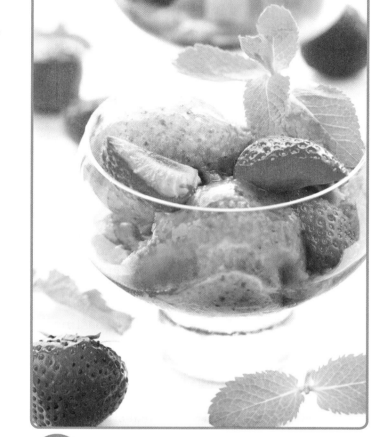

9-19 Frozen desserts must be served quickly to prevent melting.

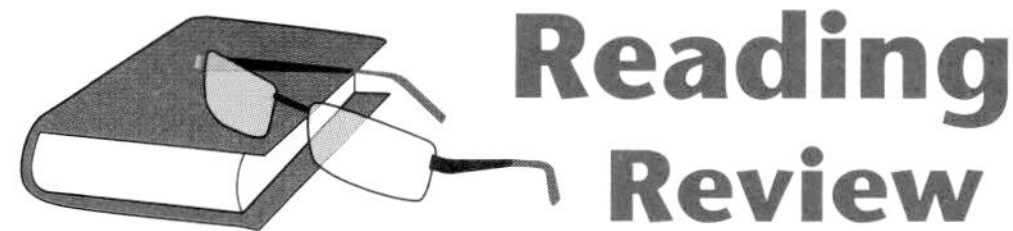

Reading Review

1. Why should desserts not be a large part of your diet?
2. Why do you need to follow recipes carefully when preparing desserts?

Section Summary

- Fruits and vegetables can be eaten raw or cooked. Always wash them before eating.
- The two types of bread are quick breads and yeast breads.
- Cook cereals, pasta, and rice in the right amounts of water at the correct temperatures to achieve the best results.
- Milk and other dairy products should be cooked on low heat to prevent curdling.
- Moist-heat and dry-heat methods are used to cook meat, poultry, and seafood, depending on their tenderness.
- Desserts should always be prepared according to the recipe.

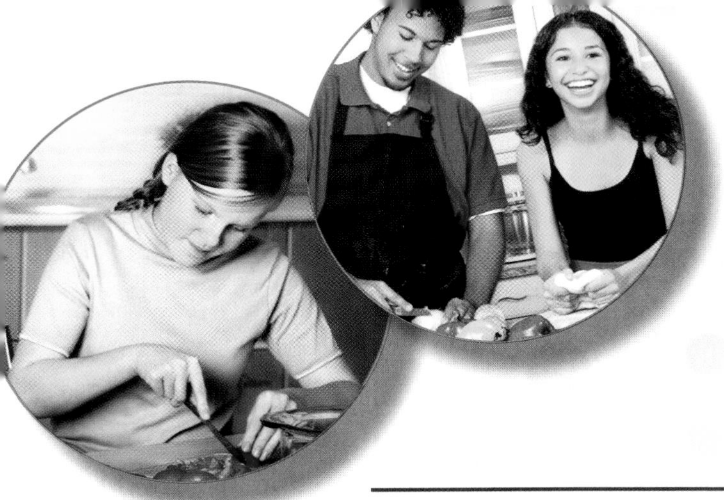

Section 9-6 Making Meal Preparation Easy

Objectives

After studying this section, you will be able to

- **define** *time schedule*, *multitasking*, and *work center*.
- **describe** how to use a time schedule to make meal preparation easier.
- **state** how to organize your kitchen.

Key Terms

time schedule: a written plan for a person that lists when tasks should be started and completed.

multitasking: doing more than one task at a time.

work center: an area of a kitchen designed around a specific activity or activities.

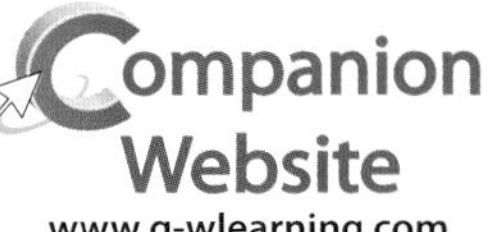

Study the Key Terms by completing crossword puzzles, matching activities, and e-flash cards at the website.

Main Ideas

- Using a time schedule can make meal preparation easier.
- It is important to plan your kitchen so meal preparation is easy.

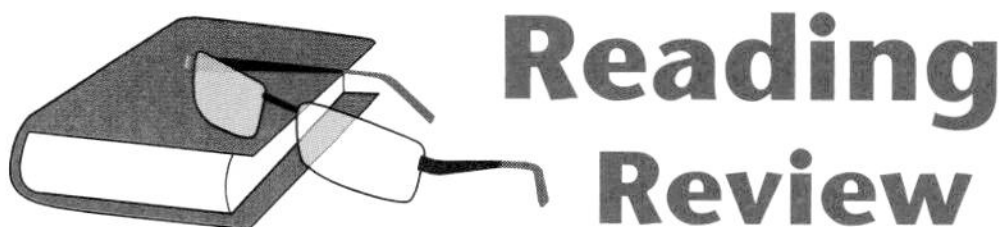

1. Which cooking methods are best for less tender cuts of meat? Which cooking methods are best for tender meats?
2. Why is it important to cook eggs before you eat them?

Desserts

Cakes, cookies, pastries, and doughnuts are just a few types of desserts. You probably like desserts. Their rich flavors often come from fat and sugar. Desserts, however, should not be the main part of your diet. Most are high in calories. Eat small servings.

Each type of dessert is prepared differently from the others. Therefore, follow the recipe carefully when making a dessert. Make sure you combine the ingredients properly. Use the right size pan. Cook at the correct temperature. Follow directions for storing and serving desserts. See **9-19**. By doing so, you can prepare a tasty dessert.

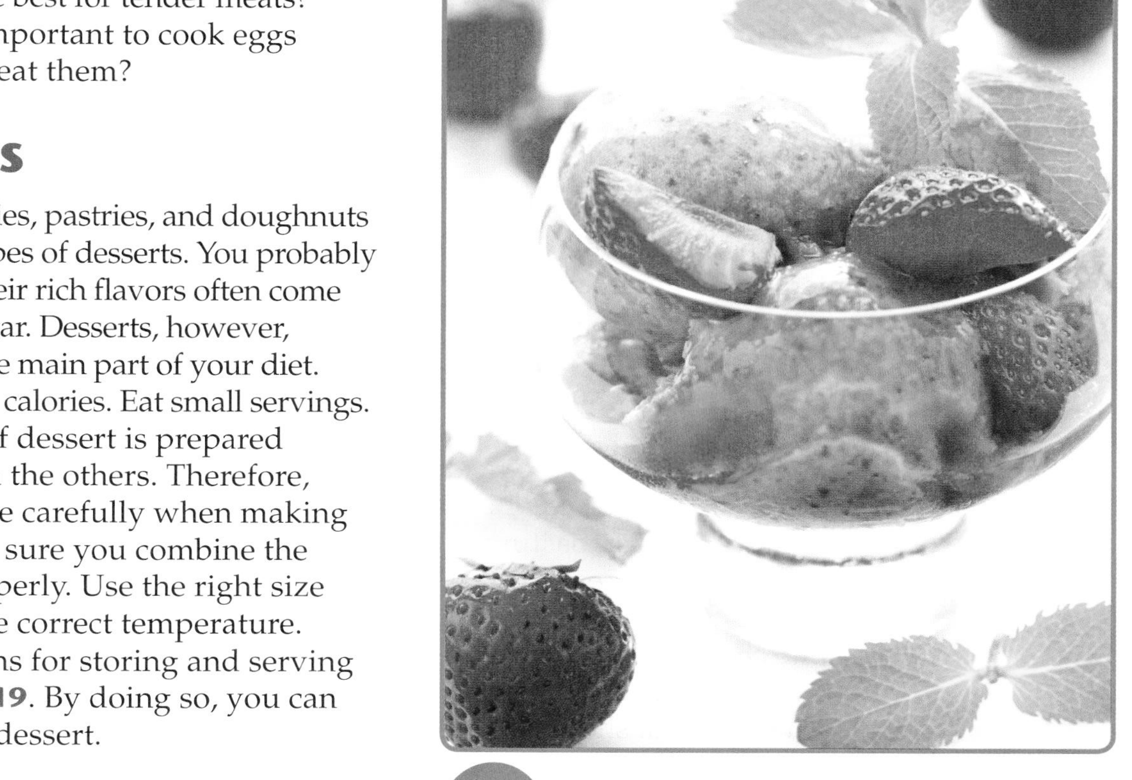

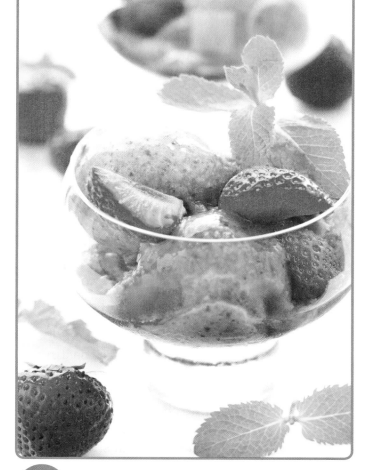

9-19 Frozen desserts must be served quickly to prevent melting.

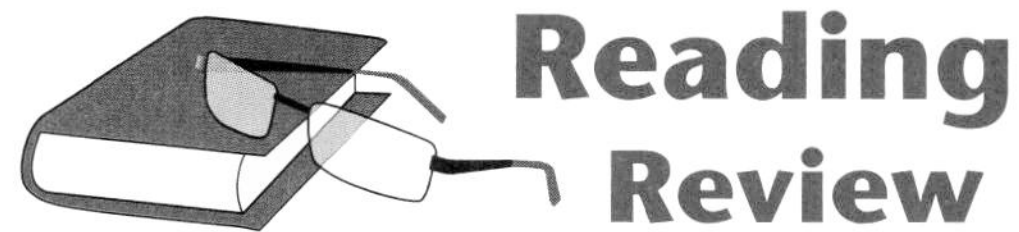

1. Why should desserts not be a large part of your diet?
2. Why do you need to follow recipes carefully when preparing desserts?

Section Summary

- Fruits and vegetables can be eaten raw or cooked. Always wash them before eating.
- The two types of bread are quick breads and yeast breads.
- Cook cereals, pasta, and rice in the right amounts of water at the correct temperatures to achieve the best results.
- Milk and other dairy products should be cooked on low heat to prevent curdling.
- Moist-heat and dry-heat methods are used to cook meat, poultry, and seafood, depending on their tenderness.
- Desserts should always be prepared according to the recipe.

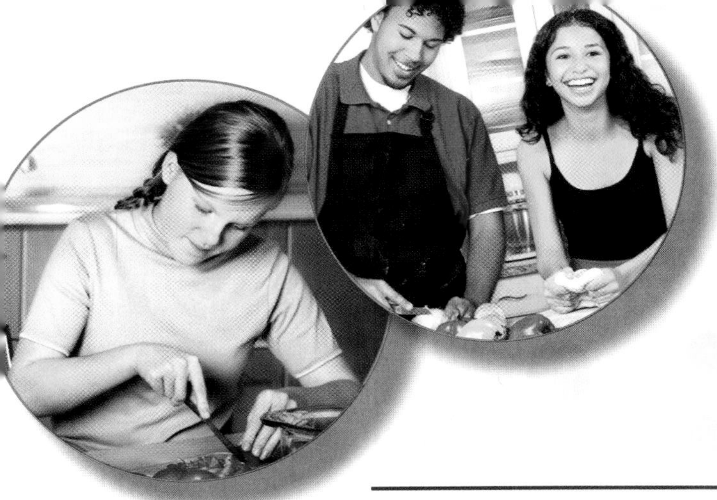

Section 9-6 Making Meal Preparation Easy

Objectives

After studying this section, you will be able to
- **define** *time schedule*, *multitasking*, and *work center*.
- **describe** how to use a time schedule to make meal preparation easier.
- **state** how to organize your kitchen.

Key Terms

time schedule: a written plan for a person that lists when tasks should be started and completed.

multitasking: doing more than one task at a time.

work center: an area of a kitchen designed around a specific activity or activities.

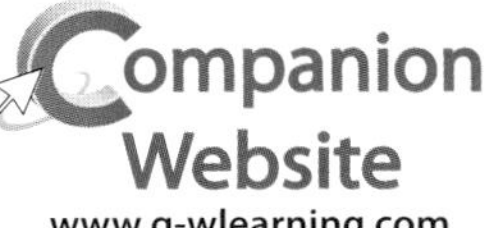

Study the Key Terms by completing crossword puzzles, matching activities, and e-flash cards at the website.

Main Ideas

- Using a time schedule can make meal preparation easier.
- It is important to plan your kitchen so meal preparation is easy.

You may have heard the saying, "If you want to get something done, give it to a busy person." People who plan and organize their work often get much done. Planning and organizing are important in meal preparation. They will save you both time and energy. This section will help you plan your meal preparation and organize your kitchen in the school lab and at home.

Meal Preparation Planning

Meal preparation planning takes both time and energy. To have successful meals, however, you should take the time to plan for them. You may already help to plan and prepare meals at home. See **9-20**. You need to do the same at school. Because class time is limited, a time schedule will help. A **time schedule** is a written plan for a person that lists when tasks should be started and completed. This helps prevent a last-minute rush.

For instance, you and your classmates are planning a class project to serve lunch to a small group of invited guests. Your goal is to have the food prepared well and served on time. Follow these steps:

1. Decide on the time you want to serve the meal.
2. Choose the menu and recipes. Keep them simple, since time is limited. Read all the recipes. Decide how long it will take to prepare, cook, and serve each food. Identify any preparation you can do ahead of time.
3. Make sure you have all the ingredients and tools you need. If not, prepare a shopping list and buy them.
4. Prepare a time schedule. Make a chart showing when you will start and finish each of the tasks. Be sure to include time for setup and cleanup in your schedule.

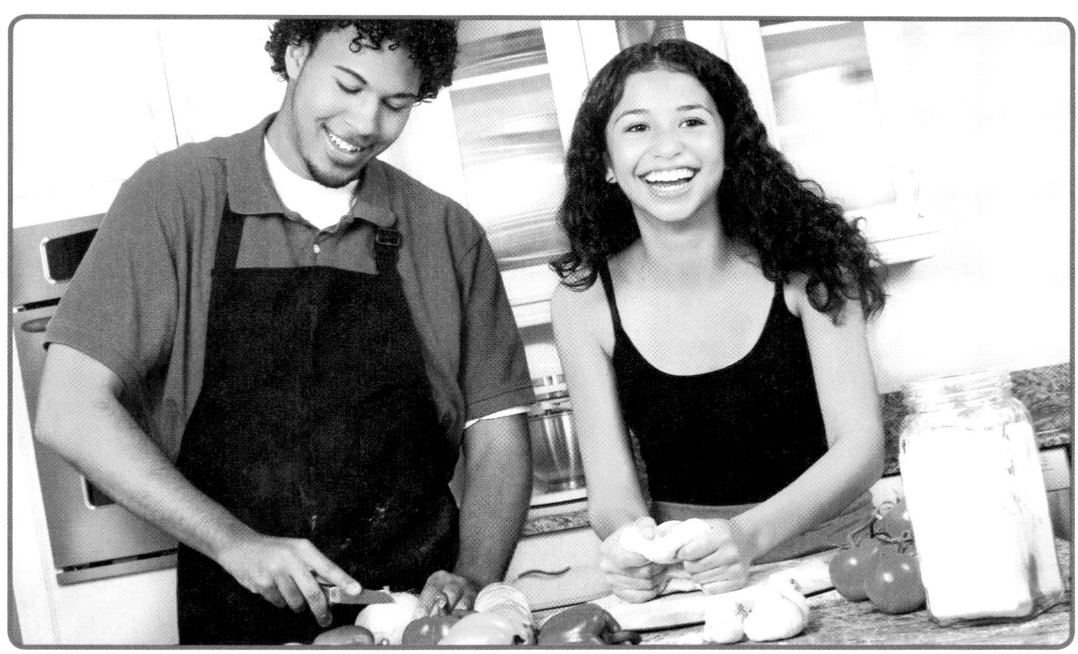

9-20 This brother and sister took the time to plan a meal, which helps them prepare it more quickly.

While following your time schedule, you can plan to multitask. **Multitasking** is doing more than one task at a time. For instance, you can prepare a tossed salad *while* the main dish is cooking.

More people are cooking meals at home instead of eating out to save money and have more nutritious foods. Preparing and serving meals at home with others can be fun, just as it is in the school lab. In the busy lives of families, eating together can be a time of pleasure and sharing daily events.

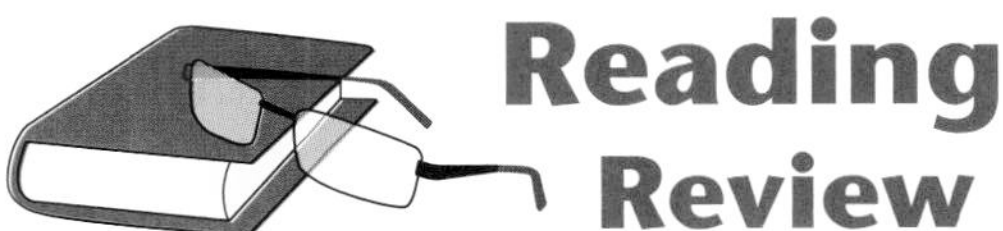

Reading Review

1. How can making and following a time schedule help you when preparing meals at school?
2. How can multitasking help you manage your time better?

Organizing Your Kitchen

Part of being a good cook is organizing your kitchen so meal preparation is easy and enjoyable. Begin by arranging the kitchen tools.

Store tools at the correct work center. A **work center** is an area of a kitchen designed around a specific activity or activities. These activities include preparing and serving food, storing food, and cleaning up.

Storing tools near where you use them can make working in the kitchen much easier. If you always have to stop and look for the tools you need, you will waste time and energy. See **9-21**.

You can store tools you often use together, such as mixing bowls and rubber scrapers, in the same place. You can also store the same type of tools in two different places. For instance, you may store mixing spoons near the cooktop and preparation area.

Succeed in Life

Making Meal Preparation Easier

There are many ways you can make meal preparation easier. Here are some ideas to consider before you begin to work in the kitchen.

- Plan meals according to other activities. On busy days, plan meals that are easy to prepare and serve. This leaves you free to do other tasks.
- Prepare food for more than one meal when you can. The extra food may be served the next day or frozen for later use.
- Store extra food in containers you can use in both the refrigerator and the microwave. This prevents unnecessary dishwashing.
- Rinse and stack tools as you finish using them. This makes dishwashing easier.
- Peel fruits and vegetables over a large piece of paper to help keep your work area clean.

Storing Ingredients and Kitchen Tools
In the preparation and serving area of your kitchen, you should store • cooking tools • cookware and bakeware • standard measuring tools • pot holders • serving dishes
In the food storage area of your kitchen, you should store • food storage containers • foods that do not need to be refrigerated • foil and plastic wrap • tools for serving refrigerated and frozen foods
In the cleanup area of your kitchen, you should store • knives • cutting board • tableware • flatware • cleaning supplies • wastebasket

9-21 Tools and ingredients are easy to find when they are stored in the correct work center.

Store tools you use often in easy-to-reach places. You may want to store tools you use less often in the backs of drawers and cabinets. For instance, store a can opener you use frequently in the front of a drawer in the food preparation area. Store holiday cookie cutters you use only once a year in the back of a cabinet.

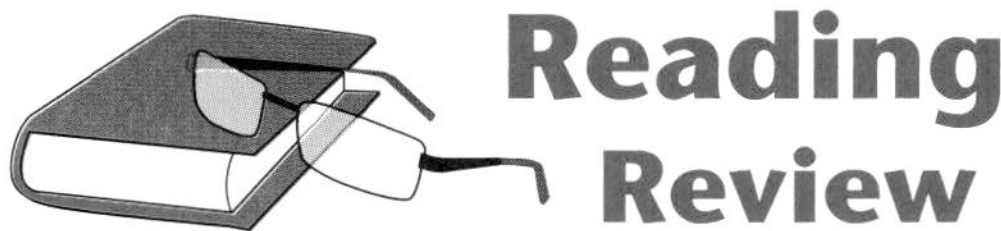

Reading Review

1. What are the three types of activities that make up work centers?
2. Why is it helpful to store tools you use together in the same place?

Section Summary

- There are many ways to make meal preparation easy.
- Making a time schedule will save you time and energy before you begin preparing food.
- Organizing your kitchen is important and will help you avoid wasting time.
- You will save time and energy when you store tools in easy-to-find places.

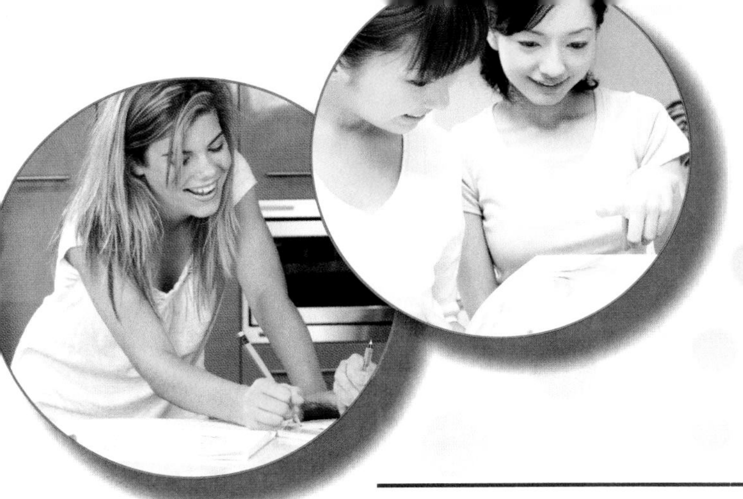

Section 9-7
Working with Others

Objectives

After studying this section, you will be able to

- **define** *work plan*.
- **demonstrate** how to work with others in the kitchen.
- **explain** how to make and follow a work plan.

Key Term

work plan: a list of tasks to be done, who is to perform them, and the tools and ingredients needed.

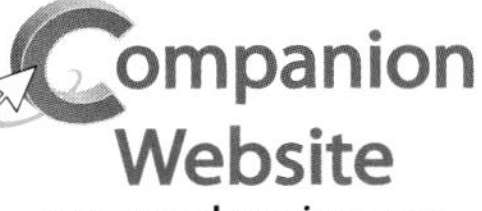

Study the Key Term by completing crossword puzzles, matching activities, and e-flash cards at the website.

Main Ideas

- You can learn to work well with others in the kitchen at home or in the school foods lab.
- A work plan can help you work with others to complete food preparation tasks.

Food preparation and cleanup tasks are shared at home or in the school foods lab.

You may prepare certain foods or an entire meal by yourself. Preparing meals can often involve more than one person. Others may help you by setting the table and cleaning up after the meal. Someone may also help you prepare the food.

Sharing in food preparation and cleanup tasks is important both at home and in the school foods lab. Knowing how to work well with others can make this work more enjoyable.

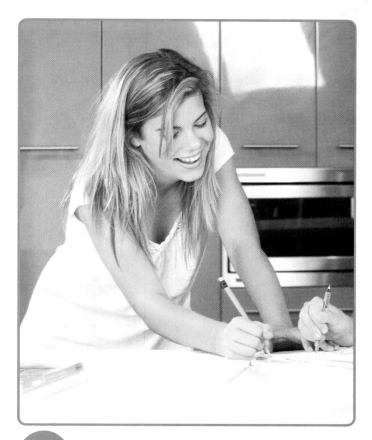

9-22 When working in the foods lab, be sure to bring the supplies you need. This will allow you to start working right away.

Ready for Class

In your foods lab, use class time wisely. Begin working right away to make good use of your time. Do not waste time standing around talking with your friends. This is not fair to the other people in your lab group.

Also, come to class prepared. See **9-22**. For some classes, you may only need a pencil and paper. For other classes, you may need your textbook, an apron, or other supplies.

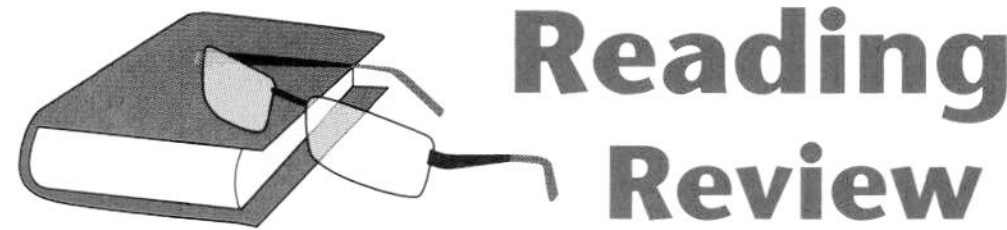

Reading Review

1. Why is wasting time in the foods lab unfair to your lab partners?
2. How can being prepared help you in class? Give examples.

The Work Plan

Preparing meals in a foods class may seem harder than at home. There are several reasons for this. There are usually fewer people working in the kitchen at home. Working with family members can be less confusing because you know one another's habits. You also have more time to prepare meals at home. Because class time is limited, schedule time more carefully.

Making plans is an important part of cooking. Plans are needed whether you cook alone or in a group. When you work alone, use a time schedule. When working in a group, use a work plan. A **work plan** is a list of tasks to be done, who is to perform them, and the tools and ingredients needed.

Work plans can help group members work well together. They let you know what is expected of you as part of the group. They also let you know whether you are completing your assigned tasks. If you are not happy

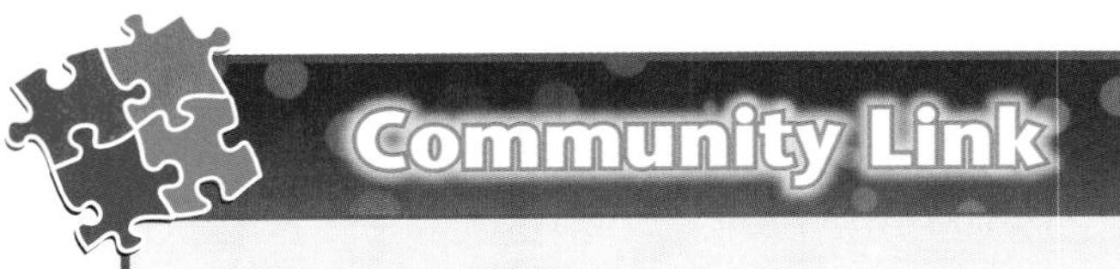

Feeding Those in Need

Every community has either a homeless shelter or another organization that provides meals for those who need them. Volunteer to help plan, prepare, serve, or deliver meals either individually or as part of a group. Helping others makes both you and them feel good. Write a short report on the experience.

with how tasks are assigned, take time to discuss your concerns and feelings with your group.

When writing a work plan, be sure to include all the tasks that must be performed. First, you must decide what foods you are going to prepare. This will be done by your teacher or by you and your lab partners. Then make a time schedule. Include what tasks must be done and in what order. Finally, decide who will perform each task. Write your work plan two or three days before you plan to cook. This will give you time to get your supplies together.

At home, you may want to make a work plan if several family members are helping in the kitchen. This work plan does not need to be as detailed as the one at school. It can list the tasks to be done and whose turn it is to do each task.

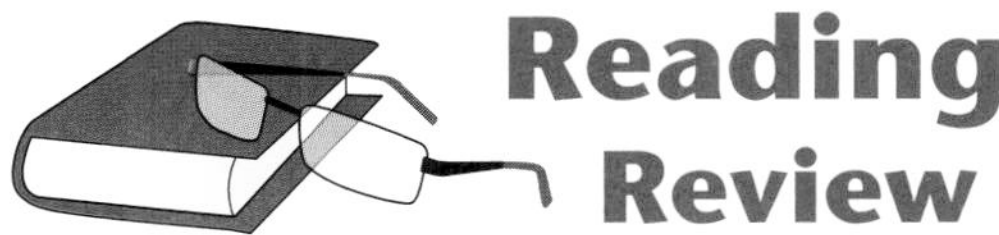

1. How can a work plan help you when you are working in the school foods lab?
2. When you are cooking with other people, why is it important to plan the tasks each person will perform?

Group Food Preparation

When tasks are divided, only one or two people in the group are responsible for the actual food preparation. The other members of the group are assigned serving and hosting tasks. See **9-23**. Each task is needed to create a successful meal. The experience you gain from performing each of these tasks will help you prepare meals in the future.

Group tasks should be rotated each time a new work plan is written. In a *rotation work plan*, you are assigned a task to perform for a day or a week. Then, you are assigned another task the next day or week. This gives you a chance to practice all the tasks involved in food preparation.

Cleanup tasks should be included in your work plan. These tasks are needed to put a room or work area in order. It is easier to work in a clean and orderly foods lab than a messy one. Know what

Food Preparation Task List

Cook: responsible for food, does most of the actual food preparation.

Assistant cook: helps the cook prepare food.

Host/food server: set table, serve food, greet any guests. There may be one student for each task or two students working together.

9-23 This is one way to divide food preparation tasks when working with others in the kitchen.

your assigned cleanup task is and do it well. The next people using the kitchen or work area will appreciate it.

You should have two goals for preparing meals in the school lab or at home . Produce foods that are nutritious, flavorful, appealing to the eye and taste buds, well prepared, and carefully served. Enjoy the experience of eating food you have prepared with your classmates, friends, guests, and family.

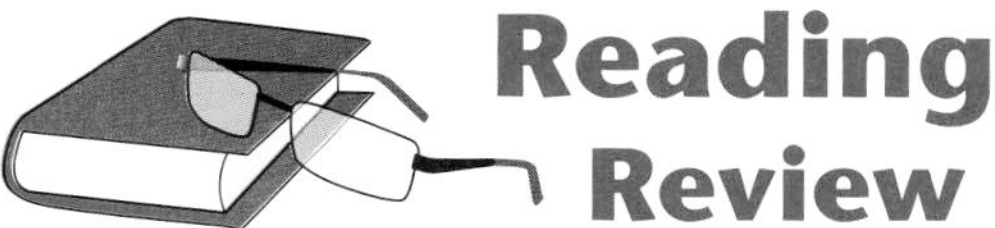

Reading Review

1. How does a rotation work plan help you learn all the tasks involved in food preparation?
2. Why should you leave your school foods lab clean and orderly?

Section Summary

- Working well with others is important whether you are working in your kitchen at home or in the school foods lab.
- Learn to use your time wisely.
- A work plan can help you complete all the tasks you are assigned.
- When working with others in the kitchen, food preparation and cleanup tasks are often rotated.

Chapter Summary

There is more involved in making food than just preparing it. There are several guidelines to follow to make sure the food turns out right. Before you begin preparing food, find out what the different kinds of tools are and how to use them. Also, follow the safety and sanitation guidelines. Otherwise, accidents and illnesses may occur.

Correctly reading and following recipes is important. Knowing how to correctly measure, cut, mix, and cook different foods are also necessary skills. Use the right tools and follow the correct methods when preparing food.

To prepare food, there are simple rules to follow. They are different for each type of food. Follow these guidelines carefully to prepare food that is nutritious, attractive, and tasty.

Meal preparation can be made easier by making a time schedule and organizing your kitchen. This will help you save time and energy. These same guidelines apply when you are working with others. Make a work plan and follow it. Work plans help you organize the work to be done and decide who will do each task.

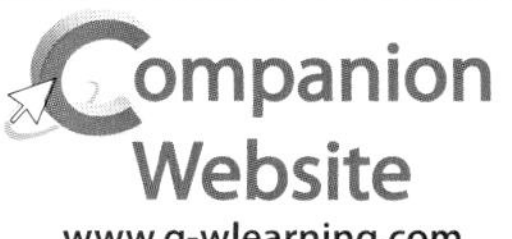

Review Key Terms and Main Ideas for Chapter 9 at the website.

Chapter Review

Write your answers on a separate sheet of paper.

1. List three reasons you should use and care for kitchen tools properly.
2. What are two benefits of using a microwave oven?
3. Give two examples of bakeware and two examples of cookware.
4. List three common kitchen accidents. Give two hints for preventing each accident listed.
5. What are five ways to prevent foodborne illnesses?
6. List four pieces of information that should be included in recipes.
7. List the steps for measuring dry ingredients.
8. Fill in the blanks.
   A. _____ teaspoons = 1 tablespoon
   B. _____ tablespoons = 1 cup
   C. _____ ounces = 1 pound
   D. _____ quarts = 1 gallon
9. Why is it important to understand the measuring, cutting, mixing, and cooking terms used in recipes?
10. Why do you need to cook food at the correct temperature?
11. What is the difference between moist-heat cooking methods and dry-heat cooking methods?
12. List hints for cooking foods from each food group.
13. What should you do to prevent a banana from turning brown after it has been sliced?
14. What is the first step in making a time schedule?
15. Perry is making dinner tonight. While the potatoes bake, he is preparing the salad and making the main course. This is called _____.
16. True or false. Your kitchen should be organized according to work centers.
17. True or false. Work plans are used when cooking by yourself.

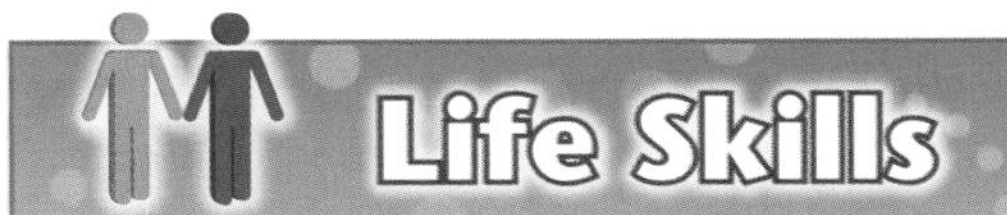

Life Skills

18. A manager of a local small restaurant is a friend of your family. The restaurant offers meals served in the restaurant and carryout food. She heard you had been studying safety and sanitation in the kitchen. She has asked you to visit her restaurant and check the safety and sanitation practices and to prepare a report for her. She will use the report to train her staff in the restaurant. Review Section 9-2 to develop your plan. Write the section's four headings at the top of one or two pages, then list the points under the heading you will look for on your visit. Turn in your final report. What have you learned that you might use in your family's kitchen?

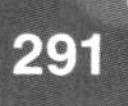

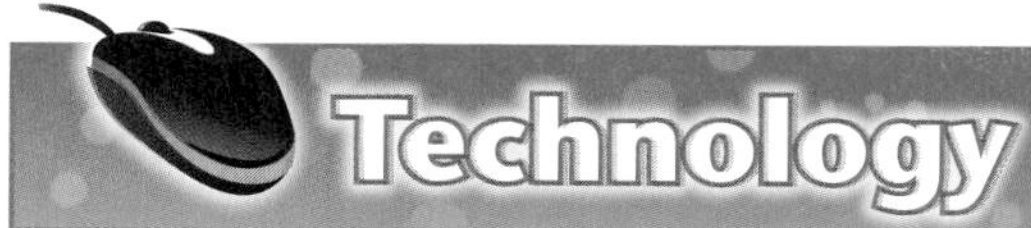

19. Research the Internet for information about food safety education. Use a key term like food safety. The fightbac.org website offers simple, practical advice to keep food safe from harmful bacteria. Use word processing software to prepare a report with suggestions to help keep food safe in food preparation class and in the school cafeteria. Share this information with your classmates, teachers, and cafeteria manager.

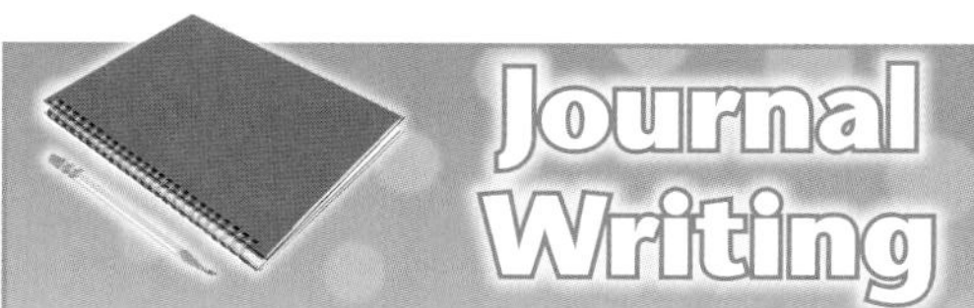

20. Plan to make a meal for your family. Choose the foods you want to prepare. Then make a schedule to follow when preparing the meal. After you have prepared your meal, write a short journal entry describing the event.

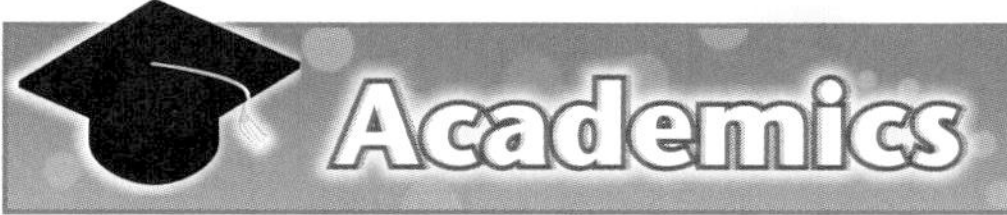

21. **Science.** Research which nontoxic, common household products can be used instead of cleaners with toxic chemicals. Those chemicals are unsafe and can cause pollution. Make a list of the environmentally friendly materials and substances that can be used for different kitchen cleaning tasks. Turn in a one-page report.
22. **Math.** In the school foods lab or at home, practice measuring 1 cup and 1 tablespoon of each of the following ingredients: milk, flour, brown sugar, and butter. Be sure to follow the directions given in the chapter.
23. **Writing.** In your food preparation class, write a work plan for a nutritious meal your group is going to prepare. Follow the work plan as your group prepares and serves the meal and cleans up. Discuss any problems that may have occurred after the event. Brainstorm ideas for how to solve these problems in the future.

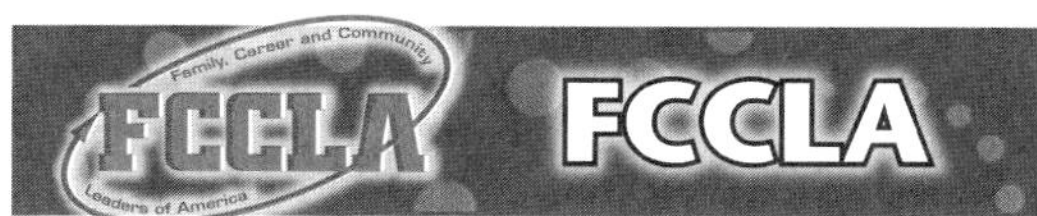

24. Set up a family dinner night, where your family gathers at least one evening a week for dinner together. Work with your family to decide the night and the menus to be planned. Set up a work plan. Then develop an FCCLA *Family Ties* project for the *Power of One* program. Obtain further information about this program from your FCCLA advisor.

Unit 4
You and Your Clothes

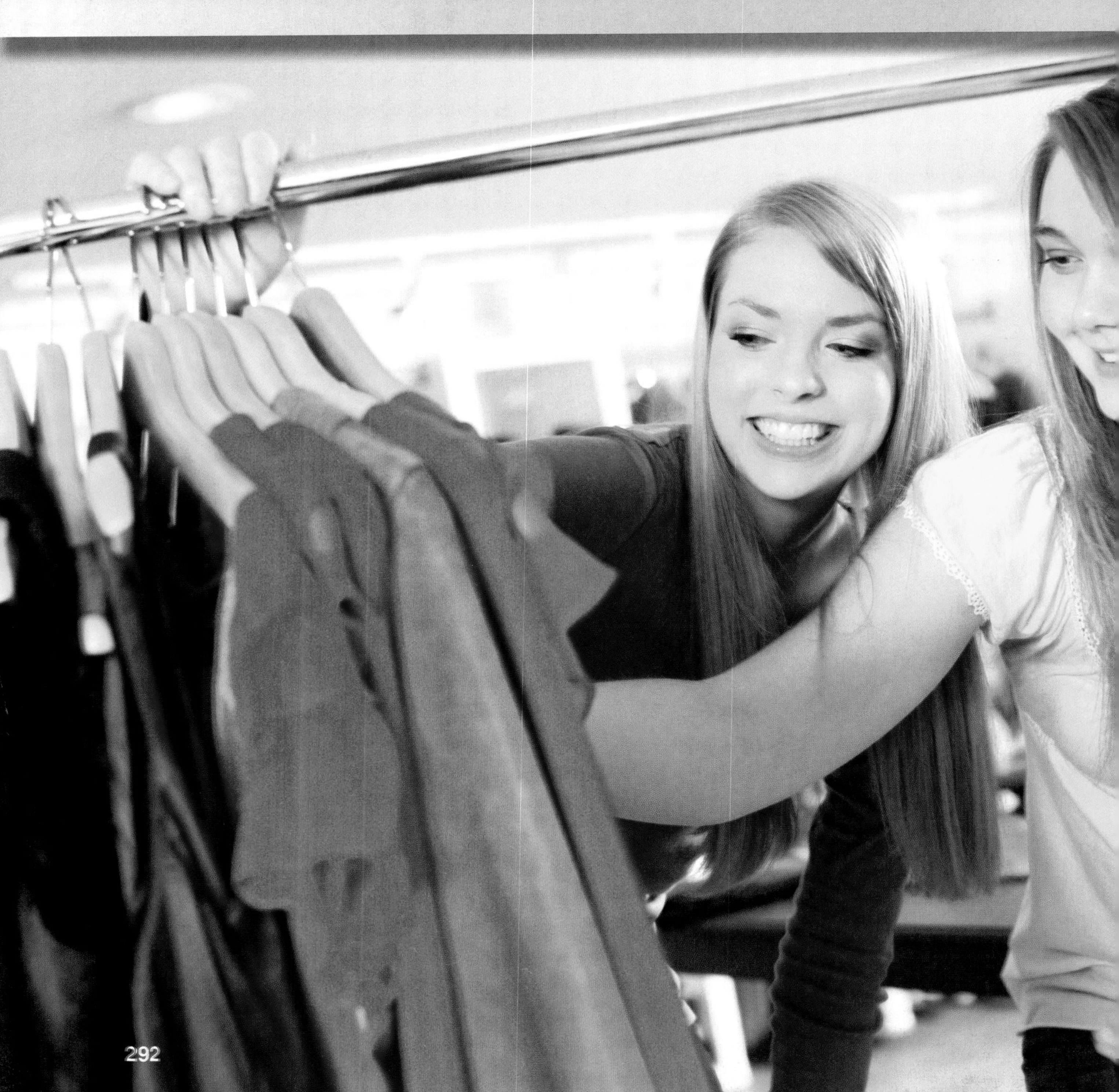

Chapter 10 Buying and Caring for Clothes

Chapter 11 Learning to Sew

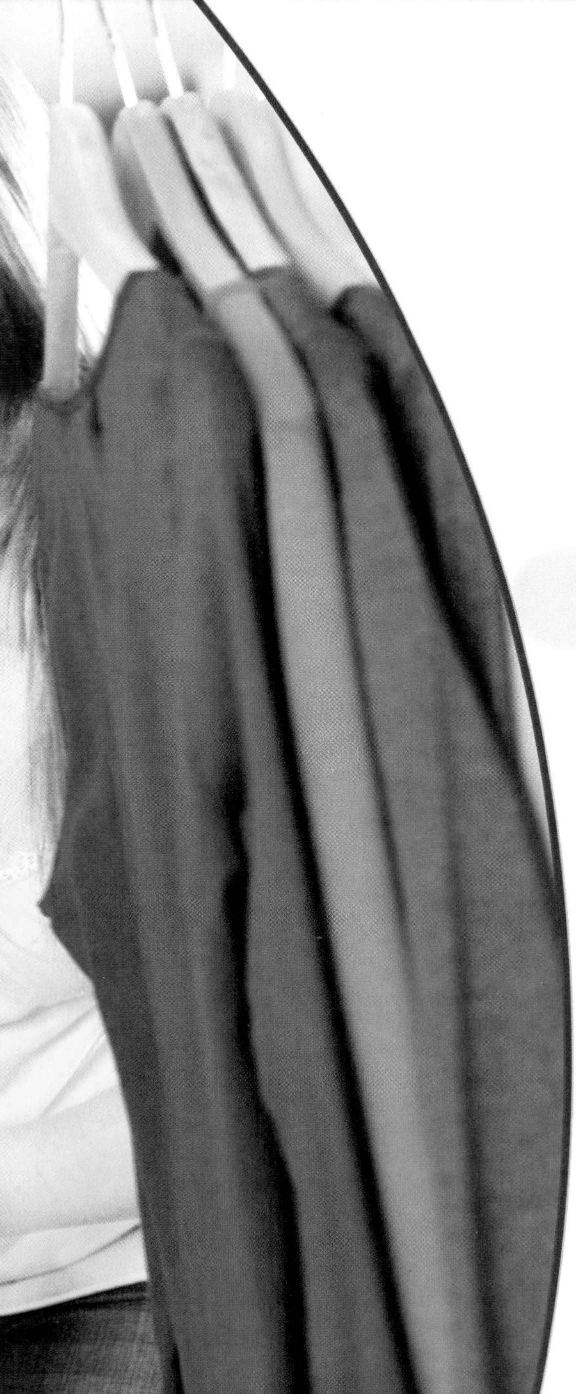

Exploring Careers

The following careers relate to the information you will study in Unit 4. Read the descriptions and then complete the activity to learn more about the careers that might interest you.

Career	Description
Tailor	Sews and alters garments
Buyer	Responsible for choosing and purchasing goods for companies to sell at a profit
Fashion illustrator	Draws garments that have been designed and produced by others
Merchandiser displayer	Creates a store's look, including the window and interior displays
Fashion photographer	Takes pictures that show fashionable clothes and accessories attractively using merchandise or live models
Fashion designer	Creates designs for clothing and accessories
Textile designer	Creates designs for knitted, woven, or printed fabrics
Patternmaker	Turns designs into patterns for various items to be mass-produced

Activity: Take a few minutes and list your top ten current interests. Which of these careers might be good fits with some of your interests? Why?

Chapter 10
Buying and Caring for Clothes

Sections

10-1 Building Your Wardrobe
10-2 Shopping for Clothes
10-3 Inspect Before You Buy
10-4 Fibers and Fabrics
10-5 Caring for Your Clothes

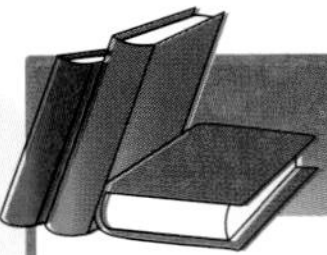

Sharpen Your Reading

Think of a movie you have seen that relates to this chapter. Sketch a scene from the movie or write a brief description. As you read the chapter, visualize the characters in the movie. How would the scene be different if the characters had read this chapter?

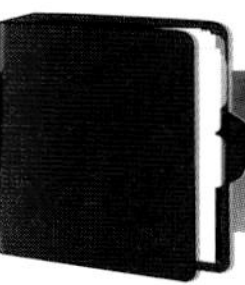

Concept Organizer

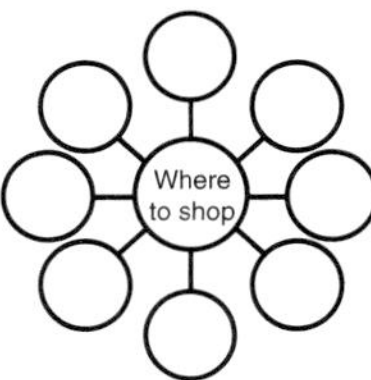

Use a star diagram like the one shown to identify the many different choices consumers have for where they shop.

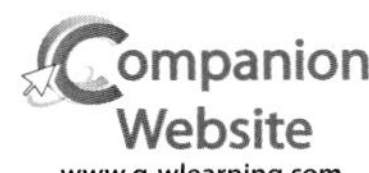

Print out the concept organizer at the website.

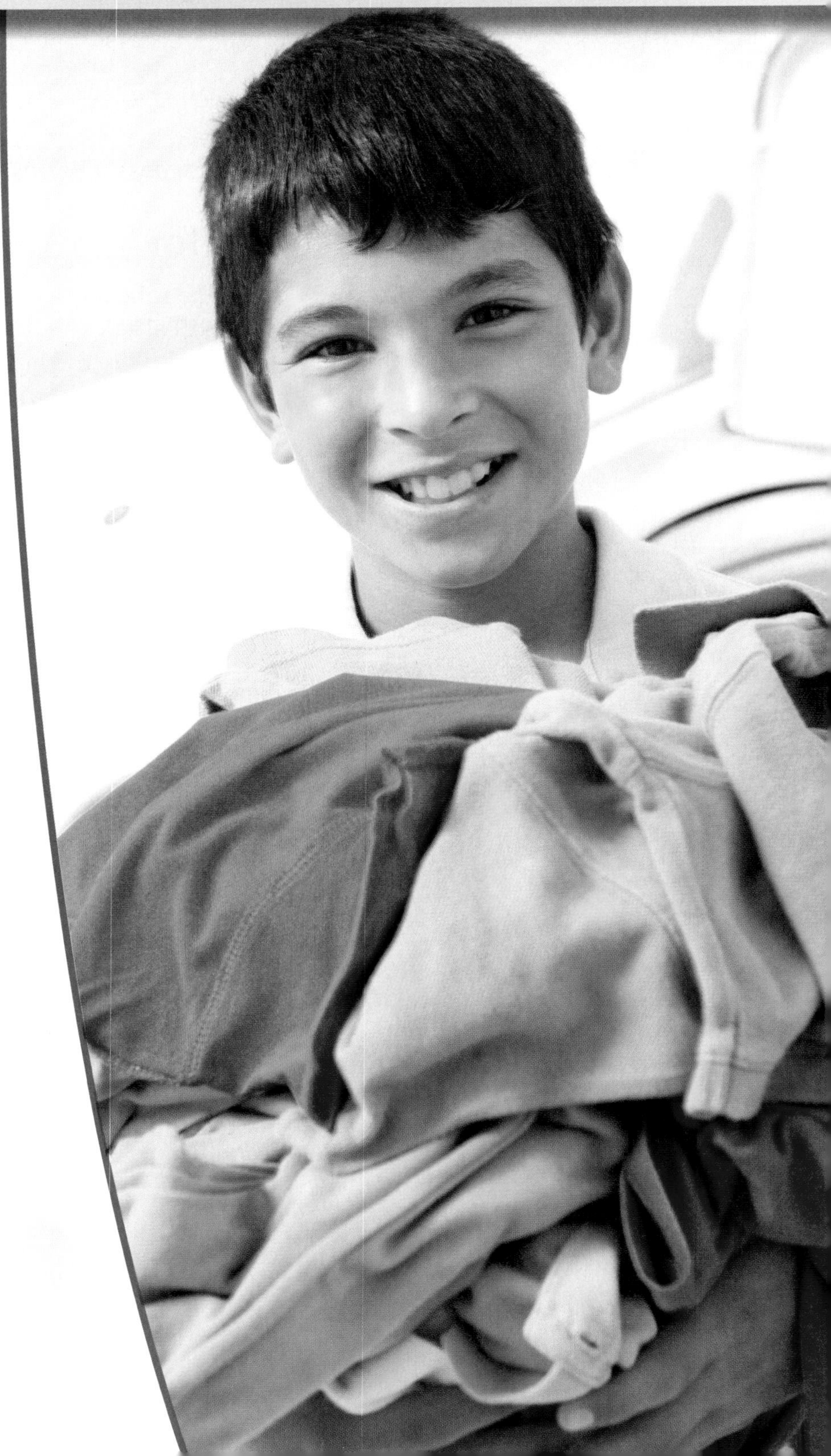

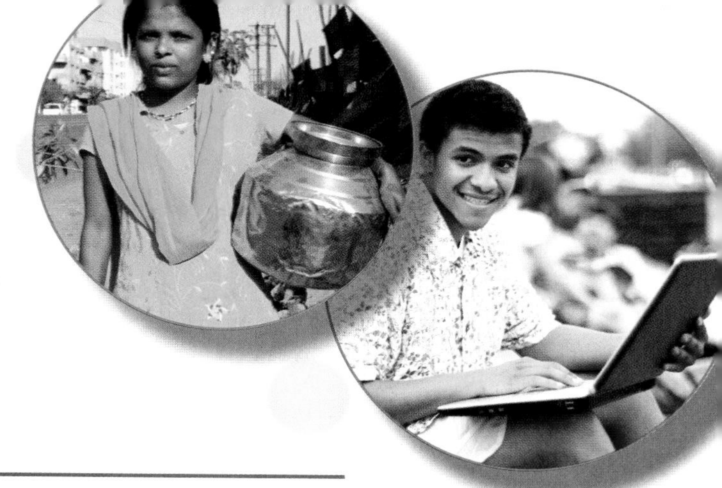

Section 10-1
Building Your Wardrobe

Objectives

After studying this section, you will be able to
- **define** *wardrobe*, *style*, *fashion*, *classic*, *fad*, *accessories*, *inventory*, and *consignment store*.
- **give examples** of factors that affect clothing needs.
- **explain** the importance of completing a wardrobe inventory.

Key Terms

wardrobe: all the clothes and accessories you have to wear.
style: a distinctive form of dress or the design of a garment.
fashion: styles that are popular at a given time.
classic: a style that stays in fashion for a long time.
fad: a new style that is popular for only a short time.
accessories: items worn to accent clothing.
inventory: a list of clothing items you have on hand.
consignment store: a store that sells pre-owned clothing and other items where the original owner receives part of the selling price.

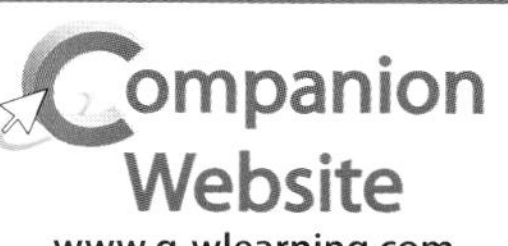

Study the Key Terms by completing crossword puzzles, matching activities, and e-flash cards at the website.

Main Ideas

- Clothing needs are affected by your climate, standards of dress, and activities.
- Knowing fashion terms can help you plan your clothing purchases.
- Taking a wardrobe inventory lets you know exactly what clothes you have.

You may spend a lot of time thinking about your clothes. It is natural to be interested in clothes. They can express your personality. Certain clothes can make you feel good about yourself.

You often are not able to buy all the clothes you might want. This section will help you learn how to build your wardrobe without spending a lot of money. A **wardrobe** is all the clothes and accessories you have to wear.

Clothing Needs

As you build your wardrobe, think about your clothing needs. There are three factors that affect clothing needs. They are standards of dress, activities, and climate. See **10-1**. Your needs may be very much like those of your friends and other people in your community. If you move to another city or state, your clothing needs may change.

Your *standards of dress* are the clothes that are acceptable in your country and community. Your school is a community. Students at your school probably dress in a similar fashion. In some schools, students tend to wear casual clothing. In other schools, students may dress up or wear uniforms.

Think about your activities when choosing your clothing. If you play sports, you need clothes that let you be active. You may own a lot of swimsuits if you live near a beach.

Perhaps you live in a part of the country that has definite seasons—winter, spring, summer, and fall. Your clothing needs would not be the same as those of a person who lives where it is warm or cold for most of the year. He or she would mainly need clothes for only warm or cold weather. On the other hand, you would need clothing for both types of weather.

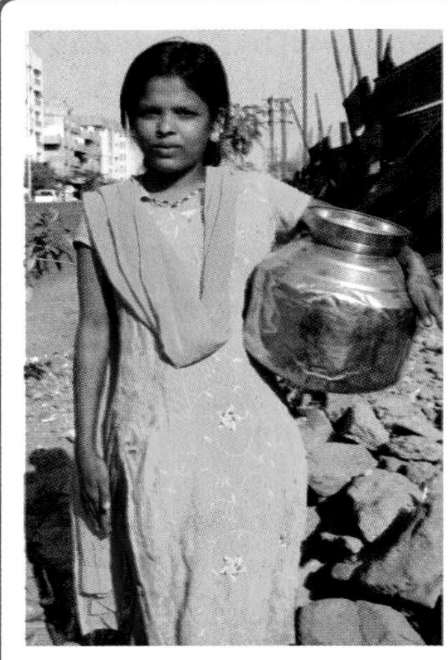
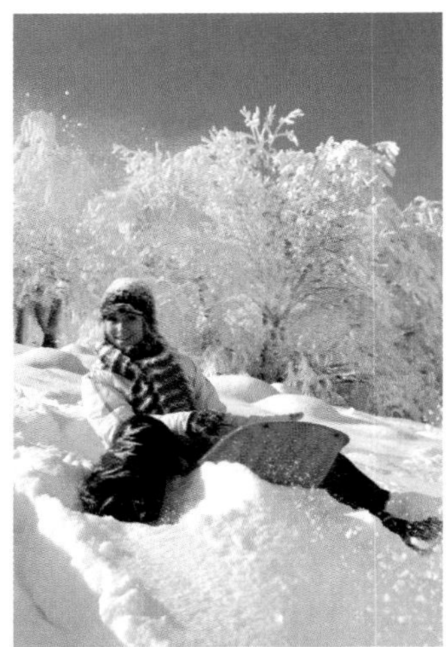
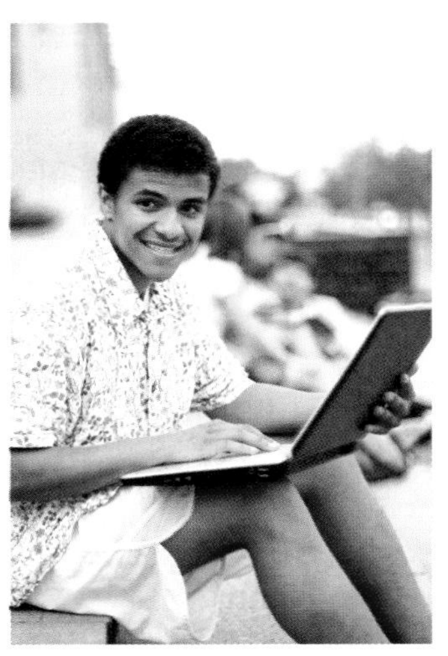

10-1 Clothing needs differ throughout the world, based on standards of dress, activities, and climate.

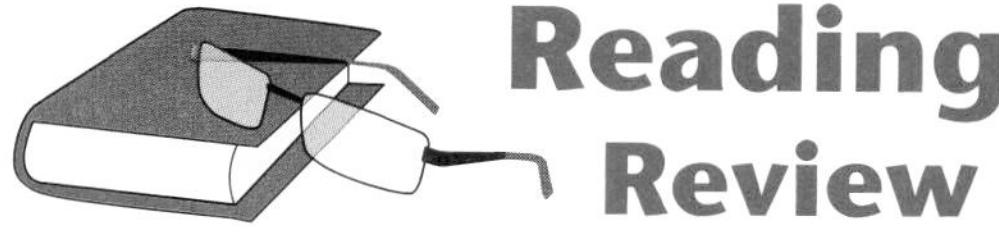

1. How do your friends and community affect your clothing needs?
2. How do your activities affect your clothing needs? Give examples.

Planning Your Wardrobe

To build a wardrobe, make a plan. First, determine your clothing needs. Then consider your wants. What kind of clothes do you want to wear? What makes you feel good about yourself? You may be influenced by what your friends like to wear.

Some people like to wear clothes that have a certain look. **Style** is a distinctive form of dress or the design of a garment. Various styles can be identified by their distinctive looks. *Hippie*, *punk*, and *retro* are names for different styles. Can you think of others? You can create your own unique style through your clothing choices. A style can also refer to the design of a garment. For instance, corduroys and blue jeans are two different styles of pants.

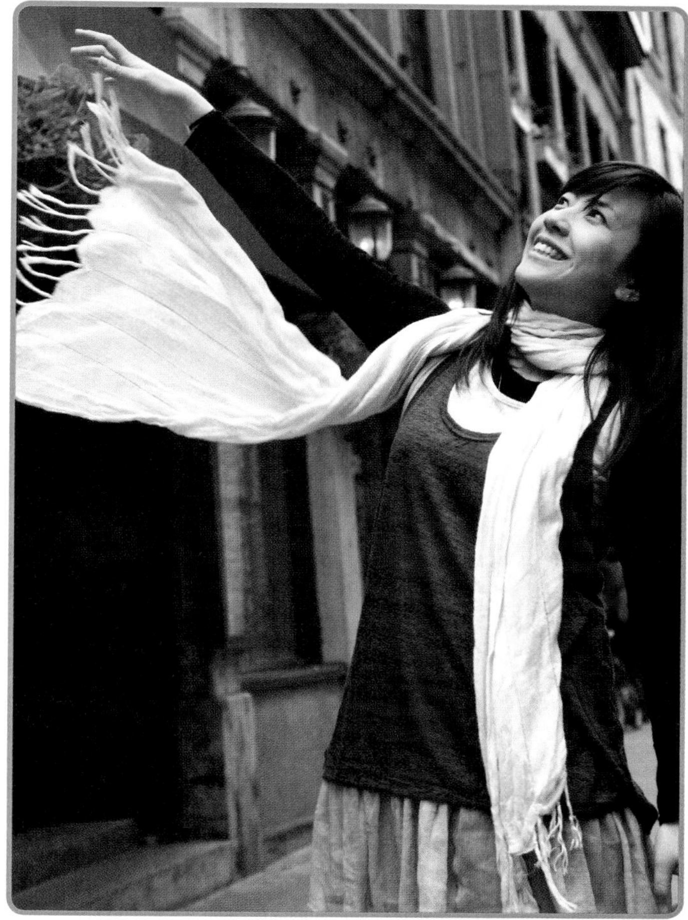

10-2 Accenting with fashionable accessories is an easy way to stay in style.

A **fashion** is a style that is popular at a given time. The legs of your blue jeans may have been wide last year, while this year, they may be narrower.

There are two types of fashions. One is a classic. A **classic** is a style that stays in fashion for a long time. Khaki pants are a good example of a classic. A **fad** is a new style that is popular for only a short time.

Because fads go out of style quickly, it is smart to spend most of your clothing money on classics. To keep your wardrobe up-to-date, you can buy **accessories**, or items you can wear to accent your clothing. See **10-2**. Examples of accessories include jewelry, ties, belts, hats, and scarves. This is one way to wear the latest fads without spending a lot of money.

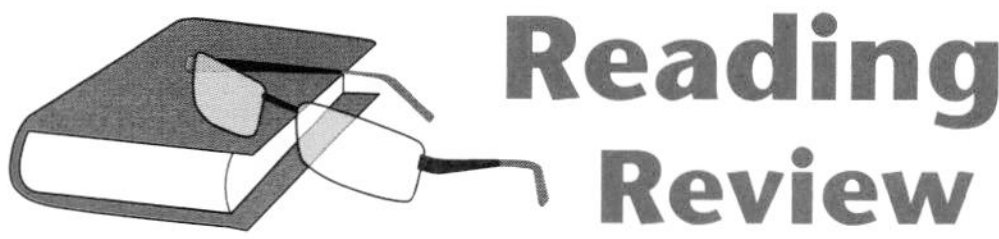

1. Why should you limit the fad clothing you buy?
2. How can you increase your wardrobe? Give examples.

Succeed in Life

Increase the Size of Your Wardrobe

You can increase the size of your wardrobe through buying clothes that can be worn with those you already have. You will be able to mix and match your clothes to create more outfits. You can also increase the size of your wardrobe by sharing clothes, such as sweaters or jackets, with your brothers or sisters. Always ask permission before borrowing another person's clothes. Some people have large wardrobes because they make and repair their own clothes. Others may find inexpensive clothing at yard sales, thrift shops, or consignment stores.

A Wardrobe Inventory

When you plan your wardrobe, you must know what clothes you have. This can be done by taking an inventory. An **inventory** is a list of the clothing items you have on hand. First, remove all your clothing from dresser drawers and closets. Put them on your bed, or another place that will give you room to work. Then divide your clothing in groups such as jeans, sweaters, and shirts. This makes it easier for you to check and list each item.

Inspect each item of clothing. Set aside all the clothes you no longer wear. Think about why you no longer wear them. If the clothes are damaged or the wrong size, you can mend or possibly alter them. You may also decide to give away clothes that do not fit. Consider selling the clothes at a consignment store. A **consignment store** is a store that resells pre-owned clothing and other items. If the clothes sell, you would receive part of the selling price.

Then take an inventory of the clothing and accessories you still wear or plan to keep. See **10-3**. List all the items you have under different headings. If an item of clothing must be repaired or altered, note this on your list. This will remind you to make these repairs.

Based on your inventory, decide which clothes and accessories you might acquire to complete your wardrobe. Consider how your wardrobe satisfies your climate, activity, and style needs. Have your parents help you decide how you will buy these clothes. You may have to buy some of these clothes yourself.

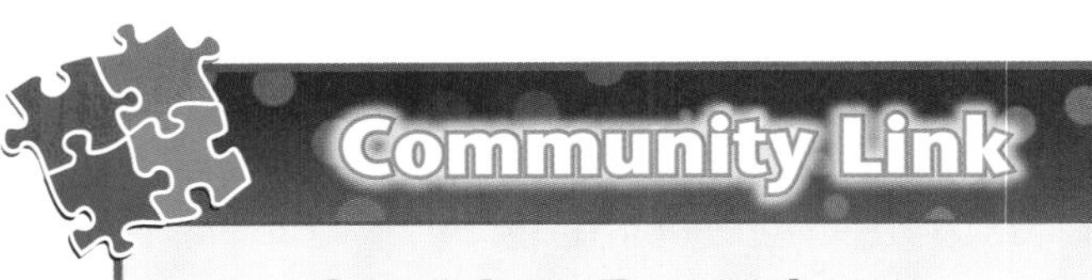

Clothing Donations

Make a list of all the places in your community where you could donate pre-owned clothing. Create a flyer for your school suggesting ways to donate clothing to charities or thrift shops. Donated clothes should be clean and free of rips and stains.

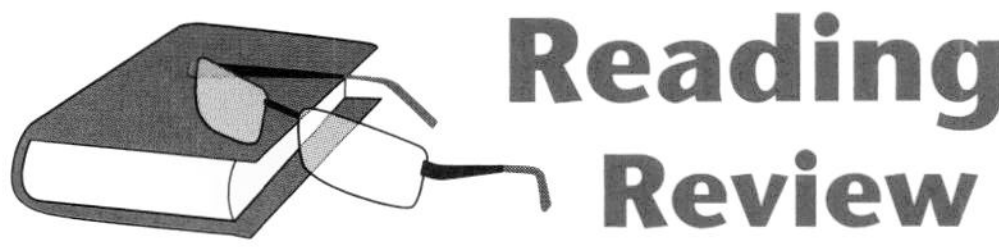

1. Why is it important to know exactly what clothes you own?
2. How does taking a wardrobe inventory help you plan your wardrobe?

Wardrobe Inventory			
List of My Clothes	**Description and Color**	**Condition**	**Notes**
Shirts			
Sweaters			
Suits or dresses			
Pants			
Shorts			
Undergarments			
Socks			
Coats			
Accessories			
Shoes			

10-3 Using a wardrobe inventory can help you decide what clothes and accessories you need.

Section Summary

- Planning your wardrobe is important.
- When you plan ahead, you can build a large wardrobe without spending a lot of money.
- Planning includes understanding your clothing needs, knowing the fashion terms, and taking a wardrobe inventory.

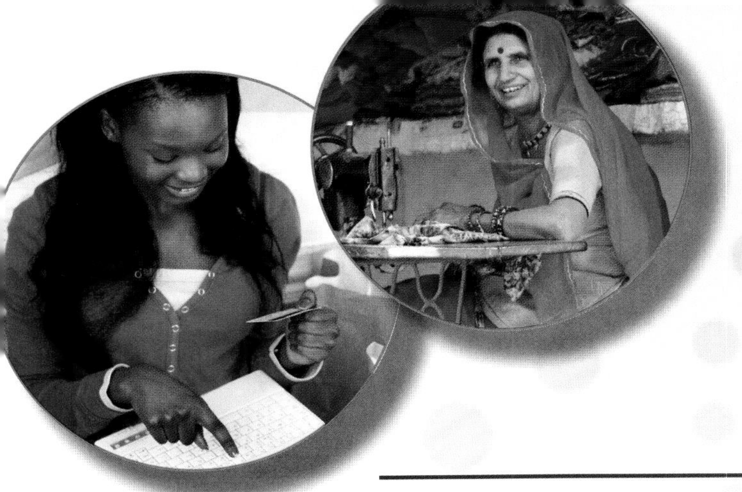

Section 10-2
Shopping for Clothes

Objectives

After studying this section, you will be able to
- **define** *virtual fit* and *value*.
- **explain** how to decide where to shop.
- **give examples** of how to save money when shopping for clothes.
- **explain** how to behave when shopping.

Key Terms

virtual fit: a method of using a person's body measurements to show that body image with clothing on the computer.

value: buying the highest quality of clothing for the lowest prices.

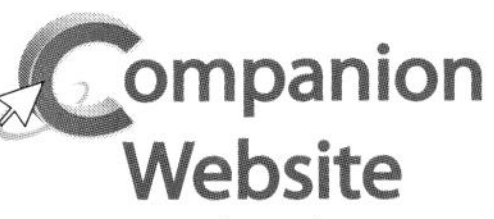

Study the Key Terms by completing crossword puzzles, matching activities, and e-flash cards at the website.

Main Ideas

- Variety, quality, price, service, and location should all be considered when deciding where to shop.
- There are many ways to save money when shopping for clothing.
- Using good manners can make shopping more pleasant for everyone.

After you have decided the clothes you need to complete your wardrobe, make a buying plan. Your buying plan should include where you are going to shop and how you are going to pay for your clothes. When you make a plan and follow it, you will be more organized and have more time to shop. This will give you a chance to find the best buys possible.

Deciding Where to Shop

Before deciding where to shop, consider your ethics and values. Think about who made the clothes and where they were made. See **10-4**. Were they made in countries that allow child labor? What are the environmental effects that come from making the clothes?

Think about where you are going to shop. There are many types of clothing stores. Each type offers different varieties, quality of goods, prices, and services. Some examples of services offered by stores are parking, fashion consultants, credit plans, alterations, gift wrapping, and free shipping.

Store location is another factor when deciding where to shop. Convenience, variety, and price should be considered when choosing among stores located in malls, your neighborhood, or downtown areas. Shop around to find the location that best meets your needs.

Department Stores

Department stores have a wide variety of clothing. The quality and prices are often higher, unless you are able to take advantage of special sales or coupons. Some department stores offer special services. Many are part of national store chains.

Discount Stores

Discount stores can also offer a wide variety of clothing. The quality of the clothes can range from low to high. The prices are generally lower than department stores. Discount stores have fewer salespeople and offer little customer service.

Factory Outlet Stores

Factory outlet stores are owned by manufacturers to sell only their merchandise brands. The prices may be less since items come directly from their factories. The outlets also sell *overstock* clothing, or items produced, but not ordered by retail stores. Sometimes outlets sell clothing

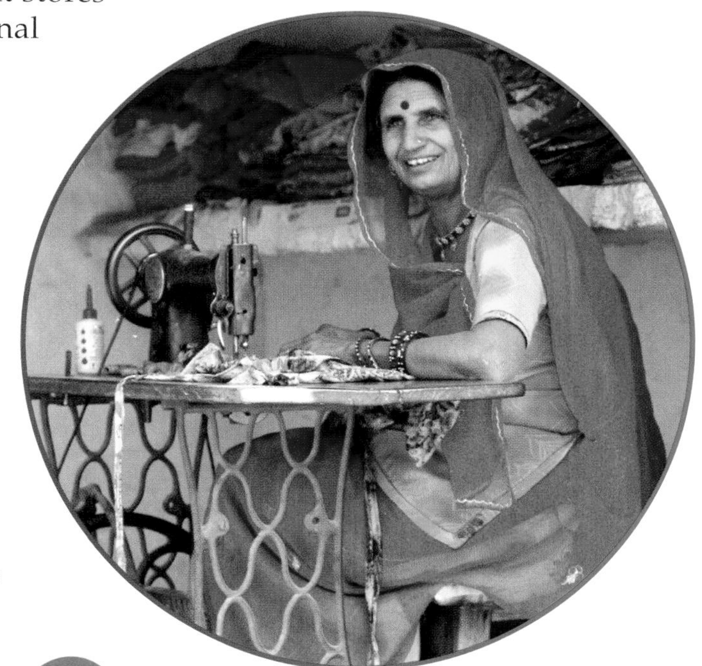

10-4 All countries do not have the same laws as the United States to protect workers. Some even allow children to work in factories.

that may not be perfect or did not pass the first quality inspection at the factory. These products are sold at reduced prices. Services at these stores are often limited, and some stores do not allow returns.

Mail-Order Catalogs

Mail-order catalogs let you buy a wide variety of clothing through the mail, by phone, online, or fax. Pictures and descriptions of the clothing are given. You are not able to try on the clothing, however, to check for fit before ordering. Prices vary, and a delivery charge is often added.

Specialty Stores and Boutiques

Specialty stores sell a limited type of goods, such as shoes, and they can be part of national chains. Sometimes small specialty stores are called *boutiques*. They may specialize in gifts, fashionable clothes, accessories, or food. There can be a wide variety available and quality varies. Prices are sometimes higher than other stores. The services offered depend on the pricing of the merchandise.

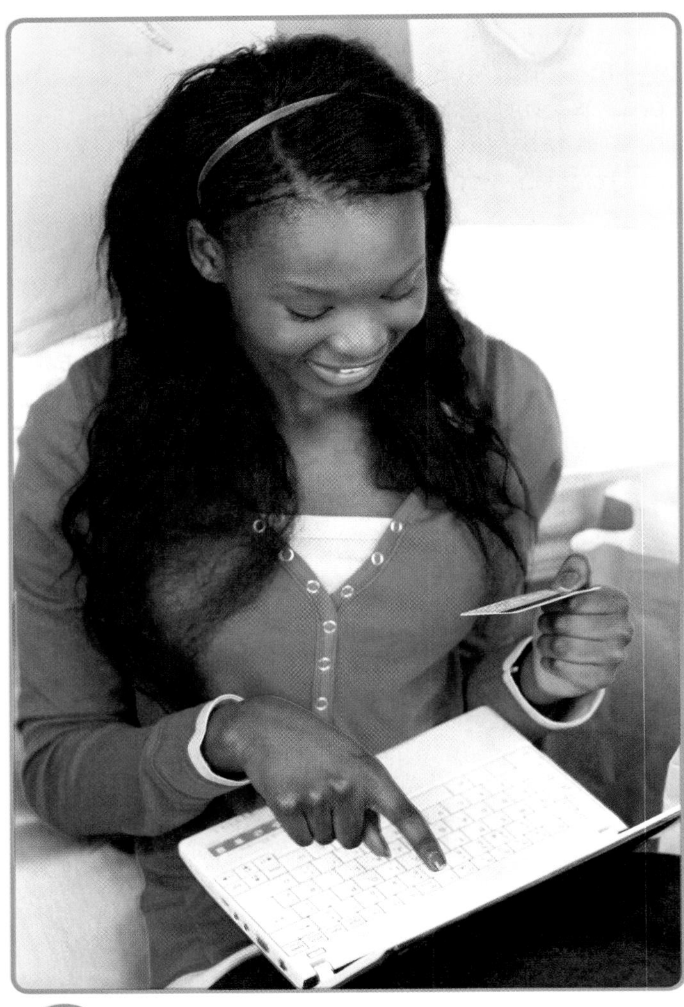

10-5 Ordering clothes online lets you shop without leaving your home.

Off-Price Discount Stores

Off-price discount stores offer brand name merchandise at lower prices. These stores buy overstock clothing from factories at a discount, which is passed on to consumers. Sometimes, they buy from other stores at the end of the season. The prices are less than retail, and there is limited customer assistance.

Online Shopping

You can shop online through the Internet. See **10-5**. You search for an item, see a photo, read a description, and place an order. Most companies require you to use a credit card to place an order. The item is mailed to you. As with mail-order catalogs, you are not able to try the clothing on or check for quality prior to purchase. If the clothing does not fit, you can return it, but usually with additional shipping charges.

Some companies are now offering virtual fit options. **Virtual fit** is a method of using a person's body measurements to show that body image with clothing on the computer. You enter your measurements online. The company's software then generates an image on your computer to show you the fit and suggest a size to buy.

Thrift Shops, Consignment Stores, and Yard Sales

Pre-owned clothing and accessories are sold at thrift shops, consignment stores, and yard sales. The variety and quality vary. Prices can be low. Services are limited. Clothes are often donated to thrift shops to make money for a given charity. At consignment stores, a portion of the sale price is given to the original owner of the garment. Yard or garage sales are held by people at their homes for a limited time.

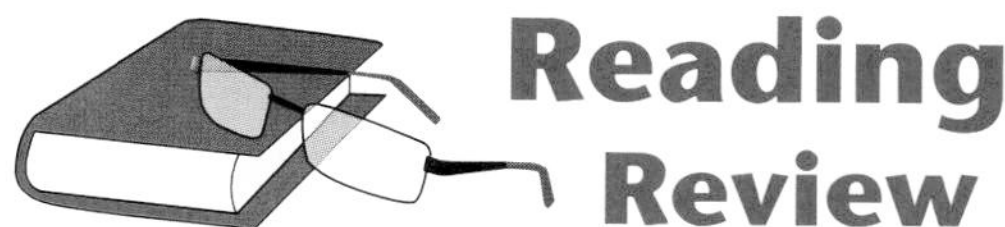

1. Why is the store location important to consider when deciding where to shop?
2. What are the advantages and disadvantages of mail-order shopping?

Shopping Wisely

There are many ways to save money when buying clothes. One way is to shop during store sales. Sales offer clothing at reduced prices. Sales are often held to make room for new merchandise. They usually take place at the end of a season or near holidays. Sales can also attract new customers and encourage current ones to return.

When you look for good buys, resist making spur-of-the-moment purchases. Consider whether you have something in your wardrobe to wear with the item. Will you have to spend more money on additional items to complete your outfit? Never buy anything you do not need just because it is on sale. It is not a good buy if you do not wear it. For instance, you may see a shirt you like on sale. Once you get the shirt home, however, you may find it does not match any of your other clothes. This shirt is not a good buy because you will not wear it. You may even have to spend additional money to buy something else so you can wear the shirt.

Buying pre-owned clothing is another way to save money. It can be a good way to recycle or discover your own fashion style without making a big investment. You can experiment with creative sewing ideas and explore retro or vintage trends. High-quality secondhand clothing is sometimes a better buy than poor-quality new clothing. Choose pre-owned clothes carefully. Buy only clothing that is clean, in good condition, and fits you well. See **10-6**.

Sale Pricing and Value

When you are shopping at sales, look for the original price of the clothing. This will help you decide whether it is a good value. For instance, if a sweater is marked $25.98 on sale, but the regular price is $33.00, you would not save much (just $7.02). If the original price is $40.00, the sweater is a better buy. You are getting more for your money by saving $14.02.

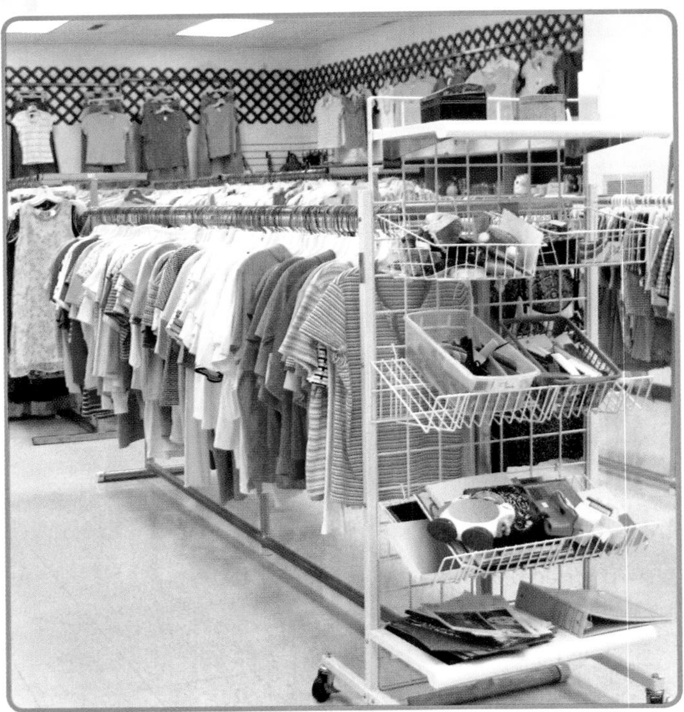

10-6 Thrift stores are good places to find pre-owned clothing for low prices.

Before you buy clothes, always compare quality and price to find a good value. **Value** means buying the highest quality of clothing for the lowest prices. Consult the garment's care label to know how you should care for the garment.

As you learned earlier, you can pay for clothes using cash, checks, and credit, debit, or gift cards. Some stores might offer layaway plans. Decide how you are going to pay and set a realistic budget before you shop. This will save you time when you get to the cash register.

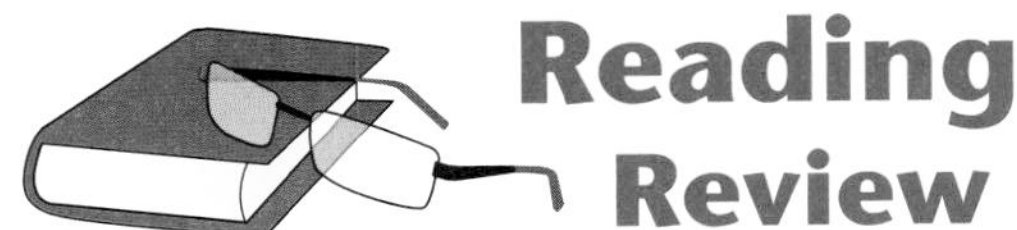

Reading Review

1. Why should you find the original price of a sale item?
2. What should you check for when buying pre-owned clothing?

Your Behavior When Shopping

Using good manners is important when you shop for clothes. It makes shopping more pleasant for everyone—you, the other customers, and the salespeople.

Succeed in Life

Shopping Manners

To make your shopping trips more pleasant for you and others, here are a few tips you can follow:

- Carry your packages low so you can see where you are walking.
- If you bump into someone, excuse yourself.
- If you stop to talk with someone, do not block aisles or doorways. Keep your voice low.
- If you shop during busy times, be prepared to wait for assistance without complaining.
- Avoid using a cell phone and texting when shopping. Be mindful of the sounds you are making with cell phones and other electronic devices when interacting with salespeople. It can be hard for them to help you and annoying to other customers.

If you are having trouble finding a garment you like, ask a salesperson for help. For instance, you may be looking for a green shirt. The salesperson may show you several green shirts. If you do not like any of them, you do not have to buy one. Say "thank you." Then explain you have not seen what you want, but plan to shop some more.

Always try on your selections before buying. This helps you determine if they fit and are flattering on you. Examine the front, sides, and back of the garment carefully for flaws.

When trying on clothes, keep them clean and in good condition. Make sure your hands are clean. If you wear makeup, wipe away any excess. If a garment feels too tight, try on a larger size. Pulling a garment to make it fit may tear it. After trying on clothes, return them to the salesperson on their hangers or folded the way you found them.

Ask the salesperson where to return your unwanted garments. Do not leave them on the floor of the dressing room. Place unwanted clothes back on the hangers or refold them.

When you buy clothing, keep your receipts. Having your receipt makes it easier for you to return or exchange an item. Always find out if the garment you want to buy can be returned or exchanged. Sometimes you will see a sign that says: *All sales final. No returns or exchanges.* Some types of clothing, such as swimsuits, cannot be returned or exchanged. Try them on before you buy them.

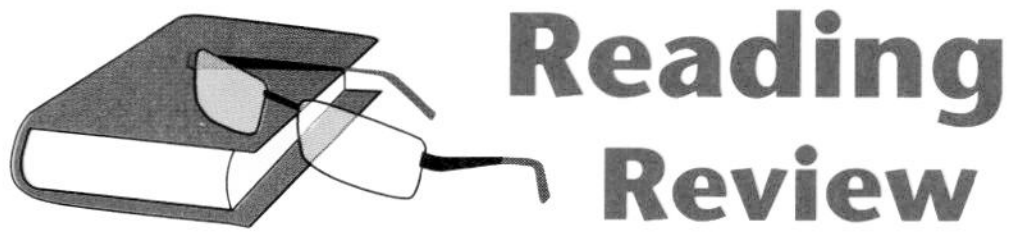

Reading Review

1. How can using good manners make shopping more pleasant for everyone?
2. Why should you keep the receipts for clothing you buy?
3. How should you handle clothes when trying them on? Give examples.

Section Summary

- Before you go shopping, make a buying plan.
- Decide where to shop and how you are going to pay for the items you buy.
- There are many kinds of stores where you can buy clothes.
- Variety, quality, price, and service vary from one store to another.
- Buying clothing on sale or less expensive pre-owned clothing can save money if you shop wisely.
- Always use good manners when shopping.

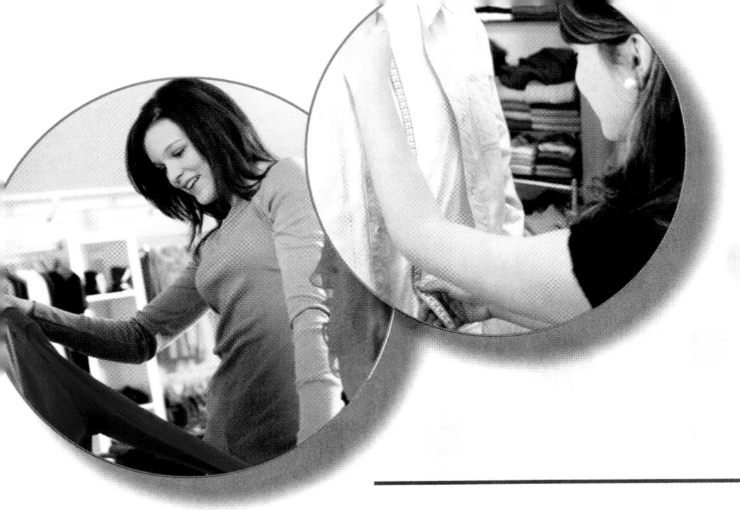

Section 10-3
Inspect Before You Buy

Objectives

After studying this section, you will be able to
- **define** *labels* and *hangtags*.
- **state** why you should read labels and hangtags.
- **show** how to check for quality in clothing.
- **select** clothes that fit correctly and look good on you.

Key Terms

labels: small pieces of cloth sewn into the garment with important information about the garment's fabric content and recommended care.

hangtags: larger tags with information about the garment or manufacturer that are attached to garments, but removed before worn.

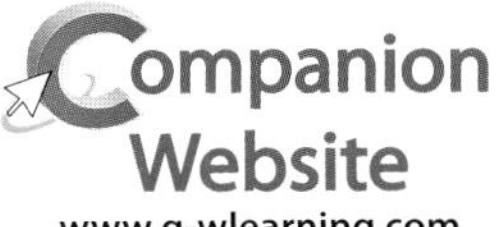

Study the Key Terms by completing crossword puzzles, matching activities, and e-flash cards at the website.

Main Ideas

- Labels and hangtags give you important information about garments.
- Check the quality of clothes before buying them.
- Clothes should fit you properly and look good on you.

When you shop for clothes, you want to get value for the money spent. Decide the quality of clothing you need and take a shopping list with you. This will make choosing clothes easier. Use your wardrobe inventory to make your list. Then add the colors and styles you need. After you find a garment that matches the qualities you desire, inspect the garment for quality. Learn about the suggested care and then try it on to check for proper fit.

Read the Labels and Hangtags

All garments have labels. **Labels** are small pieces of cloth sewn into the garment with important information about the garment's fabric content and recommended care. They are often found at the center back of necklines and waistlines or in the side seams. Sometimes the label information is actually printed on the fabric. There may be more than one label on a garment. It is important to read all of them.

Labels have important information that can help you decide which garments to buy. By law, the labels must state the fiber content, name of manufacturer, and country where the garment was made. Labels may state the size, brand name, and special finishes applied to the garment, too.

Care instructions are also required on garment labels. They must be permanently sewn on the apparel items. Shoes, hats, and gloves are not required to have care labels. A care label must list at least one safe cleaning method. In addition, the label must warn against any cleaning step—washing, bleaching, drying, or ironing—that can harm the garment. For example, if a garment cannot be bleached, the label must say so. Dry cleaning warnings must be included, too. The law requires garment manufacturers to use specific symbols to identify care instructions. See **10-7**.

Most garments have hangtags. **Hangtags** are larger tags with information about the garment or manufacturer that are attached to garments, but removed before worn. Hangtags are not required by law. They may repeat some of the information found on labels. Hangtags may also list the price, size, style number, trademark, guarantees, and any special features. They are also important to read. Extra buttons are often found on hangtags.

After you remove a hangtag, write the date, where you bought the garment, and a short description of the garment on the back. Put this in an envelope with other hangtags or make a wardrobe notebook. Refer to these when you need information about your clothes. You could use a spread sheet on a computer to record your purchases. You may want to scan the labels and take digital photos of the items. Some websites will set up this program for free.

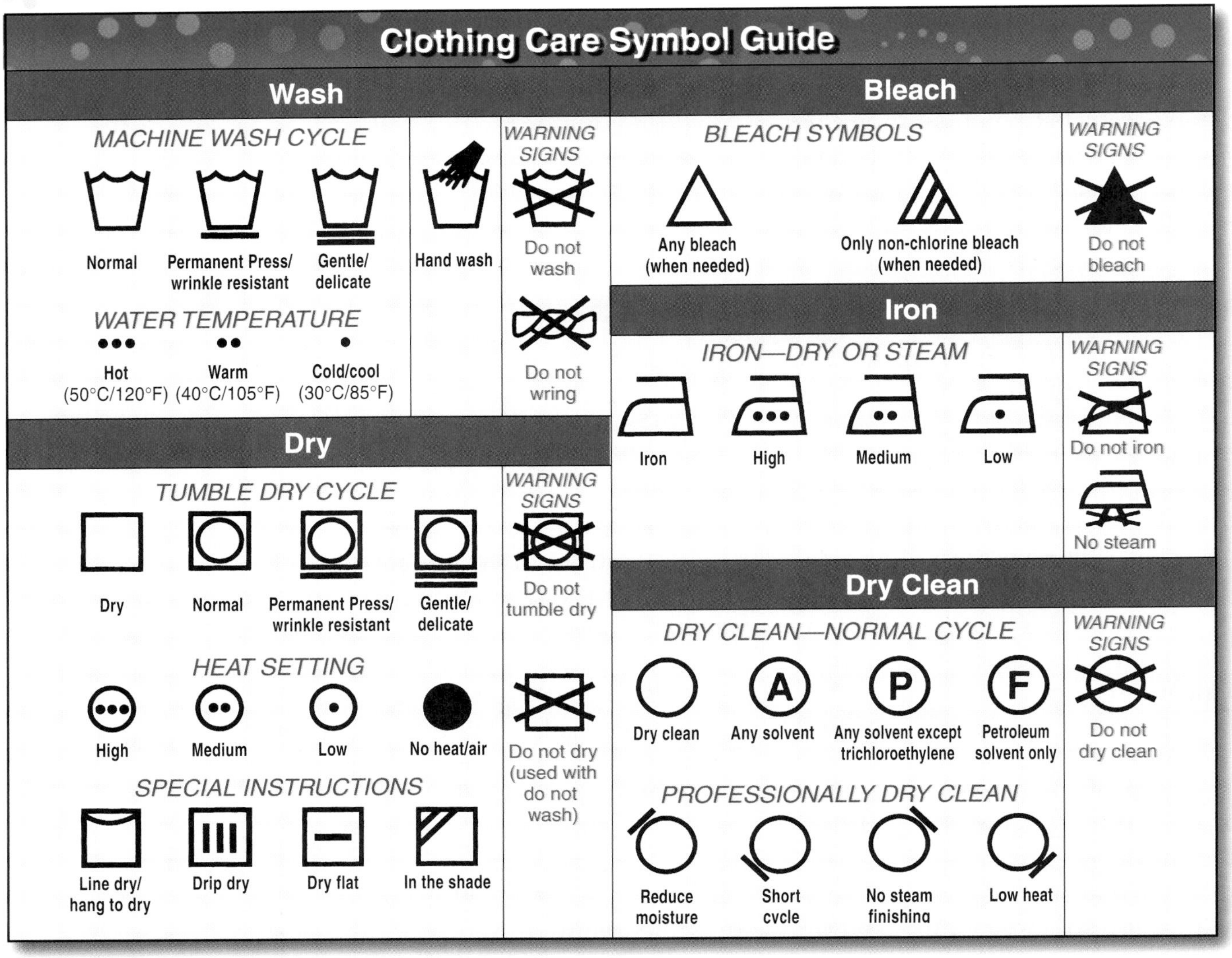

Clothing Care Symbol Guide

Wash

MACHINE WASH CYCLE

Normal | Permanent Press/ wrinkle resistant | Gentle/ delicate

Hand wash

WATER TEMPERATURE

Hot (50°C/120°F) | Warm (40°C/105°F) | Cold/cool (30°C/85°F)

WARNING SIGNS

Do not wash

Do not wring

Dry

TUMBLE DRY CYCLE

Dry | Normal | Permanent Press/ wrinkle resistant | Gentle/ delicate

HEAT SETTING

High | Medium | Low | No heat/air

SPECIAL INSTRUCTIONS

Line dry/ hang to dry | Drip dry | Dry flat | In the shade

WARNING SIGNS

Do not tumble dry

Do not dry (used with do not wash)

Bleach

BLEACH SYMBOLS

Any bleach (when needed) | Only non-chlorine bleach (when needed)

WARNING SIGNS

Do not bleach

Iron

IRON—DRY OR STEAM

Iron | High | Medium | Low

WARNING SIGNS

Do not iron

No steam

Dry Clean

DRY CLEAN—NORMAL CYCLE

Dry clean | Any solvent | Any solvent except trichloroethylene | Petroleum solvent only

PROFESSIONALLY DRY CLEAN

Reduce moisture | Short cycle | No steam finishing | Low heat

WARNING SIGNS

Do not dry clean

10-7 Variations of these symbols appear on care labels to help you know how to care for your clothes.

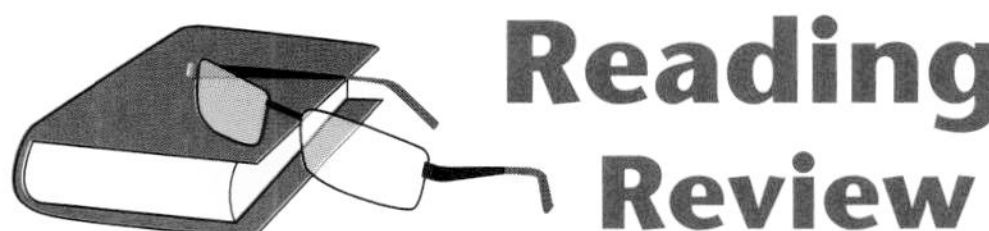

1. By law, what information must be stated on a label? What other information may be included?
2. What should you do after removing a hangtag from a garment?

Check the Quality

Quality measures how well a product is made. Garment quality varies from store to store and even within each store. Just because garments are high priced does not mean they are always of high quality. Check each garment for quality.

You can judge the quality of clothing by looking at how garments are made. Before you buy a garment, look it over carefully. See **10-8**. Look at the construction of both the inside and outside. To see how well a garment is made, check the following points:

- Stitches are small, even in length, neat, straight, and fastened at the ends.
- Thread color matches the color of the fabric.
- Seams are even and lie flat.
- Hems are even and lie flat. Stitching does not show on the outside unless it is a machine-stitched hem.
- Seams and hems are wide enough to be let out if needed.
- Crotch, armhole, and pocket seams are reinforced by extra rows of stitching.
- Openings at the side or neckline allow enough room to put the garment on and take it off.
- Zippers lie flat and zip or unzip easily.
- Hooks and eyes, snaps, buttons, and trims are sewn on firmly.
- Buttonholes fit easily over buttons. They are firmly stitched so they will not ravel or tear.

Sometimes a garment may not meet all of these guidelines. It may have hanging threads and seams that need stitching. Hooks and eyes, snaps, buttons, or trims may be sewn on loosely. The garment can still be a good buy if you are able to repair it at home. If you cannot, the garment is not a good buy. Buttons may come off and seams may rip. You may not be able to wear it and your money will be wasted.

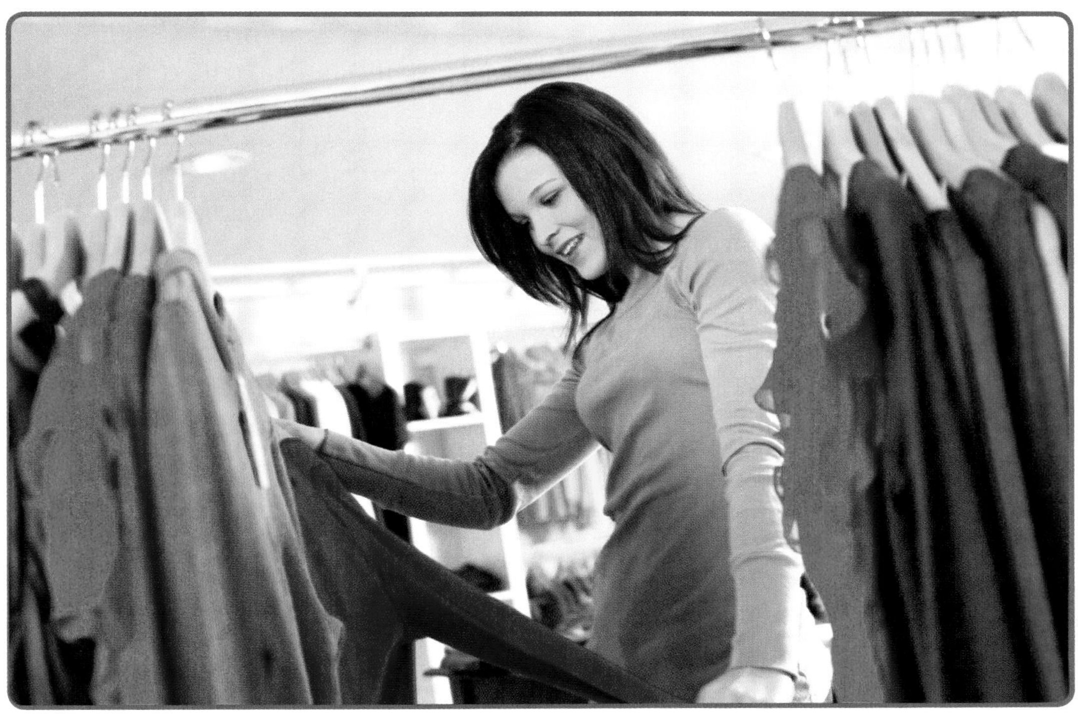

10-8 Carefully inspect a garment for quality before you decide to buy it.

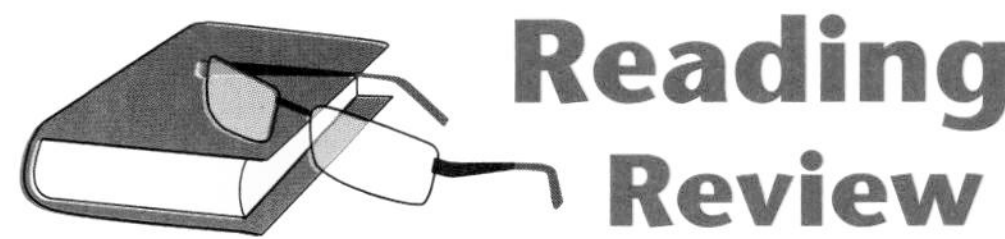

Reading Review

1. What should you check when inspecting a garment for quality?
2. When might a poorly sewn garment be a good buy? Give an example.

Check the Color and Fit

When shopping for clothes, you may notice that some colors often look better on you than others. Just because certain colors are in style does not mean everyone should wear them.

It is generally safe to stay within the color ranges of your hair, eyes, and skin tone. For instance, if you have green or hazel eyes, most shades of green may be attractive on you. If you have an olive or yellow skin tone, many warm colors might look good on you.

Think about your first reaction to the color of your clothes when looking in a mirror. Do they make you feel good? Often, the people you are shopping with can give you advice about which colors look good on you, too.

Even if a garment is the perfect color for you, it is not a good buy unless it fits properly. Good fit in a garment means it is the right size. The length is good for you if it is not too short or too long. The garment fits you properly when it is not too tight or too loose. Clothes feel comfortable when they fit you correctly.

Clothing sizes are divided into categories. The size categories for females and males are described by different names. They are based on body measurements. If you do not know the size category best for you, ask the salesperson for help.

Common size categories for females are Juniors, Misses, and Women's. Some garments are adapted to fit petite, larger, and taller females. This can help you find clothes that fit.

Common size categories for males are Young Men's and Men's. Some clothes for males are designed for different heights and builds. They may be marked *short*, *slim*, *regular*, *husky*, or *tall*.

Some clothing labels will tell you if a garment will shrink when washed or dried in certain ways. This will affect the size you choose. For instance, cotton knits will sometimes shrink when washed in

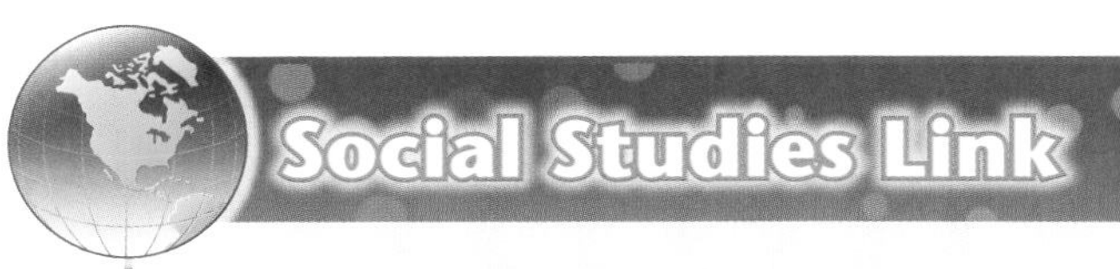

Color and Emotion

When choosing colors for your clothing, remember that color can also affect mood and emotion. For instance, *seeing red* is a common term for anger. Red is also an energetic color; it is not calm. While black tends to be a color that looks good on everyone, it also symbolizes mystery and grief. White is associated with weddings, as well as peace.

Warm, bright colors, such as yellow and orange are eye catching. They are mood lifting. Have you ever noticed that many health clinics and hospitals use subtle shades of green? That is because green often has a calming, healing effect.

hot water. If the label does not tell you, ask the salesperson.

When you shop for clothes, try them on in the store. See **10-9**. Look in a full-length mirror to get the total picture. Check to see how the garment fits in the back as well as in the front. Salespeople may tell you how perfect an outfit is for you. This may or may not be true. Only you can decide.

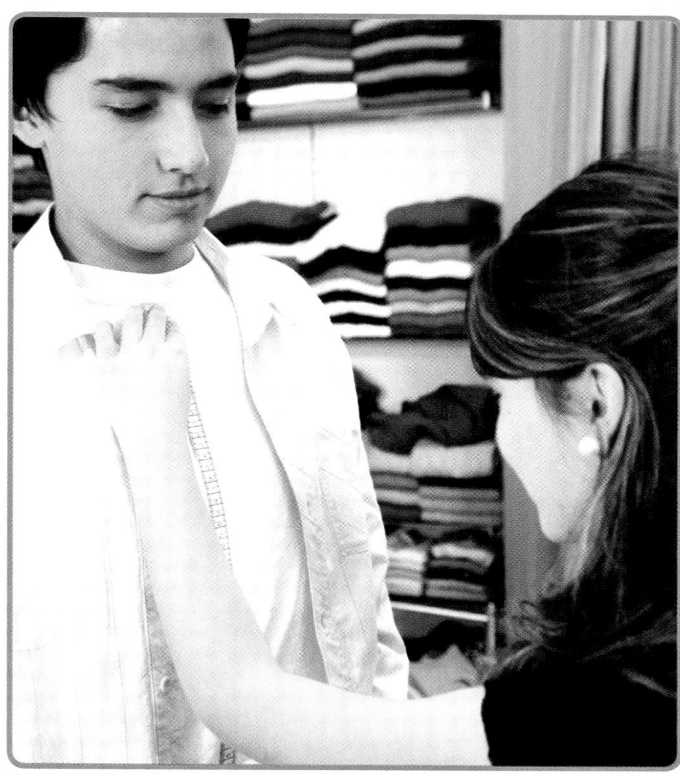

10-9 Take a parent or friend along to help you decide if the clothing you are trying on fits properly.

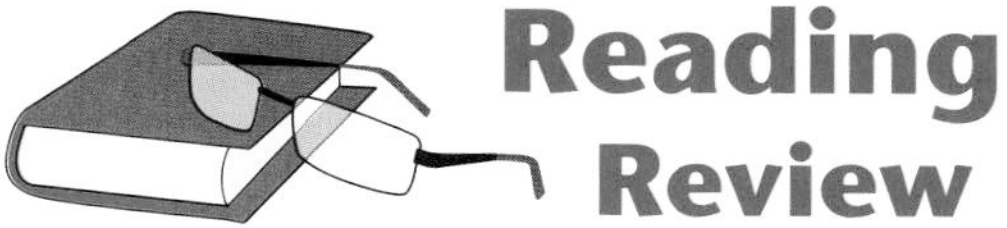

Reading Review

1. How do you know when a garment fits you? Give examples.
2. Why is color important when choosing clothes?
3. How can knowing the different clothing sizes help you find clothes that fit?
4. Why should you try on clothes in the store before you buy them?

Section Summary

- Clothing labels should be read and hangtags should be saved for reference.
- Before buying clothes, check them both inside and out.
- The quality of a garment can be determined by how well it is made.
- Check color and fit to select clothes that look better on you.

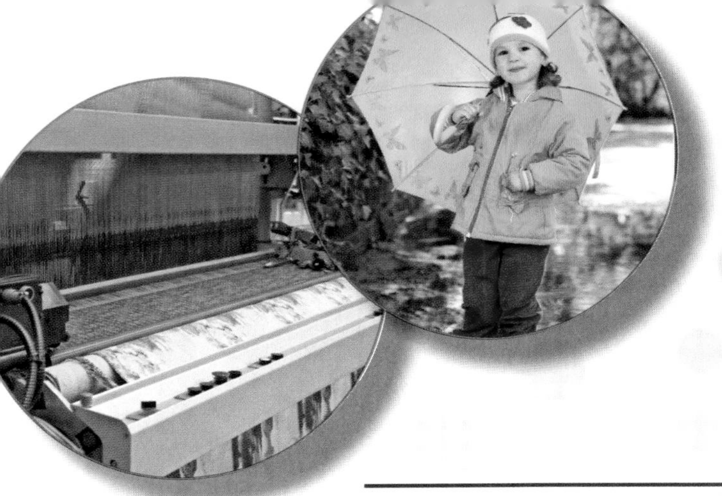

Section 10-4
Fibers and Fabrics

Objectives

After studying this section, you will be able to
- **define** *fibers*, *yarn*, *fabric*, *pilling*, *blend*, and *finish*.
- **list** traits of natural and manufactured fibers.
- **give examples** of how fabrics are made.
- **state** why finishes are applied to fabrics.

Key Terms

fibers: hair-like threads from natural materials that can be twisted together to form yarn.

yarn: a continuous strand of fibers.

fabric: cloth made by knitting or weaving yarns or by pressing fibers together.

pilling: small, fuzzy balls that form on the outside of fabric.

blend: a combination of two or more different fibers, filaments, or yarns.

finish: a treatment given to fibers, yarns, or fabric to improve the look, feel, or performance of a fabric.

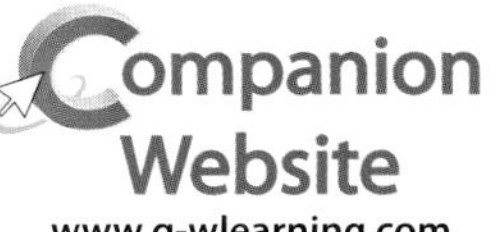

Study the Key Terms by completing crossword puzzles, matching activities, and e-flash cards at the website.

Main Ideas

- Fibers are either natural or manufactured.
- Fabrics can be made by weaving or knitting yarns or by pressing fibers together.
- Finishes are added to improve fabrics.

You may notice some of your clothes feel different from others. Some may keep you warmer or wrinkle easier than others. That is because clothes are made from different fibers, yarns, and fabrics. **Fibers** are hair-like strands that can be twisted together to form yarn. Fibers can be made from either natural substances or man-made chemicals, called *filaments*. **Yarn** is a continuous strand of fibers. **Fabric** is cloth made by knitting or weaving yarns or by pressing fibers together. See **10-10**. This section will discuss how fibers and fabrics are different.

Natural Fibers

There are two types of fibers. One type is natural fibers. These fibers come from plants or animals. The most common natural fibers are cotton, flax, ramie, wool, and silk.

Cotton comes from the fibers found in cotton plants. These fibers are spun into yarn to make fabric. Cotton accepts color dyes easily. It is a strong fiber and soft to the touch. Because it is naturally absorbent, it is cool and comfortable to wear. Cotton wrinkles or shrinks easily, unless treated with special finishes or blended with other fibers that do not shrink. Jeans, shirts, dresses, and underwear are just some of the many garments made from cotton.

Flax is the fiber that makes linen fabric. Like cotton, flax fibers are spun or twisted into yarn. Linen is cool, comfortable to wear, and strong. Without special finishes, it will shrink and wrinkle easily. Linen is used to make dresses, skirts, pants, suits, and handkerchiefs.

Ramie comes from the stems of ramie plants, also called *China grass*. China grass fibers are spun or twisted into ramie yarn. Ramie is shiny and strong. It is often combined with other fibers to add strength. Ramie accepts color dyes easily. It also absorbs moisture and dries quickly. Ramie is similar to linen and can be found in sweaters, shirts, and suits along with other fibers.

Wool comes from sheep fleece. The spinning process can make the yarns soft and fuzzy or smooth and firm. It is durable and lightweight, takes dye easily, and holds creases well. It is warm and comfortable. It also resists wrinkles and water. Wool is often made into sweaters, skirts, coats, pants, suits, and socks.

Silk comes from the cocoons of silkworms. The fibers are very long and strong. Silk is shiny and smooth and takes dye easily. It is comfortable to wear. It can, however, be damaged by sunlight and perspiration. It also needs to be treated with special finishes to resist water stains. Skirts,

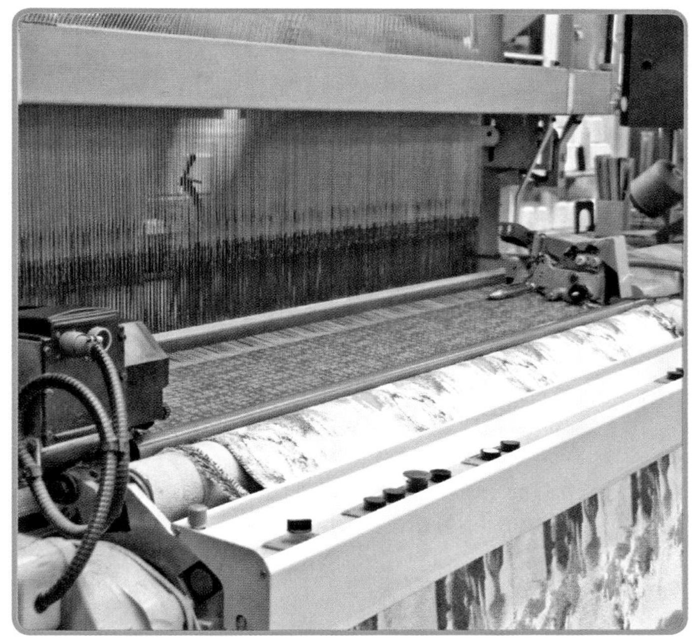

10-10 Many fabrics are woven on industrial looms in factories.

shirts, dresses, neckties, scarves, and lingerie can all be made with silk. See **10-11**.

Clothing made from different natural fibers need different kinds of care. Fabric made from cotton, linen, and ramie should be washed according to the care label instructions. Wool and silk should be dry-cleaned or hand washed.

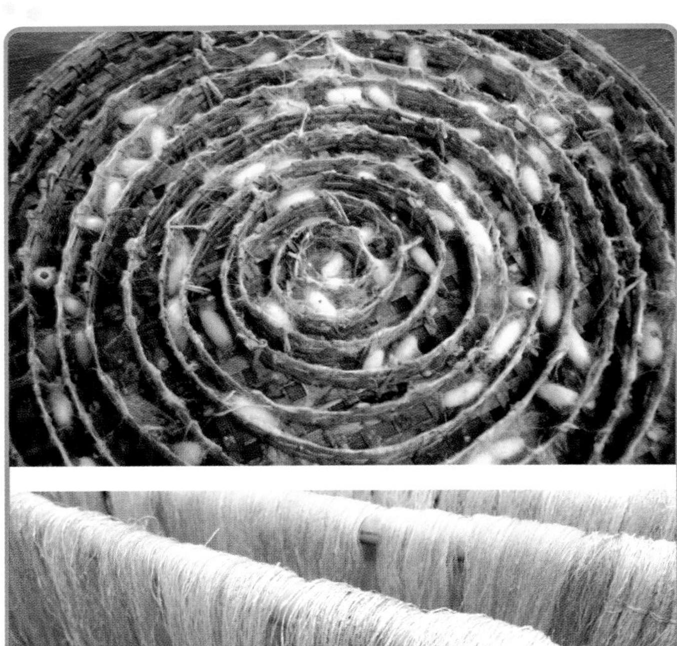

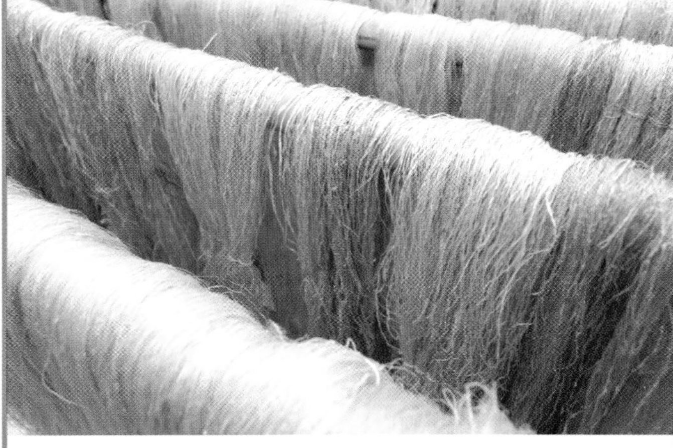

10-11 Silk fabrics start with cocoons made by silk worms. The long silk fibers taken from the cocoons are dyed and then woven into many different kinds of silks.

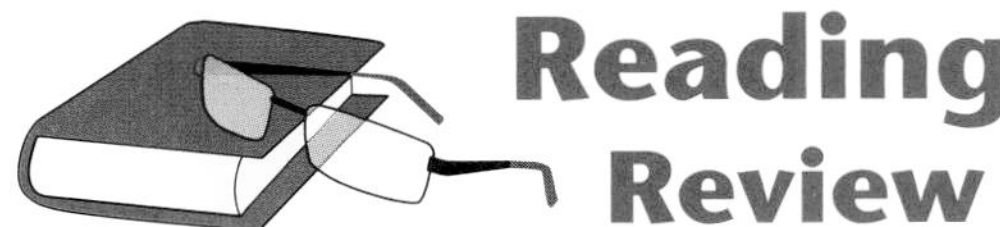

Reading Review

1. How are cotton fibers and flax fibers alike? Give examples.
2. Why do different fibers require different care methods? Explain your answer.

Manufactured Fibers

The other type of fibers is manufactured fibers, or filaments. They are made from chemicals and other raw materials put through a special process that forms hair-like threads. Some common manufactured fibers are rayon, nylon, acrylic, polyester, spandex, and lyocell. Because these fibers have a chemical source, they often feel different from natural fibers.

Rayon can look like cotton. It is soft, comfortable, and takes dye easily. Without a special finish, it can wrinkle. It can also be damaged by light and burns easily. Rayon is used to make garments such as shirts, blouses, dresses, and neckties. In many garment fiber content labels, you may see it listed as *viscose*.

Nylon is strong and holds its shape well. Nylon is uncomfortable in hot weather and can be damaged by strong sunlight. It also absorbs oily stains. Swimwear, hosiery, raincoats, and skiwear are just a few garments made from nylon.

Acrylic is softer than wool and does not feel scratchy. Acrylic resists wrinkles, damage from sunlight, and oils. It takes dye easily. It is heat sensitive and you can have trouble with pilling. **Pilling** are small, fuzzy balls that form on the outside of the fabric. Some garments made from acrylic are sweaters, skiwear, dresses, and socks.

Polyester is strong and holds its shape. It resists wrinkles. It is uncomfortable to wear in hot weather and absorbs oily stains. Pilling can occur with fabrics made of polyester. Many clothes such as shirts, blouses, dresses, suits, and neckties are made from this fabric.

Spandex stretches like rubber, but is more resistant than rubber to sunlight and oils. High temperatures can cause spandex to lose its shape and elasticity. It is often used for swimsuits, ski pants, underwear, and other garments for which elasticity is important.

Although most manufactured fibers are washable, rayon often needs to be dry-cleaned. Be sure to read the care instructions. Many manufactured fibers are sensitive to heat. Use low temperatures when drying and ironing.

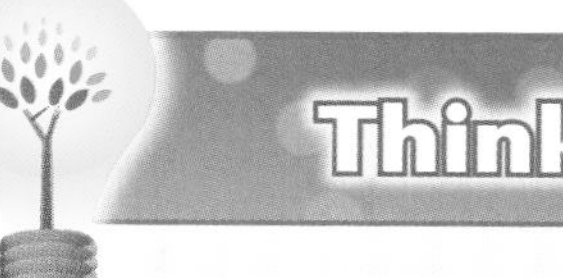

An Eco-Friendly Fiber

Lyocell is a newer manufactured fiber made from wood pulp. One trademark name of lyocell is Tencel®. It is soft to the touch, comfortable to wear, and dyes easily. The process for making lyocell is environmentally friendly. It is often called the *green fiber*. This means the manufacturing process is not toxic to the environment. Lyocell is used to make shirts, blouses, pants, and dresses.

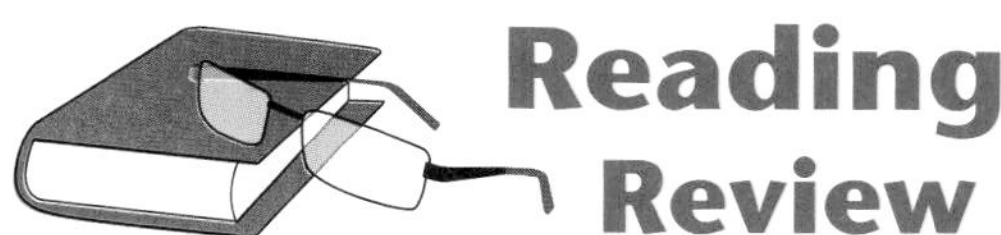

1. Why may clothing manufacturers choose to use manufactured fibers instead of natural fibers?
2. Why should you dry and iron manufactured fibers at low temperatures?

Blends

A combination of two or more different fibers, filaments, or yarns is called a **blend**. Cotton, ramie, rayon, nylon, and polyester are some fibers commonly found in blends. For instance, you may have a shirt made of 65 percent polyester and 35 percent cotton.

A blend combines the positive traits of two or more fibers and reduces the negative traits. For instance, a 100 percent cotton shirt is comfortable to wear in hot weather, but wrinkles easily. A 100 percent polyester shirt does not wrinkle. It is uncomfortable to wear in hot weather, however. A shirt made with a polyester and cotton blend is both comfortable to wear in hot weather and does not wrinkle.

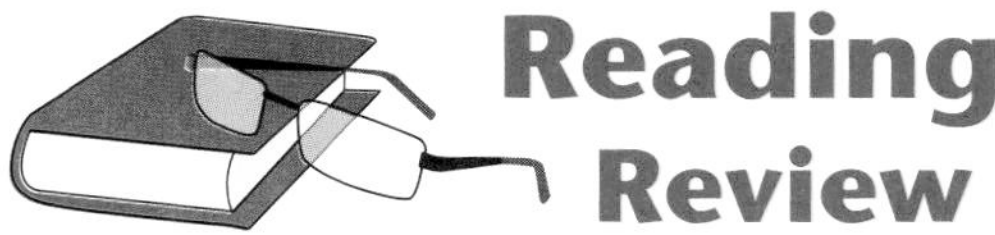

1. What are two fibers commonly found in blends?
2. What is the advantage of using blends to make fabric for clothing?

Fabrics

Fabrics can be made in a variety of ways. The most common include weaving and knitting.

Two sets of yarn are used to weave fabrics. One set of yarn, called *filling*, goes over and under the other set, called *warp*, at right angles. See **10-12**. Some different types of weaves are plain, twill, and satin. Woven fabrics are usually strong and stable. They can take a lot of stress before stretching out of shape.

Knitting is done by looping one or more yarns together on a machine or by hand. Knit fabrics are comfortable to wear. They will stretch and give. Knits are a good choice for a physical activity. Most knits are easy to care for and resist wrinkling. Knits can snag or run though. Washing and drying on high temperatures can cause knits to shrink.

Other construction methods are used to make felt, nonwovens, films, and bonded fabrics.

Short wool fibers make felt. The fibers are fused together by applying heat, moisture, and pressure. Felt can be used for decorations and hats.

Nonwovens are fabrics made from fibers that are held together with glue-like substances. Nonwovens can also be created when heat is used to melt manufactured filaments together. Some nonwoven fabrics are cheaper to make and may be disposable. For example, tea bags, disposable diapers, and some cleaning cloths are made from such nonwoven fabrics. You can also see nonwoven fabrics in the interfacing that is inside some of your garments.

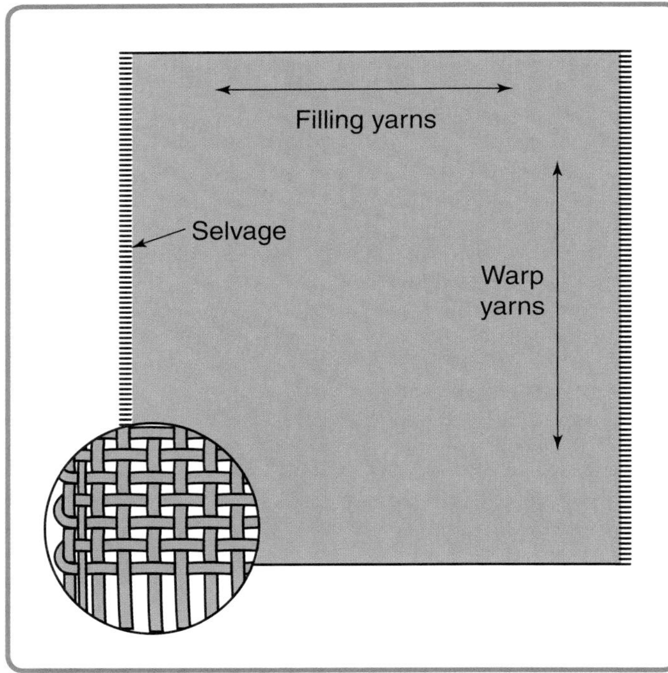

10-12 In fabric weaving, the filling yarns go over and under the warp yarns. At the end of the fabric, they turn and repeat.

Placing a thin sheet of vinyl or urethane, which are types of plastic, on another fabric forms a protective film. See **10-13**. It can make some clothing fabrics look like leather. You often see this in pants, skirts, coats, and handbags.

Bonded fabrics are made when one fabric is glued or laminated to another fabric. This process makes the finished fabric warmer without being heavy. You often see this process used on fabrics for coats and skiwear.

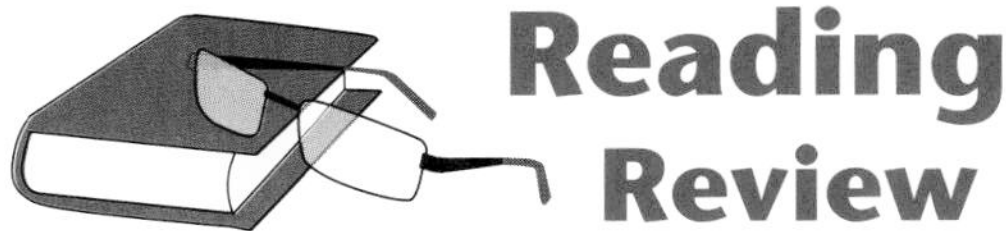

Reading Review

1. What is the difference between weaving and knitting?
2. Describe other ways to make fabrics that are not knitted or woven.

Fabric Finishes

A **finish** is a treatment given to fibers, yarns, or fabrics to improve the look, feel, or performance of a fabric. Garment labels should tell you which type of finish was used on the fabric and how to care for it. Below is a list of finishes you might find on garment labels.

- **Flame resistant:** prevents fabrics from burning easily.
- **Permanent press:** prevents fabrics from wrinkling.
- **Wash-and-wear:** lets fabrics dry without wrinkling.
- **Waterproof:** prevents water from soaking into the fabric.
- **Water-repellent:** helps fabrics resist water.
- **Preshrunk:** prevents fabrics from shrinking more than a small amount.
- **Stain resistant:** helps protect fabrics from staining.
- **Soil release:** helps soaps and detergents release soil when washing.
- **Antimicrobial:** helps protect fabrics from bacteria, mold, and mildew.

Knowing what each type of finish means can help you choose your clothes carefully. For instance, if you are buying a raincoat, make sure it is waterproof. If you are buying cotton jeans, make sure they are preshrunk.

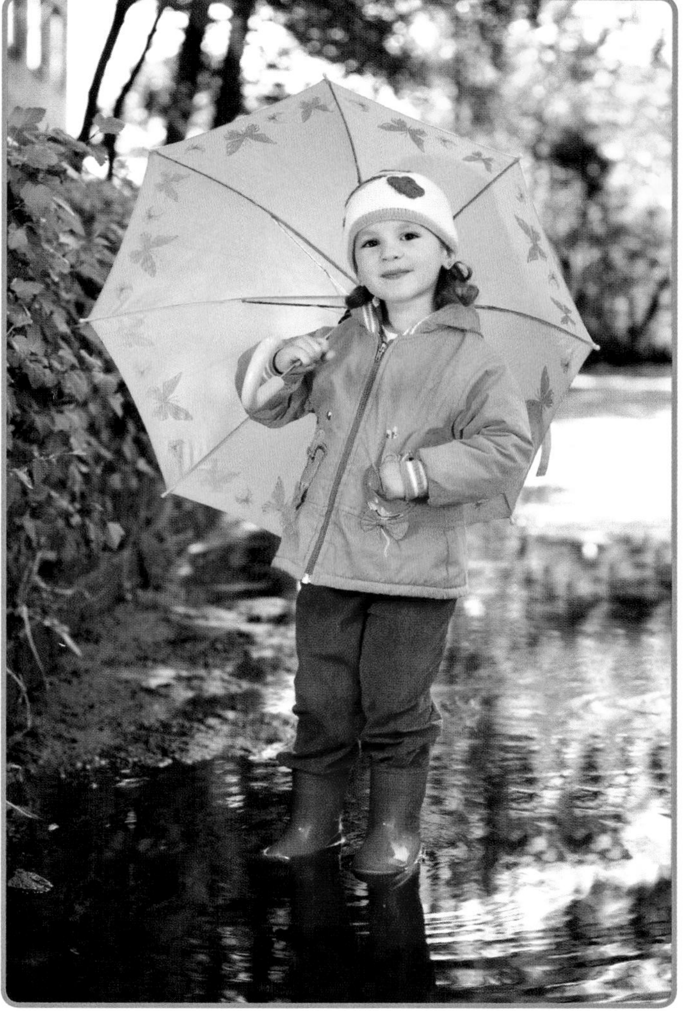

10-13 This girl's boots are water resistant due to the urethane plastic placed on the surface.

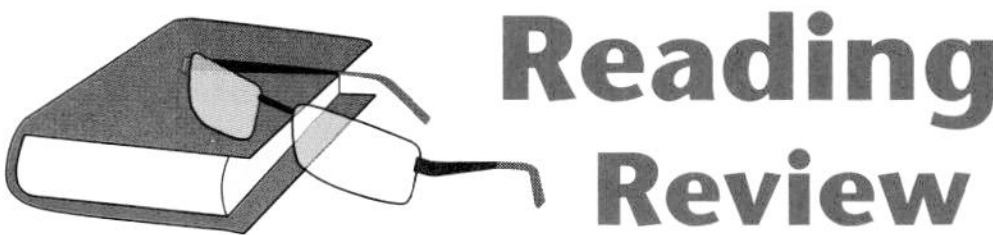

Reading Review

1. How do different finishes improve fabrics? Give examples.
2. How does knowing what each finish means help you choose clothes?

Section Summary

- The fabrics used to make clothes are different. One reason is the type of fibers used to make yarns for fabric. Another is the way those yarns or fibers are made into fabric.
- Special finishes can be added to improve fiber, yarn, and fabric performance.

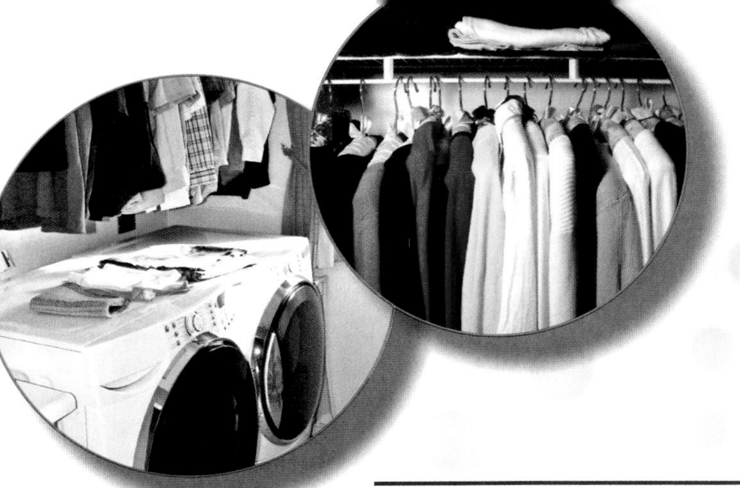

Section 10-5
Caring for Your Clothes

Objectives

After studying this section, you will be able to

- **define** *sort*, *dry-clean*, *iron*, and *press*.
- **identify** different types of laundry products.
- **state** how to wash and dry clothes.
- **explain** the difference between washing and dry-cleaning clothes.
- **demonstrate** how to iron and press clothing.
- **tell** how to store clothes properly.

Key Terms

sort: to group clothes according to the way you will wash them.

dry-clean: to clean with chemicals instead of detergent and water.

ironing: moving an iron back and forth over fabric.

pressing: lifting and lowering an iron onto an area of fabric.

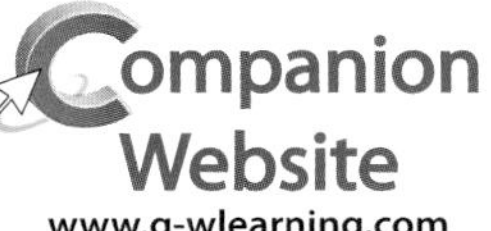

Study the Key Terms by completing crossword puzzles, matching activities, and e-flash cards at the website.

Main Ideas

- Laundry products are used to help clean clothes.
- Clothes can be cleaned by washing or dry cleaning.
- Caring for clothes after they are clean includes ironing, pressing, and proper storage.

After you spend the time to plan and build your wardrobe, take care of your investment. If you get a stain on your jeans, remove it right away. If you buy a *Dry-Clean Only* shirt and wash it, you may not be able to wear it again. When you take proper care of your clothes, they will look better and last longer. See **10-14**.

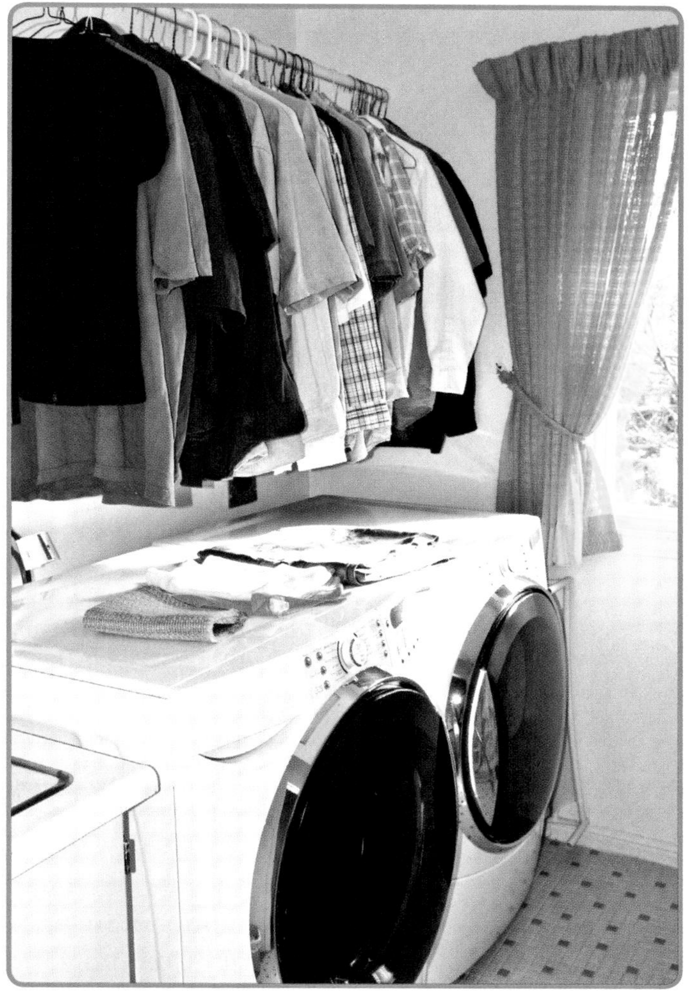

10-14 Taking care of your clothes includes using the recommended products for washing and drying them correctly, plus keeping them wrinkle free.

Laundry Products

To care for your clothing correctly, use the proper laundry products. There are many types of laundry products to clean your clothes. The type you choose depends on the fabric in the garment and the amount of dirt present.

Prewash products are used to remove oily stains and dirt from clothes before they are washed. Prewash products are rubbed into stains and hard-to-clean areas, such as collars and cuffs. They come in liquid, spray, and stick form.

To wash the clothes, you can choose from mild or all-purpose *soaps* and *detergents*. Soap is gentler on the skin than detergent. Mild soaps and detergents are best for delicate fabrics and baby clothes. Use all-purpose soaps and detergents for basic laundry needs. Be sure to use the correct amount of soap or detergent as listed on the product instructions.

Liquid and powder *bleaches* are chemicals that will lighten fabrics and sometimes remove all color. They also help remove stains. The correct amount of bleach must be used. Otherwise, it can damage or make holes in a fabric. Add bleach to the water before adding the clothes. Check the care label to make sure the garment can be bleached.

Fabric softeners are used to make fabrics feel better against your skin. They also help reduce wrinkling and static electricity. Some fabric softeners are added to the wash load during the wash or rinse cycle. Other fabric softeners come in the form of sheets to put in the dryer. Some softeners can affect the flame-retardant finish on fabrics, such as those used for children's nightwear. If you use a fabric softener, follow the directions on the package for the best results.

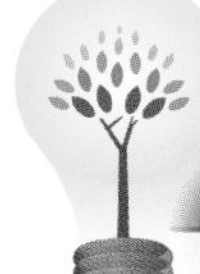

Think Green

The Eco-Friendly Laundry

Some laundry products are petroleum-based and can have negative effects on the environment. Eco-friendly products are biodegradable and contain no brighteners, dyes, or artificial fragrances. *Biodegradable* means a substance can be broken down and absorbed into the environment without harm.

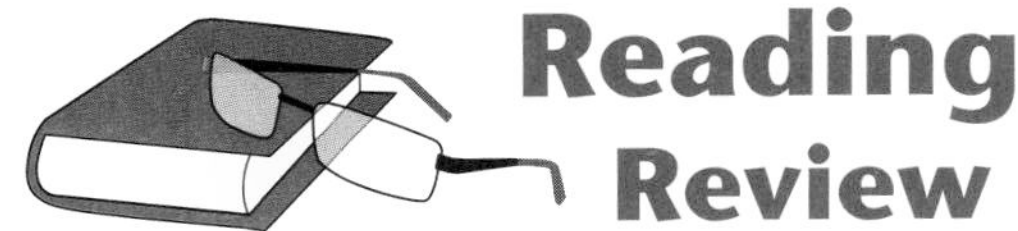

Reading Review

1. What can happen if you are not careful when using bleach?
2. What are some benefits of using a fabric softener?

Washing and Drying Clothes

To machine wash clothes, you first must sort them. **Sort** means to group clothes according to the way you will wash them. Check care labels before you sort clothes. Sort white and light-colored clothing from dark clothing. Very dark-colored clothes should be sorted into another pile. If you buy a garment with a bright or deep color, such as red, wash it by itself the first time. Some of the colored dye may come out in the water and change the colors of other items in the load. For instance, if you accidentally wash a bright red top with a load of whites, the clothes would most likely come out pink.

After you sort your clothes by color, check each pile to be sure all the clothes should be washed in the same temperature water. Care labels will show which water temperature to use. Hot water is often good for light-colored and white preshrunk, natural fabrics. Warm water is good for most fabrics. Use cold water for brightly colored and dark fabrics. Most manufactured fibers are heat sensitive and cannot be washed or dried at high temperatures.

As you are sorting the garments, look for any rips, tears, or holes in the clothing. These will need to be repaired before you wash the garment. Close all buttons, zippers, hooks and eyes, and snaps. Check pockets for any items that could ruin the garments in the wash. For instance, tissue left in a pocket can leave lint on all your other clothes.

Treat stained garments with a prewash product before washing. You can also rub soap and detergent into very dirty areas. Treat stains as soon as they occur. Otherwise, they will be difficult to remove. See **10-15**.

Wash each pile of clothes separately. Delicate fabrics need to be washed on a gentle cycle. Very dirty clothes should be washed by themselves. Baby clothes also need to be washed separately. This prevents them from coming into contact with germs from the regular family wash.

Most clothing can be dried in an automatic dryer. Check the care label to see how a garment should be dried. Use the correct setting on your dryer for the fabric. If your clothes are overdried, the fabric may be damaged. Remove clothes from the dryer as soon as they are dry to prevent wrinkling. Hang any garments you can on hangers. Then smooth out collars, cuffs, and seams with your hands to help remove wrinkles.

Stain Removal Guide

- ***Ballpoint pen ink.*** Apply rubbing alcohol or hair spray to stain until wet. Rub in detergent. Wash.
- ***Blood.*** Soak stain in cold water. Rinse. Rub detergent into stain and wash. If stain remains, apply a few drops of ammonia. Wash again.
- ***Chewing gum.*** Harden gum with ice. Scrape gum off with a dull knife. Apply a prewash product to remaining stains. Then wash in hot water.
- ***Chocolate.*** Scrape off with a dull knife. Rinse stain from the back with cold water. Rub liquid detergent on stain and let set for 5 minutes. Soak stain in cold water for 5–10 minutes. Rub stained area. Rinse. Repeat until stain is removed.
- ***Grease.*** Rub in detergent to loosen stain. Let stand. Wash in hot water. If stain remains, apply a prewash product and wash again.
- ***Ketchup.*** Soak stain in cold water for 30 minutes. Rub with detergent. Wash in hot water.
- ***Soft drinks.*** Sponge stain with cool water. Wash with bleach if safe.

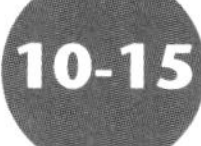

Most stains can be removed. Here are the removal methods for a few common stains.

You may need to line dry some clothes. You can do this by hanging them outdoors on a clothesline. You can also hang them indoors over a bathtub or in a shower.

Delicate and knit garments may stretch out of shape if they hang while wet. These items may need to be laid flat to dry. Make sure the surface or rack where they are laid has good air circulation and will not be harmed by the wet clothes. The garment may need to be turned occasionally so it can dry on all sides.

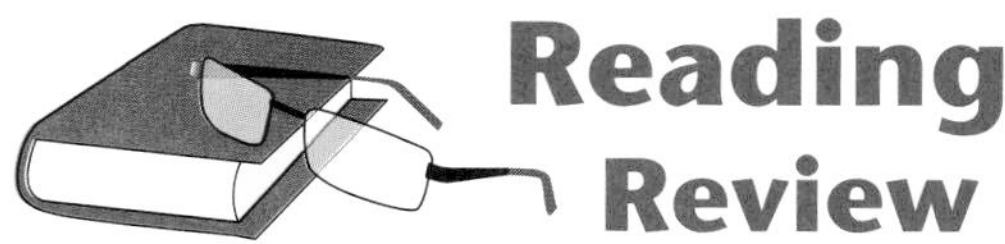

1. What are three things you should do as you sort clothes?
2. What are two ways clothes can be dried?

Dry-Cleaning Clothes

Some garments you buy may need to be dry-cleaned. **Dry-clean** means to clean with chemicals instead of detergent and water. If the care label says *Dry-Clean Only*, the garment may be ruined if machine washed.

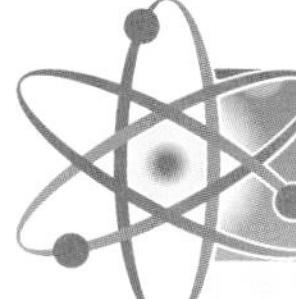

Science Link

Dry-Cleaning at Home

It is possible to dry-clean your clothes at home using a special kit and a dryer. The kit will contain a liquid stain remover, reusable bag, and premoistened cloth. You pretreat the stains and place up to four items in the reusable bag with the premoistened cloth in a dryer. The heat from the dryer activates the cloth and chemicals to remove stains and odors.

Garments made of silk or wool often need to be dry-cleaned. Garments that have decorative trims, such as beads and sequins, may also require dry cleaning.

Dry cleaning is usually done by a professional dry cleaner. Professional dry cleaners remove stains as well as provide general cleaning. If you have a stain or spot, tell your dry cleaner about it so the stain can be removed. Some fabrics, such as fur, leather, or suede, need to be dry-cleaned differently. The care label will tell you how.

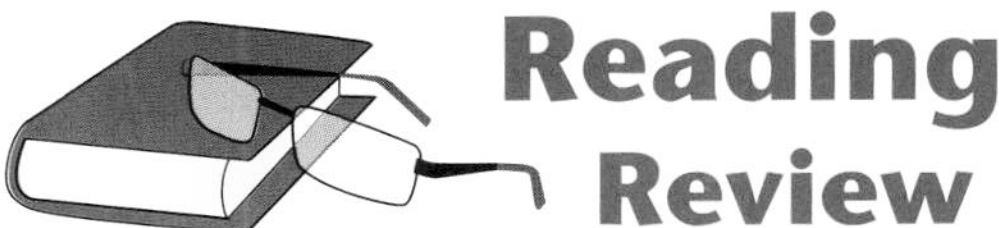

1. What is the difference between dry cleaning and washing clothes?
2. What are two ways you can dry-clean clothes?

Ironing, Pressing, and Storing Clothes

Ironing and pressing are two ways to remove wrinkles from garments. **Ironing** is moving an iron back and forth over fabric. **Pressing** is lifting and lowering an iron onto an area of fabric. Pressing is good for fabrics such as knits and wools. It prevents the fabrics from stretching.

Most irons have different temperature settings for different fabrics. Some fabrics melt or burn if the iron is too hot. If you are not sure about the right setting for a fabric, check the care label.

When removing wrinkles from a garment, first press small areas, such as cuffs and collars. Then iron the larger areas, such as shirt backs. Press dark fabrics and wools on the wrong side, meaning inside out. This will keep the fabric from developing a shiny look on the surface.

After clothes have been washed, dried, and ironed or pressed, they need to be stored properly. Hang clothes such as skirts, pants, blouses, shirts, and dresses on hangers. Clothes such as sweaters and knits should be folded and stored flat on shelves or in drawers. Do not crowd stored garments together. They may become damaged, wrinkled, or stretched out of shape. See **10-16**.

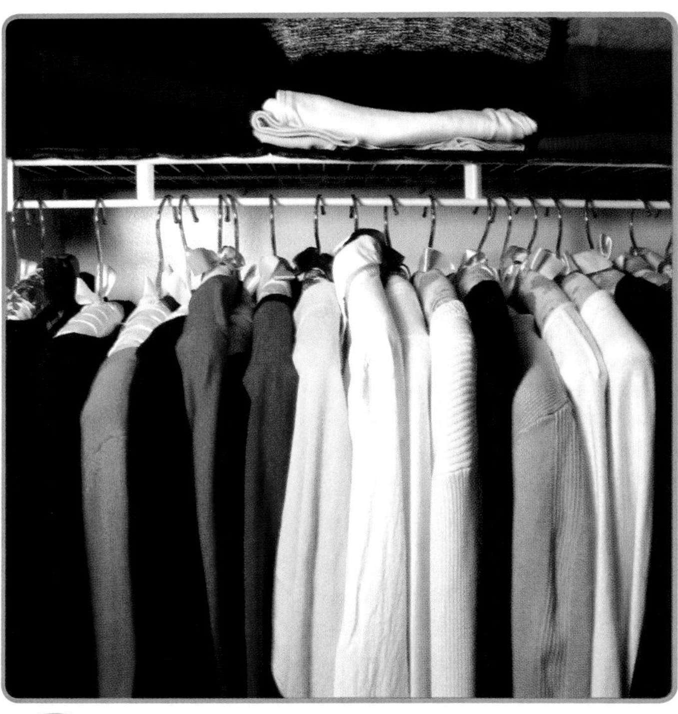

10-16 Properly stored clothes stay neat and are always ready to wear.

If you live in a part of the country where seasons change, you may need to store some of your clothes during the summer or winter. Store your clothes in dry, cool places away from sunlight. Make sure your clothes are clean before you store them. Stains you do not notice may become worse over time. You also need to be careful of insects that eat fabric. You can use moth repellents to keep them away from your clothes. You can also use natural ingredients such as cedar, cinnamon sticks, or lavender to repel insects.

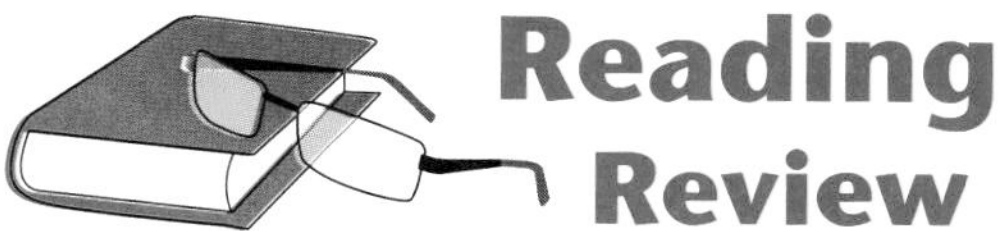

Reading Review

1. How do you know which setting to use on your iron for different fabrics?
2. How can you store clothes so they will not wrinkle or stretch out of shape?

Section Summary

- Caring for your clothes is very important.
- When you wash, dry, iron, press, and store your clothes properly, they will look better and last longer.
- Always follow the care instructions and use the right laundry products. This will prevent your clothes from being damaged and will keep them in good shape.

Chapter Summary

To build a wardrobe, first consider your clothing needs. Based on these needs, you can make a plan for purchasing them. Taking a wardrobe inventory can help you do this. The inventory will let you know what clothes and accessories you have and what you still need.

After you plan your wardrobe, make a buying plan. This consists of deciding where to shop and how to pay for your clothes. Think about variety, quality, price, service, and location.

A buying plan will help you be more organized. This gives you time to look for the best buys. Another way to get value for your money is to inspect clothes before you buy them. Read labels and hangtags. Check the quality and the fit. Clothes that fit properly and are of high quality look better and you will wear them longer.

Knowing about the different fiber and fabric choices in clothing can help you make good shopping decisions. Each fiber has a different trait. Knowing these traits can help you choose clothes that are best for you and your activities.

Taking good care of your clothes will help them look better and last longer. Caring for your clothes includes sorting, washing, drying, ironing, pressing, and storing. Be sure to follow the care instructions and use the right laundry products. This will keep your clothes in good shape and prevent damage. Some clothes may need to be dry-cleaned instead of washed. Washing can ruin these clothes.

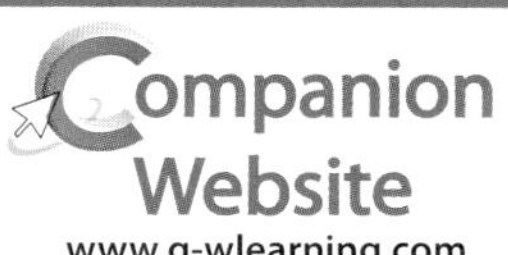

Review Key Terms and Main Ideas for Chapter 10 at the website.

Chapter Review

Write your answers on a separate sheet of paper.

1. Give one example each of a garment needed for a certain standard of dress, activity, and climate.
2. Explain the difference between a fad and a classic.
3. Name two advantages of taking a wardrobe inventory.
4. List three factors to consider when deciding where to shop.
5. List five different types of clothing stores. Name one advantage and one disadvantage of shopping at each.
6. List three ways to save money when shopping for clothes.
7. True or false. You should always keep the sales receipts for your purchases.
8. What is the difference between a label and a hangtag?
9. What are three guidelines to use when checking quality in a garment?
10. Name three natural fibers.
11. What finishes should you look for when buying rain boots, children's sleepwear, blue jeans, and clothes for working in the garden?
12. True or false. Wait several days to treat stains.
13. What could happen if you wash clothes labeled *Dry-Clean Only*?
14. (Ironing/Pressing) is moving the iron back and forth over the fabric to remove wrinkles. (Circle the correct word.)
15. List three hints for storing clothes.

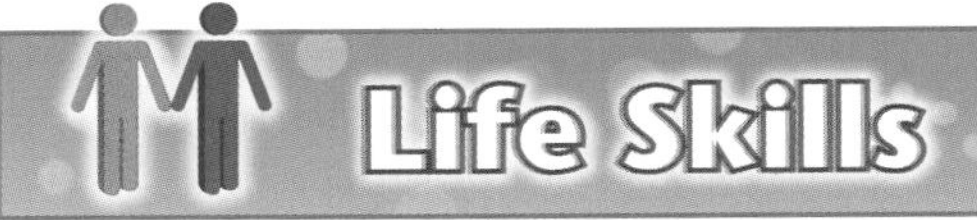

16. Complete a wardrobe inventory of your clothes and accessories. Use the suggested form in the text. Make a plan to discard the clothes you no longer wear. Then make a list of clothes and accessories you would like to add to your wardrobe. Determine the types of stores that might have the clothes you need. Also, think about ways you could save money when shopping for your clothes. Why does making a clothing plan help you be a smarter consumer?

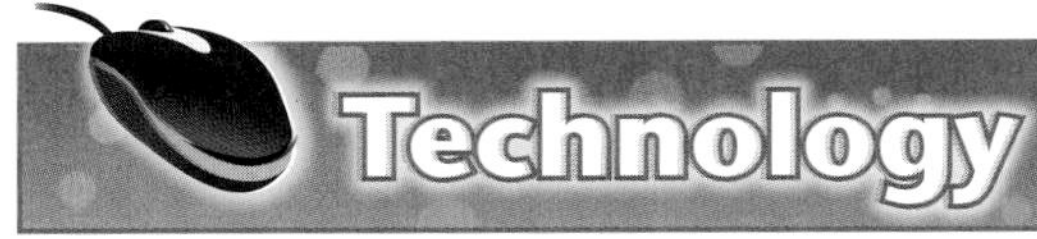

17. Using a search engine on the Internet, research ways you could conserve energy while washing and drying your clothes. Has your family used any of these conservation methods in the past? How well did they work? Discuss your research findings as a class and compare different results.

18. If you were given the opportunity to open a boutique or specialty store, what would you sell? In your journal, write about the kind of boutique you might want to own. What would it look like? Where would you get the products to sell? Who would buy your products? What kind of salespeople would you hire and why? How did your goals and values affect the kind of boutique or specialty store you wrote about? Is this a possible career for you in the future?

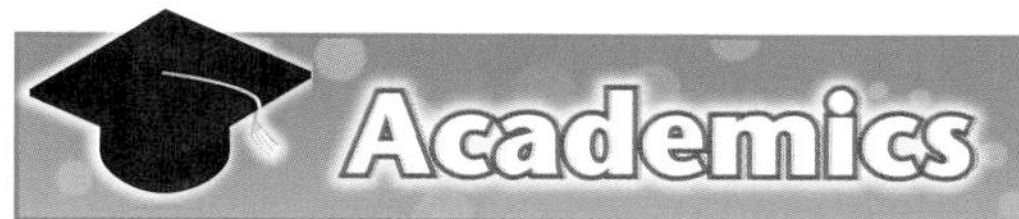

19. **Financial Literacy.** Call two local dry cleaners. Ask for the price of dry-cleaning garments, such as pants, coats, and dresses. Compare prices between the two stores. If one has higher prices, what would be the reasons?
20. **Science.** Make a chart showing the advantages and disadvantages of various types of manufactured fibers. List how they are made and the raw materials or chemicals used. Share this with your friends and family to help them make better clothing choices.
21. **History.** Interview three adults of different ages about fads that were popular when they were your age. Ask them if any of these fads have become popular again. Summarize your findings in a short report to share with the class.

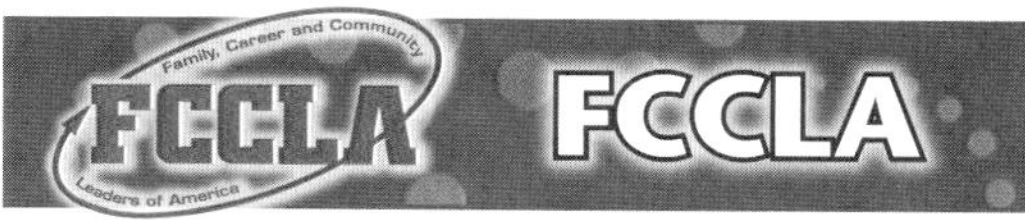

22. Have you ever bought an item, wore it once, and then had to throw it away? Why did this happen? Sometimes clothing purchased for low prices are not really a very good purchase. Pick several items of clothing or accessories you bought for various prices and compare how long they lasted (or you expect them to last). Also, determine how many times you either wore, or might wear, them. Develop a *cost per wearing* form to help you learn about price, value, and quality. Create an FCCLA *Unit Pricing* project for the *Financial Fitness* program. Obtain further information about this program from your FCCLA advisor.

Chapter 11
Learning to Sew

Sections

11-1 Sewing and Serging
11-2 Preparing to Sew
11-3 Sewing Your Project
11-4 Repairing, Altering, and Recycling Your Clothes

Sharpen Your Reading

Make a list of everything you already know about the topic of this chapter. As you read the chapter, check off the items that are covered in the chapter.

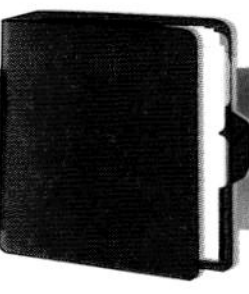

Concept Organizer

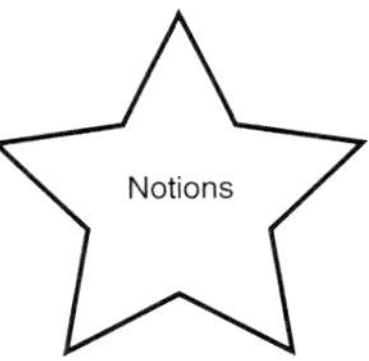

Use a star diagram like the one shown to list the five common types of notions needed for sewing projects.

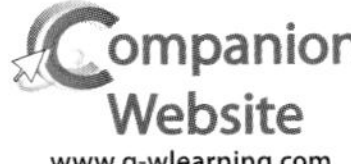

Print out the concept organizer at the website.

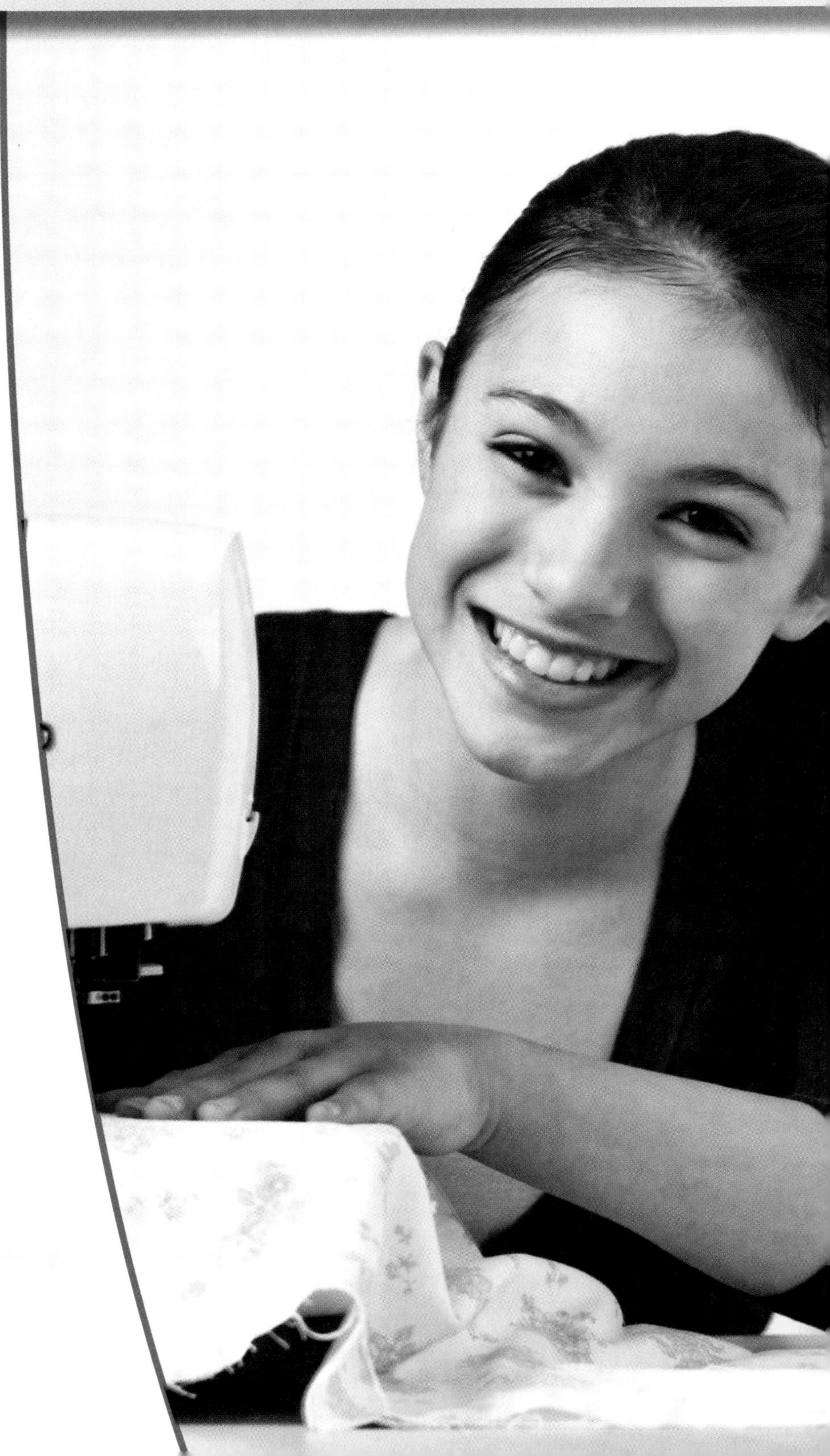

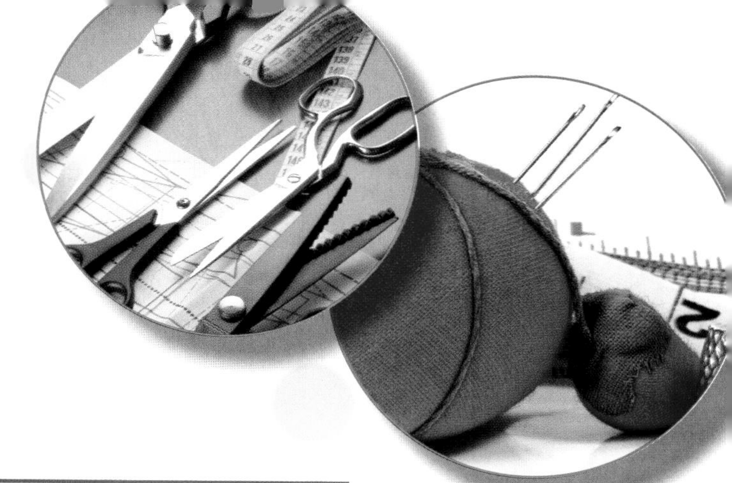

Section 11-1
Sewing and Serging

Objectives

After studying this section, you will be able to
- **define** *serger*, *overlock stitches*, and *raveling*.
- **explain** the benefits of sewing.
- **identify** the parts of a sewing machine.
- **list** the basic sewing tools.
- **describe** how to behave when you are in the sewing lab.
- **demonstrate** how to work safely with others in a sewing lab.

Key Terms

serger: a type of high-speed sewing machine that sews, trims, and finishes seams at the same time.

overlock stitches: stitching to prevent seams from raveling.

raveling: when threads pull out of the cut edges of a fabric.

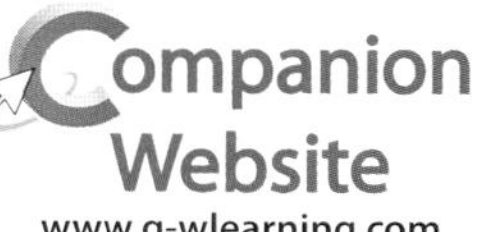

Study the Key Terms by completing crossword puzzles, matching activities, and e-flash cards at the website.

Main Ideas

- Use and care manuals tell you how to use your sewing machine properly.
- Sewing tools are used to measure, mark, cut, and sew fabric.
- It is important to help keep the sewing lab clean and neat.
- Safe sewing habits can protect you from accidents.

Sewing can be both fun and useful. You can make clothes or other items for yourself or your family and friends. You can make these special by choosing the styles and colors you want. This will save you money. You can also repair your clothes. You can change clothes you have by redesigning or recycling them.

Sewing Machines

Sewing machines make sewing easier. Before you start sewing, however, learn some basics. For instance, you will need to learn how a sewing machine works and which tools to use. Also, you should become familiar with working in a sewing lab and following the safety rules.

Sewing machines have many parts. Each of these parts performs a different task. See **11-1**. Read the *use and care manual* to locate the parts on your sewing machine. Find out how these parts work. The use and care manual will also tell you how to set up, store, and care for your sewing machine.

Before you begin a sewing project, read your use and care manual carefully. It will let you know about the different kinds of stitches your sewing machine makes. It will also provide instructions for threading the sewing machine and making stitches.

All sewing machines make straight stitches and backstitches. Conventional sewing machines also make buttonholes and can insert zippers. You will also need to learn about how to control the speed and stop at the desired point. Your teacher may show you how to do these tasks.

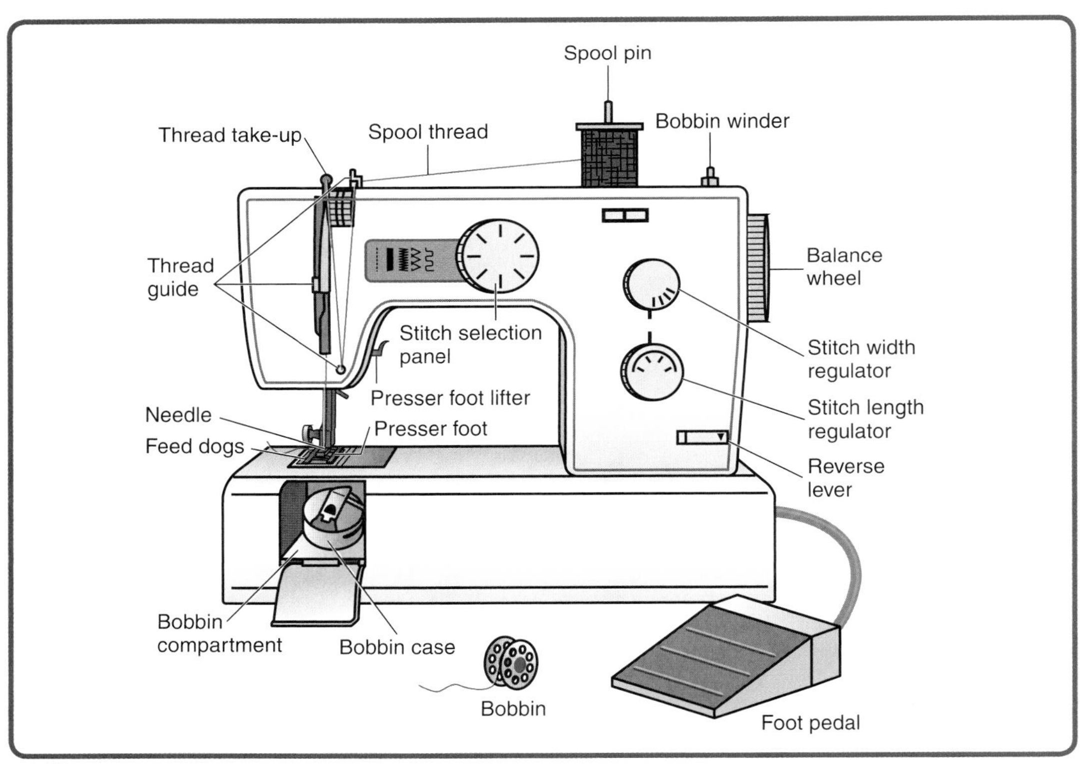

11-1 While all sewing machines are not alike, they have the same basic parts.

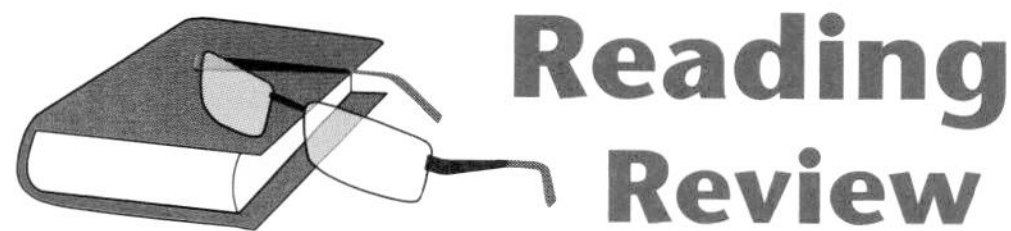

Reading Review

1. What information can you find in your sewing machine's use and care manual?
2. What are three things that can be done using a conventional sewing machine?

Sergers

A **serger** is a type of high-speed sewing machine that sews, trims, and finishes seams at the same time. Sergers use **overlock stitches** to prevent seam edges from raveling. **Raveling** is when threads pull out of the cut edges of a fabric. Different types of overlock stitches are better for different types of fabrics. When beginning a project, your teacher can help you decide which type is best for your fabric. Some overlock stitches can also be used as decorative design elements in clothing.

Sergers look and operate differently from conventional sewing machines. See **11-2**. They use up to five large, cone-shaped spools of thread, depending on the type of stitch. These spools can be different colors, and are held on *cones*, instead of bobbins.

Sergers sew much faster than conventional sewing machines, but cannot perform as many functions. Therefore, they are often used in addition to conventional sewing machines.

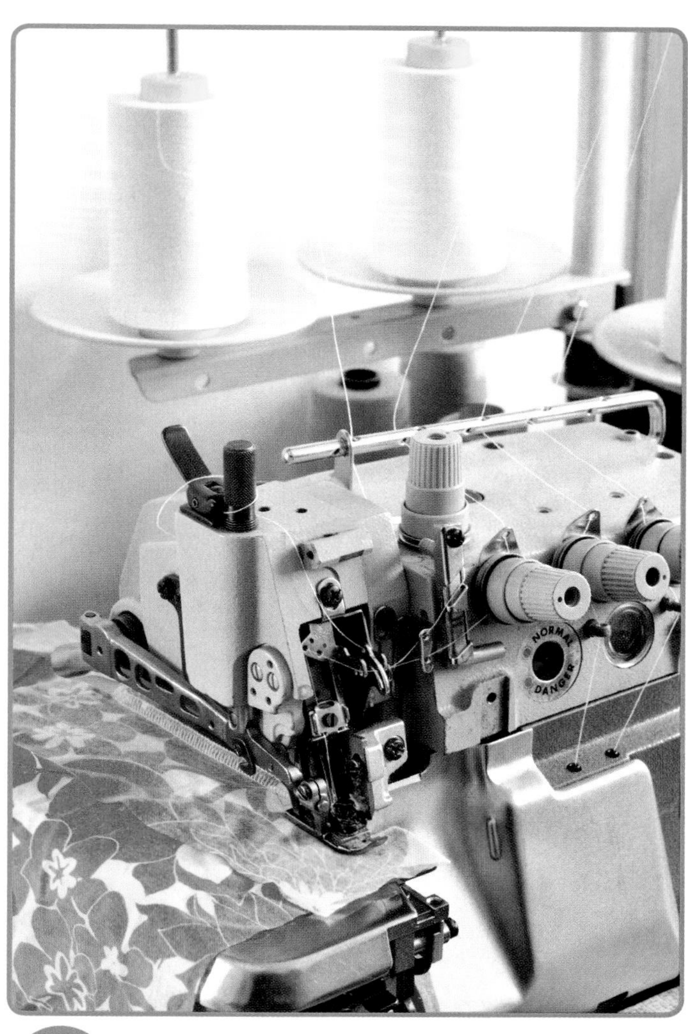

11-2 This is a home serger using two threads. Sergers used in manufacturing plants can use many, many more.

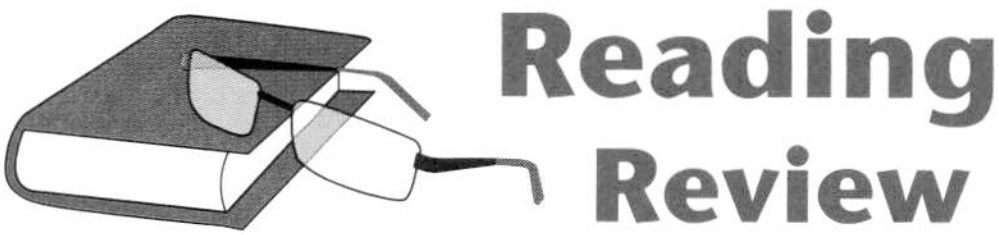

Reading Review

1. What is the difference between sergers and conventional sewing machines?
2. Why would sewers want to use overlock stitches?

The Sewing Lab

Before you begin sewing, collect the specific tools needed for your project. See **11-3**. This will save you from having to

Common Sewing Tools	
	Measuring and Cutting Tools Tape measures Sewing gauges Scissors Shears Seam rippers
	Marking Tools Tracing wheels Dressmaker's carbon Tailor's chalk Tailor's pencils Water-soluble marking pens
	Sewing Tools Needles Pins Pincushions Thimbles

11-3 Become familiar with the different sewing tools. They are used to measure, mark, cut, and sew fabric.

stop your work and look for them. When you are finished sewing, put away your tools. That way, you will know where they are the next time you sew.

When you sew at school, make the most of your time in the sewing lab. Start working when the class begins. It is important to help keep the sewing lab clean. Work neatly at your own table or desk. Label your tools and supplies to keep them from getting mixed up with those of your classmates. Also, write your name on pieces of paper and pin them to your fabric pieces.

When you are in the sewing lab, think about your classmates. Sometimes you may have to share a sewing machine with a partner. Wait patiently until he or she is done. You may be able to do other work while you wait. You may also have to wait to use the iron. When it is your turn, be sure to test the temperature of the iron on a scrap of your fabric. If you need help from the teacher, be patient. He or she may be busy helping other students.

Help clean up at the end of the sewing lab. Be sure to clean the area around your sewing machine. Pick up stray fabric scraps, threads, and pins. Return classroom tools to the proper place. Put your supplies and tools in a tote tray and store it in the assigned place.

You may also be assigned a cleanup task. You may have to put away or cover the sewing machines, sweep the floor, or put away the iron and pressing tools. These tasks help prepare the room for the next group of students.

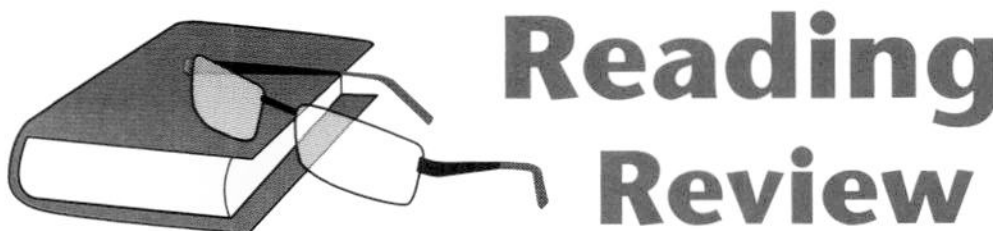

Reading Review

1. Why should you collect all your sewing tools before you begin sewing?
2. Why should you label your tools and supplies? How should they be stored?
3. Why is it important to clean your sewing area at the end of a sewing lab?

Succeed in Life

Working Safely in the Sewing Lab

There are a lot of tools in the sewing lab. To protect yourself and your classmates, use them carefully. Follow these tips for working safely both in the lab and when you are sewing at home:

- Operate sewing machines carefully. Do not operate a sewing machine if it is jammed or making unusual sounds.
- Place pins in pincushions. Do not hold pins or needles in your mouth. You could swallow them.
- Store scissors and shears in a safe place.
- Keep the blades of scissors and shears closed when you are not using them.
- Hand scissors to other people with the handle turned toward them.
- Test the temperature of an iron on a scrap of fabric. Never touch the iron with your hand. You may burn yourself.
- Rest the iron on its heel. Never rest it face down.
- Turn off the iron when you are finished using it. It might overheat and start a fire.
- Unplug the iron when you are done using it. Let it cool before you empty the water. The steam could burn you.

Section Summary

- Use the proper tools when sewing.
- Know the parts of a sewing machine and how it works.
- Sergers are a different type of sewing machine used for specific sewing tasks.
- In the sewing lab, take care of your work area, tools, and supplies. They must be carefully used, cared for, and shared.
- Safety rules must be followed to prevent accidents.

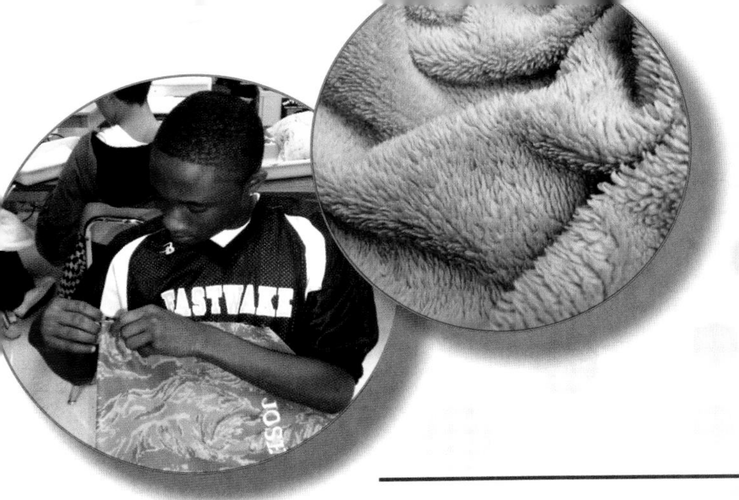

Section 11-2
Preparing To Sew

Objectives

After studying this section, you will be able to
- **define** *pattern*, *nap*, *grain*, *notions*, *guide sheet*, and *selvage*.
- **identify** your correct figure type.
- **choose** a pattern for your project.
- **explain** the information on pattern envelopes and guide sheets.
- **choose** the right fabrics and notions for your project.
- **demonstrate** how to lay out, pin, cut, and mark a pattern.

Key Terms

pattern: paper pieces to follow when cutting out fabric for making a garment or project.

nap: a layer of fiber ends above the fabric surface.

grain: the direction yarns run in a fabric.

notions: items other than fabric that become part of a garment or project.

guide sheet: step-by-step directions for cutting and sewing a project included with the pattern.

selvage: the finished lengthwise edges on a piece of fabric.

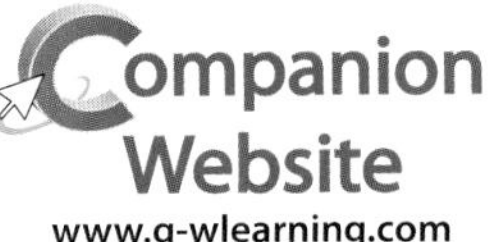

Study the Key Terms by completing crossword puzzles, matching activities, and e-flash cards at the website.

Main Ideas

- You can select a pattern suited to your figure type.
- Pattern envelopes and guide sheets give important sewing information.
- Selecting the correct fabric and notions is important.
- You need to correctly lay out, pin, cut, and mark patterns.

A sewing project should be well planned. For this to happen, certain steps must be followed. This will help you make sure your project turns out right. This section will discuss the steps to follow when preparing to sew.

Choosing a Project

The first step is to choose a project. When you are choosing a project, think about your sewing skills. Also, think about the time it will take you to make the project.

If you are a beginning sewer, choose an easy project. See **11-4**. Pillows, sweatshirts, stuffed animals, and gym bags are good ideas for first projects. They do not take long to make, and the directions are easy to follow. As your sewing skills increase, you can make more advanced projects.

You may or may not be able to choose your first project. Your teacher may decide everyone in the class will make the same project. You can make your project different from your classmates' by selecting different fabrics and designs. You may be able to add your own details.

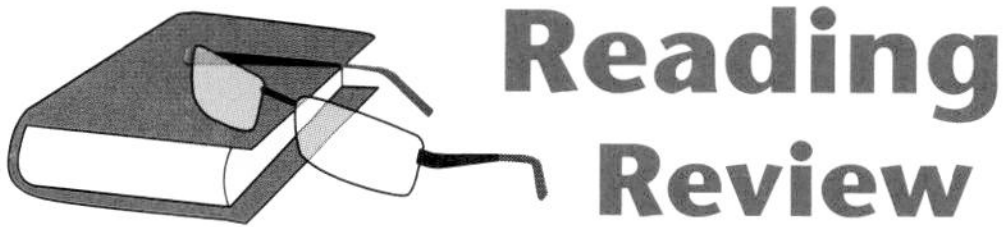

Reading Review

1. What two factors do you need to keep in mind when choosing a sewing project?
2. How can you make your project different from your classmates'? Give examples.

Choosing a Pattern

After you choose a project, select a pattern. A **pattern** contains paper pieces to follow when cutting out fabric for making a garment or project.

To find a pattern you like, look through pattern catalogs. You can find pattern catalogs in fabric stores and online. Pattern catalogs are divided into different sections. They include patterns for women, juniors, girls, men, boys, children, toys, crafts, and household items.

The front and back of the *pattern envelope* gives you a lot of information. See **11-5**. The front of the envelope shows pictures of the finished project. Sometimes more than one style or garment is shown. For instance, there may be a picture of both shorts and sweatpants.

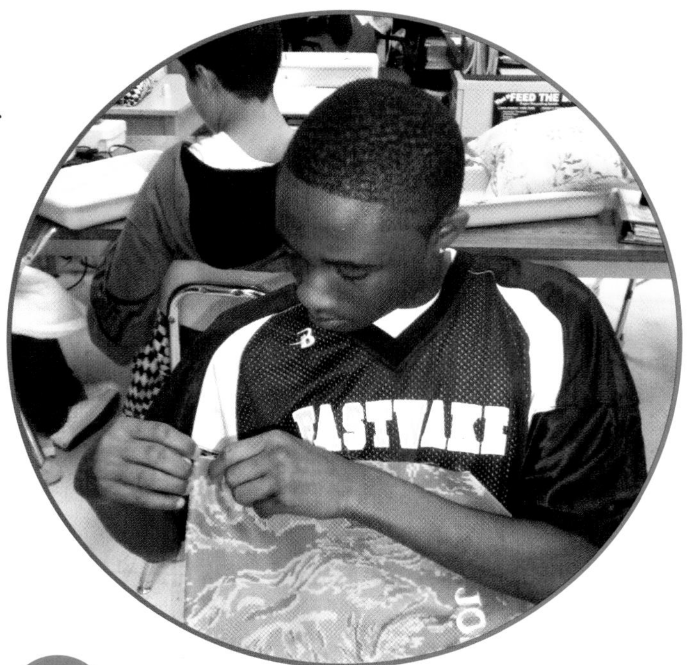

11-4 Choose an easy project, such as a pillow, for an early sewing project.

The Pattern Envelope	
Front	Size Pattern number Company name Pictures of finished project
Back	Pattern number Description of garment Type of fabric to buy Body measurements Amount of fabric needed Supplies needed Finished garment measurements Back view of the item

11-5 Always read the pattern envelope carefully before buying your sewing supplies. That way you will be sure to buy the correct amounts.

The back of the pattern envelope has more detailed information, which is useful for planning. It tells you which supplies you need and the amount of different materials to buy. The envelope back also shows you more details about the completed garment or other item. Be sure you read this information carefully before choosing a pattern.

Determining Pattern Size

If you are making a garment, you need to choose a pattern that will fit you. To do this, determine your figure type. Figure types are based on height and body measurements. Because it is hard to measure yourself correctly, have your teacher or a family member measure you. Then, compare your measurements with figure type charts in the back of pattern catalogs. Decide which figure type is most like yours.

Once you know your figure type, you can choose the correct pattern size. Compare your measurements with the different sizes for each figure type. Then choose the pattern size closest to your own measurements. Pattern sizing is not the same as the clothing you may buy in a store.

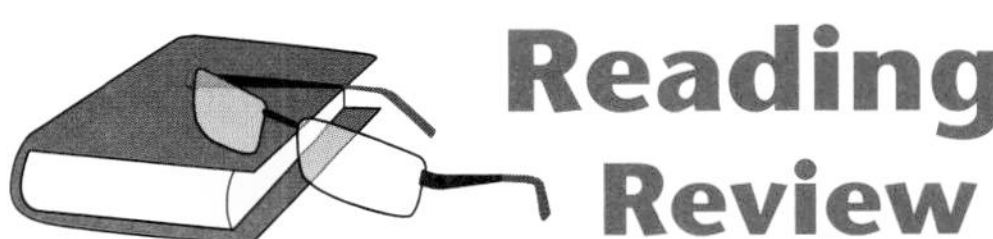

Reading Review

1. What information can you find on the front and back of a pattern envelope?
2. Why do you need to have someone else take your measurements?
3. How can you determine your figure type? How can you choose the correct pattern size?

Choosing the Fabric

Before you choose the fabric, read the back of the pattern envelope carefully. See which type of fabric is suggested. Most beginning projects will specify a *woven or knit fabric*. Select a firm weave or knit. Fabric with a loose weave or knit can easily stretch out of shape. The edges may ravel.

As a beginning sewer, there are many types of fabric you should avoid buying. Fabrics that are slippery, flimsy, stiff, or heavy may pucker, slip, or be hard to sew. Fabrics with stripes, plaids, or large prints need to be matched at the seams. Buy extra fabric for one-way designs and for fabrics with a nap. A **nap** is a layer of fiber ends above the fabric surface. It causes the fabric to look different in color and texture when viewed from different directions. See **11-6**. When you lay out pattern pieces on one-way or napped fabrics, all the pattern pieces must run the same direction.

Check whether the fabric you want to buy is preshrunk. This information can be found on the end of the fabric bolt along with the care instructions. If the fabric is not preshrunk, wash and iron it according to the care instructions before you lay it out for cutting.

Checking the Grain

Grain is the direction yarns run in a fabric. Once you have chosen a fabric, make sure the grain is straight. Fabrics should be *on-grain*. This means the lengthwise and crosswise yarns are at right angles to each other. Fabrics that are on-grain are easier to cut and sew than fabrics that are *off-grain*. See **11-7**. Finished garments will hang correctly and keep their shape.

If you buy fabrics that are off-grain, they can be straightened by pulling on the two

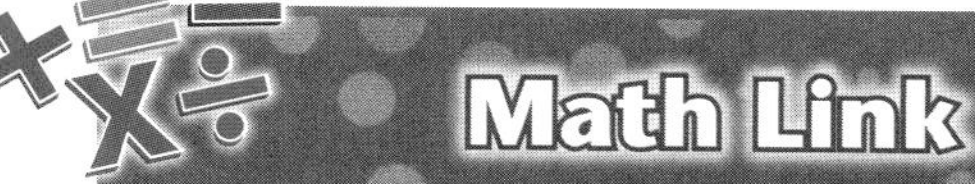

How to Take Measurements

When taking someone's measurements, use a string to tie around the body areas or to measure length. Then use a tape measure to find the string's exact length in inches.

Waist: around body at natural waistline

Chest/Bust: measure around the fullest part of bust and straight across back

Neckband (men): around base of neck or buy shirt pattern by ready-made size

Hips: at seat or fullest part of hips

Shirt sleeve: from back base of neck across shoulder around bend of elbow to wrist

Pant inseam: use a pair of pants the correct length, place on a flat surface, and measure from the bottom of the hem to where the pant legs meet

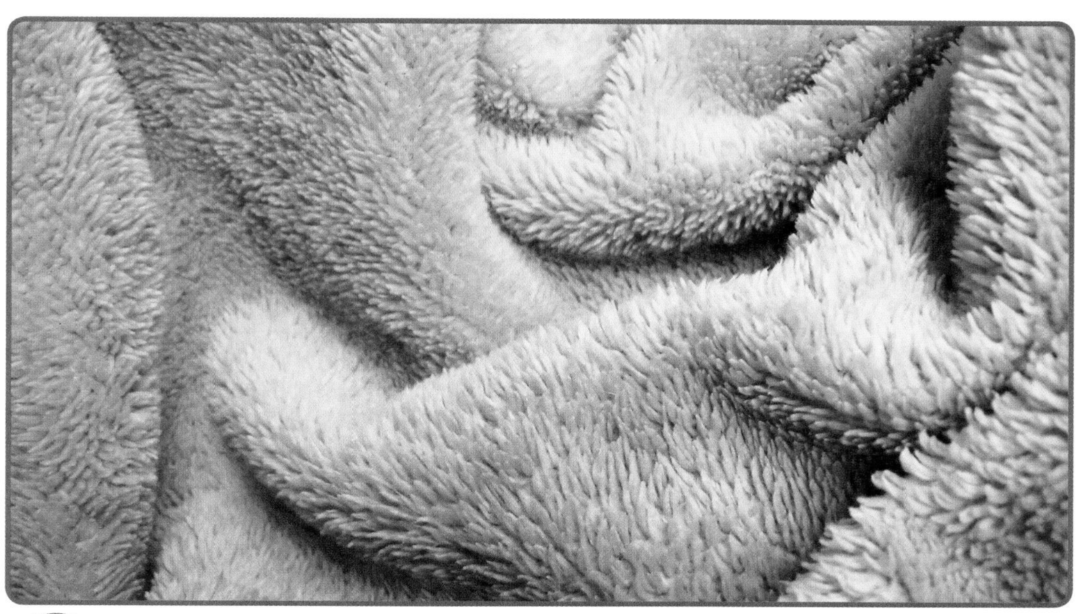

11-6 Fabrics such as terry cloth, corduroy, and velour have a nap.

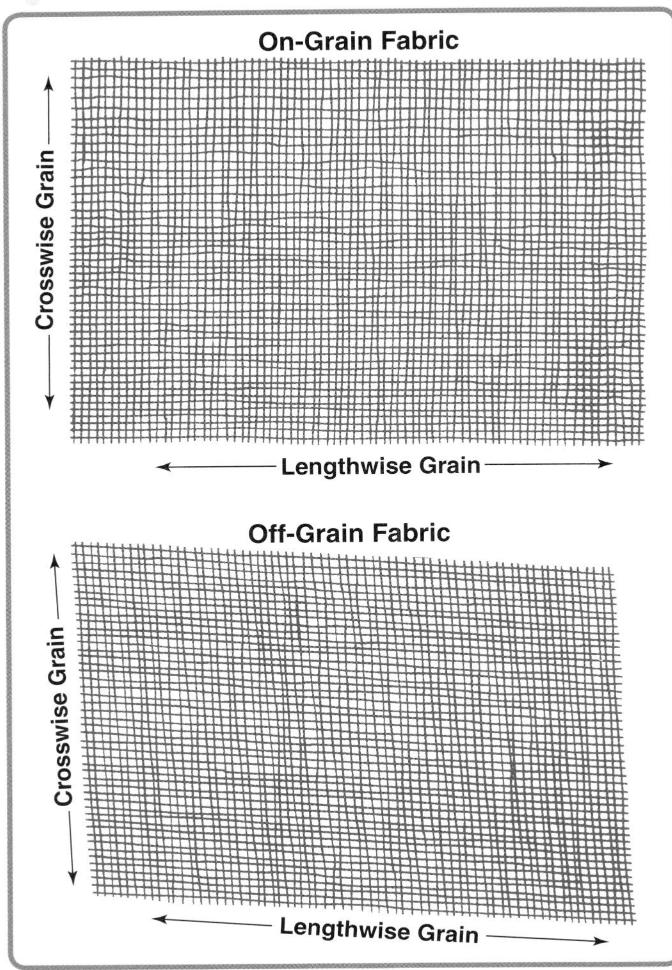

11-7 Always check to make sure the fabric you buy is on-grain.

shortest corners. Then you need to use a steam iron to press it in place. Some fabrics, however, have finishes that lock the fabric in place. These fabrics will return to their locked shape even after you straighten them. Avoid buying these fabrics.

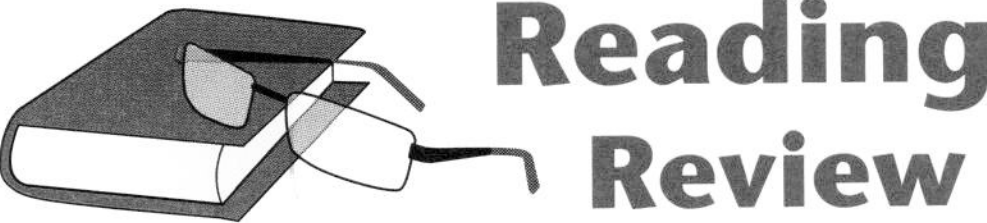

1. What factors should you consider when choosing fabric? Why?
2. Why should you choose fabrics that are on-grain?

Choosing the Notions

Notions are items other than fabric that become part of a garment or project. You also need to buy some notions to complete your project. The most common notions are

- thread
- fasteners (buttons, snaps, hooks and eyes, zippers, and hook and loop tape)
- elastic
- seam binding or hem tape
- interfacing

Buy all the fabric and notions for your project at the same time. You will then be sure the thread, buttons, zipper, and seam binding match the fabric. Also, you will not have to stop working on your project to buy extra notions.

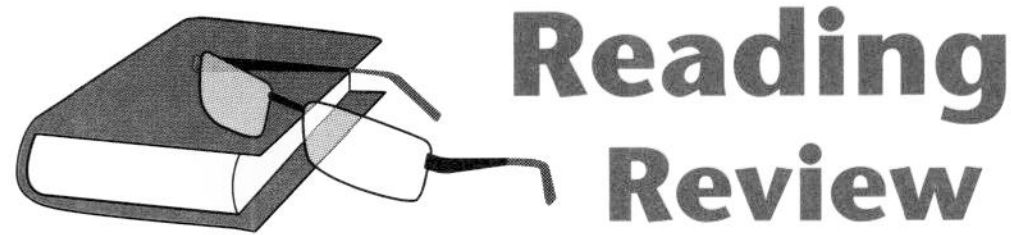

1. What are the most common notions?
2. Why should you buy fabric and notions at the same time?

Preparing the Pattern

A **guide sheet** is the step-by-step directions for cutting and sewing a project included with the pattern. The guide sheet tells you which pattern pieces you need for your project. Cut those pieces out of the paper pattern sheets. Many pattern pieces include multiple sizes. Trim the pattern to your size. Put the pattern pieces you are not using back in the envelope.

Look at the markings on the pattern pieces you are using. There are two types of pattern markings. Some help you lay out and cut the pattern. Others help you construct the project and will need to be transferred to the fabric. See **11-8**.

Pattern Guide Sheets

Your pattern's guide sheet gives you all the cutting layouts and instructions for preparing and marking your fabric. Before you start your sewing project, read these instructions very carefully and make sure you understand each step. This will save you time and prevent costly mistakes as you move through the rest of your sewing project.

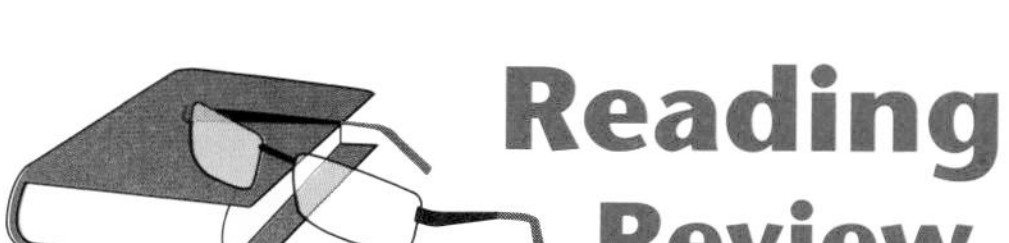

1. What information can you find on the front of a guide sheet?
2. What are two types of pattern markings? What are their functions?

Laying Out, Pinning, Cutting, and Marking

Once you have cut your pattern pieces, you can begin laying them out. Cutting layouts on the guide sheet show you where to place the pattern pieces on the fabric. There is a layout for each view, fabric width, and size. Find the layout for your garment or project. Draw a circle around it.

To lay out pattern pieces, first use a dry iron to remove any wrinkles in the paper pattern and the fabric. Place the fabric on a table and fold it according to the guide sheet directions. The fabric should be very smooth

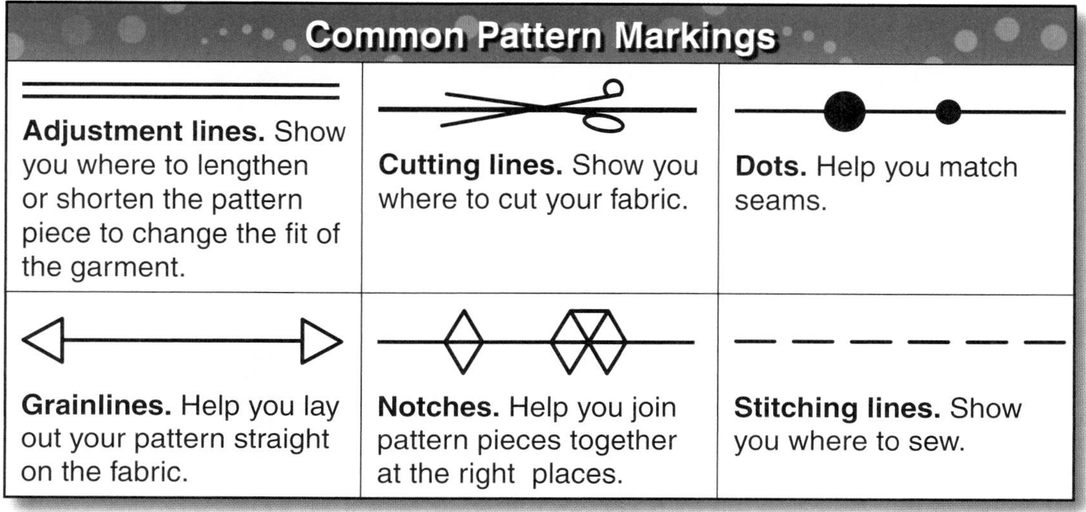

Common Pattern Markings

Adjustment lines. Show you where to lengthen or shorten the pattern piece to change the fit of the garment.	**Cutting lines.** Show you where to cut your fabric.	**Dots.** Help you match seams.
Grainlines. Help you lay out your pattern straight on the fabric.	**Notches.** Help you join pattern pieces together at the right places.	**Stitching lines.** Show you where to sew.

11-8 These are a few common markings you will see on pattern pieces.

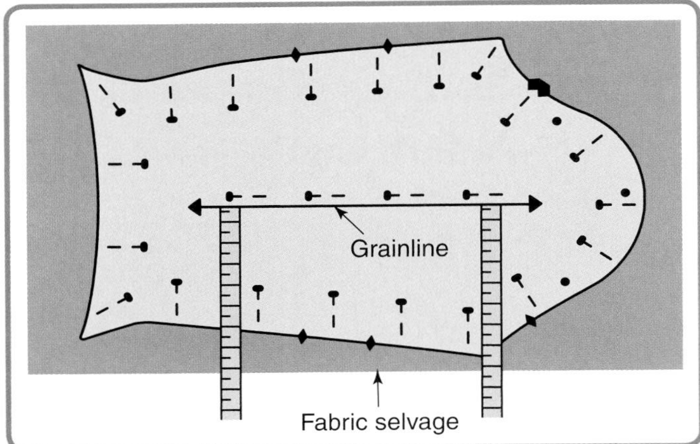

11-9 Pattern pieces need to be correctly placed and pinned.

with no wrinkles along the fold or the surface. After that, place each pattern piece on the fabric following the cutting layout. Check this carefully several times to make sure the pattern pieces have been placed correctly.

Make sure the grain lines shown on the pattern pieces are placed on the grain of the fabric. The grain line should be parallel with the selvage. A **selvage** is the finished lengthwise edges on a piece of fabric. Use a ruler or yardstick to check that the grain line is even with the selvage at each end. Make sure it is also even with the grain in the middle of the fabric. See **11-9**.

The next step is pinning the pattern pieces to the fabric. Pins should be placed along the pattern piece's grain line and diagonally on the corners. Also, place pins every three to four inches near the pattern edges. If you place pins too close together, the fabric will not lie flat. Pins placed too far apart can cause the fabric and pattern to slip while cutting. Never start cutting until all the pattern pieces are correctly placed and pinned.

To cut out pattern pieces correctly, let your scissors glide across the table. Do not pick the fabric up to cut around the pattern. Cut around notches.

Before sewing, transfer all pattern markings, such as those for darts and dots, to the wrong side of the fabric. Do this before you unpin the pattern pieces from the fabric. Be careful when marking the fabric. Mark a scrap of fabric first to make sure the marks do not show on the right side.

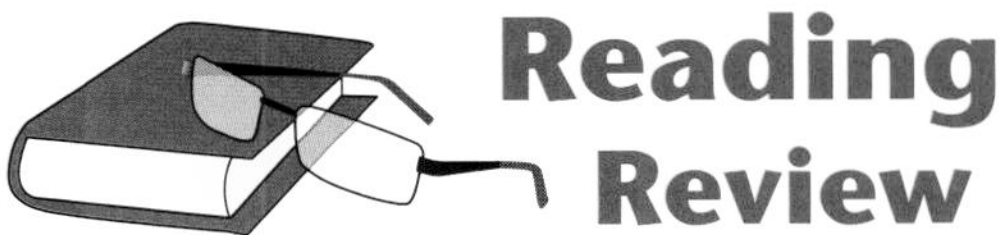

Reading Review

1. How can you make sure the grain lines are placed straight on the fabric?
2. How should pins be placed when pinning pattern pieces to fabric? Why?
3. Why should you not pick up fabric to cut around the pattern pieces?

Section Summary

- As a beginning sewer, start with a simple project. You may need to choose a pattern for this project.
- If you are making a garment, choose a pattern that will fit you.
- Make sure to read the outside of the pattern envelope for information about the project.
- After selecting your pattern, choose fabric and notions.
- Inside the pattern envelope, you will find the guide sheet and pattern pieces. Next, lay out, pin, cut, and mark the fabric.

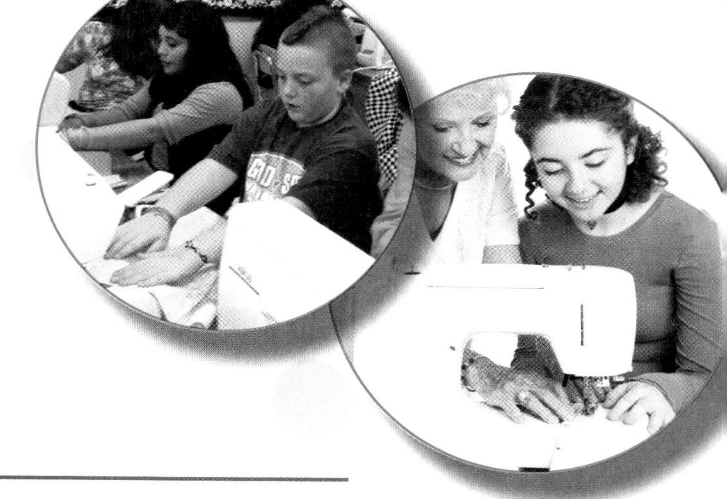

Section 11-3
Sewing Your Project

Objectives

After studying this section, you will be able to
- **define** *basting*, *seam,* and *shank*.
- **demonstrate** how to machine stitch.
- **make** different hand stitches.
- **show** how to sew seams.
- **state** how to attach different fasteners.

Key Terms

basting: sewing fabric pieces together with long, loose, temporary stitches.

seam: a row of permanent stitches used to hold two pieces of fabric together.

shank: a short stem that holds a button away from fabric.

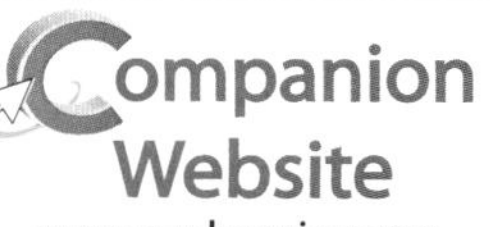

Study the Key Terms by completing crossword puzzles, matching activities, and e-flash cards at the website.

Main Ideas

- You can make stitches by machine or hand.
- Well-made seams have certain traits.
- Fasteners need to be attached securely.

After you have completed all the sewing preparation steps, you are ready to sew your project. There are certain skills you should have to make your project turn out right. They include making good stitches and seams. Attaching fasteners correctly is also important.

Making Stitches

There are two types of straight stitches. Some are temporary, while others are permanent. Both can be done by machine or by hand. Temporary stitches are removed from the fabric after a short time. **Basting** is a temporary stitch that holds fabric pieces together using long, loose stitches.

Permanent stitches are left in the fabric. They hold the fabric pieces together securely. Machine stitching is quicker and stronger than hand stitching. Your machine's use and care manual shows how to make different stitches.

Hand stitching takes longer, but gives you more control over the fabric and stitches than machine stitching. Some common hand stitches are basting, blind, catch, and slip stitches. See **11-10**. Hand stitching is used for temporary stitching, hemming, and attaching fasteners.

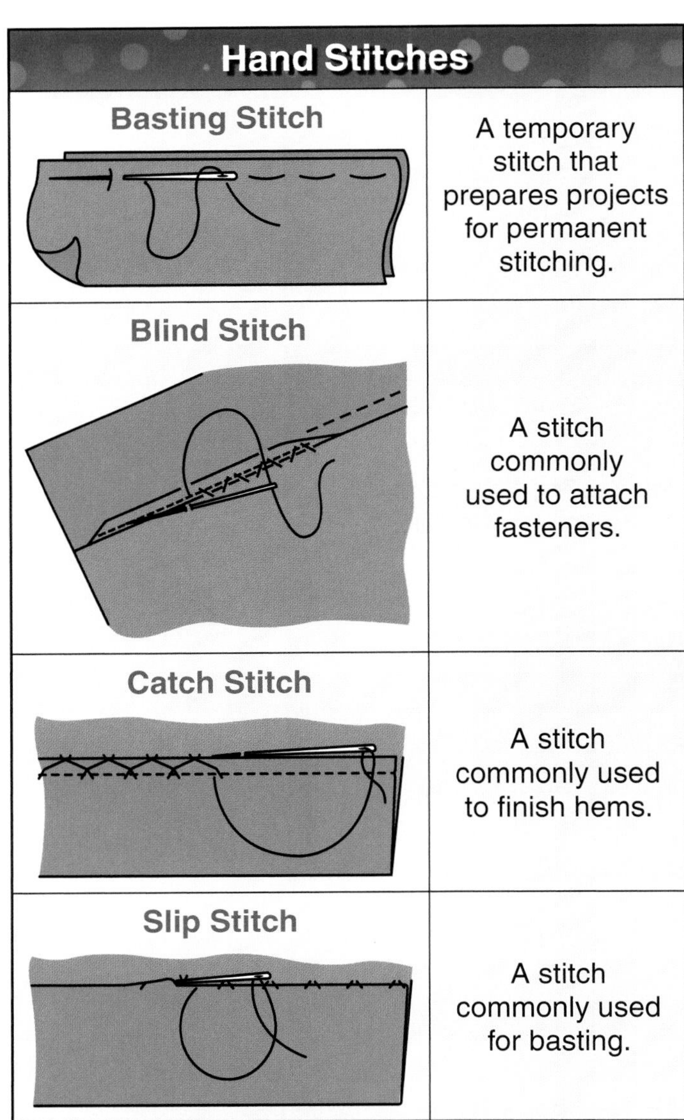

Hand Stitches

Basting Stitch	A temporary stitch that prepares projects for permanent stitching.
Blind Stitch	A stitch commonly used to attach fasteners.
Catch Stitch	A stitch commonly used to finish hems.
Slip Stitch	A stitch commonly used for basting.

11-10 Each hand stitch is sewn a little differently from the others.

1. What is the difference between temporary and permanent stitching? Which one is stronger?
2. Why do you have more control over the fabric and stitches when you hand stitch?

Seams

A **seam** is a row of permanent stitches used to hold two pieces of fabric together. Seams should have strong, even stitches that are flat, smooth, and straight.

To make a seam, place the right sides of the fabric pieces together. Match the edges and notches. Then use pins or a basting stitch to keep the pieces together while you are stitching the seam. Most pattern seams are sewn ⅝ inch (1.5 cm) from the edge of the fabric. See **11-11**. Remove the temporary basting stitches after completing the seams.

Each permanent stitch should begin and end with a few small backstitches. This secures the stitching. Reversing the stitch on the machine makes backstitches.

After seams are stitched, press or finish them according to the directions in the guide sheet. Pressing keeps the seams flat and smooth. Always press on the wrong side of the fabric.

Making straight and curved seams and knowing how to turn corners are basic stitching skills you will need to sew well.

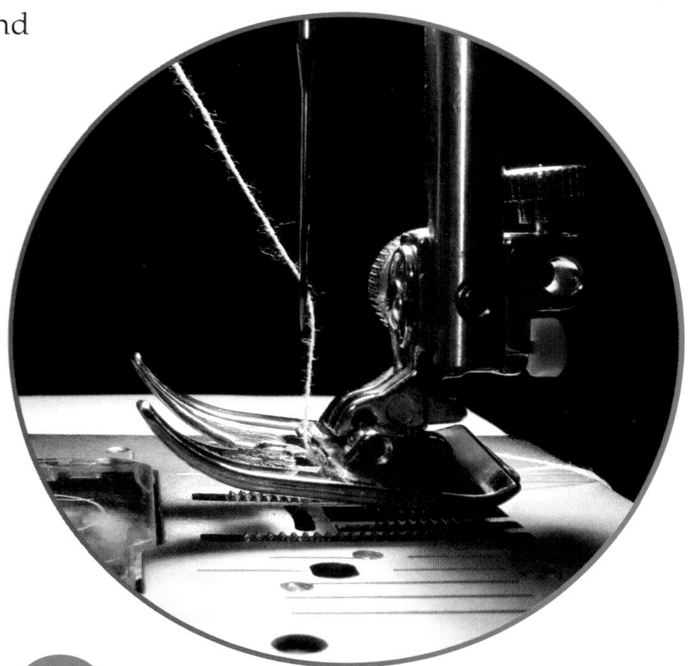

11-11 On the throat plate of the sewing machine, there is often a marking showing ⅝ inch.

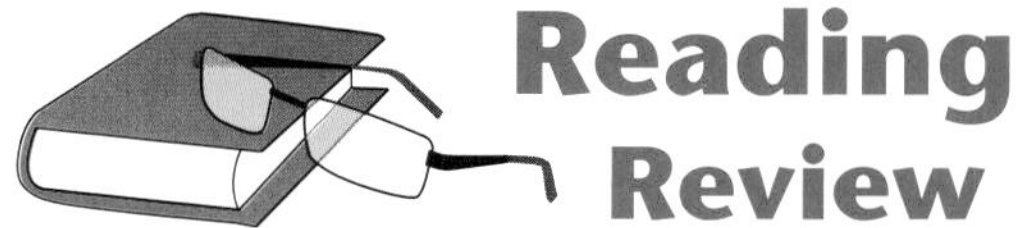

Reading Review

1. What are the traits of a well-made seam?
2. What can happen if you forget to backstitch at the beginning and end of a seam?

Attaching Fasteners

Sew fasteners on securely because much stress is placed on them. Buttons are sewn by hand. Always use a double thread with a knot at the end to attach them more securely. Make sure your buttons are the correct

Succeed in Life

How to Sew Buttons

Follow these steps for sewing buttons on your clothing:

Step 1: Make several small stitches to secure the thread in the fabric where you want to place the button. Insert the needle through one of the holes on the underside of the button. Pull the thread through to the top of the button.

Step 2: Place a pin on top of the button. If you are sewing on heavy fabric, use a toothpick. This helps produce a shank when you stitch on a sew-through button. Push the needle down through the second hole and back up the first hole. Repeat this four or five times.

Step 3: Remove the pin or toothpick when you are finished. Then pull the button up. Wrap the thread around the loose threads underneath the button four or five times. This creates the shank.

Step 4: Push the threaded needle to the back of the fabric. Make several small stitches through the thread loop. This will fasten the thread.

Step 5: If your button already has a shank, simply sew it following Steps 1 and 4.

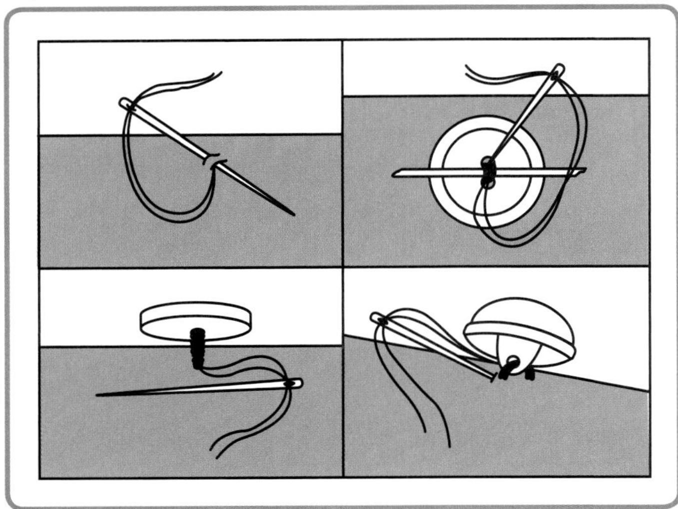

11-12 Before you sew on a button, make sure it is in line with the buttonhole.

size and color for the garment. Select thread that matches the buttons. If you are sewing a button on heavy fabric, like a coat, use button thread.

Buttons need space to lie smoothly on fabric. A **shank** is the short stem that holds a button away from the fabric. Shanks also help secure buttons more firmly. Some buttons are made with shanks. Other buttons, called *sew-through buttons,* need thread shanks to be made when they are attached. See **11-12**.

Snaps are used to hold overlapping edges flat. They do not stay fastened under stress. Hand stitch the two snap parts on with a series of small stitches. Make sure the stitches do not show on the right side of the fabric.

Hooks and eyes are used to fasten waistbands and neck edges. Hooks and eyes can take more strain than snaps. Hand stitch hooks and eyes using several short stitches. The stitches should not show on the right side of the fabric.

Hook and loop tape can be attached by following the directions on the package. Zippers should be inserted according to the directions in your guide sheet.

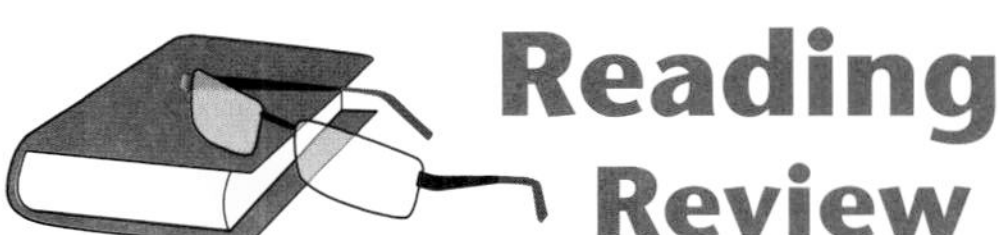

Reading Review

1. Why should you use a double thread when attaching fasteners?
2. What are the steps for sewing a button on without a shank? with a shank?

Section Summary

- Sewing projects often need to be both machine and hand stitched.
- Some stitching is temporary and some is permanent.
- Once you know how to make stitches, you can make good, strong seams. Seams hold your fabric together.
- Fasteners also need to be attached securely and correctly.

Section 11-4
Repairing, Altering, and Recycling Your Clothes

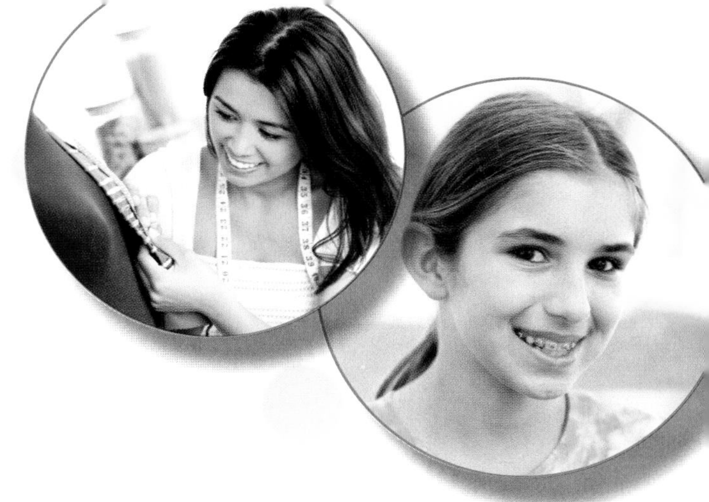

Objectives

After studying this section, you will be able to
- **define** *alterations*, *redesign*, *appliqué*, and *embroidery*.
- **explain** the advantages of repairing and altering your clothes.
- **demonstrate** how to make clothing repairs.
- **describe** how to make clothing alterations.

Key Terms

alterations: changes made in the size, length, or style of a garment so it will fit properly.

redesign: changing the appearance or function of a garment.

appliqué: smaller pieces of fabric or trim sewn on a garment.

embroidery: decorative stitching using a needle and thread.

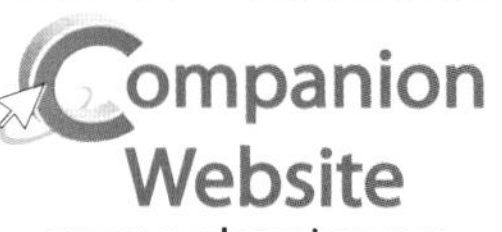

Study the Key Terms by completing crossword puzzles, matching activities, and e-flash cards at the website.

Main Ideas

- Some common clothing repairs are fixing fasteners, rips, and tears.
- You can alter hems and seams to make your clothes fit better.
- You can redesign and recycle garments to extend the use of your clothes.

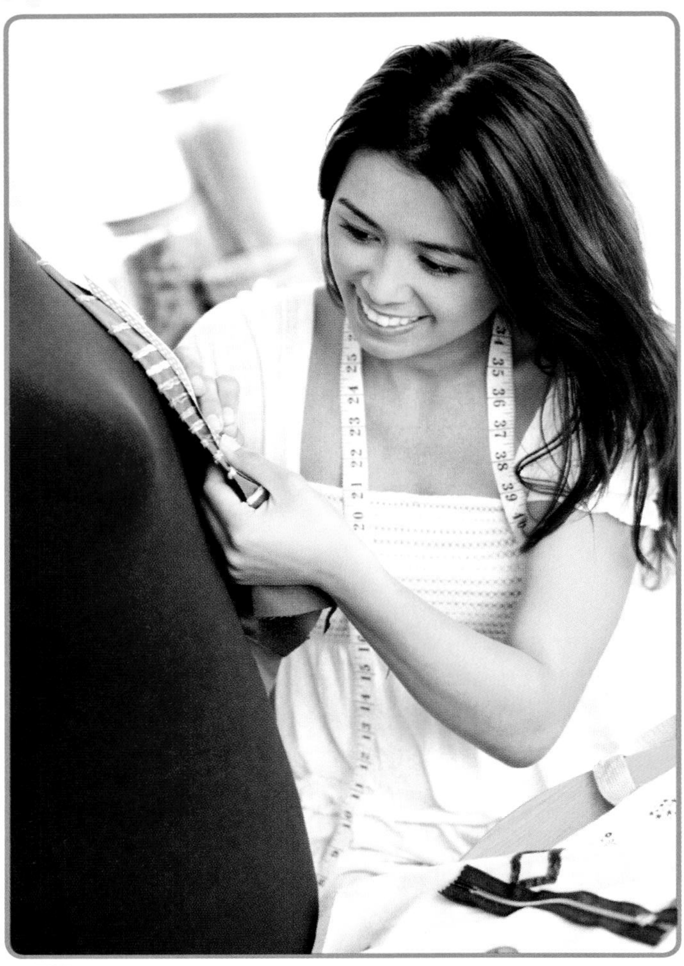

11-13 Alterations may include changing hems and seams or moving buttons.

Do you have clothes in your closet that need repair? Many times you can make these repairs yourself. When you make your own clothing repairs, your clothing will last longer.

You can stretch your clothing budget by making alterations to your clothes. **Alterations** are changes made in the size, length, or style of a garment so it will fit properly. See **11-13**.

Repairing Fasteners

Sometimes fasteners may come loose. They may also break. Resew fasteners when they loosen. If they fall off and you lose them, they will need to be replaced. Follow the previous directions for attaching fasteners.

If you lose a button, check to see if you have any extra buttons that match. Some clothes come with extra buttons when you buy them. If you cannot find an identical button, you may have to replace all the buttons on the garment. That is why you should resew loose buttons before they fall off.

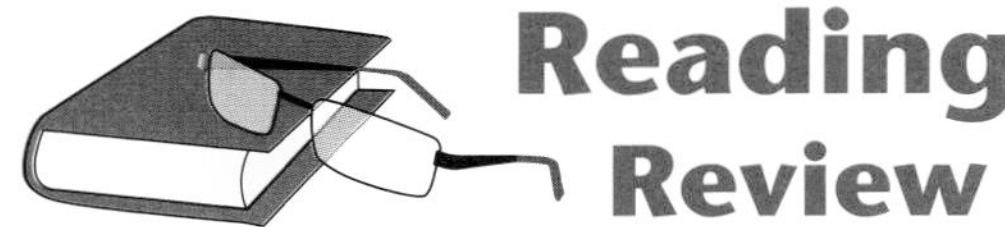

Reading Review

1. Why is it important to resew loose buttons before they fall off?
2. What steps should you take to replace a zipper in a garment?

Repairing Rips and Tears

If you notice a ripped seam, repair it right away. Rips are easier to repair when they are small. To fix a rip, turn the garment inside out and pin the seam together. Then stitch the seam, going past the ripped area a little on each end. Try to match the color of the thread to the garment. If this is not possible, use thread a shade darker.

You can repair seams by machine or by hand. If you hand stitch, make small stitches. Make sure the stitching is not too tight. This could cause the threads to break. Seams that receive a lot of stress need to be stitched twice. These seams include crotch seams in pants and armhole seams in shirts.

Succeed in Life

How to Replace Zippers

If a zipper breaks, replace it. Be sure to buy a new one that is the same color and size as the old zipper. Follow these steps to replace a zipper:

Step 1: Remove the broken zipper carefully, using a small pair of scissors or a seam ripper. Be careful not to cut the fabric. If you are replacing a zipper on a garment with a waistband, you will have to remove some of the stitching in the waistband.

Step 2: Press the zipper area flat.

Step 3: Pin the new zipper in place, following the directions on the zipper package.

Step 4: Baste and then stitch the zipper along the old stitching lines.

Step 5: Press well.

Repair tears in clothing with iron-on mending tape or material. First clip any frayed threads. Then apply iron-on mending tape or material in the correct color to the inside of the garment. Be sure to follow the directions on the package.

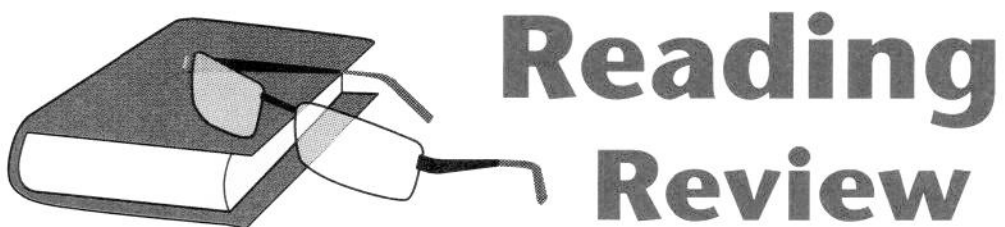

Reading Review

1. Why do you need to repair ripped seams right away?
2. What are the steps to repair torn clothes?

Altering Hems

Sometimes, you may have clothes you want to make longer or shorter. You can make these changes by altering the hems. See **11-14**.

Before you lengthen a garment, make sure there is enough fabric in the hem for the length you need to add. If not, you can buy hem facing to extend the hem. This can be sewn on the edge of the hem. To shorten a garment, you may need to trim away some of the extra fabric.

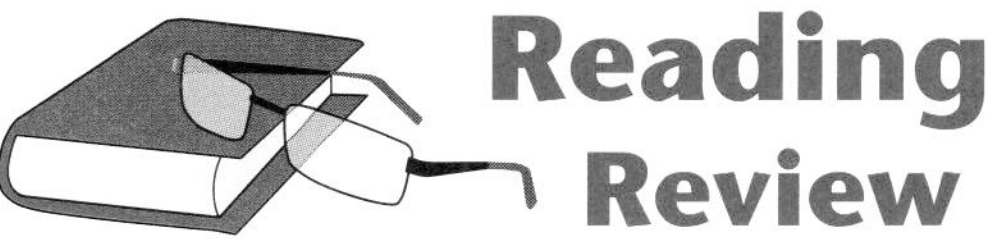

Reading Review

1. If you have a garment that is too long or short, what steps should you take to change the hem?
2. Why do you need to stitch seam tape to the edges of woven fabric that ravels?

How to Alter Garment Hems

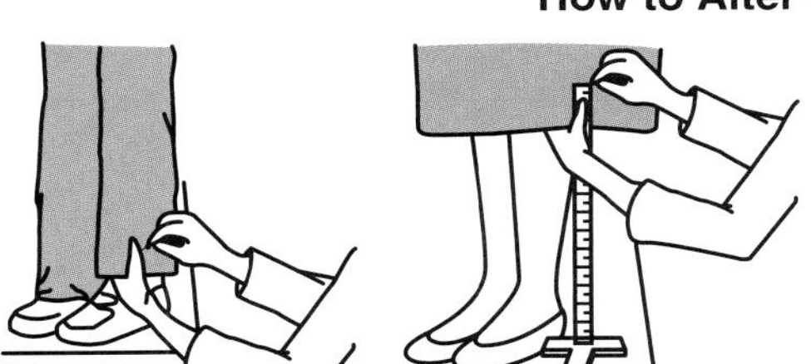

1. Remove stitching from the hem and press out the crease. Try on the garment. Have someone mark the hem with a pin line. Use a yardstick to be sure all pins are the same distance from the floor.

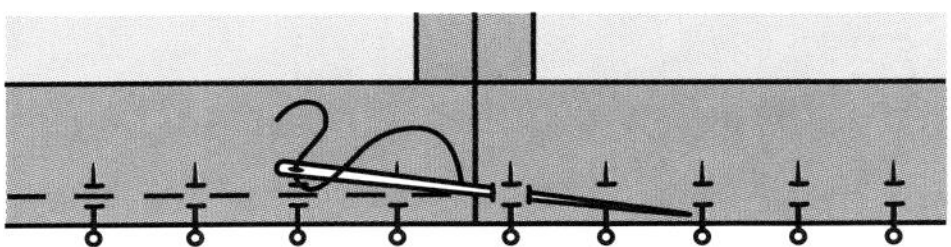

2. Turn up the hem on the pin line. Pin the hem in place and press the fold. Then baste close to the fold. Remove the pins.

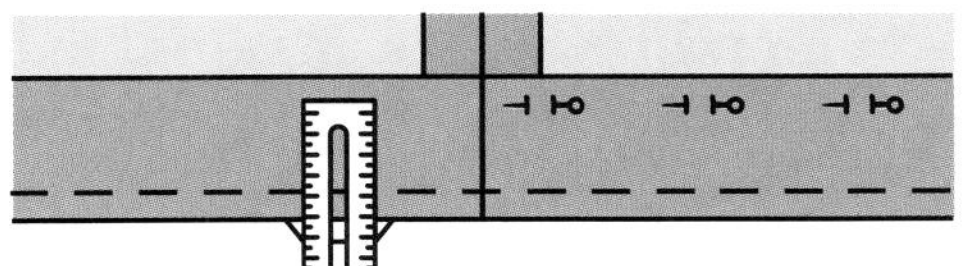

3. Measure the hem. Hems on straight skirts should be 2½ inches wide. Hems on pants and flared skirts should be 1½ inches wide. The hem should be even all the way around. If it isn't, make a pin line the same distance from the fold all the way around.

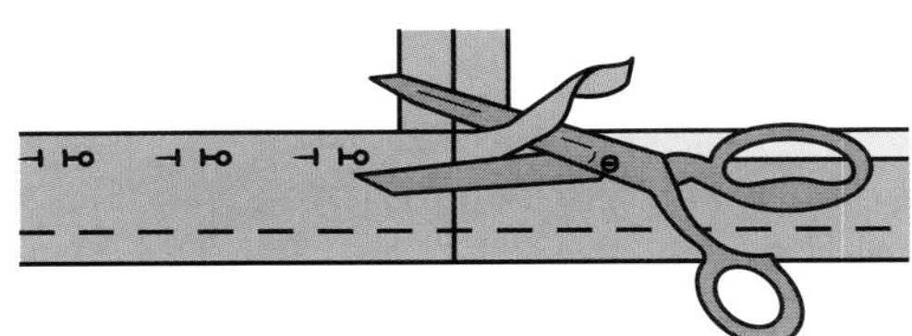

4. Cut the fabric along the pin line. Remove the pins.

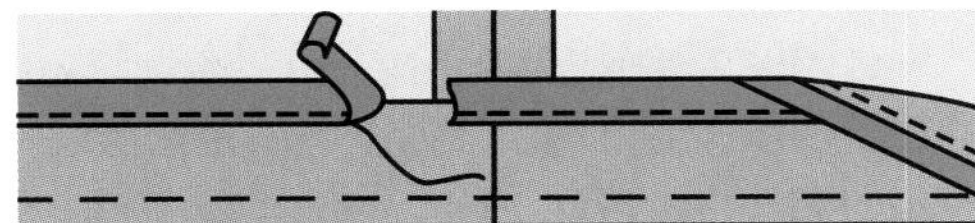

5. Machine stitch seam tape to the raw edge of woven fabrics that ravel. Knit fabrics do not need seam tape.

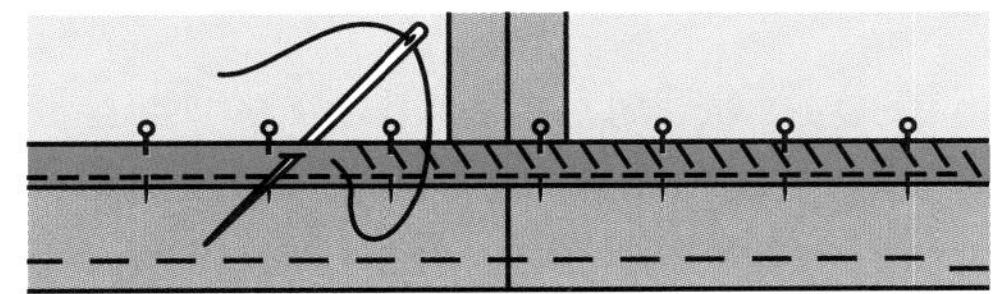

6. Pin the hem edge in place. Hand stitch the hem edge to the garment. Use the hemming stitch for hems on woven fabrics. Use the slip stitch for hems on knitted fabrics. Be careful that the stitching doesn't show on the right side of your garment.

7. Remove the pins and basting. Press well.

11-14 To make sure your new hem looks good, follow these steps very carefully.

Altering Seams

Sometimes your clothes may be too big or too small. Instead of discarding or giving them away, you may be able to make alterations. Some alterations are easy to make. You may just need to move a button or a hook. Other alterations can be more complicated. For instance, you may need to let out the seams to make the garment larger. By taking in the seams, you can make the garment smaller. These changes mean adjusting the sides or the front and back of the garment.

When altering seams, always try on the garment to check the fit and change any necessary seam widths *before* sewing permanent stitches.

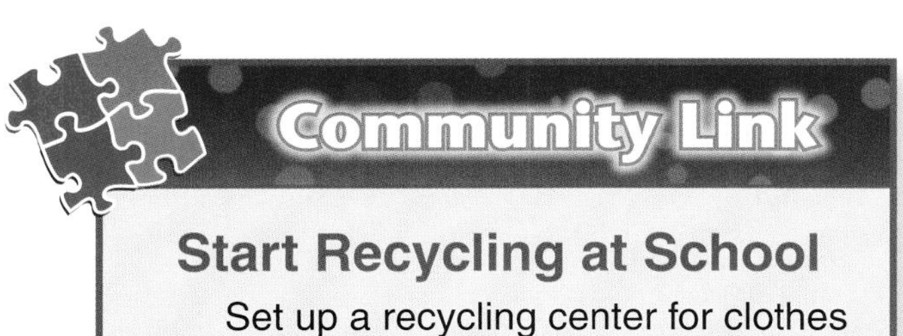

Start Recycling at School

Set up a recycling center for clothes at your school. Find agencies that will accept pre-clothing and donate them. Make sure the clothing is clean and wearable before donating.

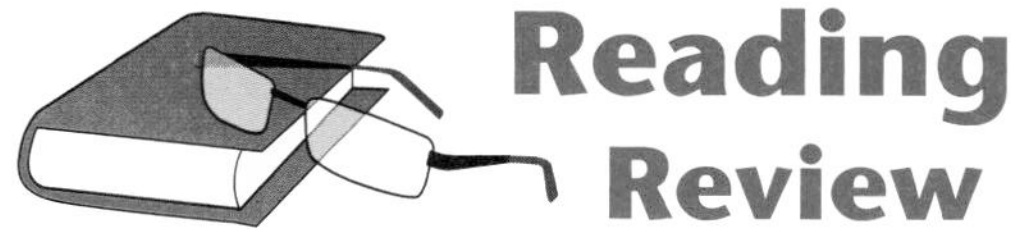

Reading Review

1. Why might you need to let out or take in a garment? Give examples.
2. Why should you check the fit of the garment before you sew the new seams?

Redesigning and Recycling Clothes

Basic sewing skills can be used to **redesign** your clothes by changing the appearance or function of a garment. For example, if you have a pair of jeans that are too short, you could redesign them into shorts.

Another example of redesigning your clothes includes using appliqués. **Appliqués** are smaller pieces of fabric or trim sewn on a garment. Colorful trims can make good appliqués. For instance, Alan used a design of his school mascot as an appliqué to his jacket.

Appliqués can also patch rips or cover stains. You can buy patches or cut them out of fabric scraps. Make sure they match the color of the fabric unless you are creating a new look. Patches are sewn on the outside of the garment by machine or by hand just like appliqués. Katie, for instance, made an appliqué for her stained jacket out of various pieces of old silk material.

You may want to add embroidery to your clothes for a new look. **Embroidery** is decorative stitching using a needle and thread. It can be done by hand or by machine. Your school might have a computerized sewing machine that can create embroidery designs.

T-shirts are fun to redesign. You can use fabric paint and create a unique shirt. You can create a special design through a process called *tie-dyeing*. See **11-15**. Tie-dyeing simply means that parts of the item's fabric are tied, to prevent the dye from reaching the fabric evenly. New patterns and designs are formed.

Finding new and different uses for old clothes is a form of *recycling*. For instance, those same too-small jeans you turned into shorts could also be turned into a backpack. To do this, cut off the legs

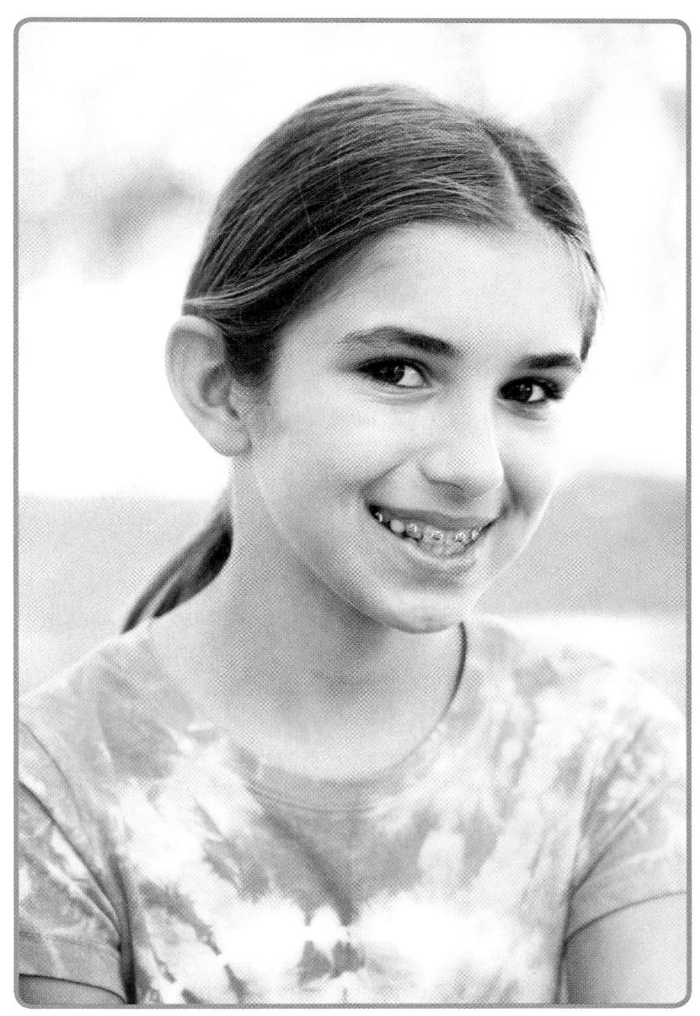

11-15 You can color a white T-shirt by tie-dyeing it.

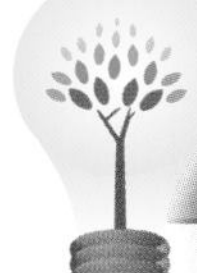

Think Green

Environmental Ideas for Old Clothes

The average American throws away 68 pounds of clothing a year. Some fabrics are not biodegradable and will take up space in a landfill for hundreds of years. You can reduce waste and extend the use of your clothes by redesigning them. You may also enjoy making creative projects with the fabric from discarded clothing. Could you use your sewing skills to help others keep their clothes longer? Donating your clothes to a charity also keeps them out of landfills. Some communities offer recycling drop-offs for pre-owned clothes. You can sell your clothing at a yard sale or in a consignment shop and receive a portion of the sale price.

below the crotch, turn the garment inside out, and sew the legs together. Use the rest of the fabric to make a top flap and straps.

You can use the fabrics of old clothes to make pillows, stuffed animals, quilts, or children's clothing. Soft cotton garments, such as T-shirts, can be used for cleaning.

The simplest way to recycle clothing is to give your outgrown garments to another person. Many families and friends give clothes that no longer fit to other family members and friends. For instance, Mary recycled her grandfather's old jacket for her own use. It fit her, so she simply added some decorative trim for style.

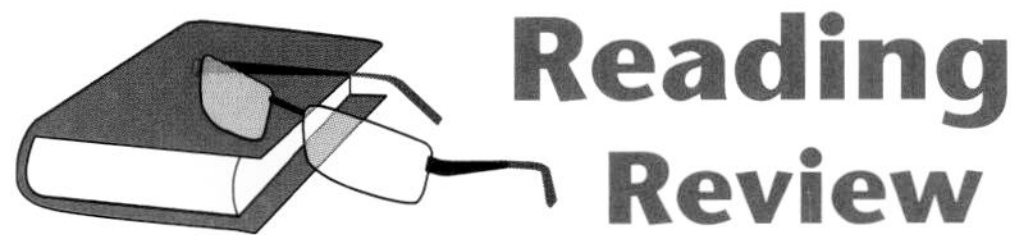

1. What is the difference between redesigning and recycling clothing?
2. Which organizations in your community accept donations of used clothing?

Section Summary

- It is important to know how to repair and alter your clothes. You can save money and make your clothes last longer.
- Repairing fasteners, rips, and tears are easy tasks.
- You can alter hems and seams to make your clothes fit better.
- Redesigning and recycling clothes can increase the amount of clothing you have and reduce waste.

Chapter Summary

Sewing can be fun. It can also save you money. You can make clothes and other items, such as gym bags or stuffed toys, for yourself. You can make gifts for family and friends. You can also repair and alter your clothes.

If you are a beginning sewer, you first need to learn the basic sewing skills. Know the parts of a sewing machine and the different types of sewing tools. When you are in the sewing lab, learn to use your time wisely and work well with others. You also need to work safely to prevent accidents.

The next step is to plan a project and prepare to sew it. Your first project should match your sewing skills. Look in pattern catalogs to find a pattern for a project you have the skills to make. If you are making a garment, make sure you choose a pattern that is the correct size.

After you have selected a pattern, choose the fabric and notions. The pattern envelope gives important information about choosing supplies and making the project. Directions in the guide sheet will tell you how to lay out, pin, cut, and mark the fabric.

When you sew, you may use machine stitching or hand stitching. Machine stitching is strong and permanent. It is good for making seams. Hand stitching is temporary and lets you have more control over the fabric and stitches than machine stitching. It is good for sewing on fasteners and making hems.

Repairing and altering your clothes will make them last longer. Some common clothing repairs include fixing fasteners, rips, and tears. You can alter hems and seams to make your clothes fit better. Redesigning and recycling clothes extend their use.

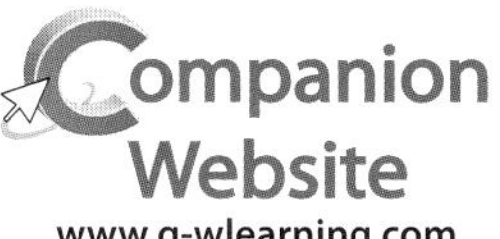

Review Key Terms and Main Ideas for Chapter 11 at the website.

Chapter Review

Write your answers on a separate sheet of paper.

1. List three benefits of sewing.
2. What are the four types of sewing tools?
3. True or false. It is easy to take your own body measurements.
4. What are two items found on the front of a pattern envelope?
5. Draw symbols for notch, grain line, and cutting line pattern markings.
6. Be sure to buy fabrics that are (on-grain/off-grain). (Circle the correct word.)
7. Which of the following are examples of notions?
   - A. zippers and seam binding
   - B. needles and pins
   - C. scissors and shears
   - D. patterns and fabric
8. What is a guide sheet?
9. How far are most seams sewn from the edge of the fabric?
10. Press seams on the _____ side of the fabric.
11. True or false. Use a double thread when sewing on a button.
12. What are two uses for appliqués?
13. True or false. Use a contrasting color of thread when sewing rips.
14. What are two alterations you can make to your clothes?
15. Finding new and different uses for old clothes is a form of (recycling/basting). (Circle the correct word.)

Life Skills

16. Participate in a service learning project with your sewing class. For instance, you might be able to make stuffed animals, pillows, or blankets for children in the hospital. Patients undergoing chemotherapy could use turbans, pillows, and lap blankets. Make a plan for this project by answering the following questions: Where could you find patterns for these items? What equipment and materials do you need? Can you obtain any of these items from donations? How can your class work together to complete this project?

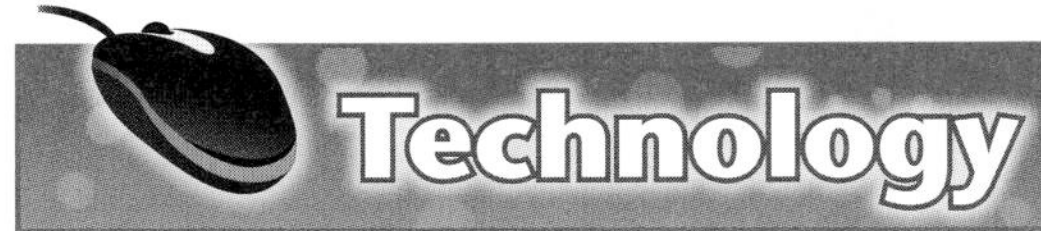

Technology

17. Research different types of sergers on the Internet. Give a short report to the class about how they differ. List a few of the projects that could be completed using them. What are the price ranges?

Journal Writing

18. Think about some different kinds of easy, inexpensive sewing projects you could make for birthday or holiday gifts.

Throughout the year, use your journal to keep track of the colors and materials your friends and family members prefer. What are some items they need? If you find fabric on sale that would be perfect for one of your gifts, buy it and keep track of how much you use and how much remains for other uses. You can even add pictures of how pleased the person is when they open your gift.

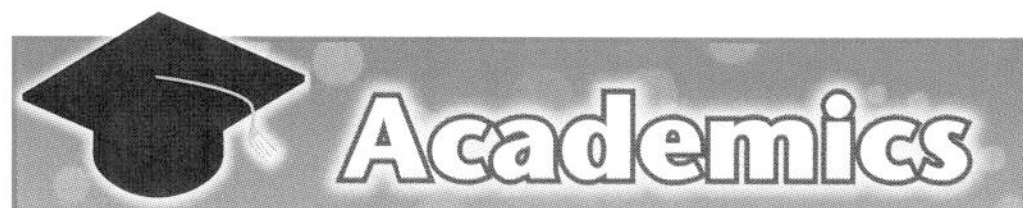

19. **Writing.** Devise a work plan for keeping the sewing lab clean at the end of each class. Make sure to include all of the tasks that must be done to prepare the lab for the next class.
20. **Financial Literacy.** Look at the back of a pattern envelope from a store—or at the directions for a free sewing project online. Pick a fabric you think would look good. Determine the amount of each material needed and the prices. How much would it cost if you decided to make two projects using the exact same materials?
21. **Speech.** In small groups, demonstrate to the class: straightening fabric, preparing fabric for layout, laying out and pinning a pattern, and transferring markings to fabric.

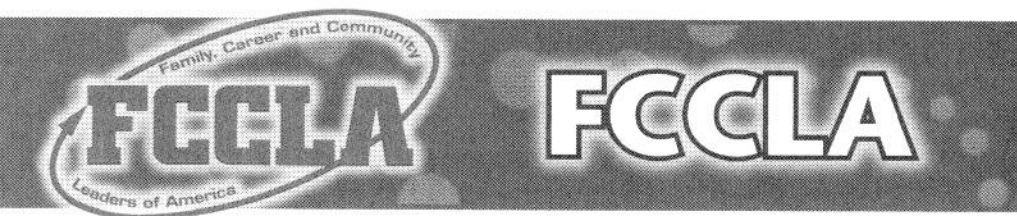

22. Choose one sewing project you made in class and another one or two that you made at home. Create a display of your items. Prepare a presentation about your sewing experience. Then develop an FCCLA *Textiles and Apparel* project for the *Career Connections* program. A garment designed for the upper and lower body (including eight different sewing techniques) can also be a *STAR Events* entry. Obtain further information about this program from your FCCLA advisor.

Unit 5
The World of Work

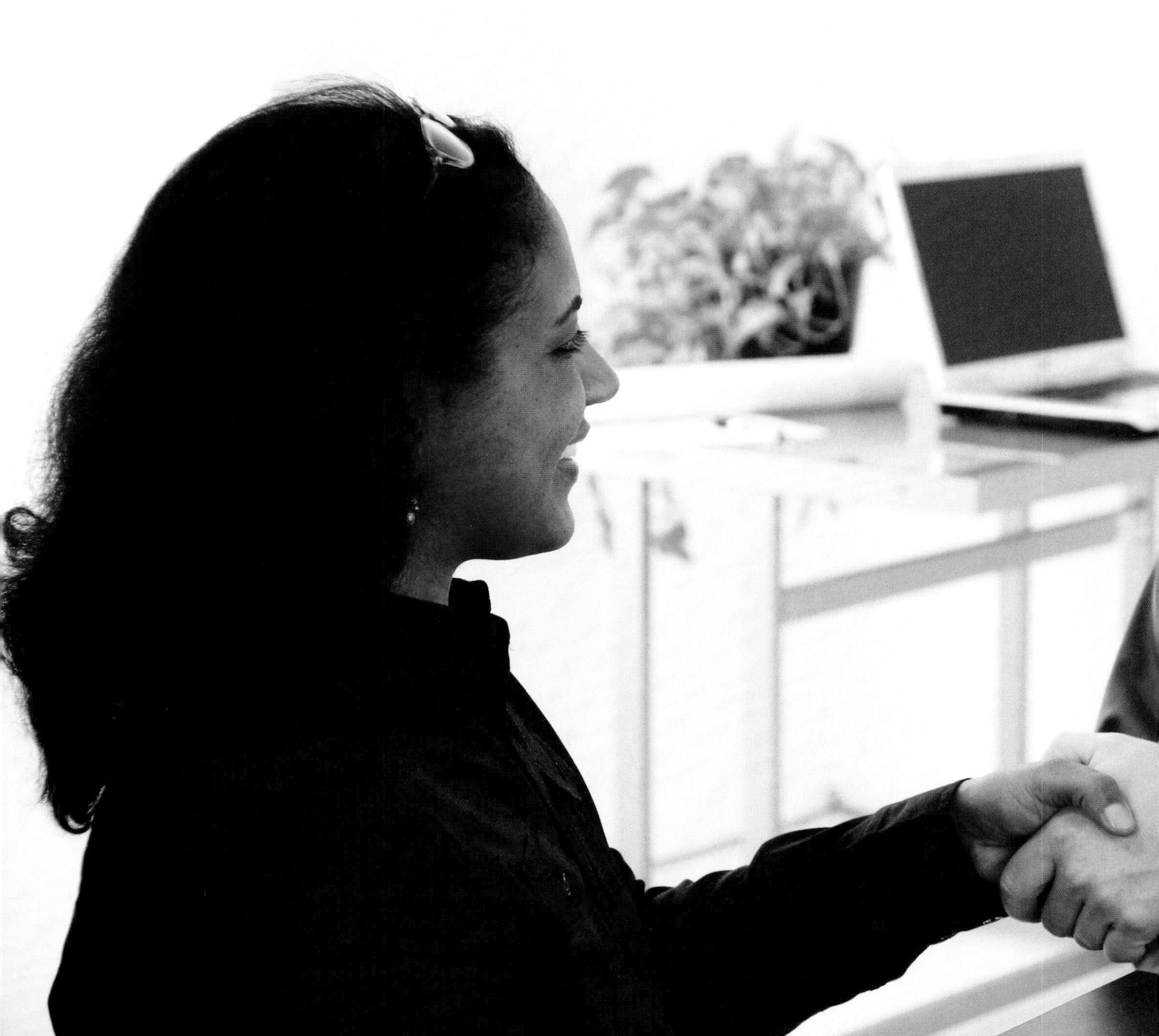

Chapter 12	Learning About Work
Chapter 13	Preparing for Work

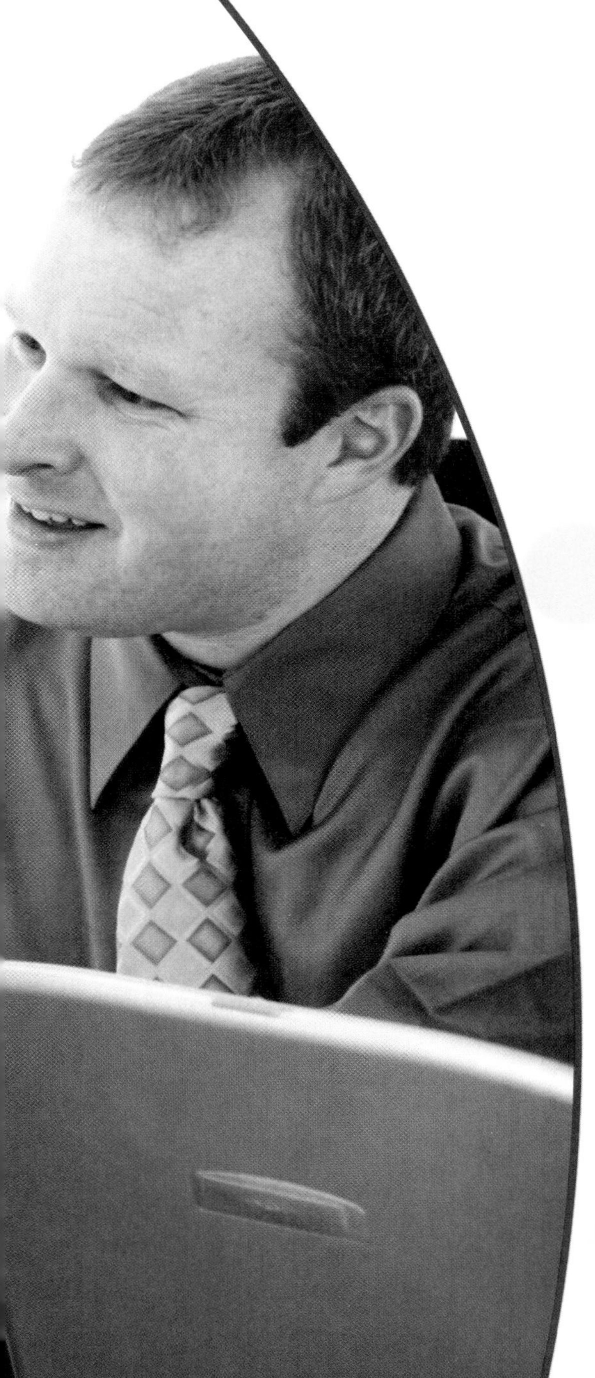

Exploring Careers

The following careers relate to the information you will study in Unit 5. Read the descriptions and then complete the activity to learn more about the careers that might interest you.

Career	Description
Teacher	Responsible for the education of students
Career counselor	Advises people about their career decisions
Lawyer	Provides advice for clients and/or represents them in court
Social worker	Assists people by helping them cope with and solve issues in their everyday lives
Technical support specialist	Provides technical assistance and support to individuals and organizations that use information technology
Marketing manager	Creates the demand for a company's products and services
Writer	Creates manuscripts, articles, or press releases on a variety of topics
Public relations specialist	Develops and executes communications efforts for clients to build and maintain positive relationships with the public

Activity: Identify a person who is working in a career you might want to pursue. Create a list of five questions about the career and conduct an interview with that person. Send a thank-you note to the person for giving you their time. Present your findings to the class.

Chapter 12
Learning About Work

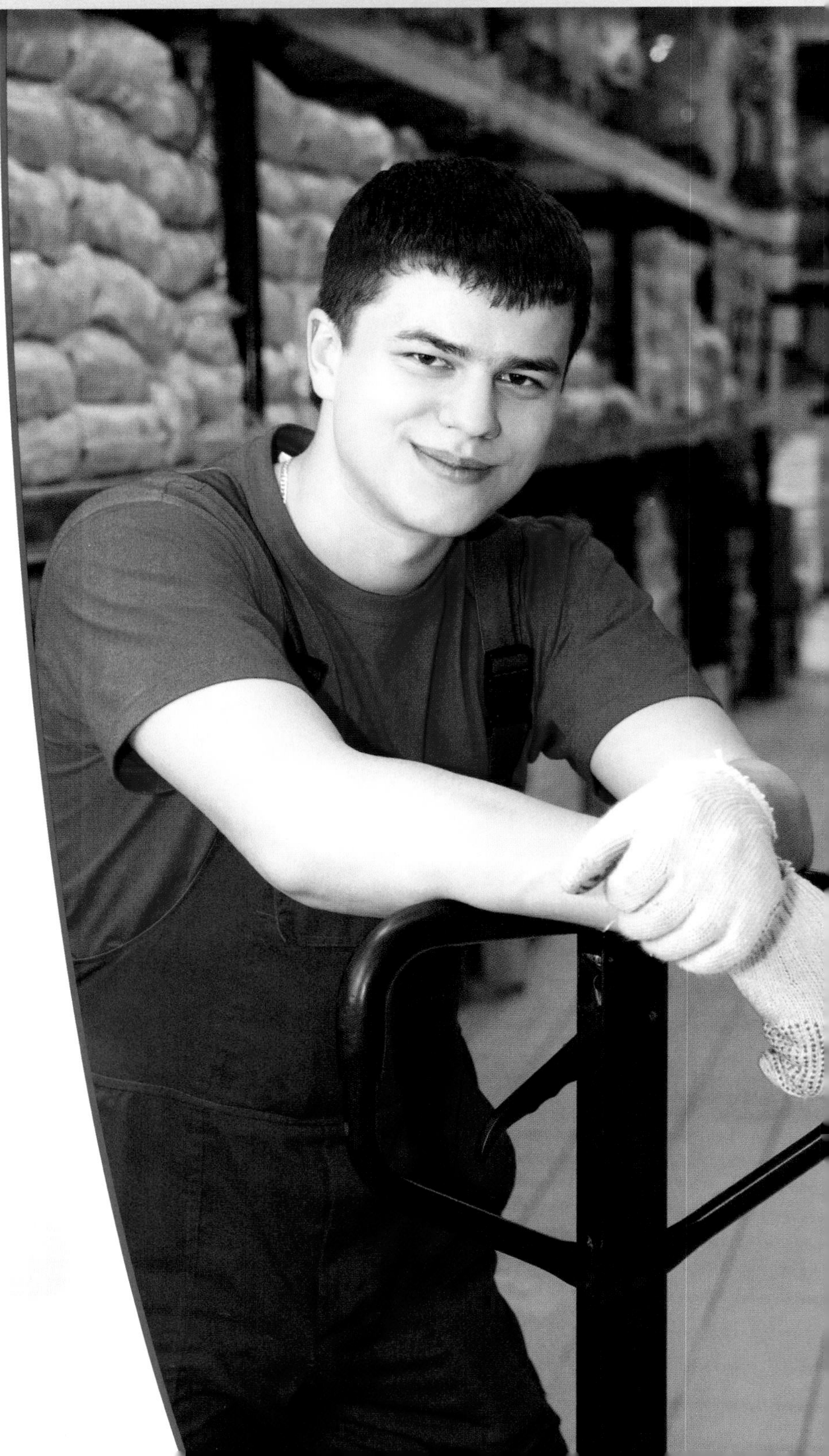

Sections

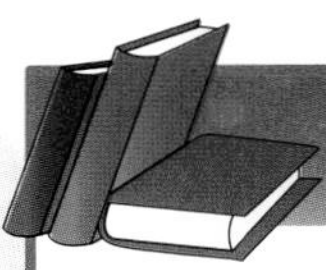

Sharpen Your Reading

Rewrite each chapter objective as a question. As you read, look for the answers to each question. Write the answers in your own words.

Concept Organizer

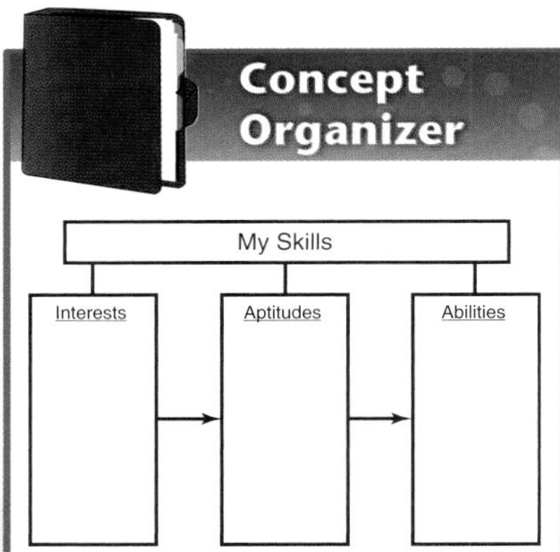

Use a chain diagram like the one shown to identify your interests, aptitudes, and abilities. What careers might you enjoy based on your list?

Companion Website
www.g-wlearning.com

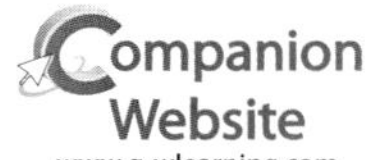

Print out the concept organizer at the website.

Section 12-1

Questions About Work

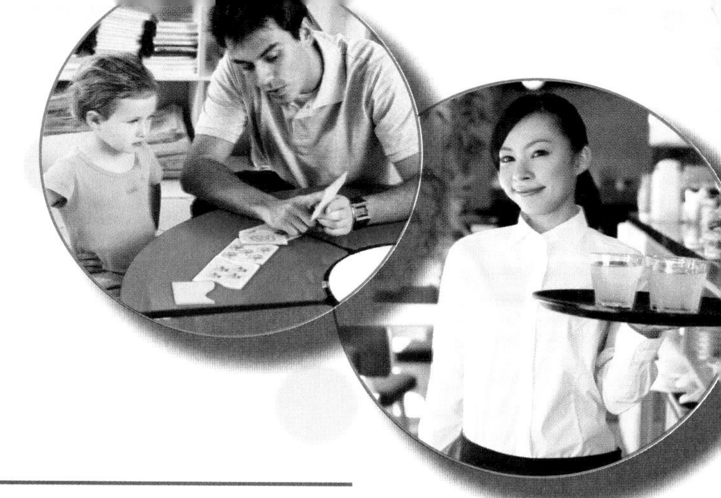

Objectives

After studying this section, you will be able to
- **define** *work*, *fringe benefits*, *job*, and *career*.
- **give examples** of how working benefits you and your community.
- **explain** the difference between a job and a career.
- **describe** how decisions about work will affect a person's future.

Key Terms

work: what a person does to earn money.

fringe benefits: rewards of a job other than income, such as paid vacation time and health insurance.

job: a position held by a worker.

career: a series of related jobs a person holds over time.

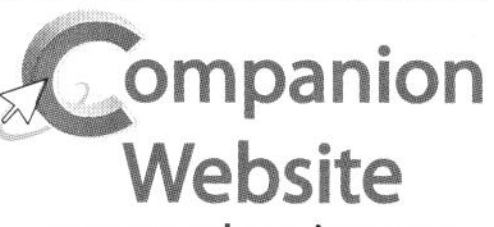

Study the Key Terms by completing crossword puzzles, matching activities, and e-flash cards at the website.

Main Ideas

- Work benefits you and your community.
- Some people have a series of jobs while others pursue a career.
- Your decisions about work will affect your future.

You see people working every day. You have probably thought about what kind of work you would like to do some day. You may, however, have a number of questions about what work will mean in your life. This section will attempt to answer some of those questions.

In this unit, **work** means what a person does to earn money. Work is also energy spent in order to complete a task. In this sense, work can mean any specific effort made to achieve a goal. For instance, you work when you mow the lawn or do homework. Jogging three miles is work.

Why Work?

One of your first questions about work may be: "Why should I work?" There are many reasons to work. Working to earn a living is only one of them. All jobs serve some purpose and are worthwhile. See **12-1**. Think of all the jobs you have seen today. Perhaps you rode the bus to school. The bus driver performed a worthwhile job. Can you think of other workers you have noticed today? Think of the reasons each job is worthwhile.

Working has many personal benefits. Work can give you a sense of *dignity*, or self-worth. It can provide you with a sense of pride, success, and independence. For instance, Lamont is a social worker who works with child abuse cases. He has a strong desire to help children. He wants to provide a service to society. The feeling that he is helping others is one reward of his job.

Working can also give you a sense of identity. Your job gives you a place in your community. You may be known as a hairstylist, doctor, dance teacher, salesperson, or some other title.

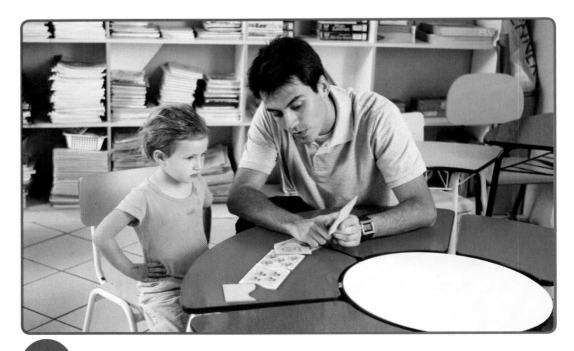

12-1 This man provides a valuable service through his job as a child care provider.

Earning an income is an important benefit of having a job. *Income* is the money you earn. You can use your income to buy items you need and want. In addition to earning an income, many workers also earn fringe benefits. **Fringe benefits** include paid vacation time, health insurance, life insurance, bonuses, and retirement funds.

Friendship can be a benefit of work, too. Sharing experiences with coworkers can give you a chance to make new friends.

You are not the only one who receives something from your work. Your community also benefits. For instance, you use the money you earn to buy products and services. Some of the money you spend is used to pay the people who make the products and offer the services. You provide work for others when you spend your money in this way. See **12-2**.

You also pay taxes on your income. These taxes help support public resources in the community. These resources include schools, fire and police protection, hospitals, and libraries.

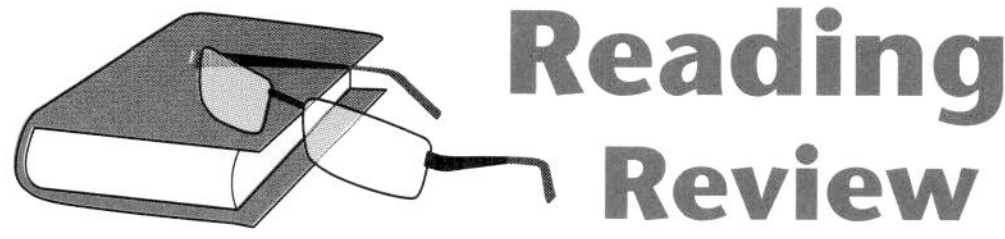

Reading Review

1. What personal benefits can you get from having a job?
2. What are two ways your community benefits by your working?

Job or Career?

A **job** is a position held by a worker. A **career** is a series of related jobs a person holds over time. Do you want to hold a series of unrelated jobs, or do you want to pursue a career?

Each job in a career builds on the knowledge and experience gained from the previous job. Suppose you decide on a career in food service. You may start with a job as a waiter. Then you may get a job as a cook. With some classes or special training, you might advance to pastry chef. Your hard work and experience may even land you a job as executive chef.

A career involves your feelings about work, as well as what you do. A career requires setting goals. You may need more training to help you get your first job. Then you have to stick with that job to gain enough experience to advance.

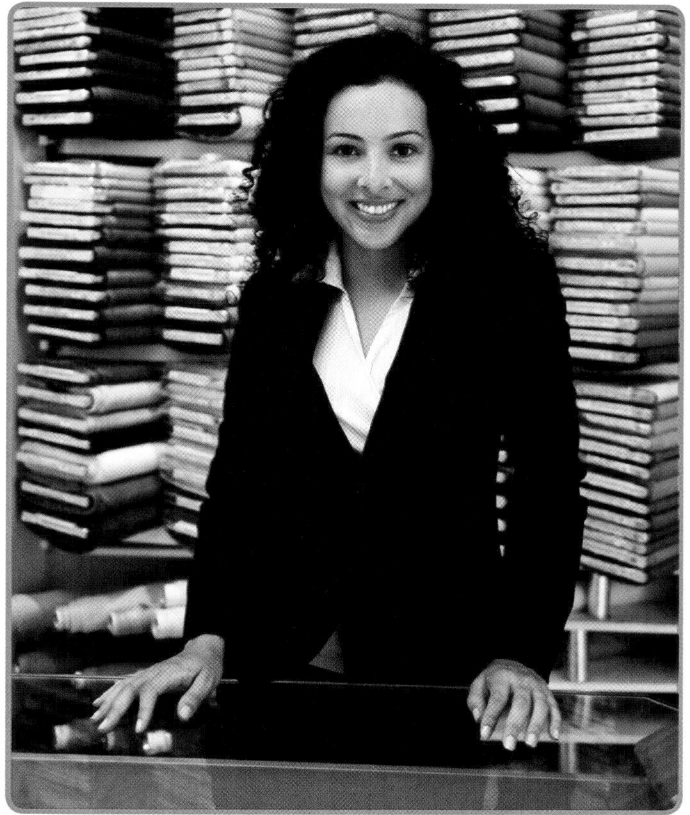

12-2 Communities benefit when people work. By buying local products, you help others in your community.

Social Studies Link

Career and Lifestyle Choices

In the past, many people had only one career. The current workplace, however, is more flexible. Many people change careers in their lifetimes. For instance, Pam's goal was to be a kindergarten teacher. She went to college for four years and got her teaching degree. After teaching for eight years, she decided to stop teaching and sell real estate. She changed her career in education to a career in sales.

Interview an older person who has a career that interests you. Ask questions to find out what jobs he or she has held. Also, find out how his or her choice of careers affected his or her lifestyle.

Pursuing a career takes dedication, time, and hard work. Advancing in a career is rewarding. You are also likely to earn more money than if you held a number of unrelated jobs.

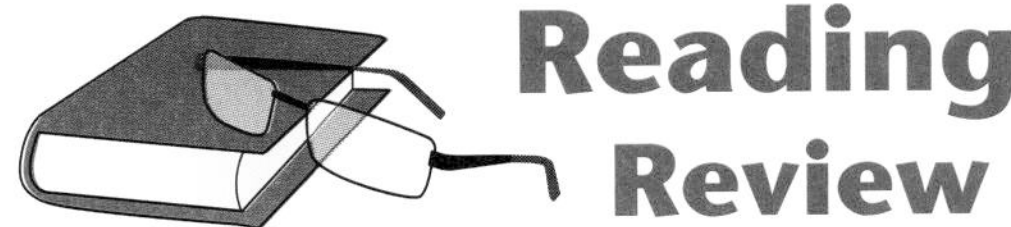

Reading Review

1. Why is your attitude important to pursuing a career?
2. What is a career that interests you? What are four related jobs that career might include?

How Will Work Affect You?

Your job decisions will affect your future *lifestyle*, or the way you live. Your job will affect your income, how you spend your time, and where you live. It will even have some effect on who will be in your circle of friends. How can a job do all this?

Your choice of jobs will affect how much money you make. The amount of income you have impacts what goods and services you buy. See **12-3**.

How often you are paid is decided by your job. You may be paid every week, every other week, or once a month. You might even be paid every time you complete a certain task. The way you are paid will affect how you budget your money.

For instance, Briana is a professional dancer in a large city. She is paid each time she performs. The number of her performances varies each month. She must plan carefully how to pay for her living expenses. When Briana is working, she must save part of her money. Those savings will cover her expenses when she is not working.

The hours you work will depend on your job. Many people work the same hours every week. Some jobs have schedules that change from one week to the next. You might work at night

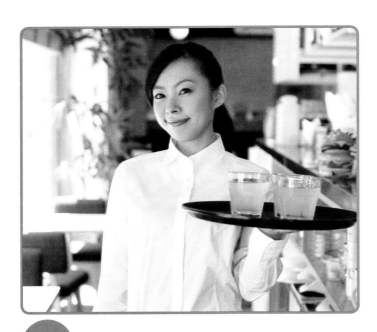

12-3 Your job will affect how much income you can save as well as how much you can spend.

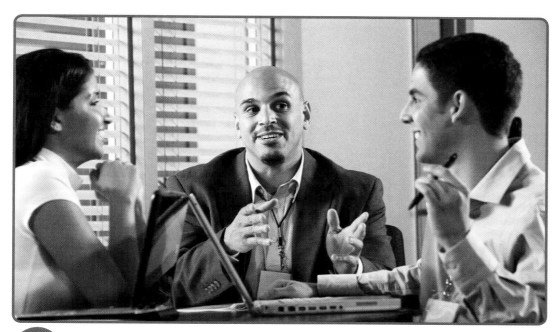

12-4 Most people form friendships with some of their coworkers.

or during the day. You may need to take work home for some jobs. The amount of time you spend working will affect how much time you can spend doing other activities.

Your work can determine where you live. Some jobs require you live in a certain area. Even if you can live anywhere, you may want to live near your job. This will allow you to avoid long drives to and from work.

You are likely to become friends with some of the people who work with you. Therefore, your job may even affect who your friends will be. See **12-4**.

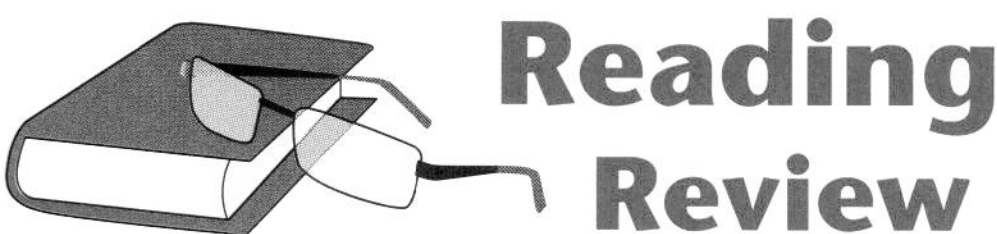

Reading Review

1. What difference might it make in your life if you are paid monthly instead of weekly?
2. How can your job affect who your friends will be?

Section Summary

- There are many reasons for working. These reasons include benefits for both you and your community.
- Decide if you would rather hold a series of unrelated jobs or pursue a career.
- Your lifestyle will be directly affected by your choice of jobs.

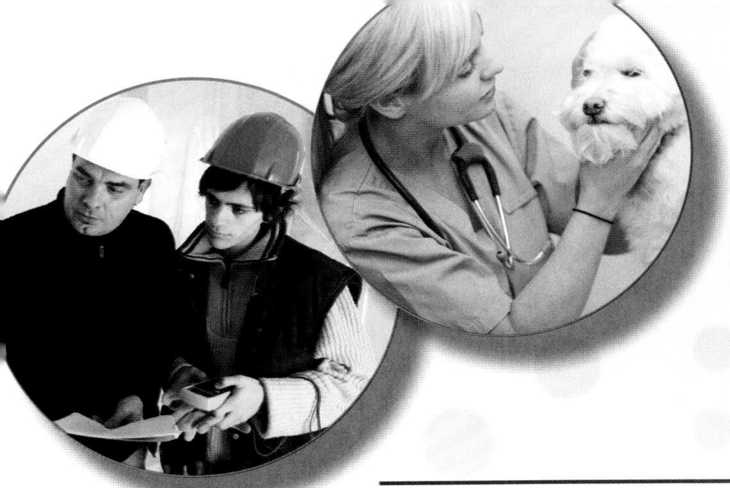

Section 12-2
Researching Careers

Objectives

After studying this section, you will be able to
- **define** *interests*, *aptitude*, *abilities*, *career clusters*, *trend*, *job shadowing*, and *mentor*.
- **give examples** of ways to learn about interests and aptitudes.
- **identify** ways to research careers.
- **explain** how you can learn more about careers through job shadowing.
- **demonstrate** how to research careers.

Key Terms

interests: the ideas and activities you like most.

aptitude: a natural skill.

abilities: skills you develop through practice or training.

career clusters: sixteen groups of career specialties.

trend: a general pattern of events.

job shadowing: following a worker on the job to observe what he or she does.

mentor: a person you trust to guide you along your career path.

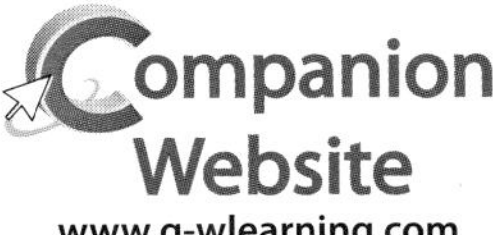

Study the Key Terms by completing crossword puzzles, matching activities, and e-flash cards at the website.

Main Ideas

- Identifying your interests, aptitudes, and abilities can help you choose a career you will enjoy.
- Learning about many careers can help you decide which one is right for you.
- There are many ways to learn about careers, such as using the career clusters and online resources.

Preparing to enter the world of work involves matching your abilities to a suitable career. Think about your interests and skills. Then find out which types of jobs would need them.

There are many resources available to help as you begin researching various careers. For instance, the career clusters can help you plan and prepare for your career. There are also many online career sources available. You can get information about careers from other sources as well.

Writing Link

Consider Your Values

In addition to your interests, aptitudes, and abilities, your values will also affect the kinds of jobs that appeal to you. Suppose you value time with your family. You may be happier in a job that does not require a lot of travel. If change is important, you may want a job with varied tasks. Think about the values that are most important to you. Then write a brief essay about how these values could influence your career choices.

Interests, Aptitudes, and Abilities

The first step in deciding on a career is learning about you. What are your interests? **Interests** are the ideas and activities you like most. What are your special talents? What are your values? What kind of lifestyle do you want to have when you are older? Answering these questions can help you decide what type of career would be right for you.

You will likely enjoy a job you find interesting. See **12-5**. To find such a job, it may help you to take an interest inventory. An *interest inventory* is a short quiz that suggests activities in which a person is most likely to excel. For instance, an interest inventory might show whether you prefer working with people, information, or objects. It may show whether you like working indoors or outdoors. Some questions reveal if you prefer working alone or with others.

You will do your best work in a job for which you have an aptitude or ability. An **aptitude** is a natural skill. For instance, suppose you have an aptitude for spelling. Working as a proofreader could be a good fit for you. A *proofreader* is someone who checks for errors in written work, such as misspelled words. You can take an *aptitude test* to show if you have a natural talent for doing certain tasks.

Abilities are skills you develop through practice or training. You can develop abilities more easily when you have related aptitudes. For instance, if

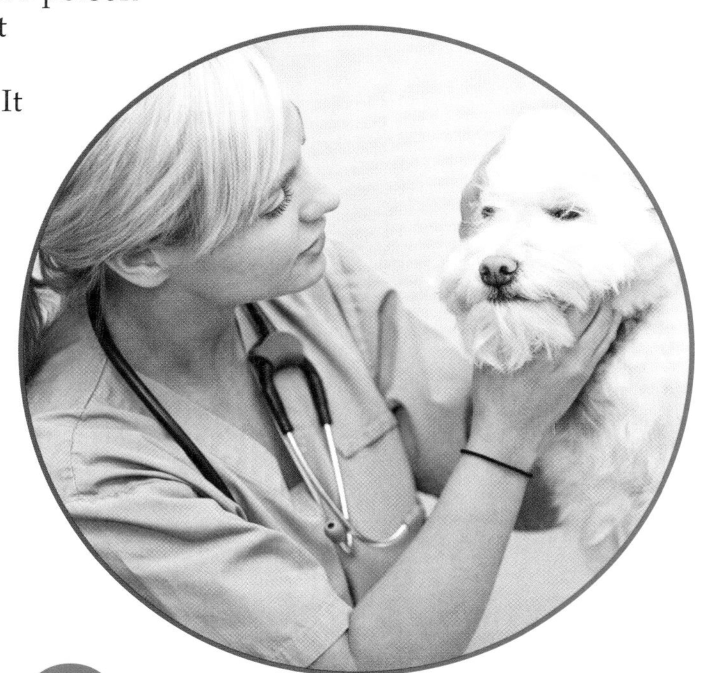

12-5 Someone who is interested in animals may enjoy working as a veterinarian.

you have an aptitude for music, you may quickly develop the ability to play an instrument. If you have a low aptitude, however, you may need to practice much more to learn the skill.

Learning about your interests, aptitudes, and abilities can point you to careers you will enjoy. Your guidance counselor can give you an interest inventory or an aptitude test. These tests are often available to take online, too.

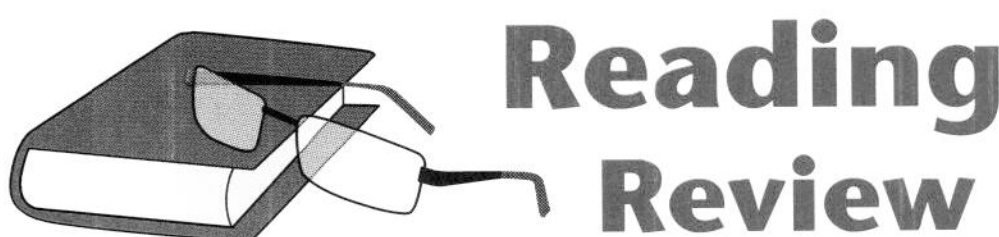

Reading Review

1. Why should learning about yourself be the first step in deciding on a career?
2. What is one of your aptitudes? What job might let you use this aptitude?

The Career Clusters

The **career clusters** are 16 groups of career specialties, **12-6**. Each cluster includes jobs that require similar knowledge and skills, or *essential knowledge and skills*. When you explore each cluster, you will find more

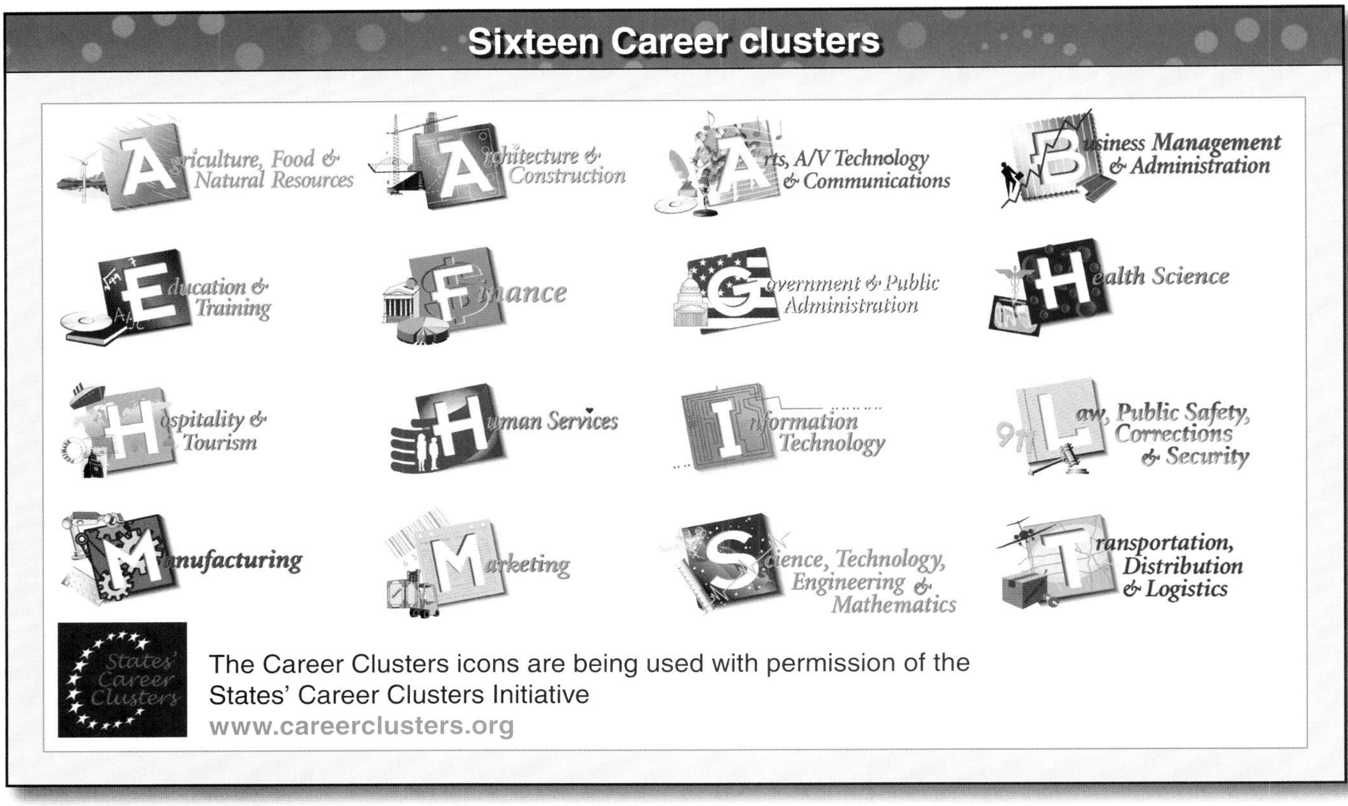

Sixteen Career clusters

Agriculture, Food & Natural Resources
Architecture & Construction
Arts, A/V Technology & Communications
Business Management & Administration
Education & Training
Finance
Government & Public Administration
Health Science
Hospitality & Tourism
Human Services
Information Technology
Law, Public Safety, Corrections & Security
Manufacturing
Marketing
Science, Technology, Engineering & Mathematics
Transportation, Distribution & Logistics

States' Career Clusters

The Career Clusters icons are being used with permission of the States' Career Clusters Initiative
www.careerclusters.org

12-6 Learning about these 16 career clusters is a good way to begin exploring careers.

groupings of jobs, called *career pathways*. Jobs in these pathways usually require more specialized knowledge and skills.

As you research jobs in a career pathway, pay attention to the skills you need for a job. You will often notice you need similar skills for another job within the same pathway. This knowledge will help as you plan your career. For instance, if you cannot get the job you want, you can use your skills to get a similar job. Learning about related jobs now can make it easier for you to adjust to job changes later.

Think Green

Green Jobs

A *green job* is loosely defined as one that promotes a clean environment. This means there are green jobs at every skill- and job-level. For instance, the U.S. Green Building Council (USGBC) posts construction and design jobs for green building projects. Renewable energy jobs include all positions working in that field, from scientists to maintenance operators. Green jobs are one of the fastest-growing areas of employment. The higher levels all require education beyond high school.

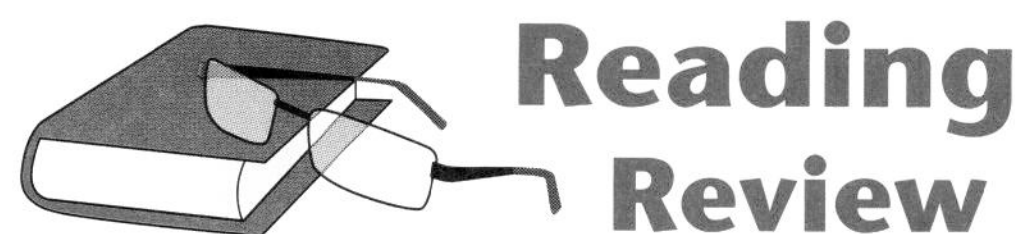

Reading Review

1. What career clusters would you like to learn more about?
2. Why is it important to pay attention to the skills you need for a job?

Online Career Sources

There are many online career sources available to help you find out about careers that interest you. The U.S. Department of Labor provides several sources that can help you gather information about *occupations*, or jobs. The *Occupational Outlook Handbook* describes many different jobs. This publication's website is bls.gov/oco. It lists job requirements, places of work, and income. It also predicts future needs for each job.

The Occupational Information Network, called O*NET™, can help you find your interests and aptitudes. You can also explore careers, job skills, and trends. A **trend** is a general pattern of events. For instance, technology is always changing. This means the jobs in technology are often changing. By studying trends that will affect jobs in the future, you can make better career choices. O*NET's website is onetonline.org. See **12-7** for a list of other online sources you can use.

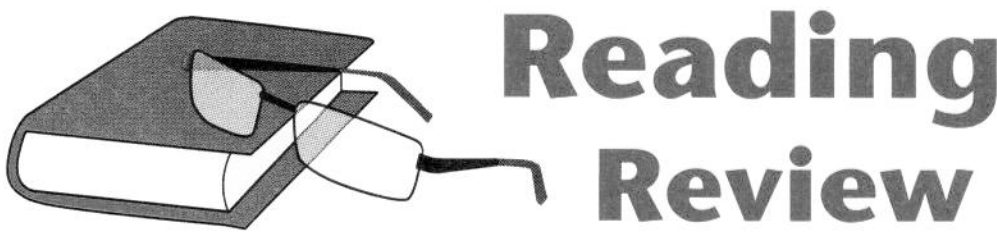

Reading Review

1. What kinds of information should you try to find out about careers that interest you?
2. How can studying job trends help you make better career choices?

Online Career Resources	
Source	**Internet Address**
USAJOBS, the official job site of the U.S. Federal Government	www.usajobs.gov
Occupational Outlook Handbook, U.S. Department of Labor	www.bls.gov/oco
U.S. Department of Labor Employment and Training Administration	www.doleta.gov
The Occupational Information Network (O*NET™)	www.onetcenter.org
CareerOneStop	www.careeronestop.org
Mapping Your Future	www.mappingyourfuture.org

12-7 These are just a few of the many websites available for researching careers.

Other Career Sources

In addition to the career clusters and online sources, you can visit your local library to check out books that describe various careers. You can also get help from your school's guidance counselor. Some classes provide job information. You can also talk to people who have jobs that interest you.

Many schools offer opportunities to observe various careers in person. **Job shadowing** is following a worker on the job to observe what he or she does. See **12-8**. You get to see what skills are needed. Observing a typical day

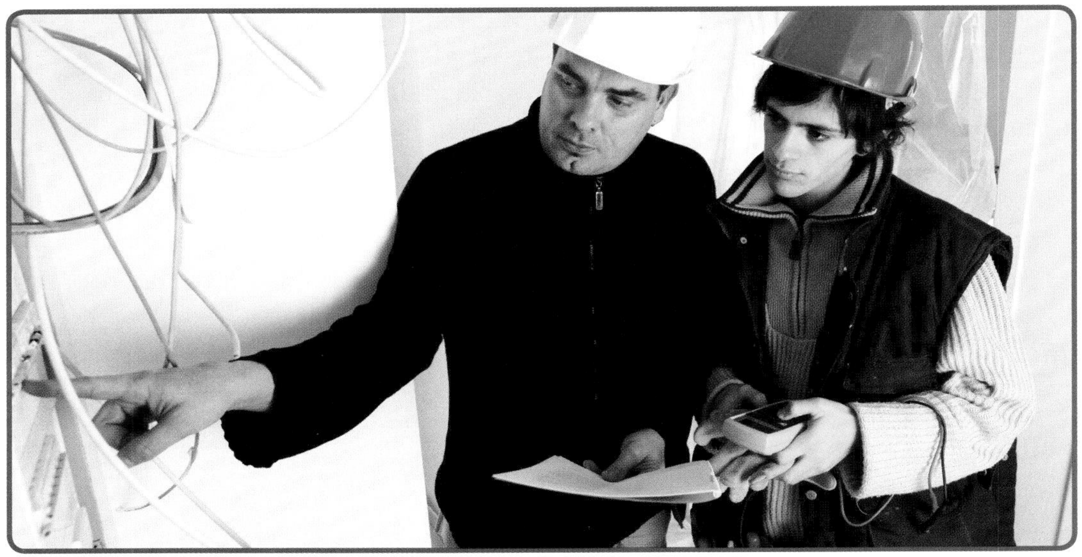

12-8 This student is job shadowing an electrician to learn more about the job.

lets you know what the job would be like for you. It is a time to ask questions about the education and experience you would need for that position.

Job shadowing can last a day or a few days. Your counselor or teacher may set up the experience. You can also create one by asking someone to allow you to shadow him or her. It would be helpful to research the job before you go. This will help you prepare meaningful questions to ask.

You may also want to consider finding a mentor. A **mentor** is a person you trust to guide you along your career path. A mentor usually has experience in a certain career field and values your skills and abilities.

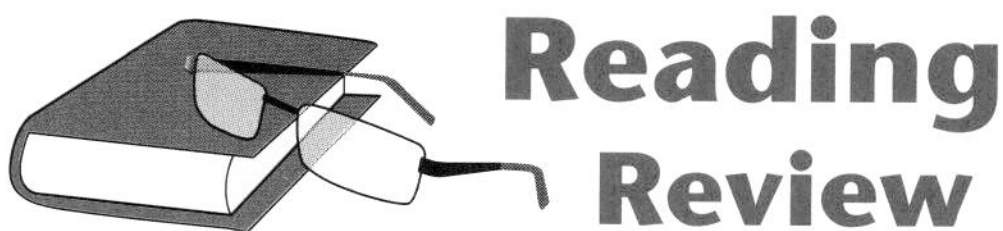

Reading Review

1. Why is it important to research careers before making any career decisions?
2. What are three occupations that appeal to you? How can you gather information on these jobs?

Section Summary

- Learning about your interests, aptitudes, and abilities can point you to careers you will enjoy.
- Researching various careers will give you information about possible careers in your future.
- Thinking about trends can help you predict future job needs.
- Some schools provide hands-on opportunities through job shadowing.

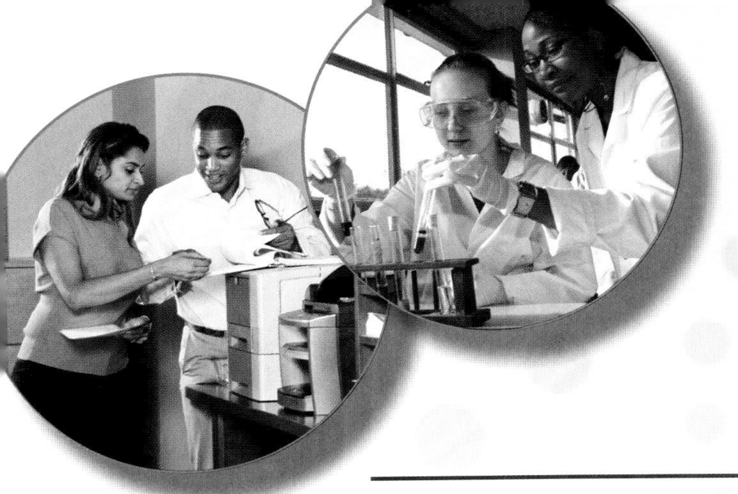

Section 12-3
Heading for a Career

Objectives

After studying this section, you will be able to
- **define** *work-based learning*, *job skills*, and *apprentice*.
- **list** three ways to get education and training.
- **explain** how setting goals can help you plan for a career.

Key Terms

work-based learning: programs in which students learn about a job through direct work experience and attend related classes.

job skills: the abilities needed for success in a certain job.

apprentice: someone who learns a job by working with a skilled worker.

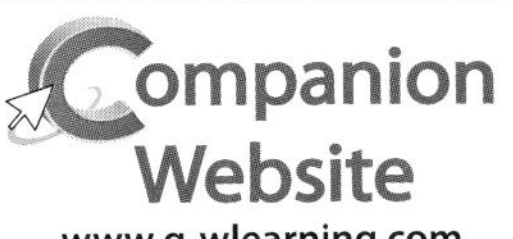

Study the Key Terms by completing crossword puzzles, matching activities, and e-flash cards at the website.

Main Ideas

- There are many ways you can get the education and training you need for a job.
- Having the right job skills can help you get and keep a job.
- Setting short- and long-term goals can help you better prepare for your career.

As you research careers, you will learn about the type of education and training needed. You will also learn about what the job is like. This information can help you set career goals and decide which jobs appeal to you. See **12-9**.

Decide on Education and Training

Your career decisions will affect the amount of education and training you need. Some jobs only require a high school diploma. Many other jobs, however, require more education. There are many ways you can get the education and training you need. For instance, you may decide to attend college after high school. You might receive training in the military. You may decide to receive training for specific job skills.

Work-Based Learning Programs

One way to get the education and training you need is to take special courses in high school. Many schools offer work-based learning programs. In **work-based learning** programs, students learn about a job through direct work experience as part of their class work. A program coordinator works with the student and the employer to make sure the experience is a success.

Some high schools offer work-based learning programs called *co-op programs*. Students in co-op programs attend classes for part of the day and then work in their field of interest the remainder of the day.

After high school, these programs are called *internships*. An internship can be either paid or unpaid. Students in an internship often earn credits toward graduation. They also learn about a job while gaining work experience.

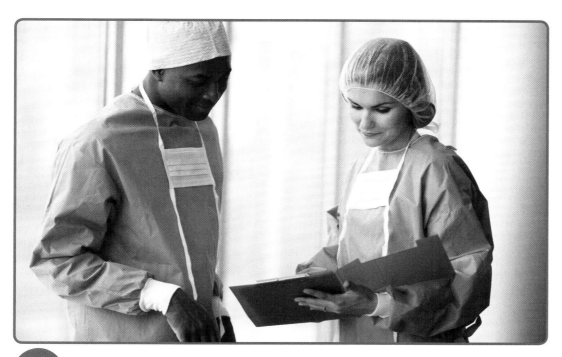

12-9 Someone who is interested in medicine may want to explore a career as a doctor.

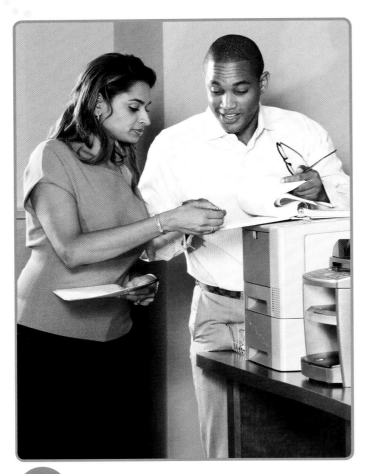

12-10 Being able to communicate clearly is a skill needed for all jobs.

Job Training

The purpose of job training is to learn job skills. **Job skills** are the abilities needed for success in a certain job. Having the right job skills can help you get and keep the job you want.

Basic skills, such as reading and writing, are required for all jobs. See **12-10**. Some jobs also require specific job skills. For instance, if you want to work as an artist, you need well-developed drawing and painting skills.

When you want to learn specific job skills, you might want to attend a technical school. *Technical schools* provide job training at both high school and college levels. Woodworking, culinary arts, and auto repair are just a few examples of programs that teach specific job skills. High school students who complete these programs often receive a certificate with their diploma.

You may also choose to be in a tech prep program. Students in *tech prep programs* complete special training for two years each of high school and college. Students who complete a tech prep program receive a certificate or a two-year college degree.

Trade schools provide training for specific jobs at the college level. Students can take up to three years of classes. When they complete the program, they receive a certificate or two-year college degree.

You might also become an apprentice. An **apprentice** is someone who learns a job by working with a skilled worker. Depending on your career goals, job training may last a few months or many years.

Colleges and Universities

Many careers require education beyond high school. Your career research can help you decide which courses you will need. For instance, suppose you want to be an engineer. Your research tells you engineers need a college degree and an aptitude in math and science. Therefore, you decide to take the math and science courses in high school to prepare for getting an advanced degree in engineering. With the help of your guidance counselor, you must also decide which college offers the best programs to become an engineer. See **12-11**.

Community colleges are two-year colleges. They are also called *junior colleges*. An *associate's degree* is a two-year college degree.

Other colleges and universities offer four-year programs. Students who complete four years of college receive a *bachelor's degree*. A *master's degree* requires another one or two years of study after a bachelor's degree.

To learn more about the colleges that might be right for you, talk to your guidance counselor. You can also find out about colleges on the Internet. Some colleges even accept courses taken in high school.

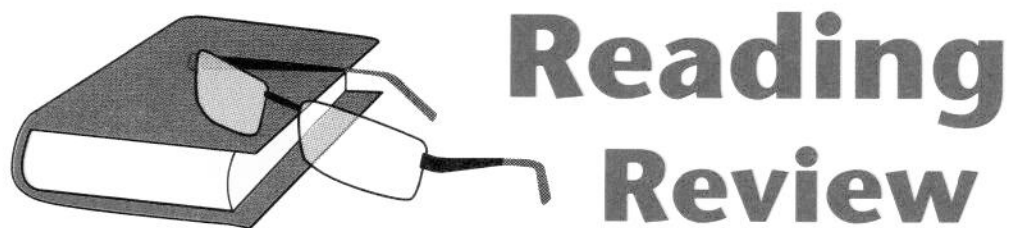

1. Why do you think it might be important to get job training before you begin looking for a job?
2. Why might you want to enroll in a high school career or technical education program?

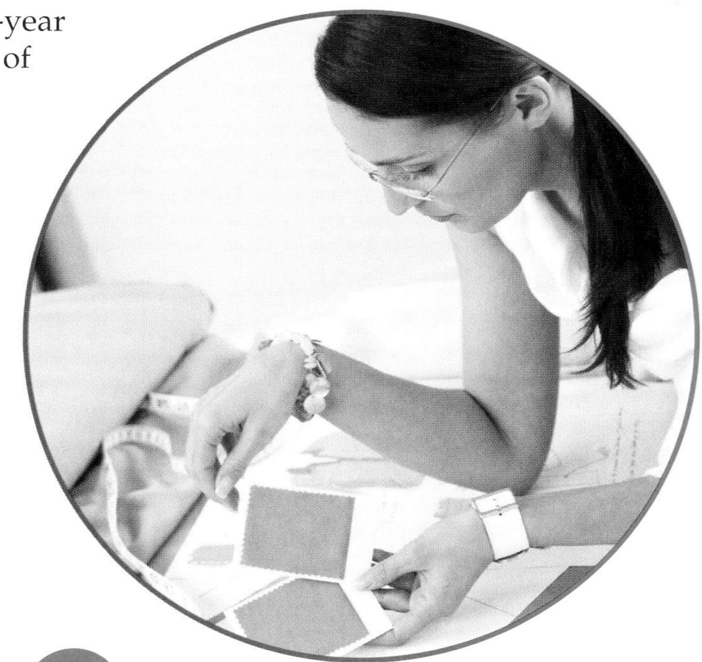

12-11 This fashion design college student took clothing and art courses in high school.

Think About Trade-Offs

Career decisions, just like other decisions, involve making trade-offs. For instance, one job that interests you may require a college degree. Another may require a two-year training program. Before you decide which area to pursue, think about the positive and negative points of each.

The first job might pay better than the second job. In order to earn the higher income, however, you have to attend school for four years instead of two. This is a trade-off. Think about trade-offs when planning your future. They will affect your decisions.

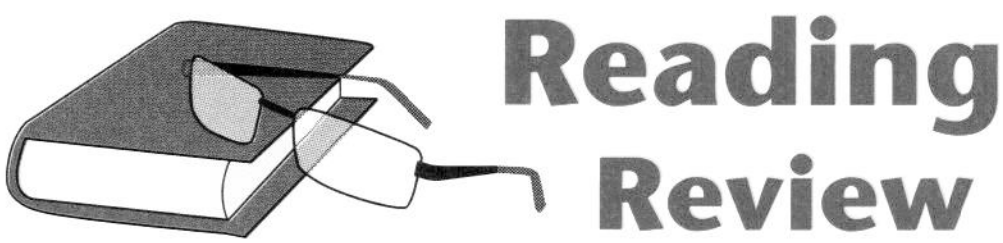

1. What is an example of a trade-off involving a job choice?
2. What trade-offs might affect your career decisions?

Financial Literacy Link

How Education Pays Off

The U.S. Census Bureau's statistics on earning show the realities of education in the job market. During a lifetime, those with just a high school diploma will make around $1.2 million. Those with a four-year college degree, however, will make $2.1 million (nearly twice the amount). People who go on to earn professional degrees, such as doctors, lawyers, and dentists, will earn around $4.4 million during their careers. Employees who continue to upgrade their skills while working also earn higher wages. Higher education and continued job training are investments in your future.

Set Career Goals

Once you have gathered facts, you will be ready to set some early career goals. Setting short-term goals is a good place to start. From the facts you have gathered, you know what type of training and background you might need. See **12-12**. You may revise your goals along the way or change your mind about possible careers.

Your goals can help you decide which of the careers you have explored could be right for you. For instance, you may have a goal to improve how some machines work. If so, you would choose a technical career. You may have a goal to help other people. In that case, you would choose a service career.

James is a forest ranger in a state park. When he was young, James always preferred being outdoors in the woods behind his home. He researched the kind of careers available for people who liked that activity. A forest ranger seemed to be a good fit for him.

He found that to become a ranger he needed a college degree in forestry. To reach his final career goal, James set some short-term goals. First, he had to finish high school. In his junior year, he found a college that offered degrees in forestry.

He applied and was accepted at that college, but had to find a way to pay for college tuition and expenses. He also had to study and pass his college courses. These are just some of the short-term goals that helped James reach his final career goal.

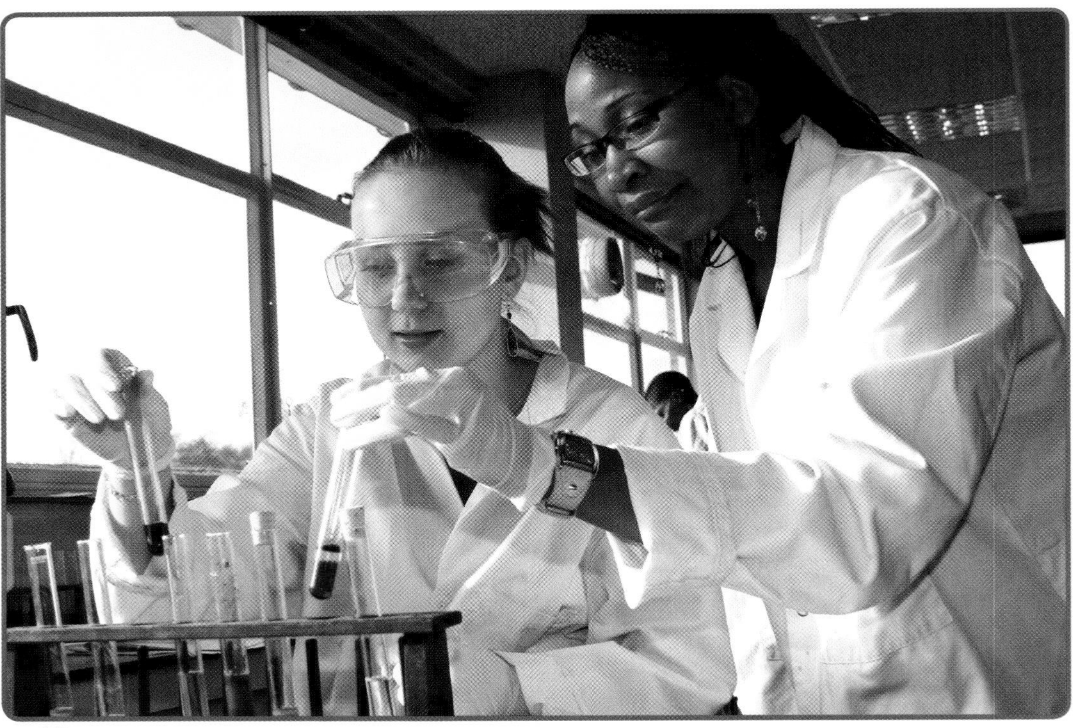

12-12 Set goals to get the education you need to achieve your career plans.

Try to set realistic career goals. Ask for help. Your counselors are trained to help you learn about jobs and their requirements.

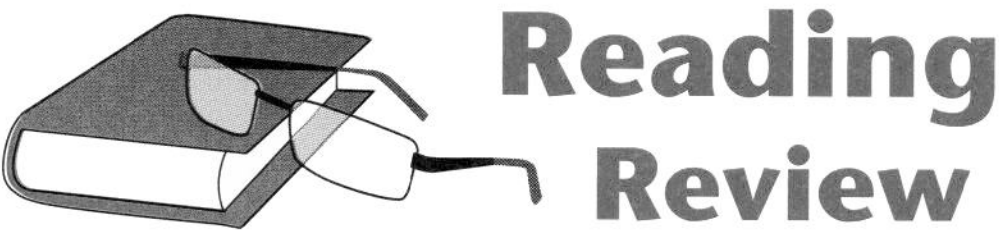

Reading Review

1. What is one of your goals for the future? What career can help you reach that goal?
2. How can setting short-term goals help you enter the career you want?

Succeed in Life

How to Set Goals

Sometimes the idea of setting personal goals seems overwhelming. How do you even start? Here are a few goal-setting tips.

- Avoid setting goals that are too broad, such as *save more money*. Set specific goals, such as *save $50 in two months*.
- Start with setting realistic, short-term goals you can reach. For instance, *take a higher-level art class before starting high school*.
- Write your plan to achieve the goal in a short, outline form. Make sure to list the specific activities you must do, or challenges to address, to reach your goal.
- Tell your family and friends when your goals are met. It is always good to have your support group recognize your achievements.
- Use the same system to set your long-term goals, too. For instance, if your goal is to *travel in Europe for six weeks after college*, there are a number of things that must be addressed over the years for you to reach that goal.
- For long-term goals, develop one or two strategies to keep your self motivated. For instance, in the case of the previous goal, one strategy might be to make a collage of the cities you want to visit. Keep it in your room where you can see it often to remind yourself of your goal.
- Celebrate when you achieve your big goals.

Section Summary

- Career decisions will affect the type and amount of education and training you need.
- Many schools offer work-based learning programs.
- Think about trade-offs as you make your career decisions.
- Setting career goals can help you decide on the right career for you.

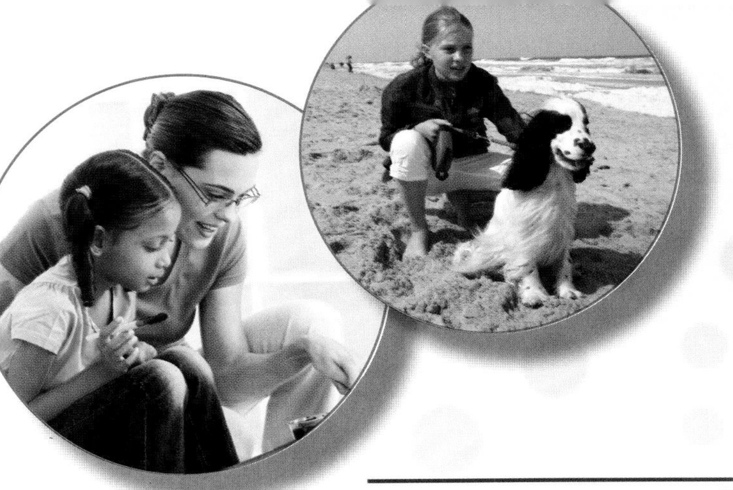

Section 12-4
Career Options

Objectives

After studying this section, you will be able to
- **define** *entrepreneur*.
- **give examples** of jobs in each of the seven areas of family and consumer sciences.
- **describe** opportunities for entrepreneurship.

Key Term

entrepreneur: a person who starts and manages his or her own business.

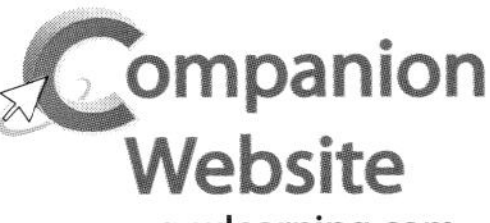

Study the Key Term by completing crossword puzzles, matching activities, and e-flash cards at the website.

Main Ideas

- Careers are available in all fields of family and consumer sciences.
- Entrepreneurship is a growing trend in the world of work.

Investigating the career clusters is one way to research careers. Another way to research careers is by looking at various fields of study. One field, family and consumer sciences, appeals to those who seek career variety. Careers in family and consumer sciences help people make informed decisions about their well-being, relationships, and resources to improve their quality of life.

Family and Consumer Sciences Careers

The field of family and consumer sciences includes careers in several areas. *Food science, nutrition and wellness, housing and interior design,* and *textiles and apparel* are part of family and consumer sciences. Other specialty areas of this field include *child and human development, family relations, personal and family finance*, and *education and communications*.

Food Science, Nutrition, and Wellness

Today, keeping fit and eating healthy is an important trend. Eating more meals away from home is also a trend. Therefore, there is a demand for people to work in food science, nutrition, and wellness areas.

Food scientists research new foods. They also work to make sure foods are safe to eat. Hospitals, advertising agencies, and food companies have jobs for people in this area, too. Dietitians plan meals for hospital patients. See **12-13**. A food stylist arranges food for ad photos. A product development specialist works in a test kitchen to refine new food products and create recipes.

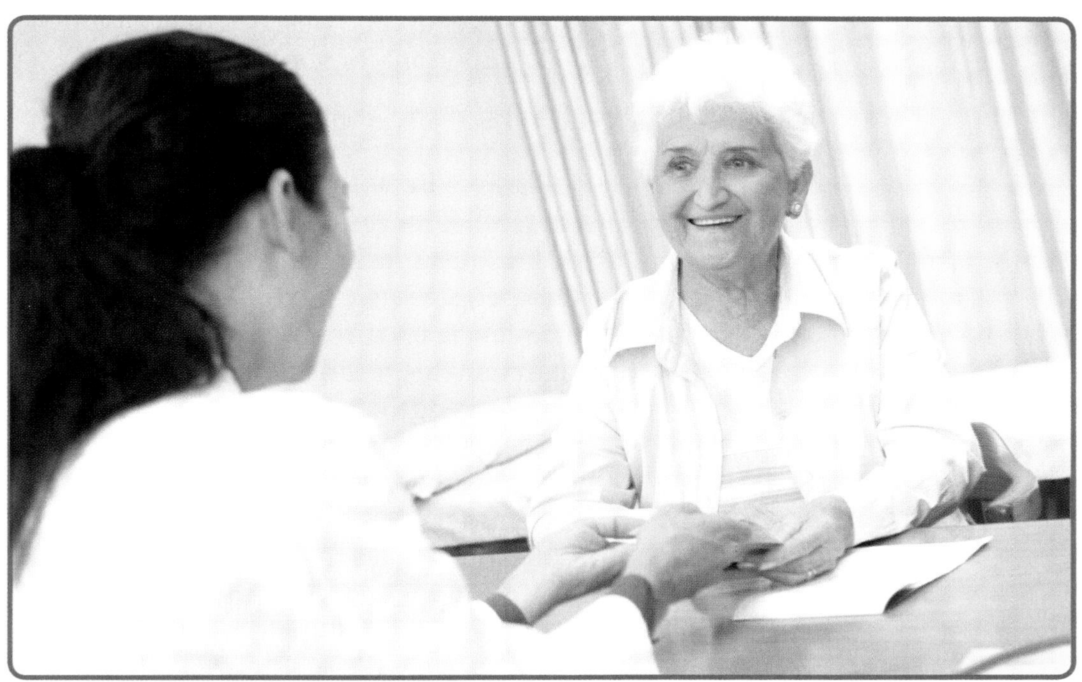

12-13 This dietitian is helping a patient make better food choices.

This area also includes food and nutrition specialists in the food service industry. Chefs and cooks prepare your food. Chefs may have helpers who specialize in preparing pastries or salads. Banquet managers prepare meals for large groups in hotels, on cruise ships, and in other settings. Caterers provide meals to homes, offices, and other places. They may be scheduled for one special meal or regularly scheduled events.

Careers in nutrition and food science demand a science background. Some jobs require math skills to figure amounts of ingredients and nutrients. Those desiring a job in this diverse area should be able to get along well with others. An interest in hospitality and different foods is also helpful. Some jobs call for artistic skill or long working hours.

Housing and Interior Design

People who work in housing might design, decorate, sell, or care for homes. Interior designers plan and decorate the interior spaces of homes and commercial buildings. See **12-14**. They suggest color schemes and furnishings to make the spaces appealing and functional. Other specialists solve complex problems with creative ideas in focused areas of the house. These include space planners, lighting specialists, and kitchen and bath designers. Real estate agents assist people in buying and selling homes. Housekeepers keep homes clean.

Housing is a basic physical need. Therefore, people will always be needed to work in housing-related careers. If you are interested in housing, learn the basic principles of art and design. An eye for detail is also important for success in this field.

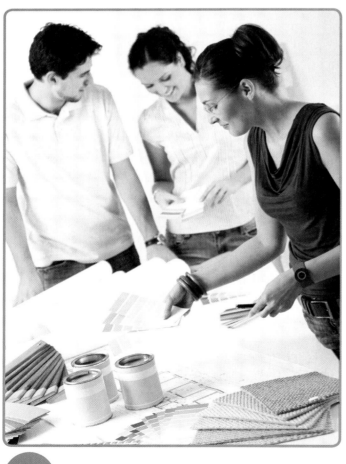

12-14 These interior design students are learning design techniques.

Textiles and Apparel

Careers in clothing and textiles deal with clothes, accessories, and fabrics. Fashion designers create the clothing styles people wear. Textile designers create fabric textures and patterns. Textile researchers test fabrics for certain qualities, such as strength. Tailors make clothes. Retail store buyers purchase garments and accessories from the manufacturers to sell to consumers. Salespeople sell clothes, and dry cleaners clean them.

Clothing, like food and housing, is a basic need. There will always be a need for people to work in this area. Many clothing and textile careers require a command of color and design. Researchers need a science background. Tailors need good hand/eye coordination. Retail store buyers and salespeople need strong communication skills.

Child and Human Development

If you babysit, you already have a job in child development. Jobs in child development involve working with children and designing products for them. Child care centers employ directors, teachers, and teaching assistants. See **12-15**. Jobs in recreation include planning and directing children's activities at camps, parks, and playgrounds. Social workers in Child Protective Services help children who are abused or neglected. People who write children's books and design children's toys also work in this field.

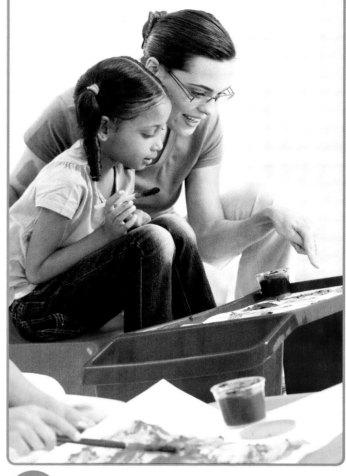

12-15 Teachers in child care centers plan and lead learning experiences for children.

With many parents working outside the home, more child care is needed. Those who work in this field need to understand how children grow and learn. They also need to enjoy helping them. You should know about nutrition and first aid. Patience and creativity are other traits that will help you care for children.

Some jobs focus on a person's development beyond childhood. These jobs are in social work, therapy, counseling, training, and education. For jobs in these areas, you should enjoy working with people. You should also be familiar with issues relating to the physical, intellectual, social, and emotional changes in life.

Family Relations

Family relations workers help people and families manage daily tasks and crises. Home companions visit people who have trouble handling day-to-day matters. Counselors and therapists help children, teens, adults, couples, or families deal with their challenges. Crisis hotline operators are trained to handle calls for help from people who are facing challenges. People who manage events at older adult living centers also work in this field.

Jobs in this area require good communication skills and a desire to serve others. You also need to get along well with people and have a warm, caring personality.

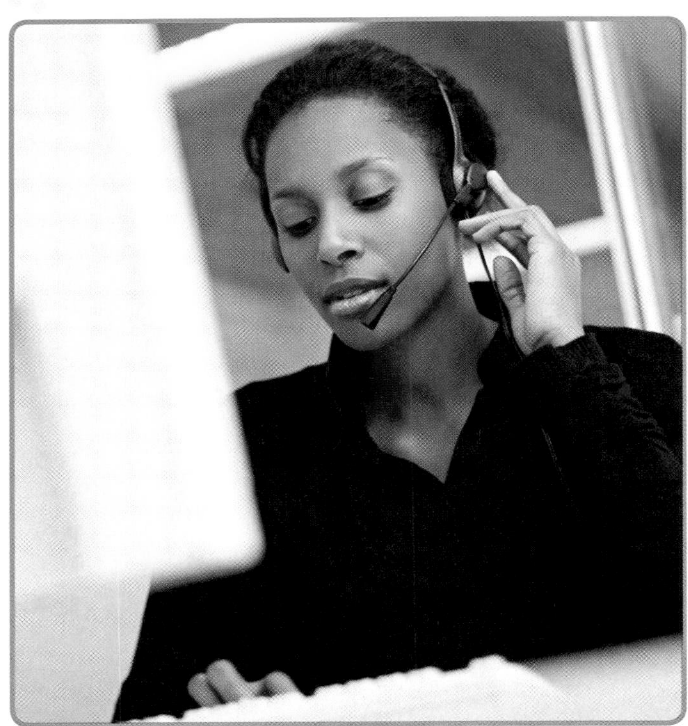

12-16 Consumer service representatives help resolve customer complaints.

Personal and Family Finance

Jobs in the field of personal and family finance teach people how to manage their money wisely. Financial planners help customers set up budgets and invest money to meet future goals.

In related money management areas, other types of jobs are available. Store credit managers approve credit applications and make sure bills are collected. Credit counselors advise families about how to pay their debts. Some stores hire comparison shoppers to check prices in competing stores. Customer service specialists handle customer complaints about prices and other matters. See **12-16**.

Many people need help managing their incomes and expenses. To succeed in this field, you need to have a business background and usually a college degree. All jobs involving finance require math skills. Communication skills are also vital in many jobs.

Education and Communications

Most careers in education and communications require a college degree. You may study some of the areas discussed in this section, but there are others. Teaching family and consumer science subjects in a middle school, high school, or college is one career path.

Another path is working as a cooperative extension agent. Some extension agents work with young people in groups such as 4-H. Others keep adults informed on important consumer issues.

The family and consumer sciences field includes a broad range of careers. See **12-17**. If any of these careers interest you, find out more about them. Ask your guidance counselor or research them online. You may decide a career in this field is right for you.

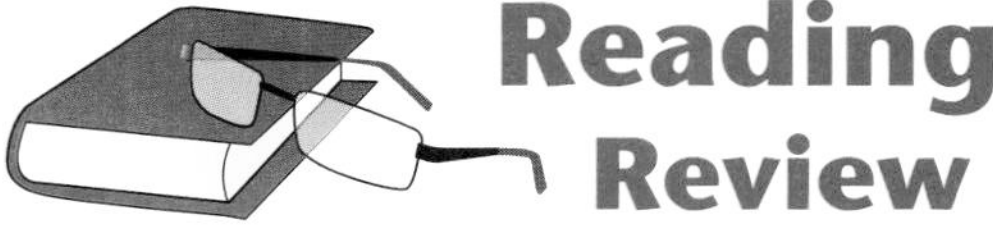

Reading Review

1. Choose one area of family and consumer sciences that interests you. What factors create a need for people to enter careers in that area?
2. What are three jobs related to that area of family and consumer sciences?
3. What traits do you need to enter a career in that area?

Family and Consumer Sciences		
Major Categories	**Postsecondary Training and / or Associate's Degree**	**Bachelor's Degree or Higher**
Food Science, Nutrition, and Wellness	Banquet manager Caterer Chef or chief cook Cook's helper Executive chef Personal trainer Restaurant owner Short-order cook	Athletic trainer Dietitian Food service manager Food technologist Product developer Quality control supervisor Sanitation supervisor
Housing and Interior Design	Designer's aide Drapery/slipcover maker Home furnishings salesperson Home lighting assistant Upholstery assistant	Facilities planner Home furnishings buyer Home lighting designer Home planning specialist Interior designer Kitchen and bath designer
Textiles and Apparel	Alterationist Clothing consultant Display artist Dry cleaner Fashion or textile designer Store manager Tailor/reweaver	Apparel historian Apparel marketing specialist Merchandise manager Textile market analyst Textile scientist
Child and Human Development	Child care teacher Designer of children's clothing, toys, or furniture Parent's helper Scout leader Teacher's aide	Child care center or preschool administrator Early childhood educator Parent educator Recreation director
Family Relations	Home companions Counseling paraprofessional Homemaker services director Hot line counselor Older adult living facilities aide	Crisis center counselor Family health counselor Family/marriage therapist Youth services specialist
Personal and Family Finance	Bank teller Collection agent Consumer product specialist Consumer service representative Credit bureau clerk Loan officer assistant	Consumer affairs director Credit counselor Financial planner Loan officer Money investment advisor Retail credit manager
Education and Communications	4-H leader Journalism intern Teacher's aide	Cooperative extension agent Family and consumer sciences teacher or college professor

12-17 Family and consumer sciences offers a wide range of job opportunities.

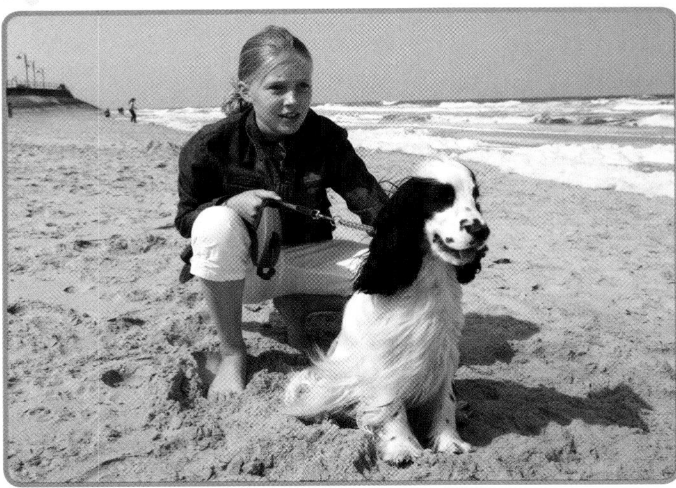

12-18 This teen started a pet-sitting service to care for animals while their owners are away.

Entrepreneurship

An **entrepreneur** is a person who starts and manages his or her own business. Entrepreneurs see the need for certain products and services, often based on new trends. Then they start businesses to supply those products and services. For instance, many adults work outside the home. One resulting need is for housecleaning services for families. A person who sees this need and begins such a service is an entrepreneur. A developing trend, however, is more businesses being operated from home. What are some new business ideas geared to help people with home-based businesses?

People choose to become entrepreneurs for many reasons. Most like being in charge and making their own business decisions. They want to benefit directly from their skills and talents. Perhaps they can make more money by working for themselves.

You do not have to be an adult to become an entrepreneur. Many teens have successfully started businesses. Lawn care services and children's party planning are just two examples. See **12-18**.

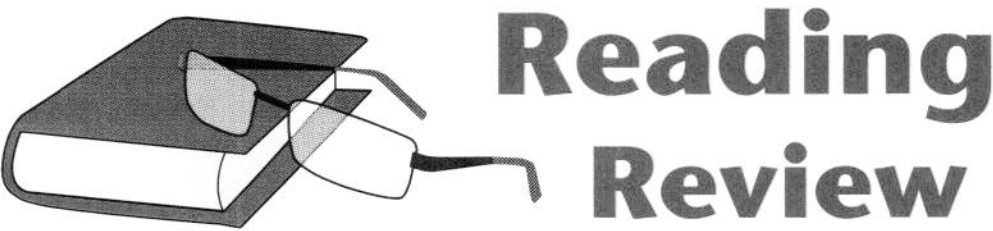

Reading Review

1. Why do some people choose to become entrepreneurs?
2. What are some examples of businesses teens can start?

Succeed in Life

Tips to Become an Entrepreneur

Do you think you might like to become an entrepreneur? If you are interested in starting your own business, keep the following tips in mind:

- Choose a business you will enjoy.
- Offer a service or product that is needed. Find out about the trends in your community.
- Research the requirements of your proposed business before you begin.
- Try to talk to people who have similar businesses.
- Decide on a fair price for your service or product. Do not undervalue yourself, but do not overcharge either.
- Assume responsibility for this job just as if you were working for someone else.

Section Summary

- Careers in the family and consumer sciences field involve helping people improve their quality of life.
- Careers in family and consumer sciences include jobs in foods and nutrition, housing, and clothing and textiles. It also includes jobs in child development, family relations, consumer education and management, and education and communications.
- Entrepreneurs start businesses to meet the need for certain products and services.

Chapter Summary

Most teens are working now or plan to work in the future. You can earn an income and receive fringe benefits. Working can give you a sense of dignity and identity. Your family and community can also benefit when you work. Decide if you want to hold a series of unrelated jobs or pursue a career. Your lifestyle will be affected by what you decide.

The job you choose will be affected by changes in society and technology. Being aware of trends in the world of work will help you follow these changes. You will be able to make better choices about a job or career.

To find the right career or job, first, identify your interests and skills. Then learn about the different types of careers and jobs available. Once you take these two steps, you can match your interests and skills to a career or job. Set goals to help you find the job or career you want.

You may choose a career in family and consumer sciences. Careers in the family and consumer sciences field help people improve their quality of life. This includes jobs in foods and nutrition, housing, and clothing and textiles. It also includes jobs in child development, family relations, consumer education and management, and education and communication.

Entrepreneurs see needs for products or services and decide to start their own businesses. You do not have to be an adult to start your own business. Teens can start businesses, too.

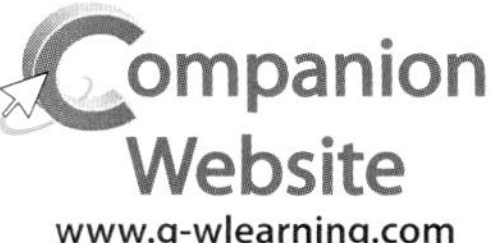

Review Key Terms and Main Ideas for Chapter 12 at the website.

Chapter Review

Write your answers on a separate sheet of paper.

1. List three reasons people work.
2. What are three examples of fringe benefits?
3. What is the difference between a job and a career?
4. How can jobs affect people's lifestyles?
5. List two ways you can learn about your interests and aptitudes.
6. An (interest inventory/aptitude test) will point out your natural skills. (Circle the correct word.)
7. True or false. The career clusters are 12 groups of career specialties.
8. True or false. The *Occupational Outlook Handbook* describes many different jobs.
9. How do trends affect future jobs?
10. What is job shadowing?
11. Give examples of two sources of job information.
12. What is the purpose of job training?
13. List the seven main areas in the family and consumer sciences field and give an example of a job in each area.
14. List three benefits of being an entrepreneur.

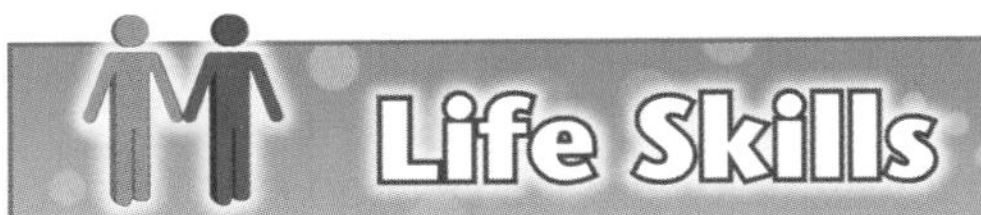

15. As a class, plan an assembly on careers related to family and consumer sciences. Use the Internet or the phone book to come up with a list of people your teacher could invite to speak. Prepare questions for the speakers to answer about their current jobs. Also, ask them about their training and past job experiences.

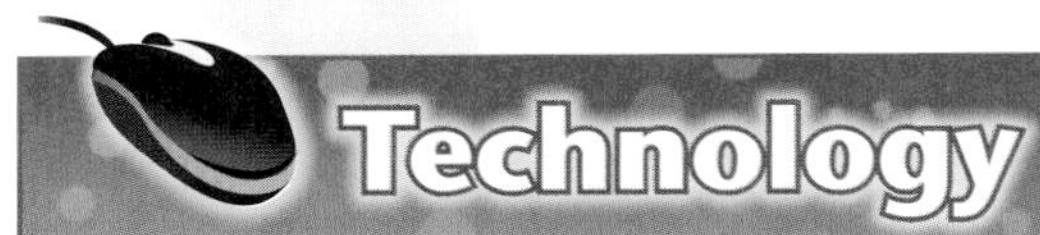

16. Conduct career research online at www.bls.gov/oco, the *Occupational Outlook Handbook* website. Find three careers that interest you. Write a short report about the information available for the most appealing job within each of those career categories.
17. Research free sources of career information online. Include a list of websites for interest inventories and aptitude tests. Share your list of websites with your classmates.

18. Write an entry in your journal about your dream job. Describe what a day at work is like. What are your favorite things about this job? What might be your least favorite activities? How did you become interested in this field? What or who was your inspiration?

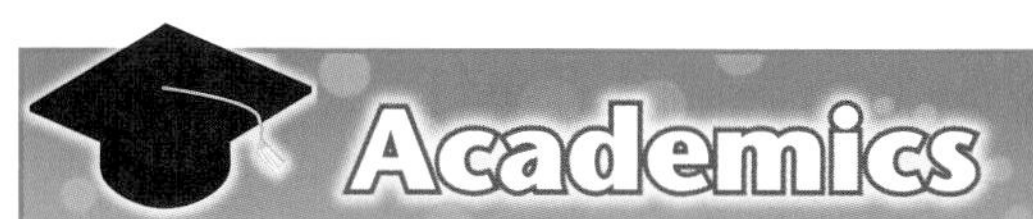

19. **Writing.** Find and complete career inventories that would identify your interests, aptitudes, and abilities. What have you learned about yourself? Write a brief essay of your findings.
20. **Speech.** Find out about work-based learning programs at a local high school. Interview a student from one of the programs that interests you. Ask the student what courses he or she must take. Ask what job skills he or she is learning. Find out how well the student feels the program is preparing him or her for a future career. Share your findings with the class.
21. **Math.** Imagine you are a financial planner for a day. You are advising a family with two very young children about planning for college. How much will they have to save for each child? How long will it take them to save that amount of money? Do they have other options?
22. **Social Studies.** Make a list of services needed in your community. Write a report on how an entrepreneur could provide one of the services you listed.

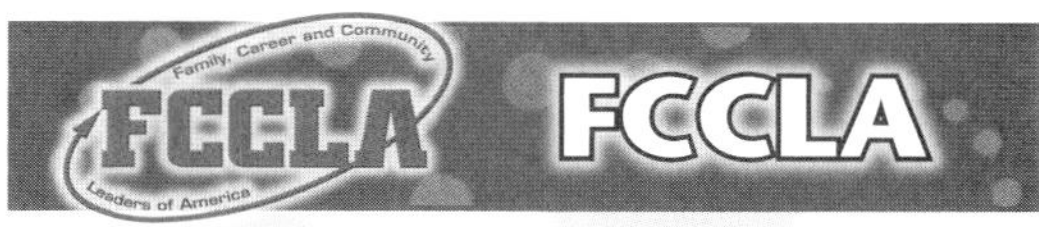

23. Your class can hold a *Career Exploration* event. In small groups, choose a career you would like to explore more. Each person will research a different aspect of that career and the education needed. Prepare a short oral presentation for the rest of the class on your research findings. Then develop an FCCLA *Career Exploration* project for the *Career Connection* program. Obtain further information about this program from your FCCLA advisor.

Chapter 13
Preparing for Work

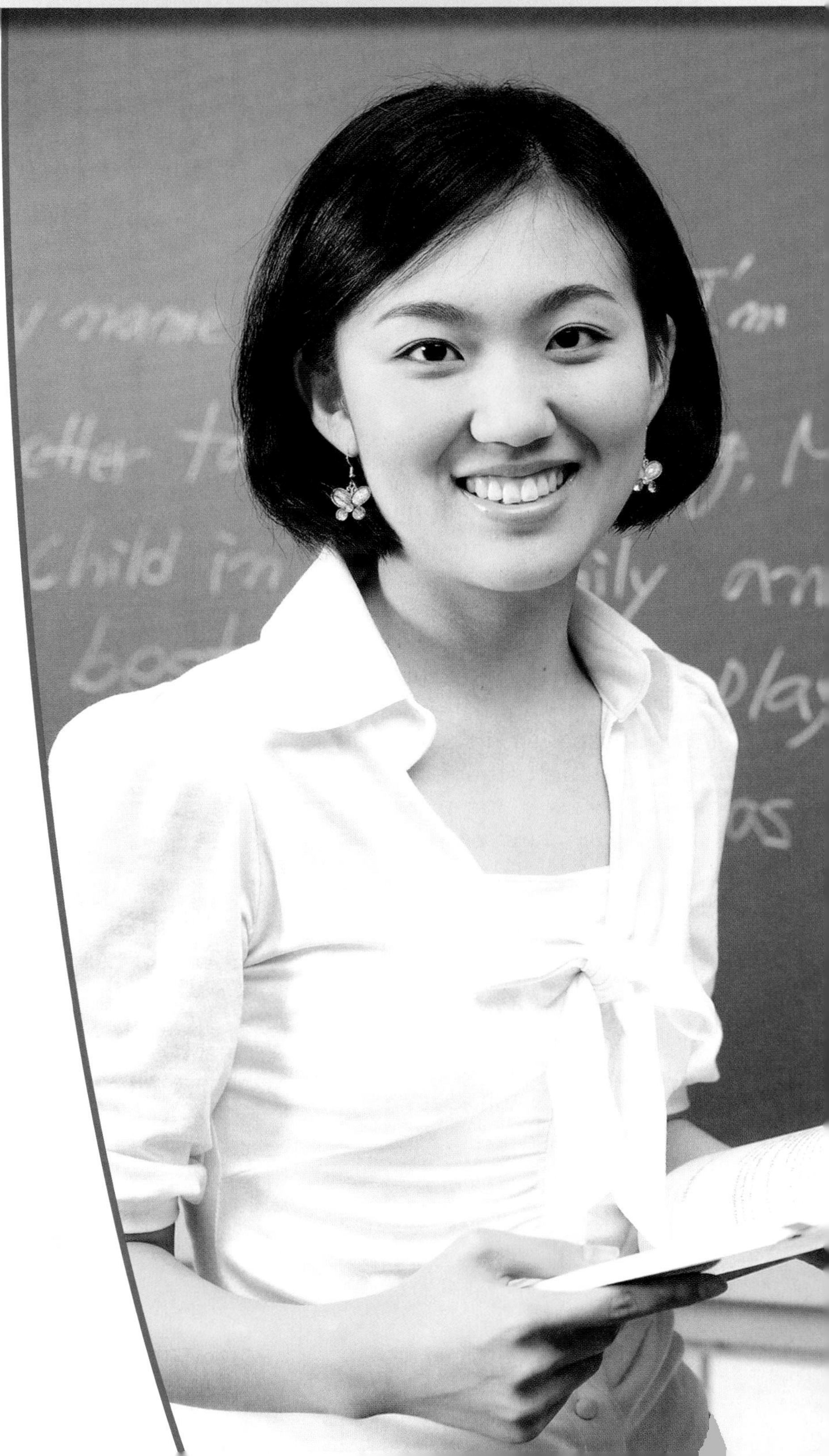

Sections

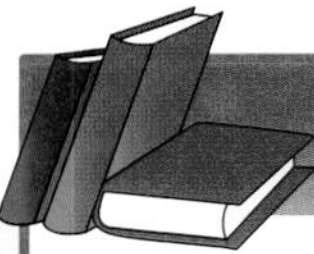

Sharpen Your Reading

As you read the chapter, write a letter to yourself. Imagine you will receive this letter when you are working at your future job. What would you like to remember from this chapter? In the letter, list key points from the chapter that will be useful in your future career.

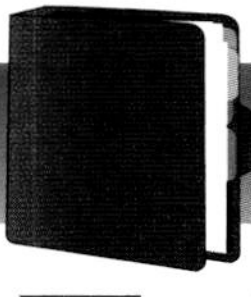

Concept Organizer

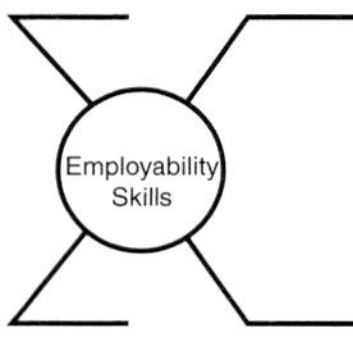

Use a spider diagram like the one shown to identify the employability skills that are required for most jobs.

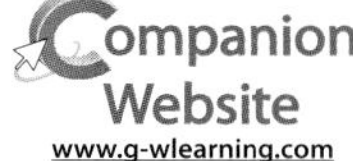

Print out the concept organizer at the website.

Section 13-1
Getting Your First Job

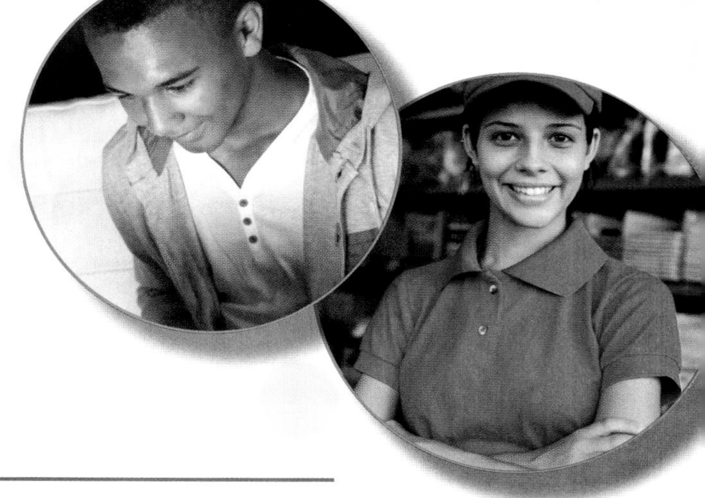

Objectives

After studying this section, you will be able to
- **define** *networking*, *résumé*, *letter of application*, and *reference*.
- **identify** sources you can use to look for a job.
- **outline** the steps in getting a job.
- **explain** the advantages and disadvantages of part-time work.

Key Terms

networking: making contacts with people who may be able to help you find jobs.

résumé: a written description of a person's education, qualifications, and work experience.

letter of application: a document you send with your résumé to give more information about your skills.

reference: a name of a person who can be contacted about you and your work habits.

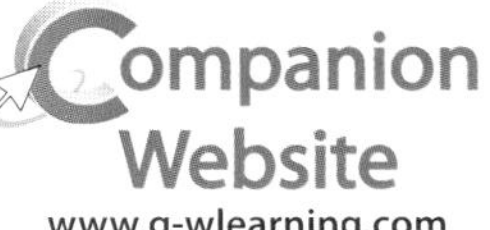

Study the Key Terms by completing crossword puzzles, matching activities, and e-flash cards at the website.

Main Ideas

- The Internet, newspaper, and family and friends are just a few of the sources you can use to find a job.
- Many employers want you to submit a résumé, letter of application, and references when applying for a job.
- First impressions are very important when interviewing for a job.
- Part-time work can help you learn job skills you can use in the future.

To find and get the job you want, you first need to develop some job-search skills. They involve knowing where to look for available jobs, placing an application, and interviewing. These important skills are also useful for finding future employment.

For many teens, their first job is often part-time work. *Part-time* work means less than 40 hours a week. The job skills learned from part-time work may be helpful in future jobs.

Finding Jobs

Where can you look for jobs? The Internet is the primary place to find every level of job. See **13-1**. Local newspapers have listings, too. Your friends and family may know of job openings. Your school guidance counselor may get calls from businesses looking for qualified teens. Some communities have youth employment agencies to help young people find part-time work.

Another way to find a job is through networking. **Networking** is making contacts with people who may be able to help you find jobs. You can develop a strong network when you participate in activities. For instance, you can meet people in your local area when you volunteer or join community groups. You can also make connections with adults as well as students your age when you join career and technical student organizations such as FCCLA.

People can also find jobs by joining *professional organizations*. There are professional organizations available for many career areas. For instance, the American Dietetic Association is the professional organization for registered dietitians. Membership in professional organizations often requires a fee. In return, members receive job listings and chances to network with other professionals in their career field.

Use your initiative to find a job. You can place a *Position Wanted* ad in the newspaper. You can call businesses and ask if there are available jobs. You can look for *Help Wanted* signs in the windows of area stores and then apply for jobs. There are many options available to you.

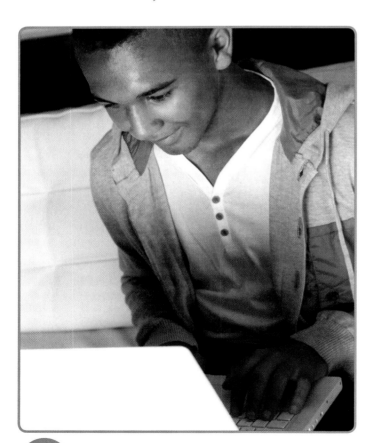

13-1 Many businesses post job listings on their websites.

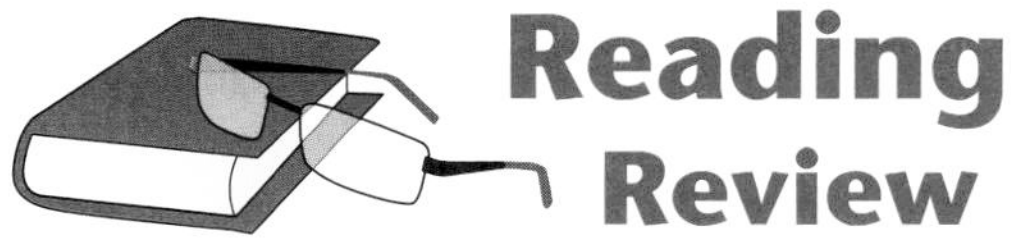

1. What is *networking*? How can you develop a strong network?
2. List three ways you can look for jobs.

Applying for Jobs

You can apply for a job in person, by telephone, by mail, or online. Carefully follow the directions given by the jobs that interest you. The employer may ask you to submit a résumé, letter of application, and references.

A **résumé** is a written description of a person's education, qualifications, and work experience. See **13-2**. Your résumé will help employers learn more about you. Some employers may want you to submit an *electronic résumé*. This is a text-only file with any special formatting removed.

Jennifer L. Wright
1603 Main Street
Parker, Iowa 50992
(555) 555-7474
jenwright@provider.com

Objective	Seeking a summer camp assistant counselor position.
Education	Parkview High School, Parker, Iowa, 20XX to present. Focus on human services, with an emphasis in child development. Graduating in June, 20XX.
Experience	Activities Volunteer, Ronald McDonald House (RMDH), 20XX to present. Responsible for preparing snacks and planning and running activities for the families staying at RMDH while their children are hospitalized far from home. Babysitter, 20XX to present. Providing quality child care for three families with children ages ten months to nine years.
Computer skills	Proficient in keyboarding and Microsoft Word, Excel, and PowerPoint.
Honors and Activities	Parkview High School honor roll, 20XX. Member, Family, Career and Community Leaders of America (FCCLA), Parkview High School chapter, 20XX to present. Member, Parkview High School creative writing club, 20XX to present. Captain, Parkview High School JV volleyball team, 20XX.

13-2 The information on your résumé helps employers decide if you will be a good fit for their company.

Sometimes when applying for a job, you may need to submit a letter of application. A **letter of application** is a document you send with your résumé to give more information about your skills. See **13-3**.

Many employers also want you to give references when applying for jobs. A **reference** is a name of a person who can be contacted about you and your work habits. Always ask people if they will give you

1603 Main Street
Parker, Iowa 50992
April 10, 20XX

Ms. Britta Nelson
Program Director
Twin Pines Camp
Rural Route 1
Big Bear Lake, Iowa 51119

Dear Ms. Nelson:

I am interested in working as a counselor-in-training at Twin Pines this summer. My guidance counselor at Parkview High School, Mr. Brandon, suggested I write you and explain my qualifications. I am currently a junior and have already taken two child development classes, with another planned next year.

I went to Twin Pines' camp for three years and really loved it. So I am very familiar with the camp and its policies and procedures. In addition to babysitting for the past five years, I also volunteer four hours a week at the Ronald McDonald House, a charity through McDonald's Corporation that keeps families together while their child is receiving critical medical treatment far from home. My duties involve planning a variety of activities for the families, such as crafts, games, and snacks. I enjoy being with children and helping them learn. My long-term career goal is to open my own child care center when I graduate from college.

I have enclosed my résumé and would appreciate the opportunity to meet for an interview. Please contact me at (555) 555-7474 or at jenwright@provider.com. I look forward to further discussion about Twin Pines' counselors-in-training program. Thank you for your time and consideration.

Sincerely,

Jennifer L. Wright

Jennifer L. Wright

13-3 A letter of application introduces your résumé and highlights specific skills.

a recommendation before you list their names. References should be people who know about you and your work. Do not use relatives. Former employers are good choices. Teachers, counselors, and religious leaders also make good references.

Some employers may ask you to fill out a *job application*. The application often asks for similar information that is on your résumé. Be neat and accurate when completing an application. Avoid making mistakes, such as spelling errors. Provide all the requested information.

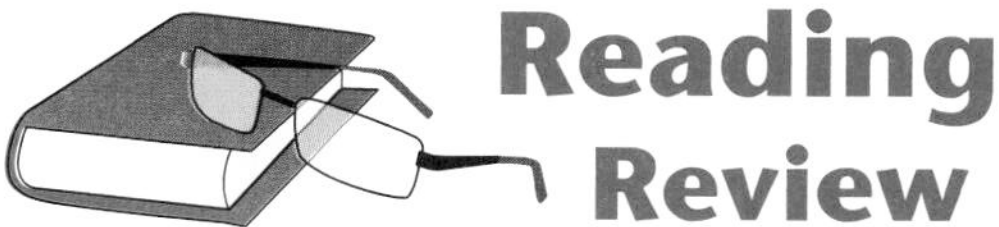

Reading Review

1. What information should you include in a résumé?
2. Why do employers often want references from a job applicant?

Interviewing for Jobs

Most employers interview potential workers before they decide which person to hire. See **13-4**. First impressions are very important. Dress appropriately. Make sure you look clean and well groomed. Have a positive attitude. Smile and shake the interviewer's hand when you arrive. Maintain good posture. Be on time and show good manners. Thank the person for his or her time.

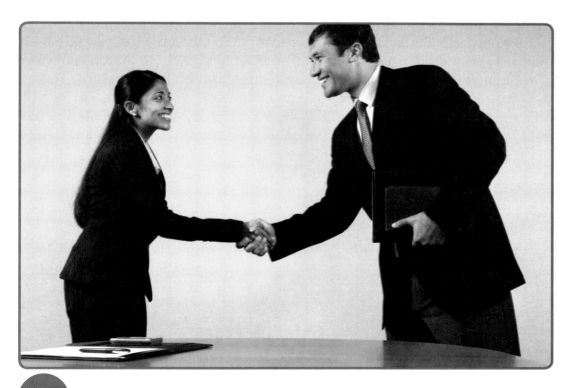

13-4 Learning interviewing skills will help you get the job you want.

Succeed in Life

Creating a Portfolio

Many people prepare portfolios to show to potential employers. A *portfolio* is a collection of materials that showcase your skills. A portfolio can include

- samples that show specific skills, such as drawings or writing samples
- summaries of volunteer experiences
- a résumé
- a cover letter
- letters of recommendation
- a list of references
- awards or special honors
- certifications, such as first-aid or CPR

Gather samples for your portfolio over time. Keep your portfolio organized and up-to-date. Consider your career goals as you prepare your portfolio. For instance, if you want to go to college, you can have your portfolio align with admission requirements. When you are ready to apply for a job, update your portfolio to include samples that relate to the job.

Learn as much as possible about the company so you can appear knowledgeable and ask good questions. Have a family member or friend practice asking you some standard interview questions. You can obtain many examples of interview questions on the Internet.

After the interview, send a *follow-up letter* thanking the interviewer for his or her time. In the letter, be sure to express your interest in the job.

Try not to get discouraged if you are not offered the job. Most people have more job rejections than job offers. It takes a lot of trying to get the job you want.

When you do receive a job offer, consider your options carefully. You can accept or reject the offer. If you are unsure you want the job, ask for a little more time to decide. Whether you accept or reject the offer, always be polite and courteous and thank the interviewer for his or her consideration.

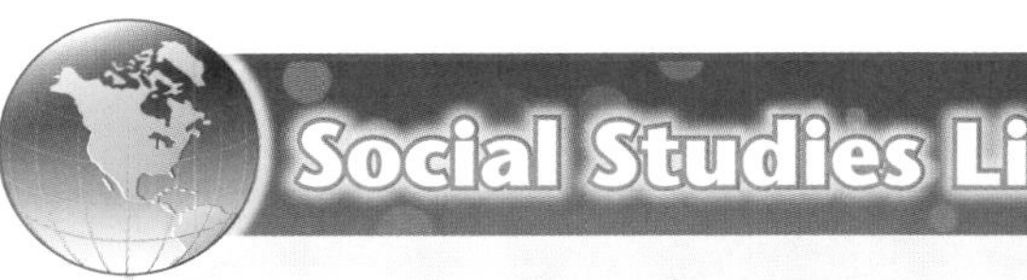

Labor Laws

When you get your first job, you must show your Social Security card. Child labor laws affect the work you can do when you are under age 18. The types of jobs, hours, and work settings may be restricted. You might be required to get a work permit. Your guidance counselor can tell you about the laws in your state.

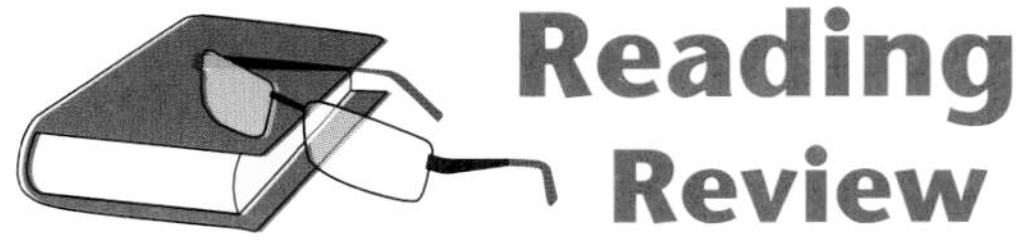

1. What skills are involved in getting a job?
2. What are three hints for interviewing successfully?

Working Part-Time

Many teens choose to get a part-time job while they are in high school. See **13-5**. Part-time jobs have many advantages. You learn how to be a responsible employee. You learn job skills you can use in the future. You learn how to handle an income. A part-time job can also lead to other jobs.

There are some disadvantages to working part-time while in school. You will have less time to do your schoolwork. You may not be able to participate in many after-school activities such as sports and clubs. When you work, you will not have as much time with your friends. Deciding to work part-time requires a look at both the advantages and disadvantages.

Try to find a part-time job related to a career that appeals to you. This will give you a chance to see if you like that field. You may choose another career if you do not like the job.

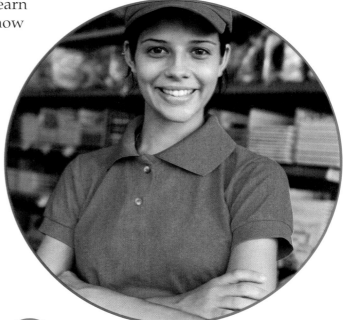

13-5 Teens who have part-time jobs may work during evenings and on weekends when they are not in school.

Some teens do volunteer work instead of getting a part-time job. Although you will not receive an income, you learn many of the same job skills. For instance, if you volunteer in a health clinic, you will learn skills you can use in a medical career. The skills you learn may be more helpful to your future than the income you earn.

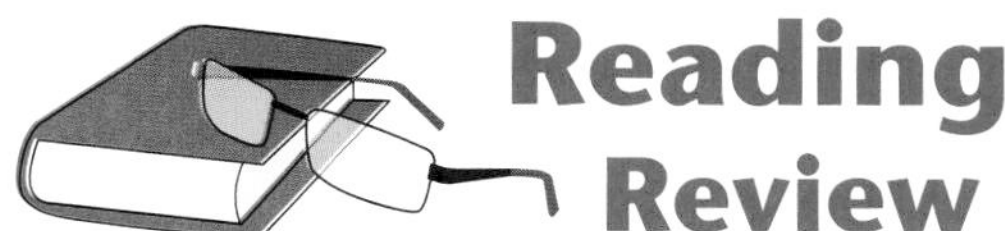

Reading Review

1. What does working part-time mean? Why do you think some students have part-time jobs?
2. What are two advantages and two disadvantages of having a part-time job or doing volunteer work?

Section Summary

- You can learn job-search skills to help you get your first job. These skills include finding available jobs, applying for the position, and interviewing.
- There are many sources you can use to look for jobs. The Internet, newspaper, and family and friends are just a few.
- When applying for a job, many employers want you to submit a résumé, letter of application, and references.
- A part-time job or volunteer work can help you prepare for a career.

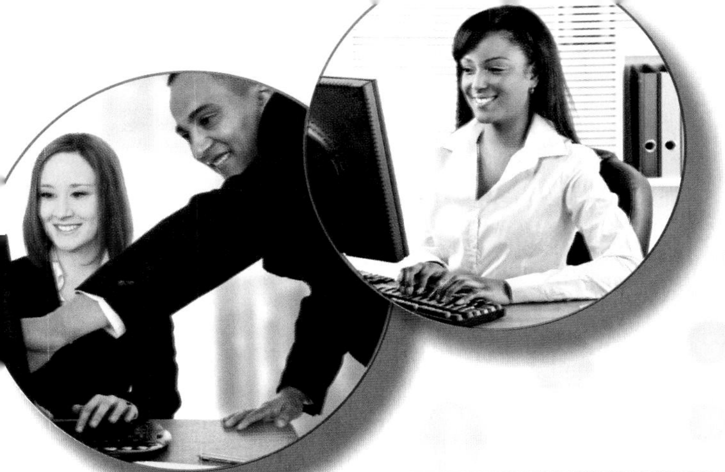

Section 13-2
Getting Ready for Job Success

Objectives

After studying this section, you will be able to
- **define** *employability skills*, *thinking skills*, *work ethic*, and *criticism*.
- **give examples** of how employability skills are used on the job.
- **describe** the importance of getting along with others on the job.
- **list** traits of a successful worker.
- **explain** why successful workers must continue to learn.

Key Terms

employability skills: the basic skills you need to get, keep, and succeed on a job.

thinking skills: the ability to think creatively and critically, make decisions, and solve problems.

work ethic: the employee values of working hard and showing dedication.

criticism: a judgment.

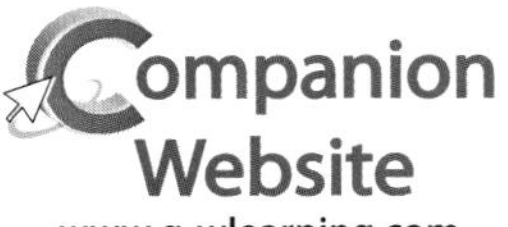

Study the Key Terms by completing crossword puzzles, matching activities, and e-flash cards at the website.

Main Ideas

- You need employability skills to get, keep, and succeed on a job.
- Your ability to get along with others can affect your career success.
- You can develop certain traits that will help you be a successful worker.
- Continuing to learn on the job will help you advance in your career.

Some people are successful in their work. They receive more responsibility and more pay. They may have other job offers, too. To be successful on the job, you need to develop and improve the basic skills you need to become a good employee. They will be useful throughout your life. See **13-6**.

Boost Your Reading Skills

You can develop your reading skills by reading a variety of books and magazines. As you read, take time to review what you have read and make sure you understand the material. If there are words you do not know, look them up in the dictionary. Improving your reading skills now will help you at home, school, and work.

Employability Skills

Few jobs are open to workers without employability skills. **Employability skills** are the basic skills you need to get, keep, and succeed on a job. They include academic skills such as reading, writing, math, and science. Most jobs require basic computer skills. Communication and thinking skills are needed, too.

Academic Skills

You need *reading skills* to function effectively on the job and in life. Without reading skills, you would not be able to check a work schedule. You could not read e-mails from your coworkers. You would not be able to read directions for your school or work assignments.

You need to have effective *writing skills* to fill out a job application or prepare a résumé. Employers expect workers to use writing skills to create

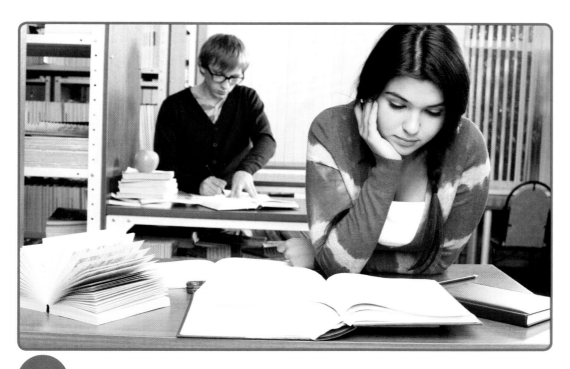

13-6 Developing employability skills will help you succeed in the world of work.

reports and to communicate with others. If you cannot write a message clearly, others will not understand what you are trying to say. Therefore, it is important to always use correct spelling, grammar, and punctuation.

Math skills and *science skills* are also needed every day at home and in the workplace. You use math skills to manage your income and spending. Taking measurements requires the use of math skills. You use science principles when you examine a problem, conduct research, and analyze possible solutions. Demonstrating an understanding of cause and effect also uses science principles.

You use academic skills every day. When you complete a homework assignment, read a book, or count change from a purchase you are developing your academic skills. Practicing the skills you already have and learning new skills will help you now and in the future.

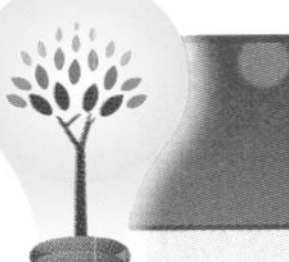

Think Green

Saving Paper in the Office

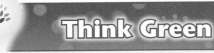

To help save trees and reduce costs, most businesses want their employees to waste less paper. E-mails and other documents can be saved on computers. One of the best rules to remember for saving paper is to think twice about whether you really need to print something. If printing is necessary, make sure you print on both sides—this is an easy way to cut paper use in half. You can use this tip at home, too.

Technology

In today's workplace, most employers expect their workers to have basic computer skills. This means you need to know how to use a computer and access the Internet. You should also be able to adjust quickly to new responsibilities as technology continues to change. Your ability to adapt and learn new technology will help you succeed on the job.

13-7 Being able to communicate clearly is a skill needed for all jobs.

Communication

The ability to clearly communicate with others is always needed on the job. See **13-7**. Therefore, you need to have good listening and speaking skills. To become a good listener, focus on what is being said. Then make sure you understand the message. You are more likely to make mistakes when you do not listen carefully to every word.

Expressing your ideas to supervisors and coworkers requires good speaking skills. You need to be clear and concise so others can understand what you are saying. Having good communication skills is necessary for job success.

Thinking Skills

Thinking skills are the ability to think creatively and critically, make decisions, and solve problems. When you are creative, you can come up with new solutions to a problem. You develop many ideas. Employers value creative people.

Critical thinking means you can look at all the sides of a problem. You can understand different points of view. You are able to reason and analyze situations.

Decision making is an important skill, both in life and on the job. Making good decisions means weighing alternatives and picking the best one. It involves thinking through all possible consequences to determine the pros and cons. This process helps individuals and teams make good decisions.

Employers need workers who can solve problems. You gather facts and suggest practical solutions. You are able to solve problems calmly and quickly. For instance, parents like to hire Rashad as a babysitter. In his neighborhood, he is known for using good problem-solving skills with children. He also handles emergencies well. These skills are important in every job.

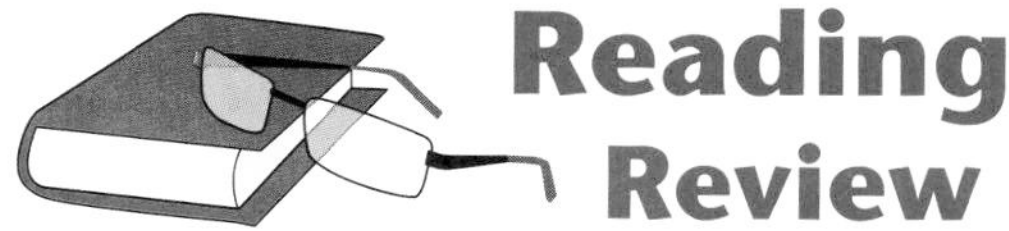

Reading Review

1. How can you develop your reading, writing, math, and science skills now?
2. Give one example of how each of the employability skills might be needed on the job.

Getting Along with Others

The ability to get along with others is required in all jobs. If you cannot get along well with others, employers will not want to hire you. Other people will not want to work with you.

Getting along with your supervisor is important. Obeying company rules will help you get along. Following your supervisor's instructions is important. If you disagree with your supervisor, follow his or her decisions anyway. Realize that you are new to the workplace and have a lot to learn.

You will need to get along with your coworkers, too. See **13-8**. Working together requires *teamwork skills*. It requires patience and understanding. Other workers may be different from you. Do not allow these differences to keep you from getting along with others. Recognize, too, that your employer values their ideas as well as yours.

How to Get Along with Coworkers

- Listen to what your coworkers have to say. This will help you know them.
- Take part in group discussions. This involves listening as well as offering ideas.
- Take part in group decision making. Do your part after the decision is made, even if the decision is not what you wanted.
- Avoid blaming coworkers for your problems. Talk about conflicts. Try to reach agreements that will let you get along in the future.

13-8 Getting along with coworkers is a requirement of all jobs.

Your job may also require you to work with customers. Be friendly, helpful, and polite when dealing with customers. You are representing your company. How you treat customers will affect whether they do business with your company again.

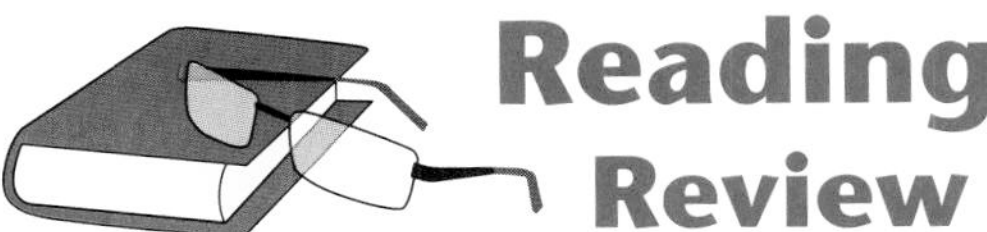

Reading Review

1. How can getting along with others affect your job success?
2. Why is it important to be friendly, helpful, and polite when dealing with customers?

Being a Successful Worker

Successful people have common traits that help them do their jobs well. They have positive attitudes. They manage their time well. They are also loyal, honest, and trustworthy. They demonstrate a strong work ethic. A **work ethic** is the values of hard work and dedication held by employees. This is reflected by the effort you put into your job and how you feel about it.

One of the biggest factors affecting your job success is your attitude. See **13-9**. Have a positive attitude about yourself and your work. This means you believe in your skills as a worker. A positive attitude gives you confidence and helps you do a good job. If you like your job, you tend to perform better.

Your attitude is seen by others in how you act and what you say. If you have a positive work attitude, you will be cheerful and confident. Employees enjoy being around a coworker with a positive attitude.

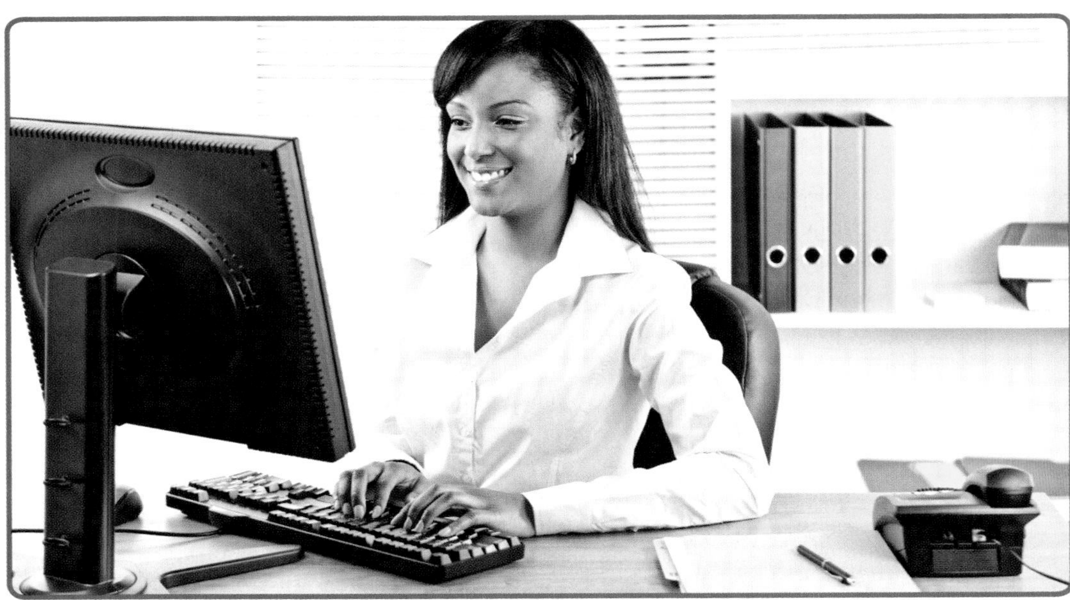

13-9 Having a positive attitude toward work contributes to a strong work ethic.

To be successful, use your time wisely. Arrive for work on time. Avoid leaving work early. Use your time at work for company business, not private business. Do not take more than the allowed amount of time for breaks. Do not waste time on the telephone or computer.

Successful workers are loyal. As a loyal worker, do not gossip or make unkind remarks about your coworkers. Do not complain about the job or your supervisor either. Above all, never discuss private company information outside work.

You must be honest to be successful on the job. You may handle money or work with costly products. Employers need to be able to trust you. If you are suspected of stealing or cheating, you will be closely watched. You may even lose your job.

It is always best to work hard to complete your assigned tasks on time. When you make a mistake, be willing to admit it. Learn from it so you will not make the same mistake again. See **13-10**.

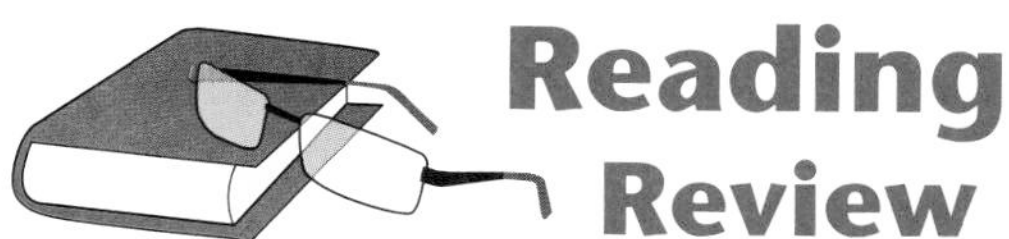

Reading Review

1. How do workers with a strong work ethic feel about themselves and their jobs?
2. Why should you not gossip about coworkers and complain about your supervisor?
3. What are three jobs in which a worker's honesty is the most important trait?

Guidelines for Success

- Arrive on time.
- Use work time for work, not for personal matters.
- Take only the amount of time that is allowed for breaks or lunch.
- Do not leave work early.
- Ask for vacation time only after it is earned.
- Use sick time for illness only.
- Use the telephone for business only. Do not use a personal cell phone while on the job.
- Be cheerful.
- Show interest in the job and the company.
- Ask intelligent questions.
- Get along with other workers.
- Accept suggestions from others.
- Be willing to learn new skills as the job demands.

13-10 Following these guidelines will help you be a successful worker.

Continuing to Learn

In order to advance in your career, keep learning and developing new skills. Tools, materials, and methods change. As you advance, your responsibilities will change, too. You must be willing and able to keep up with changes. This often means learning new skills.

How can you continue to learn? Reading can help you stay informed. Many businesses offer classes to help workers stay informed. You can take adult education classes. Professional organizations provide workers with up-to-date information that relates to their career area.

Another way to learn is through criticism. **Criticism** is a judgment. Criticism is not always negative. When used in a kind way, it is constructive and helpful. Your supervisor or coworkers may make you aware of errors through criticism. You should use it to improve your work in the future.

You can also learn by asking questions. When you are given new tasks, ask for help when you need it. Be willing to learn from other workers and your employer.

Learning is a lifelong process. You cannot learn everything you need to know in school. By continuing to learn, you will help ensure your job success.

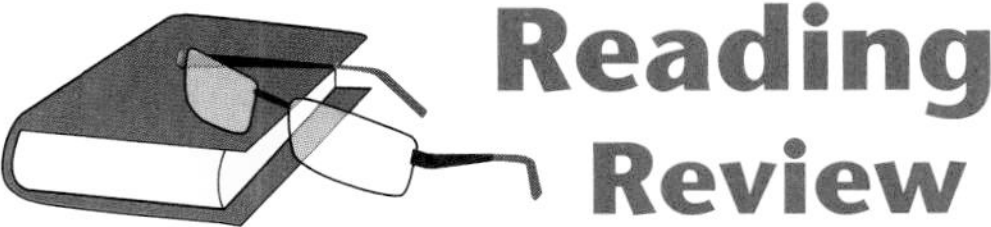

Reading Review

1. Why is it important to continue learning even after you get a job?
2. What are three ways you can continue to learn after you finish school?

Leaving a Job

Most people do not stay at the same job their entire life. You may start with a part-time job while in school and get a full-time job with another company later. You may get a different job because you are moving to a new location. Whatever the reason, you should always try to have a positive attitude and leave a job on good terms. Quitting suddenly is not fair to your employer. You may also have more difficulty getting a good reference from your employer for future jobs.

Most employers expect a worker to give at least a two-week notice in writing before they leave a job. This gives the employer a chance to hire someone new. Your written notice should also state your last day of work. If a job requires a lot of responsibility, you may want to give your employer more than a two-week notice.

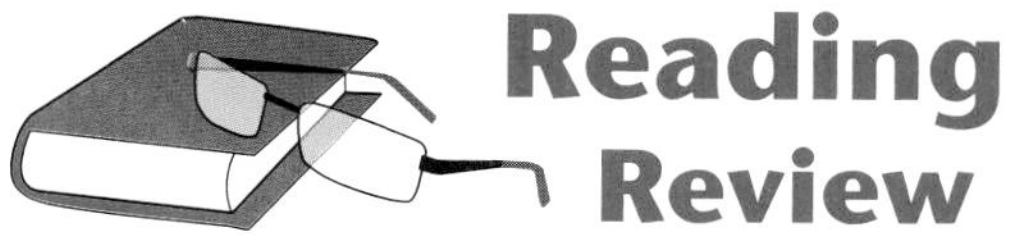

Reading Review

1. What are some common reasons people leave jobs?
2. Why is it important to give a two-week notice when leaving a job?

Section Summary

- Employability skills are needed to get, keep, and succeed on a job. These skills include academic skills, technology, communication, and thinking skills.
- You must be able to get along with others. Have a positive attitude and manage your time well.
- Being honest, loyal, and hardworking will help you be successful, too.
- Your success in the workplace is also affected by your willingness to keep developing new skills and learning.

Chapter Summary

To find and get the job you want, you need to know where to look for available jobs. The Internet, newspaper, family or friends, and networking are some sources you can use. You need to know how to place an application. You also need to make a good impression during an interview.

Working part-time is another way to prepare for a career. You learn how to behave properly in a work setting. Part-time jobs and volunteer work also give you the chance to explore careers in fields that interest you.

Having employability skills will help you be successful in a job. Developing your reading, writing, math, and science skills now will help you in future jobs. Employers expect employees to have basic computer skills. Communication and thinking skills are also necessary for job success.

Other important traits include having a good attitude; managing time well; and being loyal, honest, and hardworking. You must also be willing to learn new skills.

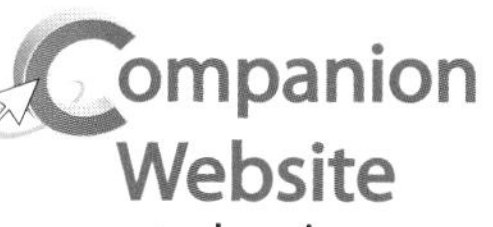

Review Key Terms and Main Ideas for Chapter 13 at the website.

Chapter Review

Write your answers on a separate sheet of paper.

1. True or false. When you work part-time, you work more than 40 hours a week.
2. List three ways you can look for a job.
3. What is a résumé?
4. List three benefits of working part-time.
5. List four employability skills you need to succeed on the job.
6. What does *critical thinking* mean?
7. Why is it important to get along with others on the job?
8. List four hints for getting along with others at work.
9. True or false. Your attitude affects your success on the job.
10. How can you learn from criticism?
11. Why is learning a lifelong process?
12. Most employers expect employees to give at least a _____-week notice before leaving a job.

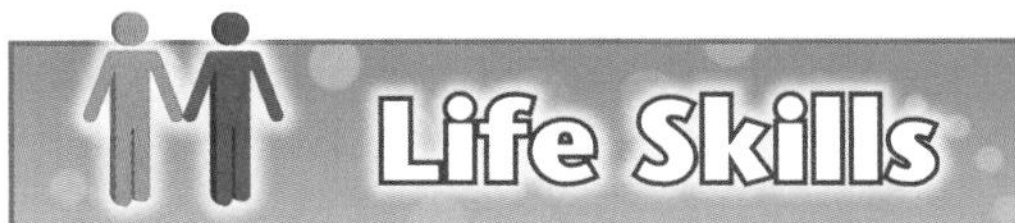

Life Skills

13. Help your class prepare a *jobs survey*. Each student should interview five people who are currently employed. Try to interview people in a variety of jobs. Ask each worker how he or she uses employability skills on the job. What computer skills are required? How important are decision-making and problem-solving skills on the job? What are some creative ways they have solved problems? Does the employer offer special classes or workshops to attend? When you finish your survey, compile the results and discuss your findings in class.

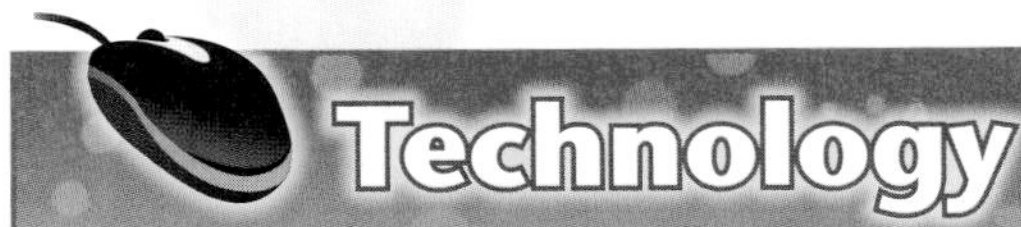

Technology

14. Look at want ads on the Internet. Print any ads for part-time jobs that teens might be able to fill. Make a collage or bulletin board display with the ads.
15. Use a software program of your choice to create a sample letter of application and a résumé for one of the part-time jobs you found on the Internet. You can use the samples in the chapter as a guide. Be sure to check your work for correct spelling, grammar, and punctuation.

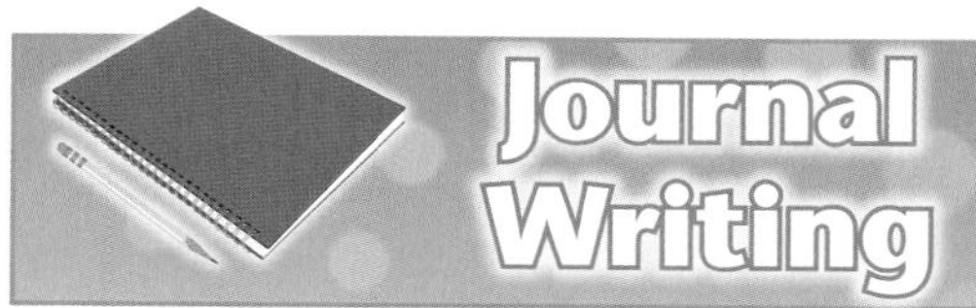

16. Taking a few minutes every day to write in your journal will help develop your writing skills. Think about other ways you can develop your writing skills and write about it in your journal. Review your journal entries every couple months and note any changes in your writing style.

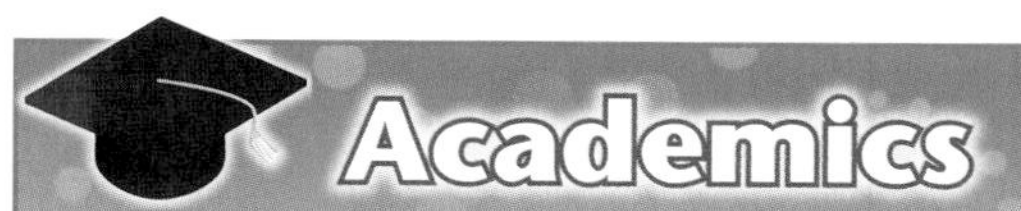

17. **Social Studies.** Use online or print sources to find samples of five standard interview questions. Think about how you would respond to each of the questions. Share possible responses with the class.
18. **Speech.** Pretend you are working as a salesperson in a local store. Role-play a situation showing poor skills in getting along with others on the job. Then repeat the role-play showing good skills in getting along with others.
19. **Writing.** Conduct an interview with a person who is a job supervisor. Ask the supervisor to describe traits of a successful worker. Ask him or her to discuss the most common reasons workers are fired. Write a one-page report of your findings.

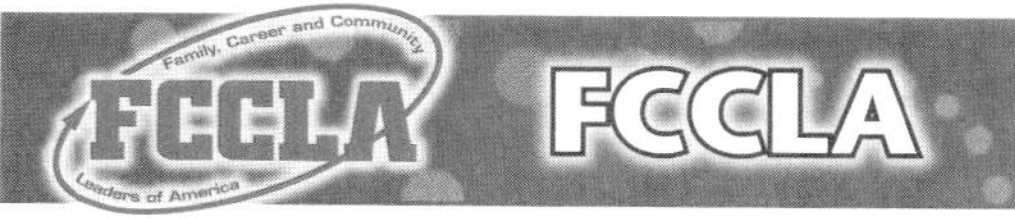

20. In small groups, list ways teens can learn about job openings. Talk to your school guidance counselor and teachers of career courses to find out about options within the community. Use the FCCLA *Job Source Directory Form* or create your own form to collect information for a job directory. Then prepare a flyer to let other students know this information is available. You can take it a step further by completing a *LINK UP* project for the *Career Connection* program. Obtain further information about this program from your FCCLA advisor.

Appendix

On Your Own—A Lesson in Self-Care

Now that you are older, your family may decide you can be left for short periods of time, either alone or with siblings. This may be because the adults in your family need to be away from home at the same time. They may have jobs and cannot be home with you. You may have to take care of yourself while they are away. This could be in the morning before you leave for school or after you get home. You may also need to stay by yourself for a few hours during the evening. Do you know how to behave and what to do when adults are not home? Do you know how to handle situations that might come up?

Some of the situations you should be prepared for are described here. Tips for handling them are also given. You may want to think about these ideas and talk about them with your family before you stay by yourself or babysit younger children. Your parents may have their own ideas about what they want you to do.

Coming and Going

When you are the first one home, check to see that everything looks normal before you enter the house or apartment. Signs that an intruder might be present are

- lights are on when they should be off
- a car you do not recognize in the driveway
- a broken or open window
- an open or unlocked door

If you notice any of these signs, take the following steps:

- DO NOT GO INSIDE.
- Go to a neighbor's house and call home. Maybe another family member came home early.
- If no one answers the telephone, call a parent. Ask what you should do. Perhaps a family member came home during the day and then left.
- If you cannot reach a parent, call 911 or the police. Give your complete name and address. They will come and check the house for you.

If you arrive home and everything looks normal, enter your house or apartment. Be sure to lock the door behind you. If you have lost your key, go to a neighbor's home. Your parents may want to leave a spare key with the neighbor. If they do not have a key, call a parent for instructions.

You may be the last one to leave your home in the morning. If so, there are some tasks you must remember to do.

- Make sure the windows are closed and locked.
- Turn off all the lights.
- Check the weather. Decide if you need a coat, boots, raincoat, hat, or gloves.
- Make sure you have your house key.
- Lock all doors.

Using the Phone

When you are home alone, your phone (or computer) can keep you from getting lonely. Your parents can text, call, or leave messages for you. If you have a problem, you can call someone for help.

You should make a list of important telephone numbers. Keep this list by the phone at all times—or have them programmed into speed dial, if available. The list should include the following telephone numbers:

- parents' work numbers
- neighbor or relative who is home most of the time
- police and fire (if 911 is not available in your community)
- family doctor
- ambulance
- poison control

If you are talking on the phone too long, however, a parent may not be able to get important messages to you. Strangers may call. You need to discuss with your parents what to do if a stranger calls your home phone. Keep the following points in mind:

- Always answer the phone. If you do not answer, potential intruders may think no one is home and it might be a good time to break in.
- If the caller asks for your parents, do not say you are home alone. Instead, tell the caller that your parents cannot come to the phone right now. Keep the conversation brief. Hang up if you need to.
- Ask the caller if you can take a message. Be sure to write the caller's name and telephone number.
- Do not give the caller your name or address.

Answering the Door

If you are by yourself, you should always be cautious when someone comes to the door. Do not open the door until you know who is there. Look through a window or peephole. If you cannot see the person, ask for a name. It may be a friend or neighbor.

If the person is a stranger, keep the following rules in mind:

- Keep the door locked.
- Talk only briefly and then go away from the door.

- If the person asks to use your telephone, offer to make the call yourself.
- Do not let the person know you are alone.
- Do not let anyone inside your home unless you have a parent's permission. Your family may have rules about when you can have friends over if you are alone. Know your family's rules. Let your friends know, too. Do not let your friends pressure you into breaking those rules. You are the one who will experience the consequences, not them.
- If someone is delivering a package, tell them to leave it outside.

What to Do If...

There are many situations that could happen while you are on your own. Many of these have already been discussed. There are others, however. Some situations may be serious. You and your parents should talk about what to do if

- you or a sibling gets hurt or very sick
- you smell smoke or a smoke alarm goes off
- the electricity goes out
- there is a severe weather warning
- a stranger offers you a ride home (*Hint:* never get into the car of someone you do not know well)
- You should also talk about what to do when
- you have homework
- you are taking care of younger brothers or sisters
- you get hungry
- you get bored
- you feel lonely
- you feel afraid

Being on your own is a big responsibility. If you and your parents think you can handle these situations, then you are ready.

Glossary

A

abbreviation. Shortened form of a word. (9-3)

abilities. Skills you develop through practice or training. (12-2)

accept. View as normal or proper. (1-2)

accessories. Items worn to accent clothing. (10-1)

accidents. Unexpected events causing loss or injury. (5-2)

acrylic. Manufactured fiber that is softer than wool and does not feel scratchy. (10-4)

active listening. Being focused on the communication process. (1-5)

addiction. A physical dependency on a substance. (4-2)

adolescence. The stage of growth between childhood and adulthood. (1-2)

adoptive family. A couple, or a single person, chooses to raise another person's child as their own. (1-3)

adulthood. The stage of growth following adolescence. (1-2)

advantages. Positive points. (3-4)

advertising. The process of calling attention to a product or a business through the mass media. (4-5)

affection. A feeling of fondness. (1-3)

à la carte. A menu term meaning each food or course is listed and priced separately. (8-5)

allergens. Substances that cause an allergic response in people that can be fatal. (8-2)

alterations. Changes made in the size, length, or style of a garment so it will fit properly. (11-4)

alternative energy sources. Energy from renewable resources, such as the sun or wind. (6-1)

alternatives. Options available to choose from when making a decision. (3-4)

anorexia nervosa. An eating disorder in which the fear of weight gain leads to poor eating patterns, malnutrition, and excessive weight loss. (7-3)

antiperspirant. A product that helps control wetness and covers unpleasant body odor. (4-3)

appearance. The way you look. (4-2)

appetite. The desire to eat. (7-3)

appetizer. Light food or drink served before the meal. (8-1)

appliance. A tool run by electricity or gas. (5-2)

applications software. Computer programs you use to do work or other activities. (6-3)

appliqué. Smaller pieces of fabric or trim sewn on a garment. (11-4)

apprentice. Someone who learns a job by working with a skilled worker. (12-3)

aptitude. A natural skill. (12-2)

aptitude test. A test taken to show if you have a natural talent for doing certain tasks. (12-2)

associate's degree. Degree from a two-year college. (12-3)

B

babysitting. Caring for children, usually during a short absence of the parents. (2-1)

bachelor's degree. Degree from a four-year college. (12-3)

bakeware. Pots and pans used in conventional ovens. (9-1)

balance. A principle of design using equality in size. (5-1)

balanced diet. A diet that provides all the nutrients your body needs for good health. (7-2)

basting. Sewing fabric pieces together with long, loose, temporary stitches. (11-3)

batter. Thin mixture of ingredients for baking quick breads. (9-5)

binge eating. An eating disorder in which people eat large amounts of food in a short time without taking measures to rid the body of unwanted food. (7-3)

biodegradable. Capable of decomposing under natural conditions. (5-3)

bleaches. Chemicals that will lighten fabrics and sometimes remove all color. (10-5)

blend. A combination of two or more different fibers, filaments, or yarns. (10-4)

blended family. See stepfamily. (1-3)

blog. An online journal. (6-3)

body language. Nonverbal communication, such as facial expressions and gestures. (1-5)

boutiques. Small specialty stores. (10-2)

budget. A plan for spending. (4-4)

buffet service. A style of meal service where people help themselves to food set out on a serving table. (8-4)

bulimia. An eating disorder in which people eat large amounts of food and then purge themselves of the food. (7-3)

bully. A person who uses strength or power to persuade or pressure others (force or fear) to do something. (1-5)

burners. Gas cooktop cooking units. (9-1)

C

calorie information. The number of calories in one serving of the food on the nutrition label. (8-2)

calories. Units of energy provided by proteins, carbohydrates, and fats. (7-3)

carbohydrates. Nutrients needed by your body for energy. (7-1)

career. A series of related jobs a person holds over time. (12-1)

career clusters. Sixteen groups of career specialties. (12-2)

career pathways. Groupings of jobs in each career cluster. (12-2)

caregiver. A person who takes care of children. (2-1)

casual dating. Dating as part of a couple. (1-4)

centerpiece. A decorative object placed in the middle of the table. (8-4)

challenge. A demanding or difficult task or situation that can be a source of distress. (1-6)

character. The traits that guide you in deciding right from wrong. (1-2)

childhood. The stage of growth from birth to adolescence. (1-2)

child labor. Children under a legal age are forced to work long hours in harmful conditions. (3-5)

childless family. A couple without children. (1-3)

childproof. To make an area safe for children by keeping potential dangers away from them. (2-2)

cholesterol. A fatty substance found in foods from animal sources. (7-2)

citizen. A member of a community. (3-5)

citizenship. The ways in which citizens handle their responsibilities. (3-5)

civic engagement. Actions that individuals and groups take to identify and solve the problems of their communities. (3-5)

classic. A style that stays in fashion for a long time. (10-1)

clutter. When personal belongings are unorganized. (4-1)
color. Element of design using color for effect. (5-1)
communication. Sending or receiving information, signals, or messages. (1-5)
community resources. Resources shared by everyone and paid for through taxes. (3-2)
comparison shopping. Finding the price of a product at different stores. (4-4)
compost. A mixture of decaying organic matter used to improve soil structure and provide nutrients. (5-3)
compromise. An agreement in a conflict in which both sides are willing to give up a little of what they wanted. (1-6)
cones. Spools of thread used on sergers instead of bobbins. (11-1)
confident. Being sure of yourself. (2-3)
conflict. A disagreement between two or more people. (1-6)
conflict resolution. The process of finding a solution to a disagreement. (1-6)
consequences. What happens as a result of your decisions. (3-4)
conserve. To save. (6-1)
consignment store. A store that sells pre-owned clothing where the original owner receives part of the profits. (10-1)
consumer. A person who buys or uses goods and services. (4-4)
consumer decisions. Decisions you make about how to spend your money. (4-5)
convenience stores. Small stores offering little selection, but open long hours. (8-2)
cook. To prepare food for eating using heat. (9-1)
cookware. Pots and pans used on the cooktop. (9-1)
cool colors. Blues, greens, and purples. (5-1)
cooperate. To act or work together with others. (2-4)
co-op programs. Work-based learning programs. (12-3)
cotton. Natural fiber from cotton plants used to make cotton fabric. (10-4)
course. All the foods served as one part of a meal. (8-1)
cover. The table space in front of a person's seat. (8-4)
credit. A way to pay that lets you buy now and pay later. (4-4)
crisis. Affects the functioning of a family. (1-6)
critical thinking. The ability to look at all sides of a problem. (13-2)
criticism. A judgment. (13-2)
culture. The beliefs and customs of a certain racial, religious, or social group. (1-3)
curdling. Lumping of milk proteins caused by cooking with high heat. (9-5)
cut. To divide foods into small pieces. (9-4)
cyberbullying. When a person is negatively targeted by another through technology. (6-3)

D

Daily Values (DV). Percentage figures on nutrition labels that help consumers see how food products fit into a total daily diet. (8-2)
dandruff. Excessive scalp flaking. (4-3)
debit card. A card issued by banks that allows the user to deduct money electronically from the user's bank account. (4-4)
decision. A choice you make about what to do or say in a given situation. (3-4)
decision-making process. A set of six basic steps to help you make decisions, solve problems, or reach goals. (3-4)
deodorant. A product that helps destroy or cover unpleasant body odors. (4-3)
dependent. Relying on another for support. (2-2)
dermatologist. A doctor who specializes in treating the skin. (4-3)

development. Age-related changes that are orderly and directional (moves toward greater complexity). (1-2)

developmental tasks. Skills or behavior patterns people should accomplish at certain stages of their lives. (1-2)

diet. The food and beverages consumed each day. (7-1)

dietary components. A list of nutrients found in each serving of the food product on the nutrition label. (8-2)

Dietary Guidelines for Americans. Document developed by experts to promote a healthful lifestyle through improved nutrition and physical activity. (7-2)

dignity. Feeling of self-worth. (12-1)

disadvantages. Negative points. (3-4)

discipline. The use of various methods to help children learn to behave in acceptable ways. (2-1)

displayed storage. Space for storing items in view. (5-1)

dough. Thick mixture of ingredients for baking yeast breads. (9-5)

dry-clean. To clean with chemicals instead of detergent and water. (10-5)

Dry-Clean Only. Product care label instructions; the garment may be ruined if machine washed. (10-5)

dry-heat cooking. Methods for cooking foods without liquids. (9-5)

dry measuring cups. Standard measuring tool used to measure dry ingredients, such as flour and sugar. (9-4)

E

early adolescence. The ages between eleven and fourteen. (1-2)

eating disorders. Abnormal, unhealthy eating patterns. (7-3)

ecology. The study of all living objects in relation to each other and the environment. (6-1)

efficiency. Working in the best possible manner with the least amount of waste. (6-2)

elements. Electric cooktop cooking units. (9-1)

embroidery. Decorative stitching using a needle and thread. (11-4)

emotional growth and development. Recognizing and accepting your feelings. (1-1)

emotional needs. Safety, being liked by others, gaining recognition, feeling good about yourself, and reaching your potential. (3-1)

emphasis. A principle of design having area as the visual center. (5-1)

employability skills. The basic skills you need to get, keep, and succeed on a job. (13-2)

energy. The capacity for doing work. (7-3)

enriched. To have nutrients added to a product to replace those removed during processing. (7-2)

entrepreneur. A person who starts and manages his or her own business. (12-4)

environment. The conditions, objects, places, and people that are all around a person. (1-1)

environmentally friendly products. Products that are effective and safe for the environment. (5-3)

environmental resources. Assets found in nature. (3-2)

equivalent measures chart. Chart showing how much of one measure equals a larger measuring amount. (9-4)

ethical decision making. Applying ideas of right or wrong to specific situations. (3-4)

ethics. Your strong beliefs about right and wrong that guide your conduct. (1-3, 3-4)

etiquette. Proper behavior in social settings. (8-5)

evaluate. To judge an entire plan of action. (4-1)

F

fabric. Cloth made by weaving or knitting yarns or by pressing fibers together. (10-4)

fabric softeners. Chemicals used when washing or drying to make fabrics feel better against your skin. (10-5)

fad. A new style that is popular for only a short time. (10-1)

family. A group of people related to one another by blood (birth), marriage, or adoption. (1-3)

family and consumer sciences careers. Careers in the areas of food science, nutrition and wellness, housing and interior design, textiles and apparel, child and human development, family relations, personal and family finance, and education and communications. (12-4)

family council. An informal meeting called to talk over issues concerning family members. (1-6)

family counseling agency. Group that works with family members to help them deal with changes and challenges. (1-6)

family service. A style of meal service where people serve themselves as dishes are passed around the table. (8-4)

family type. The makeup of a family. (1-3)

fashion. Styles that are popular at a given time. (10-1)

fatal. Deadly. (5-2)

fats. Nutrient needed by your body for energy. (7-1)

feedback. A response that lets the speaker know you received and understood the message. (1-5)

fibers. Hair-like strands that can be twisted together to form yarn. (10-4)

Fight BAC. Government program to educate consumers about preventing foodborne illnesses. (9-2)

filaments. Long, continuous fibers made from chemicals. (10-4)

filling. Horizontal set of yarn when weaving. (10-4)

finish. A treatment given to fibers, yarns, or fabric to improve the look, feel, or performance of a fabric. (10-4)

fixed expenses. Costs that remain the same on a regular basis. (4-4)

flatware. Forks, knives, and spoons used for serving and eating. (8-4)

flax. Natural fiber used to make linen fabric. (10-4)

flexible expenses. Costs that may change from month to month. (4-4)

follow-up letter. Letter sent by a job applicant thanking the interviewer for his or her time. (13-1)

foodborne illnesses. Illnesses caused from toxins produced by harmful bacteria in food. (9-2)

food processors. Electric kitchen appliances that cut ingredients in different forms and mix them. (9-4)

food shortage. A condition in which there is not enough to meet the demand. (8-2)

fossil fuels. Coal, oil, and natural gas. (6-1)

foster family. Family that cares for children who are not related to other family members. (1-3)

friend. Someone you care about, trust, and respect. (1-4)

fringe benefits. Rewards of a job other than income, such as paid vacation time and health insurance. (12-1)

G

generation. All people who are born and live in about the same time span. (1-3)

gifted. A child who has developed more quickly than other children the same age. (2-1)

goals. What you want to achieve. (3-3)

grade labeling. A rating of quality determined by the USDA for meats, poultry, and eggs. (8-3)

grain. The direction yarns run in a fabric. (11-2)

grooming. Cleaning and caring for your body. (4-3)
group dating. When several people of both sexes meet for an activity. (1-4)
growth. Specific body changes that can be measured. (1-2)
guardian. Person chosen by a family to take responsibility for a child if the parents are no longer able to provide care. (1-3)
guidance. Everything parents do and say to affect their children's behavior. (2-1)
guide sheet. Step-by-step directions for cutting and sewing a project included with the pattern. (11-2)

H

habit. A repeated pattern of behavior. (4-1)
hangtags. Larger tags with information about the garment or manufacturer that are attached to garments, but removed before worn. (10-3)
heredity. The result of receiving traits from parents or ancestors. (1-1)
hidden storage. Space for storing items out of sight. (5-1)
home. Any place people live. (5-1)
homogenization. A process in which milk fat is broken into tiny pieces and spread throughout the milk. (8-3)
hot line. A telephone service that offers immediate information to people who need help. (1-6)
house. A freestanding, single-family dwelling. (5-1)
human resources. The qualities and traits people have within themselves to get what they need or want. (3-2)

I

image. The mental picture others have of a person. (4-3)
implement. To carry out a plan of action. (4-1)
impulse buying. Making an unplanned or spur-of-the-moment purchase. (4-5)
income. The money you earn. (4-4, 12-1)
independence. The freedom to decide, act, and care for yourself. (1-2)
infant. A child under one year of age. (2-2)
ingredients. Food items needed to prepare a food product. (9-3)
ingredients labeling. Food products must list all ingredients, including allergens. (8-2)
inherited. Physical traits from your parents and grandparents. (1-1)
insulation. Material used to prevent the transfer of heat or cold. (6-2)
integrity. A commitment to do what is right. (3-5)
intellectual disability. A condition that limits a person's ability to use his or her mind. (2-1)
intellectual growth and development. Learning. (1-1)
interest inventory. A short quiz that suggests activities in which a person is most likely to excel. (12-2)
interests. The ideas and activities you like most. (12-2)
internships. Work-based learning program after high school. (12-3)
inventory. A list of items you have on hand. (10-1)
ironing. Moving an iron back and forth over fabric. (10-5)

J

job. A position held by a worker. (12-1)
job application. Personal information of potential employees required by companies. (13-1)
job shadowing. Following a worker on the job to observe what he or she does. (12-2)
job skills. The abilities needed for success in a certain job. (12-3)
junior colleges. Two-year colleges providing associate's degrees. (12-3)

L

labels. Small pieces of cloth sewn into the garment with important information about the garment's fabric content and recommended care. (10-3)

layaway plan. An arrangement in which you place a small deposit on an item so the store will hold it for you. (4-4)

leadership. The ability to inspire others to meet goals. (3-5)

learning. Gaining information or skills through engaging in play that provides hands-on materials. (2-5)

learning style. The conditions under which you learn best. (4-1)

leavening agent. An ingredient that causes foods to rise during baking. (9-5)

letter of application. A document you send with your résumé to give more information about your skills. (13-1)

lifestyle. The continuing way in which a person lives. (4-2, 12-1)

limits. Boundaries or restrictions. (2-1)

line. Element of design using straight or curved lines for effect. (5-1)

liquid measuring cups. Standard measuring tool used to measure liquid ingredients, such as milk, water, and oil. (9-4)

long-term goals. What you hope to accomplish at a later date. (3-3)

M

management. Using resources to reach goals. (4-1)

management process. A series of steps for reaching a goal. They are setting goals, planning, implementing, and evaluating. (4-1)

manicure. A method of caring for hands and fingernails. (4-3)

manners. Guidelines for behavior. (8-5)

mass media. A means of communicating to large groups of people. (4-5)

master's degree. Advanced degree after a bachelor's degree. (12-3)

material resources. The objects you own. (3-2)

meal patterns. The number of times and types of foods you eat daily. (8-1)

measure. To determine the amount of an item. (9-3)

measuring spoons. Standard measuring tools in teaspoon and tablespoon sizes. (9-4)

mediator. A person not involved in the conflict, but helps settle the conflict. (1-6)

mentor. A person you trust to guide you along your career path. (12-2)

menu. A list of foods to be prepared and served. (8-1)

microwave cookware. Items safe to use in microwave ovens. (9-1)

microwaves. High-frequency energy waves often used to cook food. (9-1)

minerals. Nutrient needed by your body to regulate body processes. (7-1)

moist-heat cooking. Methods for cooking foods in which water or other liquids are added. (9-5)

money management. The process of planning and controlling the use of money. (4-4)

multitasking. Doing more than one task at a time. (9-6)

MyPlate. The United States Department of Agriculture's (USDA) new food guidance system. (7-2)

N

nap. A layer of fiber ends above the fabric surface. (11-2)

natural cheese. Cheese made from milk. (8-3)

natural resources. Substances that are supplied by nature and needed for survival. (6-1)

needs. The basic items you must have to live. (3-1)

negative peer pressure. When peers influence you to do something that is not right for you. (1-4)

netiquette. Proper etiquette on the Internet. (6-3)
networking. Making contacts with people who may be able to help you find jobs. (13-1)
newborn. A term used to describe a baby from birth to one month of age. (2-2)
nonhuman resource. Objects and conditions available to people to help them meet needs and fulfill wants. (3-2)
nonverbal communication. The sending and receiving of messages without the use of words. (1-5)
***no* stage.** Toddler stage when they answer *no* to almost everything. (2-3)
notions. Items other than fabric that become part of a garment or project. (11-2)
nuclear family. A married man and woman and their biological children. (1-3)
nutrient-dense. Foods that provide vitamins, minerals, and other substances that have positive health effects, with relatively few calories. (7-2)
nutrient-poor. Foods that have few nutrients, but are high in calories. (7-1)
nutrients. Chemicals and other substances from foods needed for the body to function. (7-1)
nutrition. The study of how your body uses food. (7-1)
nutrition label. A panel on a food product package with information about the nutrients the food contains. (8-2)
nylon. Manufactured fiber that is strong and holds its shape well. (10-4)

O

occupations. Jobs. (12-2)
off-grain. Fabrics with the lengthwise and crosswise yarns not at right angles to each other. (11-2)
on-grain. Fabrics with the lengthwise and crosswise yarns at right angles to each other. (11-2)
ounce equivalent. Measurement of grain food products. (7-2)
overlock stitches. Stitching to prevent seams from raveling. (11-1)
overstock. Items produced, but not ordered by retail stores. (10-2)

P

Palmar (grasping) reflex. When babies grasp any object placed in their hands. (2-2)
parallel play. Type of play in which toddlers play near, but not with, one another. (2-3)
pasteurization. A process in which a liquid such as milk is heated to destroy harmful bacteria. (8-3)
pattern. Paper pieces to follow when cutting out fabric for making a garment or project. (11-2)
pedicure. A method of caring for feet and toenails. (4-3)
peer pressure. The influence people's peers have on them. (1-4)
peers. People who belong to the same age group. (1-4)
perishable foods. Foods that will spoil if not kept cold. (9-2)
personality. The group of traits that makes each person a unique individual. (1-1)
personal resources. See human resources. (3-2)
personal responsibility. Accepting the consequences of your decisions. (3-4)
physical disability. A condition that limits a person's ability to use part of his or her body. (2-1)
physical growth and development. Body changes. (1-1)
physical needs. Food, clothing, and shelter. (3-1)
physical traits. The distinguishing characteristics of your body. (1-1)
pilling. Small, fuzzy balls that form on the outside of fabric. (10-4)
plate service. A style of meal service where plates are filled in the kitchen. Then they are carried to the table and served to each person. (8-4)

pollution. The action or process of making natural resources unsafe or unusable. (6-1)
polyester. Manufactured fiber that is strong and resists wrinkles. (10-4)
pores. Tiny openings in the skin. (4-3)
positive peer pressure. When peers influence you to do something that is good for you. (1-4)
posture. The way you hold your body when standing, walking, or sitting. (4-2)
precycling. Buying products that reduce waste. (6-1)
preschooler. A child between the ages of three and five years. (2-4)
pressing. Lifting and lowering an iron onto an area of fabric. (10-5)
prewash products. Chemicals used to remove oily stains and dirt from clothes before they are washed. (10-5)
priorities. Goals that are more important to you. (3-3)
prioritize. To list or rate in order of importance. (3-3)
private resources. Resources owned and controlled by a person or a family. (3-2)
private space. An area that is yours alone. (5-1)
process cheese. Cheese made by melting and blending natural cheeses. (8-3)
procrastinate. To put off difficult or unpleasant tasks until later. (4-1)
produce. Fresh fruits and vegetables. (8-3)
professional organizations. Associations of members in a certain profession. (13-1)
proofreader. Someone who checks for errors in written work, such as misspelled words. (12-2)
proportion. A principle of design showing the relation of objects' sizes. (5-1)
proteins. Nutrients found in meat and meat substitutes needed by your body for growth and repair of tissue. (7-1)
public resources. See community resources. (3-2)
purging. Ridding the body of unwanted food by self-induced vomiting or taking too many laxatives. (7-3)

Q

quality. How well a product is made. (4-4)

R

ramie. Natural fiber used to make ramie fabric. (10-4)
raveling. When threads pull out of the cut edges of a fabric. (11-1)
rayon. Manufactured fiber that looks like cotton. (10-4)
recipe. A set of directions used to prepare a food product. (9-3)
recycling. Turning a used product into a product that can be reused. (6-1, 11-4)
redesign. To change the appearance or function of a garment. (11-4)
reference. A name of a person who can be contacted about you and your work habits. (13-1)
reflex. A natural, unlearned behavior. (2-2)
relationship. A pattern of interaction with one or more persons over time. (1-3)
reputation. What others think of a person. (1-4)
resources. Assets that can be used to meet needs and fulfill wants. (3-1)
respect. A high or special regard for someone. (1-3)
responsibility. A task you are expected or trusted to do. (1-2)
résumé. A written description of a person's education, qualifications, and work experience. (13-1)
rhythm. A principle of design showing patterns of space. (5-1)
ripe. Fully grown and developed. (8-3)
role. A person's place in a group. (1-3)
rooting reflex. When you touch babies around their mouths, their heads turn, and their mouths search for food. (2-2)
rotation work plan. Task plan for a day or a week, then rotated through group members. (9-7)

S

sanitation. The process of making conditions clean and healthy. (9-2)

saturated fat. A fat that is solid at room temperature. (7-1)

scale floor plan. A drawing that shows the size and shape of a room. (5-1)

scarce. A resource that is limited in supply. (3-2)

schedule. A written plan for reaching goals within a certain period of time. (4-1)

scum. Film that forms on the surface of heated milk. (9-5)

seam. A row of permanent stitches used to hold two pieces of fabric together. (11-3)

self-concept. The way a person sees himself or herself. (1-1)

self-confidence. The feeling of being sure of yourself and your abilities. (1-1)

self-esteem. The way a person feels about his or her self-concept. (1-1)

selvage. The finished lengthwise edges on a piece of fabric. (11-2)

separation anxiety. A child's fear that if parents leave, they will not return. (2-2)

serger. A type of high-speed sewing machine that sews, trims, and finishes seams at the same time. (11-1)

service learning. A strategy where students use their academic skills to provide services for their community. (3-5)

serving size. The amount a person would normally eat; found on the nutrition label. (8-2)

servings per container. The number of portions that are in the food package listed on the nutrition label. (8-2)

sew-through buttons. Buttons that need shanks added with thread. (11-3)

shank. A short stem that holds a button away from fabric. (11-3)

shape. Element of design using geometric shapes for effect. (5-1)

share. To experience or enjoy with others. (1-4)

shared space. Areas shared with other family members. (5-1)

shelter. A place that offers housing and food to people who have nowhere else to go. (1-6)

shortage. When a demand for something is greater than the supply. (6-1)

short-term goals. What you plan to get done soon. (3-3)

siblings. Brothers and sisters. (1-3)

silk. Natural fiber from the cocoons of silk worms used to make silk fabric. (10-4)

single-parent family. One adult who is raising one or more children. (1-3)

smart phones. Phone that access the Internet and have other uses. (6-3)

social entrepreneurs. Individuals who identify the problems of societies and develop plans to change the world in positive ways. (3-5)

social growth and development. Forming friendships and getting along well with others. (1-1)

socialization. Teaching the ways and customs of a culture to others. (1-3)

SoFAS. Foods high in solid fats and/or added sugars. (7-2)

software. A set of instructions that tells a computer what to do. (6-3)

solar energy. Energy from the sun's rays. (6-2)

solution. An answer to a problem. (1-6)

sort. To group clothes according to the way you will wash them. (10-5)

spacing. Element of design using space between objects for effect. (5-1)

spandex. Manufactured fiber that stretches like rubber. (10-4)

specialty food stores. Store offering one type of food. (8-2)

standard measuring tools. Specially marked cups and spoons used to measure ingredients. (9-4)

standards. A means of measuring how well you achieve your goals. (3-3)

standards of dress. The clothes that are acceptable in your country and community. (10-1)

stepfamily. The husband, the wife, or both have children from other marriages. Also called *blended family*. (1-3)

stress. Emotional, mental, or physical tension felt when faced with change. (4-2)

style. A distinctive form of dress or the design of a garment. (10-1)

sucking reflex. When newborns find objects with their mouths. (2-2)

Sudden Infant Death Syndrome (SIDS). The sudden, unexpected death of a baby who seems healthy. (2-2)

supermarkets. Chain stores offering a large selection of products. (8-2)

support group. A group of people with a similar challenge who provide support and help each other cope. (1-6)

sustainability. Using a natural resource so that it is not depleted or permanently damaged. (6-1)

systems software. Everything that makes your computer run and keeps it working. (6-3)

T

tableware. Dishes, flatware, and glassware. (8-4)

teamwork. Work done by a group in a cooperative manner. (3-5, 13-2)

teamwork skills. Working well with other members of a team. (13-2)

technical schools. Schools providing job training at both high school and college levels. (12-3)

technology. Use of new knowledge, tools, and systems to solve problems and make life easier. (6-3)

thinking skills. The ability to think creatively and critically, make decisions, and solve problems. (13-2)

tie-dyeing. Parts of the item's fabric are tied to prevent the dye from reaching the fabric evenly. (11-4)

time management. The skill of organizing your time so you can accomplish tasks. (4-1)

time-out. A guidance technique in which a child is moved away from others to a place where he or she must sit quietly. (2-5)

time schedule. A written plan for a person that lists when tasks should be started and completed. (9-6)

toddler. A child between the ages of one and three years. (2-3)

top priorities. The most important goals. (3-3)

toxic. Poisonous. (5-2)

toxins. Poisonous substances. (9-2)

trade-off. The giving up of one thing for another. (3-4)

trade schools. Schools that provide training for specific jobs at the college level. (12-3)

traditions. Customs passed from one generation to another. (7-1)

traffic pattern. A path people follow as they move within a room. (5-1)

traits. Distinguishing characteristics of a person. (1-1)

trans fat. A type of fat found in vegetable shortening, some margarine, baked goods, and many processed foods. (7-1)

trend. A general pattern of events. (12-2)

trust. To believe a person is honest and reliable. (1-4)

trustworthy. A quality of being a friend. (1-4)

U

unit pricing. Cost for each unit of measure or weight. (4-4)

unity. A state of being in agreement, not being divided. (1-6); A principle of design. (5-1)

universal design. The concept of designing homes and environments to be flexible and functional for all residents, including those with disabilities. (5-1)

universal product code (UPC). A group of bars and numbers found on packages. This code provides pricing and other product information to a computer scanner. (8-2)

use and care manual. A booklet of instructions for a tool. (9-1, 11-1)

utensil. Nonelectric, handheld kitchen tool used when preparing food. (9-1)

V

value. Buying the highest quality of clothing for the lowest prices. (10-2)

values. Strong beliefs or ideas about what is important. (3-3)

verbal communication. The use of words to give or receive information. (1-5)

virtual fit. Method of using a person's body measurements to show that body image with clothing on the computer. (10-2)

vitamins. Nutrient needed by your body for growth and repair of tissue. (7-1)

W

wants. The extra items you would like to have, but are not necessary to live. (3-1)

wardrobe. All the clothes and accessories you have to wear. (10-1)

warp. Vertical set of yarn when weaving. (10-4)

warranty. A written guarantee on a product from the manufacturer. (4-4)

water. Carries nutrients needed to your body cells and removes waste. (7-1)

webcams. Small video cameras showing live images through the Internet. (6-3)

wellness. State of physical, emotional, and mental well-being. (4-2)

whole grains. Grains in food that retain their natural fiber. (7-2)

wool. Natural fiber from sheep's fleece used to make woolen fabrics. (10-4)

work. What a person does to earn money. (12-1)

work-based learning. Programs in which students learn about a job through direct work experience and attend related classes. (12-3)

work center. An area of a kitchen that has been designed around a specific activity or activities. (9-6)

work ethic. The values of hard work and dedication held by employees. (13-2)

work plan. A list of tasks to be done, who is to perform them, and the tools and ingredients needed. (9-7)

Y

yarn. A continuous strand of fibers. (10-4)

Index

A

B

C

F

G

H

J

K

L

M

I

H

I

J

Y